VULNERABILITY TO PSYCHOPATHOLOGY

©2001 The Guilford Press
A Division of Guilford Publications, Inc.
72 Spring Street, New York, NY 10012
www.guilford.com

Printed in the United States of America

This book is printed on acid-free paper.

Last digit is print number: 9 8 7 6 5 4 3 2 1

Library of Congress Cataloging-in-Publication Data

Vulnerability to psychopathology : risk across the lifespan / edited by Rick E. Ingram and Joseph M. Price.
    p. cm.
  Includes bibliographical references and index.
  ISBN 1-57230-603-3 (hardcover)
  1. Schizophrenia—Risk factors. 2. Affective disorders—Risk factors.
3. Child psychopathology—Longitudinal studies. 4. Schizophrenia—Prevention—Longitudinal studies. I. Ingram, Rick E. II. Price, Joseph M.

RC455.4.R56 V85 2001
616.89′82—dc21

00-059265

VULNERABILITY TO PSYCHOPATHOLOGY

Risk across the Lifespan

Edited by
RICK E. INGRAM
JOSEPH M. PRICE

THE GUILFORD PRESS
New York   London

About the Editors

Rick E. Ingram, PhD, is Professor of Psychology at Southern Methodist University. His research program focuses on cognitive functioning in emotional disorders and the association between cognitive functioning and vulnerability to depression. He is currently the editor of *Cognitive Therapy and Research*, and serves on the editorial boards of the *Journal of Abnormal Psychology*, the *Journal of Consulting and Clinical Psychology*, and the *Journal of Social and Clinical Psychology*. Along with Jeanne Miranda and Zindel V. Segal, he is coauthor of *Cognitive Vulnerability to Depression*, and with C. R. Snyder, he is the coeditor of the *Handbook of Psychological Change: Psychotherapy Processes and Practices for the 21st Century*. He has received the Distinguished Scientific Award of the American Psychological Association for Early Career Contributions to Psychology, as well as the New Researcher Award of the Association for the Advancement of Behavior Therapy.

Joseph M. Price, PhD, is Associate Professor of Psychology at San Diego State University, and a core faculty member in the San Diego State University/University of California at San Diego Joint Doctoral Training Program in Clinical Psychology. He is also an Associate Director at the San Diego Center for Child and Adolescent Mental Health Services Research. The author of articles on the psychosocial development of maltreated children, his current research interests include the prevention of behavior and adjustment problems in maltreated children and children in foster care.

Contributors

Patricia A. Brennan, PhD, Department of Psychology, Emory University, Atlanta, Georgia

Kelly D. Brownell, PhD, Department of Psychology, Yale University, New Haven, Connecticut

Laurie Chassin, PhD, Department of Psychology, Arizona State University, Tempe, Arizona

R. Lorraine Collins, PhD, Research Institute on Addictions, University at Buffalo, State University of New York, Buffalo, New York

Nicki R. Crick, PhD, Institute of Child Development, University of Minnesota, Minneapolis, Minnesota

Cynthia Flynn, MA, Department of Psychology and Human Development, Vanderbilt University, Nashville, Tennessee

Michelle Fortier, MA, Department of Psychology, San Diego State University, San Diego, California

Jayne A. Fulkerson, PhD, Department of Epidemiology, University of Minnesota, Minneapolis, Minnesota

Judy Garber, PhD, Department of Psychology and Human Development, Vanderbilt University, Nashville, Tennessee

Tasha C. Geiger, MA, Institute of Child Development, University of Minnesota, Minneapolis, Minnesota

Constance Hammen, PhD, Department of Psychology, University of California, Los Angeles, California

Ingunn Hansdottir, MA, Department of Psychology, San Diego State University, and Department of Psychiatry, University of California at San Diego, San Diego, California

Philip D. Harvey, PhD, Department of Psychiatry, Mt. Sinai School of Medicine, New York, New York

Rick E. Ingram, PhD, Department of Psychology, Southern Methodist University, Dallas, Texas

Pamela K. Keel, PhD, Department of Psychology, Harvard University, Cambridge, Massachusetts

Jennifer Lento, MS, Department of Psychology, San Diego State University, and Department of Psychiatry, University of California at San Diego, San Diego, California

Gloria R. Leon, PhD, Department of Psychology, University of Minnesota, Minneapolis, Minnesota

Vanessa L. Malcarne, PhD, Department of Psychology, San Diego State University, San Diego, California

Richard J. McNally, PhD, Department of Psychology, Harvard University, Cambridge, Massachusetts

Joseph M. Price, PhD, Department of Psychology, San Diego State University, San Diego, California

Jennifer Ritter, MS, Department of Psychology, Arizona State University, Tempe, Arizona

Marlene B. Schwartz, PhD, Department of Psychology, Yale University, New Haven, Connecticut

Mariela C. Shirley, PhD, Department of Psychology, University of North Carolina at Wilmington, Wilmington, North Carolina

Elaine F. Walker, PhD, Department of Psychology, Emory University, Atlanta, Georgia

Preface

For many mental health professionals, understanding causality represents something of the holy grail of psychopathology research. And among the multitude of concepts that characterize the study of psychopathology, nothing brings us closer to understanding causality than the idea of vulnerability. This desire to understand vulnerability can be seen in the growing number of research articles on different disorders that focus on vulnerability markers or processes. Similarly, theories are beginning to appear with increasing regularity that focus on understanding the nature of psychological distress from the perspective of the processes that place people at risk for this distress. These theories, and the research that stems from them, span numerous disorders and include the psychological problems of both childhood and adulthood. Regardless of whether the focus is on children or adults, however, there is little doubt that the future of clinical research and treatment efforts lies in the study of vulnerability processes.

Even though the importance of vulnerability is widely recognized by both childhood and adulthood researchers, for most disorders there has been little overlap between these two broad categories of the lifespan. Hence, we strongly believe that a volume that brings together the major work on vulnerability and risk across the lifespan is needed. Yet, as we planned this volume we soon found that the very reason such a volume was needed also presented a unique challenge: there is little cross-collaboration among adult and childhood psychopathology researchers. Hence, too few researchers (including ourselves) can claim an adequate understanding of vulnerability to a disorder as it occurs across the lifespan. It was thus not possible to invite authors who could write a comprehensive chapter on the major vulnerability theories, data, and implications of vulnerability for both childhood and adulthood versions of a disorder. Together with Seymour Weingarten at The Guilford Press, we grappled with this issue, and with the aid of several thoughtful reviews of our initial prospectus, we decided to structure the volume according to each of the major syndromes specified by the fourth edition of the American Psychiatric Association's *Diagnostic and Statistical*

Manual of Mental Disorders (DSM-IV). Accordingly, we invited one chapter on the childhood and adolescent form of a major disorder and then a chapter on the corresponding adult form of the disorder.

This structure helps to ensure that the adult and childhood ends of lifespan vulnerability are covered in this volume. Moreover, we believe that the side-by-side appearance of chapters on adult and child vulnerability to a given disorder should help stimulate the integration of theory and research across the lifespan; our assumption is that those interested in adults will also learn from the corresponding childhood chapter and vice versa. Yet, organizing chapters side by side was not a completely satisfactory solution to the lack of theory and data across the lifespan. We therefore asked the respective authors of the childhood and adult chapters to collaborate on a brief summary chapter that would examine the points of contact and the points of departure between childhood and adulthood vulnerability and then point to future conceptual and research directions that might help bridge the gap between these different aspects of the lifespan. Thus, our hope is that each of these chapters—adult, child, and a summary—will help stimulate the eventual integration of our knowledge of vulnerability across the lifespan.

The organization of this volume proved to be challenging in other respects. For example, we were faced with a decision of which disorders to cover. DSM-IV lists hundreds of disorders, suggesting that if we were to attempt to cover each officially recognized disorder we would be able to devote approximately half a page to each. We chose instead to cover the major families of Axis I disorders: alcohol/substance abuse, depression, anxiety, schizophrenia, and eating disorders. We acknowledge that some important conditions may not be included in this list, but we nevertheless believe that the list covers the bulk of psychopathological states that afflict people.

An additional challenge concerned coverage of personality disorders. This is a particularly thorny issue inasmuch as the precise diagnosis of these disorders in adulthood is difficult. Similarly, personality disorders for the most part lack childhood counterparts even though they are recognized as having their roots in childhood through personality development. Moreover, even though DSM-IV specifies 10 different personality disorders, differentiating among these can be extremely difficult. It would have been easy to omit coverage of these disorders, yet we believe that they are an extremely important set of disorders that, if nothing else, are frequently comorbid with other disorders. We therefore decided to include one chapter that examined possible childhood precursors to adult personality disorders. The rationale for this decision was that although personality disorders are not typically diagnosed until late adolescence or early adulthood, the key elements of these disorders form in early childhood and rarely, if ever, in adulthood. Although, of necessity, the format for this chapter differs from the others in the volume, our goals for this chapter are the same as our goals for the others: to stimulate theory and research to incorporate a lifespan approach to understanding vulnerability to psychopathology.

Our final challenge was to recruit a group of authors who could cover these various disorders. There are a number of outstanding theorists and researchers who are doing superb work, and we were extremely pleased to be able to entice a stellar group of authors from among this group. From our perspectives as editors we were pleased not only with the timeliness of their submissions, but also with the outstanding quality of their contributions. Moreover, they took on the difficult and sometimes arbitrary task of dividing theory and research into respective childhood and adulthood literatures, and they did a marvelous job. Any credit this book may receive toward fueling an integration of adulthood and childhood vulnerability to psychopathology belongs squarely with our contributors. It was a pleasure to work with each of them.

The book is organized into four parts. Part I includes three chapters that are intended to provide a broad introduction to the concepts of vulnerability as they pertain to both childhood and adulthood disorders. Chapter 1, by Ingram and Price, provides a broad overview of the concept of vulnerability to psychopathology in general; Chapter 2, by Price and Lento, examines child psychopathology vulnerability constructs and issues; and Chapter 3, by Ingram and Fortier, explores these constructs and issues within the adult literature.

As we noted, personality disorders provided a unique challenge in that these disorders are rarely, if ever, believed to form in adulthood, instead having their origins firmly in the development of personality in childhood. Moreover, although there are a number of officially recognized personality disorders, it was not possible to cover each disorder. Therefore, in Part II, Geiger and Crick (Chapter 4) examine the overall idea of personality from the perspective of childhood development, and then address the corresponding implications for adult personality disorders.

DSM-IV roughly divides psychopathology into personality disorders and clinical syndromes. In Part III we cover the major clinical syndromes. As we noted, vulnerability is respectively examined for childhood/adolescence disorders and then for adult psychopathology, followed by a summary. To begin Part III, Chassin and Ritter (Chapter 5) examine childhood vulnerability to alcohol and substance abuse and Collins and Shirley (Chapter 6) examine the adult counterpart. The next chapters examine depression, with the childhood and adolescence chapter by Garber and Flynn (Chapter 8) and the adulthood chapter by Hammen (Chapter 9). Anxiety comes next, with Malcarne and Hansdottir (Chapter 11) focusing on childhood and adolescence and McNally (Chapter 12) focusing on adulthood. These chapters are followed by vulnerability theory and research on schizophrenia. Here again we faced a challenge in organizing these chapters because schizophrenia typically emerges in late adolescence or early adulthood. Thankfully, we could rely on the expertise of our authors to determine how best to organize the vulnerability research in this area. Thus, Brennan and Walker (Chapter 14) discuss developmental approaches to understanding

7. Vulnerability to Substance Use Disorders   165
        across the Lifespan
        LAURIE CHASSIN, R. LORRAINE COLLINS, JENNIFER RITTER,
        AND MARIELA C. SHIRLEY

Depression

8. Vulnerability to Depression in Childhood and Adolescence   175
        JUDY GARBER AND CYNTHIA FLYNN

9. Vulnerability to Depression in Adulthood   226
        CONSTANCE HAMMEN

10. Vulnerability to Depression across the Lifespan   258
        CONSTANCE HAMMEN AND JUDY GARBER

Anxiety Disorders

11. Vulnerability to Anxiety Disorders   271
        in Childhood and Adolescence
        VANESSA L. MALCARNE AND INGUNN HANSDOTTIR

12. Vulnerability to Anxiety Disorders in Adulthood   304
        RICHARD J. McNALLY

13. Vulnerability to Anxiety Disorders across the Lifespan   322
        RICHARD J. McNALLY, VANESSA L. MALCARNE,
        AND INGUNN HANSDOTTIR

Schizophrenia

14. Vulnerability to Schizophrenia: Risk Factors   329
        in Childhood and Adolescence
        PATRICIA A. BRENNAN AND ELAINE F. WALKER

15. Vulnerability to Schizophrenia in Adulthood   355
        PHILIP D. HARVEY

16. Vulnerability to Schizophrenia across the Lifespan   382
        PATRICIA A. BRENNAN AND PHILIP D. HARVEY

Eating Disorders

17. Vulnerability to Eating Disorders in Childhood and Adolescence 389
PAMELA K. KEEL, GLORIA R. LEON, AND JAYNE A. FULKERSON

18. Vulnerability to Eating Disorders in Adulthood 412
MARLENE B. SCHWARTZ AND KELLY D. BROWNELL

19. Vulnerability to Eating Disorders across the Lifespan 447
PAMELA K. KEEL AND MARLENE B. SCHWARTZ

IV. SUMMARY AND FUTURE DIRECTIONS OF THE VULNERABILITY APPROACH

20. Future Directions in the Study of Vulnerability to Psychopathology 455
JOSEPH M. PRICE AND RICK E. INGRAM

Index 467

VULNERABILITY TO PSYCHOPATHOLOGY

Part I

FOUNDATIONS OF THE VULNERABILITY APPROACH TO PSYCHOPATHOLOGY

do not, relapse and recurrence rates will be high because the processes that place the individual at risk are, by definition, still operative or, at least, still available.

Issues of initial onset and relapse or recurrence suggest other ways that causality can be conceptualized and, by extension, reasons that it is important to understand vulnerability. As Ingram, Miranda, and Segal (1998) have noted, many researchers differentiate between the onset of a disorder and the maintenance of a disorder and tacitly suggest that the onset or appearance of psychopathology is synonymous with causality. Correspondingly, because they are not viewed as causal, relatively little importance is ascribed to the factors that help maintain the state (see Barnett & Gotlib, 1988). Indeed, such factors are frequently dismissed as epiphenomena or consequences of the disordered state with no corresponding causal relevance.

We believe, however, that this is too narrow a conception of the construct of causality. In particular, we argue that causality is not synonymous with onset. Consider the case of depression: By virtually all estimates depression is a persistent disorder with symptoms lasting months and in some cases years (e.g., dysthymia). Indeed, there is a fair degree of consensus that untreated depression lasts between 6 months to 1 year or, depending on the severity of the episode, possibly up to 2 years (Goodwin & Jamison, 1990). Thus, the factors associated with the perpetuation of depression can be considered to have real causal significance—not for the onset of the disorder but for its maintenance. Although we focus on depression in this example, virtually all psychopathological states are problematic not only because they occur but because they occur and are maintained over time. We can thus legitimately ask whether the causes of this occurrence over time are any less important than causal onset perspectives. Indeed, from a causality standpoint the entire distinction between onset and maintenance may be more artificial than is genuinely helpful. Thus, from a vulnerability perspective we believe that understanding vulnerability not only elucidates the factors that bring about a disordered state but similarly elucidates the factors that bring about the continuation of this state. Moreover, the concept of causality is not limited to just onset and maintenance or to effective recovery through treatment or through natural means but also to residual symptoms after recovery. We therefore suggest that the vulnerability construct pervades all aspects of psychopathology—from onset to maintenance to recovery to postrecovery.

Of course, these issues leave open what researchers believe constitutes vulnerability, and for that matter what they believe constitutes psychopathology. Hence, this chapter begins by briefly examining some of the various definitions of psychopathology. We then turn to a discussion of some of the core features that appear to characterize the concept of vulnerability. We also note some distinctions between vulnerability, risk, and resilience. We end the chapter with a brief examination of how childhood/adolescence is differentiated from adulthood.

WHAT IS PSYCHOPATHOLOGY?

In many cases we know psychopathology when we see it; most (although not all) individual cases are clear-cut. Yet, such clear-cut cases do little to help us define the notion of disorder itself. It thus seems reasonable that any book addressing vulnerability to disorder must make some effort to at least address the issue of what constitutes a disorder. Furthermore, because it is our goal to examine vulnerability across different developmental periods, it is important that we examine what constitutes disorder at different points in the lifespan.

A variety of definitions have been offered on what is the appropriate manner in which to define psychopathological functioning. However, as with many if not most constructs in the psychological sciences, there is also little professional consensus on exact definitions (Neale, 1997). Moreover, reflecting the current state of the field, each of the contributors to this volume may have somewhat different definitions of psychopathology. We therefore do not intend here to attempt to resolve various disputes or differing perspectives on how psychopathology is to be defined, either by this volume's contributors or in the field itself. Rather, we seek merely to mention the disagreement over definitions in order to alert readers to this issue, note briefly some of the major definitions, and then offer a broad working model that we hope, at minimum, will provide at least a framework for conceptualizing psychopathology and thus, vulnerability.

The definition of psychopathology is one that baffles virtually all undergraduates in abnormal psychology courses, perhaps because they are forced to think about it (at least early in the term). Mental health professionals, of course, have easy access to a definitive source of psychopathology definitions (Nathan, 1997): the American Psychiatric Association's *Diagnostic and Statistical Manual of Mental Disorders* (DSM) currently in its fourth edition (DSM-IV; American Psychiatric Association, 1994). DSM is a remarkable source of data and information on a variety of disorders, including criteria that we use to define and diagnosis disorders and to differentiate one disorder from another. Yet, we suggest that the DSM does not represent in and of itself a satisfactory definition of psychopathology per se; that is, it does not reflect a clear indication of what differentiates the state of abnormal functioning from the state of normal functioning. To arrive at some perspective on this differentiation, we must look elsewhere.

The issue of how to define psychopathology has been debated by a number of theorists, most offering a somewhat unique perspective. For example, Wakefield (1992, 1999) suggests that a disorder is defined by the concept of "harmful dysfunction," in which harm is defined as a condition that creates distress or problems for the individual as determined by the values and norms of the larger community. In this sense, harm is a socially constructed variable that is not possible to define without reference to a community framework. Dysfunction is defined as the failure of mechanisms to perform at a particular developmental period as it was "intended" by evolution.

Alternatively, building on earlier proposals by Ossorio (1985), Bergner (1997) argues that psychopathology should be viewed as "significant restriction in the ability of an individual to engage in deliberate action, and equivalently, to participate in available social practices" (p. 246). Such a definition differs from Wakefield's in that it does not incorporate the notion of evolutionary intent, a notion that Bergner (1997) and Lilienfeld and Marino (1995) describe as problematic (e.g., there is little consensus on the definition and nature of these evolutionary mechanisms or on whether these mechanisms are evolutionary adaptations or evolutionary by-products).

Earlier definitions by Spitzer and Endicott (1978) formed the foundation of what was to become the modern versions of DSM. In particular, Spitzer and Endicott suggested that disorder could be defined as distinct problems arising from "organismic dysfunction" that is associated with significant distress or disability. Such a definition is firmly rooted in a medical model approach to psychological (or psychiatric) disorders. For instance, in arriving at this definition, Spitzer and Endicott (1978) explicitly argued that "a mental disorder is a medical disorder whose manifestations are primarily signs or symptoms of a psychological (behavioral) nature" (p. 18), leaving little doubt on what basis psychological disorders should be considered.

In contrast, Lilienfeld and Marino (1995) argue that psychological dysfunction is best viewed as a Rochian concept in which it is not possible to clearly distinguish between normal and abnormal functioning and, hence, in any absolute fashion, to define psychological dysfunction. Lilienfeld and Marino's (1995) perspective suggests that whereas some conditions will clearly be considered abnormal (e.g., schizophrenia with florid symptoms), the exact boundaries between disorder and nondisorder are too fuzzy to clearly distinguish or to use to make a decision as to when normal behavior crosses the line into abnormal functioning.

As can be seen from these various perspectives, there is little professional consensus on how to define psychopathology, or at least on how to arrive at a clear definition of where to draw the line between normal and abnormal functioning. Indeed, where this line will be drawn in any individual case will depend on a number of factors that include both microfactors (e.g., the particular individual who assigns diagnosis or makes a decision about abnormality) and macrofactors (e.g., cultural factors that broadly influence definitions of psychopathology). For our purposes, however, we suggest a working definition that relies on practical criteria. Specifically, we assume that psychopathology can be broadly defined by impairment in the individual's established, or expected, roles at a given developmental period, and that it is typically accompanied by reports of emotional distress. We acknowledge that situations will arise in which it will be difficult to differentiate between normal and abnormal functioning using this definition but argue that such a definition will be comprehensive enough in most circumstances. Indeed, the disorders examined in this book unambiguously meet these criteria.

WHAT IS VULNERABILITY?

As with definitions of disorder, a volume on vulnerability to psychopathology must offer, at minimum, some working ideas on how to define the vulnerability construct. Hence, to arrive at a framework for defining vulnerability, we examine what we believe characterizes the core features of vulnerability that, cumulatively, should offer a reasonable definition. Ingram et al. (1998) provide an in-depth discussion of these core features.

As Ingram et al. (1998) note, the vulnerability approach to psychopathology is at least several decades old. Yet, similar to definitions of psychopathology, little consensus exists on what constitutes an adequate definition of vulnerability. Such definitional impoverishment is the case even though the notion of vulnerability has generated a significant body of theory and research. It is, however, possible to derive the core characteristics of the construct from previous theory and research on child and adult vulnerability. These characteristics appear to constitute the common themes that emerge in virtually all discussions of vulnerability and can thus help establish a consensus for what vulnerability is and what it is not.

CORE FEATURES OF VULNERABILITY

Examination of the literature suggests that several themes tend to appear repeatedly in discussions of vulnerability. These themes focus on vulnerability as a trait, the endogenous and latent nature of vulnerability, and the role of stress in actualizing vulnerability. We turn now to a brief examination of each of these features.

Vulnerability as a Stable Trait

Researchers tend to regard vulnerability as an enduring trait. Among the originators of vulnerability theory and research, Zubin and Spring (1977) were perhaps the most specific about the trait nature of vulnerability: "We regard [vulnerability] as a relatively permanent, enduring trait" (p. 109); "the one feature that all schizophrenics have . . . is the everpresence of their vulnerability" (p. 122). Other investigators have tended to not be quite as specific, but the enduring trait nature of vulnerability is implicit in many of their discussions of vulnerability. Such assumptions of permanence are likely rooted in the genetic level of analysis employed by researchers who pioneered this concept. For example, most schizophrenia researchers point to the genetic endowment of individuals who are at risk for this disorder. Meehl's (1962) concept of schizotaxia represents an inherited neural deficit, whereas other researchers such as Zubin and Spring (1977) and Nicholson and Neufeld (1992) are quite explicit that genetic factors determine level of vulnerability (at least to schizophrenia).

Such conceptualizations tend to posit that no decrease in absolute vulnerability levels is possible. This is not to suggest, however, that functional vulnerability levels cannot be attenuated by several factors, such as those that affect neurochemistry. This may very well be the case for medications such as lithium carbonate, which alter the likelihood of developing the symptoms of a bipolar episode by presumably controlling the neurochemistry of the underlying vulnerability. Similar diminishment of functional vulnerability may be seen in the actions of psychopharmacological treatments for depression with medications such as the various generations of tricyclic agents and the more recent selective serotonin reuptake inhibitors. Even though functional vulnerability may be altered and individuals are less likely to develop the disorder, the vulnerability persists; for example, the probability of episode is increased if the medication is discontinued. Thus, even though the vulnerability may be controlled, the vulnerability trait itself remains.

The trait nature of vulnerability is perhaps most clearly seen in contrast to the state or episodic nature of psychological disorders. For instance, Zubin and Spring (1977) clearly distinguish between an enduring vulnerability trait and episodes of schizophrenia which "are waxing and waning states" (p. 109). Hollon, Evans, and DeRubeis (1990) and Hollon and Cobb (1993) also distinguish between (1) stable vulnerability traits that predispose individuals to the disorder but do not constitute the disorder and (2) state variables which represent the occurrence of the symptoms that reflect the onset of the disorder. Thus, while predisposing factors are enduring traits, virtually all investigators characterize the disorder as a state. Disordered states can therefore emerge and decline as episodes cycle between occurrence and remission, but the traits that give rise to vulnerability for the disordered state are typically thought to remain constant.

Although vulnerability is assumed by many theorists to be permanent and enduring, this need not always be the case. This is especially true when the level of vulnerability analysis is psychological rather than genetic in nature. As we have noted, assumptions of genetic vulnerability offer little possibility for modification of vulnerability characteristics. Most psychological approaches, however, rely on assumptions of dysfunctional learning as the genesis of vulnerability. Given these assumptions, not only functional but actual vulnerability levels may fluctuate as a function of new learning experiences that influence the particular vulnerability factor. For instance, Hollon et al. (1990) have reported data suggesting that depressed patients treated with cognitive therapy, or combined cognitive therapy and pharmacotherapy, are less likely than patients treated with pharmacotherapy to experience recurrence of the disorder over a 2-year period, presumably because the underlying vulnerability has been at least partially altered. In this vein, Hollon et al. (1990) and Hollon and Cobb (1993) argue that the effects of pharmacological treatments may be largely symptom suppressive, but that psychological interventions such as cognitive therapy are designed to alter dysfunctional cognitive structures and, to the extent that genuine vulnerability is rooted in such structures, may lessen susceptibility to psychopathology. Fewer recurrences of the disorder over time may reflect decreased vulnerability. It is certainly possible that factors other than vulnerability reduction may be at the heart of cognitive therapy prophylactic effects, but this example does illustrate how, theoretically at least, actual vulnerability levels might be altered.

Of course, from the viewpoint of a psychological level of analysis, vulnerability may *decrease* with certain corrective experiences, or, alternatively, it may *increase* over time. This latter possibility would be the case if continued exposure to aversive experiences and stressful life events served the function of enhancing the factors that contribute to vulnerability. Some perspectives have suggested that frequent experiences with the disorder itself may increase vulnerability for future onsets. For example, in describing the idea of *kindling*, Post (1992) has proposed such a process in the area of affective disorders. Post suggests that each episode of an affective disorder leaves a residual neurobiological trace that leads to the development of pathways by which increasingly minimal stress becomes sufficient to activate the mechanisms that result in a disorder. Such a process thus leads to increased vulnerability.

Stability versus Permanence

The possibility that psychological vulnerability levels can be altered (up or down) suggests a subtle but potentially important distinction between stability and permanence. Stability and permanence are likely to be viewed as synonymous. However, even though the concept of stability clearly suggests a resistance to change, it does not presume that change is never possible. Under the right circumstances, positive changes in an otherwise stable variable may very well occur. Indeed, the entire notion of psychotherapy is based on just this premise. Without intervention or the introduction of other significant life experiences, however, little change in stable psychological variables should occur. On the other hand, variables that are considered to be enduring, particularly biological processes emanating from genetic processes, imply a permanence or immutability that is not only resistant to change under ordinary circumstances but is assumed to offer virtually no possibility of change.

Vulnerability Is Endogenous

Another core feature that is possible to glean from vulnerability work is that vulnerability represents an endogenous variable. This is perhaps most clearly seen in genetic conceptualizations of vulnerability but is equally relevant for psychological conceptualizations. That is, whether stemming from inborn characteristics or acquired through learning processes, the vulnerability resides within the person. This can be contrasted to other levels of analysis that might, for example, focus on environmental or external sources of stress that initiate a disorder, or perhaps a focus on interpersonal styles that may lead to aversive interactions (e.g., Coyne, 1976). We discuss this distinction more fully in the section differentiating vulnerability from risk. For now it is important to note that although these "external" variables are clearly important, the locus of vulnerability processes is within the person.

Vulnerability Is Latent

In line with the idea that vulnerability is an endogenous process, and that vulnerability remains stable even though observable states of psychopathology arise and then (in many cases) diminish, some investigators have suggested that vulnerability is not easily observable and can thus be conceptualized as a latent process. From a research perspective, this can perhaps be seen most clearly in the empirical search for observable markers of vulnerability; numerous investigators have sought to find reliable empirical indicators of the presence of the vulnerability. There are a variety of research strategies for identifying markers, but in each case they operate with the assumptions that (1) vulnerability processes are present in individuals who have few or no outward signs of the disorder, (2) these processes are causally linked to the appearance of symptoms, and (3) they are not readily observable and are therefore difficult to assess. This is particularly the case in investigations that rely on some kind of stressful or challenging event that makes detection of the vulnerability factor possible (see Shelton, Hollon, Purdon, & Loosen, 1991 for a discussion of the challenge paradigm as it pertains to the conceptualization of vulnerability and dysregulation). The search for vulnerability markers is thus the search for predictors of the disorder in the absence of symptoms of the disorder, an empirical strategy reflecting a conceptual judgment that vulnerability is present and stable but not easily observable.

Stress

We have alluded to the importance of stress in the various features of vulnerability, and it is therefore important to note that although stress may not be a core feature of vulnerability in the sense that it is stable and endogenous, it nevertheless is an important enough variable to be included within any discussion of the core features of vulnerability. We thus examine stress as it pertains to conceptualizations of vulnerability.

To comprehensively examine definitions of stress would necessitate an entire volume, and indeed entire volumes have been devoted to this topic (for classic examples, see Brown & Harris, 1989; Cohen, 1988). In general, however, stress can be understood as falling into several broad categories. A number of investigators (e.g., Luthar & Zigler, 1991; Monroe & Simons, 1991) note that a major category of stress is conceptualized as the occurrence of significant life events which, in the case of psychopathology, are interpreted by the person as undesirable or aversive. Another kind of stress can be seen as the accumulation of minor events, hassles, or challenges (Lazarus, 1990).

Although the definitions of stress can be numerous, we can view stress generally as the life events (major or minor) that disrupt the mechanisms maintaining the stability of an individual's physiology, emotion, and cognition. Classic descriptions of stress suggest that such events represent a strain on the person's adaptive capability that initiate an interruption of the person's routine or habitual functioning. As such, stress interferes with the system's physiological and psychological homeostasis and is thus seen as a critical variable in a multitude of models of psychopathology (Monroe & Simons, 1991) regardless of whether these models focus explicitly on (endogenous) vulnerability factors.

The problems with conceptualizing and adequately assessing stress have been well documented, as have concerns about separating concepts of stress from concepts of psychopathology (e.g., Hammen, 1991; Kasl, 1983; Monroe, 1989; Monroe & Simons, 1991). Nevertheless, we argue that at a purely conceptual level it makes sense to separate stress from vulnerability and psychological disorder. Such a conceptual separation recognizes the possibility that stress can exist independently of appraisal processes and can be consensually defined and objectively measured; everyone would agree, for instance, that a car accident resulting in permanent confinement to a wheelchair will be stressful for everyone regardless of their appraisal processes. Moreover, separation of the stress and vulnerability constructs facilitates communication about the variables potentially operating in psychopathology; that is, it is possible to talk about stress without frequent qualifications due to appraisal processes.

The Diathesis–Stress Relationship

By conceptually separating stress and vulnerability, examining the diathesis–stress relationship becomes possible. As Ingram et al. (1998) have noted, the diathesis concept has a long history in medical terminology. In tracing this history, Monroe and Simons (1991) note that the concept dates back to ancient Greeks, and as early as the late 1800s was ensconced in the psychiatric vernacular of the day. Diathesis refers to a predisposition to illness and has evolved from its original focus on constitutional, biological factors to presently also encompassing psychological variables such as cognitive and interpersonal susceptibilities. Moreover, such diatheses are typically considered to be latent and, as we have noted, must be activated in some fashion before psychopathology can occur. In line with this concept, many models of psychopathology are explicitly diathesis–stress models. Thus, although there is general agreement that vulnerability constitutes an endogenous process, most models also recognize that events perceived as stressful act to trigger vulnerability processes that are linked to the onset of the disordered state. In many cases, psychopathology is therefore the interactive effect of the (latent and endogenous) diatheses and events perceived as stressful. Framed within the context of a diathesis–stress conceptualization, stress is integral to virtually all extant conceptualizations of vulnerability.

Summary of Core Features of Vulnerability

In sum, a review of the extant literature on vulnerability suggests a number of essential features that characterize the construct of vulnerability. Perhaps the most fundamental of the core features of vulnerability is that it is considered a trait as opposed to the kind of a state that more accurately characterizes the actual appearance of the disorder. It is also important to note that even though vulnerability is conceptualized as a trait according to some conceptualizations, vulnerability is not necessarily permanent or unalterable (although psychological vulnerability is nevertheless stable and relatively resistant to change). Corrective experiences can occur that may attenuate the vulnerability, or, alternatively, certain experiences may increase vulnerability factors. In addition, vulnerability is viewed as an endogenous process that is typically conceptualized as latent. Finally, although conceptually distinct from vulnerability, stress is a critical "feature" of vulnerability in that many models postulate that vulnerability cannot be realized without stress. This latter feature of vulnerability represents the essence of the diathesis–stress approach that is common among many current models of psychopathology.

THE RELATIONSHIP BETWEEN VULNERABILITY, RISK, AND RESILIENCE

Terms such as "vulnerability," "risk," and, to a lesser degree, "resilience" tend to be used interchangeably. Such usage is understandable; clearly the ideas of vulnerability, risk, and resilience refers to similar phenomenon and share a number of features. Nevertheless, we believe that these terms, and the constructs they represent, are not interchangeable and should be clearly distinguished in any discussion of vulnerability. We therefore examine the association between vulnerability and risk and vulnerability and resilience.

Vulnerability and Risk

Vulnerability and risk are not synonymous. We argue, as have others, that the concept of risk refers to any variables that are empirically associated with an increased likelihood of experiencing a disorder (e.g., poverty and stress related to social injustice). Risk thus serves to predict the likelihood of dysfunction. However, relative to the absence of risk factors, the presence of risk suggests only an increased probability of the occurrence of a disorder but is not necessarily informative about the *mechanisms* of a disorder. Thus, risk refers to correlational or *descriptive* variables rather than to causal variables per se. Moreover, to the extent that any variable is empirically shown to be related to an increased probability of onset, the variable can be considered a risk factor.

Because risk factors are generally uninformative about the actual mechanisms that bring about a state of psychopathology, knowledge about risk factors is not necessarily helpful with regard to psychosocial intervention strategies. Presumably the most effective treatment for a disorder targets not only the symptoms of the disorder but the mechanisms that helped to bring it about. However, some authors have suggested that the only effective treatment is one that alters broadly defined risk factors. For example, Albee (2000) argues that until risk factors such as poverty and social injustice are changed, individual treatment is likely to be ineffective and inefficient—akin to putting on a Band-aid to stop a hemorrhage.

It should be noted that although risk and vulnerability are conceptually separate, these variables are not necessarily empirically unrelated. In pointing out a similar distinction, Rutter (1987) and Luthar and Zigler (1991) have argued that these variables interact with each other to produce the onset of a disorder. Thus, the person who is "at risk" because he or she lives, for example, in a particularly stressful environment will see this risk realized in disorder if he or she *also* possesses the vulnerability mechanisms. For example, the circumstances of living in poverty may trigger the dysregulation mechanisms that are at the heart of the onset of the disorder. This is the essence of the diathesis–stress interaction that characterizes numerous models of psychopathology.

We have argued that risk represents a descriptive factor rather than a causal one, and that as an endogenous factor, only vulnerability can play a causal role. Yet, data have shown that risk variables both can predict the

suggests that "there is no clear distinction between 'childhood' and 'adult' disorders" (p. 37). Nevertheless, when age is mentioned at all in diagnosing *Disorders Usually First Evident in Infancy, Childhood, or Adolescence* (the general category that covers all these disorders), the maximum ages vary from 18 to 21 for disorders appearing in adolescence. Likewise, most assessment methods for children and adolescence (e.g., the Diagnostic Interview for Children and Adolescents) define their top range at around age 17, and corresponding assessment methods for adults typically define a minimum age of 18 (e.g., the Structured Clinical Interview for DSM-IV Disorders; SCID). The current diagnostic approach thus appears to have adopted a legal standard, although perhaps for different reasons.

Another, and more comprehensive, approach focuses on theory and research on developmental processes. The developmental approach does not rely on arbitrary ages and legal standards but instead considers the biological, emotional, and psychological maturation processes that occur as individuals progress from childhood to adulthood. Not surprisingly, there is no single age at which an individual crosses into adulthood. From a biological perspective, physical maturation (e.g., maximum height and the development of secondary sexual characteristics) has occurred in both boys and girls by roughly age 16, although some physical change will continue (e.g., adding strength and muscle mass through the mid to late 20s). But, physical maturation alone is not sufficient to differentiate between adolescence and adulthood in a psychological or emotional sense.

The determination of adulthood is complicated by other matters. For example, cultural differences can vary widely; more primitive cultures typically have a shortened adolescence and a more clear-cut entry into adulthood (e.g., performance of rituals that signify entrance into adulthood). On the other hand, more developed Western cultures have the longest period of adolescence with fewer and less well-defined rituals of passage into adulthood. Moreover, there are considerable individual differences in attaining adulthood. For instance, some who are considered to be adolescents based on their age may be wise and experienced beyond their years and would thus be considered to be adults significantly before their similar-age peers. At the other end of the spectrum, maturational deficits in adulthood may place some adults more appropriately in an adolescent than an adult category.

It is clear that any approach to defining adulthood must take into account a wide range of psychological, physiological, and cultural factors. Certainly the boundary between adolescence and adulthood is a gradual transition rather than a clear-cut boundary; there is no precise age at which adolescence ends and adulthood begins. In general, however, at least in Western societies it seems safe to conclude that between the ages of 18 to 20 is a reasonable place to begin to differentiate adolescence and adulthood, recognizing that some individuals will fall on the "wrong" side of this line.

In fact, each of the approaches we have briefly examined to determine these boundaries (legal, psychiatric, and developmental) converges on this time frame. Although it would be the unusual 15-year-old who would be considered an adult, or the unusual 30-year-old who would still be considered an adolescent (barring organic dysfunction), the ages between 18 and 20 appear to be a convenient place to mark the transition from adolescence to adulthood. Indeed, even a cursory review of the published research on child and adult psychopathology supports this age period as the typical line of demarcation between adolescence and adulthood.

UNDERSTANDING PSYCHOPATHOLOGY
AND VULNERABILITY: A BRIEF SUMMARY

In this chapter we have noted some definitions of psychopathology and some core features that appear to characterize vulnerability constructs. Although frequently used interchangeably, risk and vulnerability refer to different constructs. In particular, we argued that vulnerability refers to the relatively stable causal mechanisms of psychopathology that are endogenous to the individual. We suggested a preference for conceptualizing vulnerability and resilience on different ends of the vulnerability continuity and noted that resilience implies a resistance but not an immunity to disorder. We briefly reviewed some different perspectives on differentiating adolescence and adulthood and noted that they tend to converge on the ages of 18 to 20 as defining the transitional phase into adulthood. We also noted the distinctions between biological and psychological levels of analysis that are applied to various disorders.

As should be at least implicit in this discussion, we believe that vulnerability research not only represents the current cutting edge of psychopathology research but also the future for psychopathology research. Not that psychopathology research which focuses on describing the operation of various processes *in* the disordered state will be unimportant, but rather the clearest advances in understanding the causes of psychopathology will come from research that focuses explicitly on vulnerability. Not only will this approach bring us closer to understanding causal processes, but in so doing it will bring us closer to understanding the mechanisms that must be therapeutically addressed once a disorder has occurred. An adequate understanding of vulnerability can also aid in preventing the onset of psychopathology, or at the least attenuating the duration and intensity of disorders along with their damaging effects (e.g., deficits in interpersonal functioning). Moreover, although still separated by a gulf between childhood/adolescence and adulthood theory and research, we believe that the surest road to understanding vulnerability and prevention will come from research that considers vulnerability from a lifespan perspective.

REFERENCES

Albee, G. W. (2000). Critique of psychotherapy in American society. In C. R. Snyder & R. E. Ingram (Eds.), *Handbook of psychological change: Psychotherapy processes and practices for the 21st century* (pp. 689–706). New York: Wiley.

American Psychiatric Association. (1994). *Diagnostic and statistical manual of mental disorders* (4th ed.). Washington, DC: Author.

Barnett, P. A., & Gotlib, I. H. (1988). Psychosocial functioning in depression: Distinguishing among antecedents, concomitants, and consequences. *Psychological Bulletin, 104*, 97–126.

Bergner, R. M. (1997). What is psychopathology?: And so what? *Clinical Psychology: Science and Practice, 4*, 235–248.

Brown, G. W., & Harris, T. O. (Eds.). (1989). *Life events and illness.* New York: Guilford Press.

Cohen, L. (Ed.). (1988). *Research on stressful life events: Theoretical and methodological issues.* Newbury Park, CA: Sage.

Coyne, J. C. (1976). Toward an interactional description of depression. *Psychiatry, 39*, 28–40.

Goodwin, F. K., & Jamison, K. R. (1990). *Manic–depressive illness.* New York: Oxford University Press.

Hammen, C. (1991). The generation of stress in the course of unipolar depression. *Journal of Abnormal Psychology, 100*, 555–561.

Hollon, S. D., & Cobb, R. (1993). Relapse and recurrence in psychopathological disorders. In C. G. Costello (Ed.), *Basic issues in psychopathology* (pp. 377–402). New York: Guilford Press.

Hollon, S. D., Evans, M. D., & DeRubeis, R. J. (1990). Cognitive mediation of relapse prevention following treatment for depression: Implications of differential risk. In R. E. Ingram (Ed.), *Contemporary psychological approaches to depression: Theory, research, and treatment* (pp. 117–136). New York: Plenum.

Ingram, R. E., Miranda, J., & Segal, Z. V. (1998). *Cognitive vulnerability to depression.* New York: Guilford Press.

Kasl, S. V. (1983). Pursuing the link between stressful life experiences and disease: A time for reappraisal. In C. L. Cooper (Ed.), *Stress research.* New York: Wiley.

Lazarus, R. S. (1990). Theory-based stress management. *Psychological Inquiry, 1*, 3–13.

Lilienfeld, S. O., & Marino, L. (1995). Mental disorder as a Roschian concept: A critique of Wakefield's "harmful dysfunction" analysis. *Journal of Abnormal Psychology, 104*, 411–420.

Luthar, S. S., & Zigler, E. (1991). Vulnerability and competence: A review of research on resilience in childhood. *American Journal of Orthopsychiatry, 61*, 6–22.

Meehl, P. E. (1962). Schizotaxia, schizotypy, schizophrenia. *American Psychologist, 17*, 827–838.

Monroe, S. M. (1989). Stress and social support: Assessment issues. In N. Schneiderman, S. M. Weiss, & P. G. Kaufman (Eds.), *Handbook of research in cardiovascular behavioral medicine* (pp. 511–526). New York: Plenum.

Monroe, S. M., & Simons, A. D. (1991). Diathesis–stress theories in the context of life stress research: Implications for the depressive disorders. *Psychological Bulletin, 110,* 406–425.

Nathan, P. E. (1997). In the final analysis, it's the data that count. *Clinical Psychology: Science and Practice, 4,* 281–284.

Neale, J. M. (1997). Psychopathology as disability. *Clinical Psychology: Science and Practice, 4,* 288–289.

Nicholson, I. R., & Neufeld, R. W. J. (1992). A dynamic vulnerability perspective on stress and schizophrenia. *American Journal of Orthopsychiatry, 62,* 117–130.

Ossorio, P. G. (1985). Pathology. *Advances in Descriptive Psychology, 4,* 151–201.

Post, R. M. (1992). Transduction of psychosocial stress into the neurobiology of affective disorder. *American Journal of Psychiatry, 149,* 999–1010.

Rutter, M. (1987). Psychosocial resilience and protective mechanisms. *American Journal of Orthopsychiatry, 57,* 316–331.

Rutter, M. (1988). Longitudinal data in the study of causal processes: Some uses and some pitfalls. In M. Rutter (Ed.), *Studies of psychosocial risk: The power of longitudinal data* (pp. 1–28). Cambridge, UK: Cambridge University Press.

Rutter, M. Maughan, B., Mortimore, P., & Ouston, J. (1979). *Fifteen thousand hours: Secondary schools and their effects on children.* London: Open Books.

Shelton, R. C., Hollon, S. D., Purdon, S. E., & Loosen, P. T. (1991). Biological and psychological aspects of depression. *Behavior Therapy, 22,* 201–228.

Spitzer, R. L., & Endicott, J. (1978). Medical and mental disorder: Proposed definition and criteria. In R. L. Spitzer & D. F. Klein (Eds.), *Critical issues in psychiatric diagnosis* (pp. 1–17). New York: Raven Press.

Wakefield, J. C. (1992). The concept of mental disorder: On the boundary between biological facts and social values. *American Psychologist, 47,* 373–388.

Wakefield, J. C. (1999). Evolutionary versus prototype analyses of the concept of disorder. *Journal of Abnormal Psychology, 108,* 374–399.

Zubin, J., & Spring, B. (1977). Vulnerability: A new view of schizophrenia. *Journal of Abnormal Psychology, 86,* 103–126.

portant influence of the context of development, it is also important to understand the contextual variables that can affect both the nature of the developmental tasks and extent to which these tasks are successfully negotiated. Clearly, this particular view of psychopathology suggests that atypical development can only be understood in relation to normal development. As becomes evident in a later section of this chapter, the increasing influence of a developmental psychopathology perspective on theory and research in child and adolescent psychopathology has played an instrumental role in the adaptation of this particular conceptualization of psychopathology.

PREVALENCE OF PSYCHOPATHOLOGY IN CHILDHOOD AND ADOLESCENCE

Despite the challenges to defining psychopathology in childhood and adolescence, over the past two decades a surge of studies has addressed the prevalence of psychopathology in the developmental periods prior to adulthood. This research was facilitated by the development of a wide range of measures for assessing child and adolescent psychopathology that occurred during the 1980s and 1990s. These prevalence studies used a range of assessment strategies and tended to focus on various symptom clusters and diagnostic categories of disorder. Despite the fact that these studies were conducted across a wide range of geographically diverse populations (e.g., Australia, Canada, the United States, New Zealand, and Puerto Rico) and using differing types of assessment strategies, there is an amazing degree of consistency across studies. To begin, prevalence rates range from 14% to 20%, with most studies reporting overall rates somewhere between 17% and 20% (see Schwab-Stone & Briggs-Gowan, 1998, for a review of this literature). In general, within these percentages, 2% were found to have serious disorders, 7% to 8% had moderately severe disorders, and the remainder displayed milder forms of psychopathology.

Another consistent finding in these prevalence studies was high rates of comorbidity, which tend to be in the 50% range. Not only was comorbidity found within the internalizing and externalizing clusters, but overlap was also found between these two clusters of symptoms. This consistent and striking degree of comorbidity presents challenges to understanding vulnerability processes in childhood and adolescence. As mentioned earlier, one of the unresolved issues in defining child and adolescent psychopathology is whether there are clearly identifiable categories of psychopathology or whether psychopathology represents a configuration of co-occurring disorders. If distinct homogeneous disorders do exist, then research on the vulnerability processes associated with these disorders could progress toward identifying and understanding the specific vulnerability processes associated with specific types of disorders. However, if psychopathology during childhood and adolescence is best represented by a constellation of comorbid conditions, then the task of identifying and understanding the vulnerability processes related to these conditions becomes a vastly more complex and challenging task.

RATIONALE FOR THE STUDY OF VULNERABILITY IN CHILDREN AND ADOLESCENTS

As the prevalence estimates suggest, there is a clear need to identify and understand the causal factors underlying psychopathology that arise during childhood and adolescence. The benefits from this line of research are numerous. First, the study of vulnerability processes contributes to understanding the nature of the development of psychopathology in children and adolescence. Through the study of vulnerability, the biological and psychological processes that make children susceptible to the development of psychopathology are identified and better understood, thus increasing our understanding of the potential causes of psychopathology in children and adolescents.

Through the investigation of vulnerability factors, we learn how these vulnerability processes interact with maturational processes within the child (e.g, dopaminergic dysfunction) and the environmental context (e.g., various forms of stress) to influence the onset and maintenance of disorder in children and adolescents. For example, over the past three decades the study of vulnerability to schizophrenia has revealed both genetically based and environmentally based (e.g., neurological deficits resulting from obstetrical complications) vulnerabilities associated with the development of schizophrenia. As Brennan and Walker point out (see Chapter 14, this volume), these vulnerability processes appear to interact with hormonal changes in adolescence and with stress in adolescence and adulthood to contribute to the onset of the disorder. Although far from complete, we have a much clearer picture of the factors contributing to the emergence of schizophrenia than we did three decades earlier when vulnerability research was still in its infancy.

Second, in addition to enhancing our understanding of the processes contributing to atypical development, the study of vulnerability processes also contributes to our understanding of neurological, cognitive, and affective processes necessary for normal functioning and adjustment. Recently, the importance of the early development of perceived control was highlighted by theory and research on anxiety and depression in children. In a theoretical paper on the development of anxiety, Chorpita and Barlow (1998) presented theoretical and empirical support for a model that proposes that early life experiences with diminished control may foster the development of cognitions that certain events may be out of one's control. These cognitions then represent a psychological vulnerability for both anxiety and depression. Given that perceptions of a "lack of control" contribute to maladjustment and psychopathology, it can be inferred that the converse is also true. That is, the development of a sense of control over one's internal states and environmental events contributes to the development of adjustment and competence, a notion that is supported by theory and research on mastery learning (e.g., Dweck, 1991) and on perceived competence (e.g., Harter, 1981).

Third, the study of the vulnerability factors and processes contributes to the development of efficacious treatment strategies for children who are experiencing some form of psychopathology. For example, theory and research on anxiety suggests that anxious children, like anxious adults, may have a biological vulnerability that takes the form of hypersensitivity to stress and challenge, along with a diffuse stress response involving a variety of neurobiological processes (see Malcarne & Hansdottir, Chapter 11, and McNally, Malcarne, & Hansdottir, Chapter 13, this volume). These responses are associated with anxiety-elevating cognitions (e.g., "I know I can't do this") and behavioral avoidance of the stressors. Because avoidance reduces distress and arousal, it becomes a reinforced behavioral tendency. Thus, dysfunctional anxiety results from a self-perpetuating cycle of biological arousal to stress, crippling cognitions, and avoidance of stressful situations. In an effort to alter this cycle as revealed in vulnerability research, anxiety treatment researchers have developed a set of treatment strategies that involve helping children to recognize biological arousal associated with anxious feelings, to use relaxation techniques, to confront negative self-talk, and gradually to be exposed to stressful situations. The research on vulnerability processes associated with other forms of psychopathology (e.g., depression and conduct disorders) has also contributed to the growing arsenal of efficacious treatment strategies for children and adolescents (see Kazdin & Weisz, 1996, for a review of this literature).

Finally, research on vulnerability contributes to the development of preventative intervention programs for children and adolescents at risk for psychopathology. For example, research by Dodge and his colleagues (e.g., Dodge, Bates, & Pettit, 1990) has identified a number of social–cognitive processes associated with the development of aggressive behavior and conduct disorder. These processes include hostile attributions of others' intentions, generation of aggressive solutions to social dilemma, and the endorsement of aggressive responses as being effective solutions to conflict (see Crick & Dodge, 1994). These cognitive orientations, which are hypothesized to develop in response to exposure to hostile home and community environments, in turn, serve as vulnerability processes in the development of aggressive behavior. The findings from this line of research have contributed to the development of the "Fast Track" prevention program for conduct disorder. In this intervention program, as children begin kindergarten parents are taught to respond to and interact with their children in a manner that contributes to the formation of cognitions that support prosocial and competent forms of social behavior (see Conduct Problems Prevention Research Group, 1999a, 1999b). Another key component of this preventive intervention is to teach children, within the context of interactions with peers, how to identify the intentions of others, generate prosocial solutions to social dilemmas, and understand the value of nonaggressive behavior (Conduct Problems Prevention Research Group, 1999b). The initial results from this research indicated that at the end of first grade, there were moderate positive effects of the intervention on children's social, emotional, and academic competencies and on children's peer interactions and social status. There were also reductions in the rates of children's aggressive behavior.

Although the study of vulnerability processes in children has potential benefits for understanding the development of psychopathology, for revealing essential processes for normal development and adjustment, and for the development of efficacious prevention and treatment strategies for children and adolescent psychopathology, several challenges still need to be addressed. One of the challenges is in reaching agreement on the definition and conceptualization of vulnerability in the child and adolescent literatures.

DEFINING VULNERABILITY

Perhaps the greatest challenge in defining the concept of vulnerability within the child and adolescent literatures is distinguishing vulnerability from the concept of risk. As noted by several investigators (Ingram, Miranda & Segal, 1998; Richters & Weintraub, 1990), these terms are often used interchangeably; thus the statistical risk for a disorder is assumed to imply the presence of a vulnerability factor. However, there appears to be a growing consensus that whereas risk describes a broad array of factors associated with an increased *probability* of the occurrence of a disorder, vulnerability represents a subset of risk which refers to factors endogenous to the individual that may serve as *mechanisms* in the development of the disorder.

Aside from the confusion between the terms "risk" and "vulnerability," there appears to be some agreement among those studying vulnerability to child and adolescent disorders as to the nature of vulnerability. First vulnerability factors are generally viewed as characteristics that predispose an individual to develop a particular disorder. Thus, consistent with the definition of vulnerability used in this volume, vulnerability processes are viewed as playing some sort of causal role in the development of psychopathology (Albano, Chorpita, & Barlow, 1995; Richters & Weintraub, 1990).

Second, vulnerability factors are typically conceptualized as characteristics residing within the individual that are either genetically or environmentally based. Hereditary factors include genetically determined neurobiological processes as well as various dimensions of temperament. Environmentally based factors are quite broad, ranging from central nervous system damage resulting from obstetrical and birth complications to vulnerability factors acquired through socialization and learning processes (e.g., a lack of control that might result from overprotective parenting). The extent to which genetically and environmentally based vulnerability processes have been examined in relation to a particular disorder is largely determined by the theoretical models guiding the research in that particular area. For example, research on vulnerability to schizophrenia has focused on both genetically based and environmentally based (e.g., obstetrical complications) vulnerability factors, which naturally follows the diathesis–stress models that have guided the research in this area for the past three decades (e.g., Asarnow & Asarnow, 1996). Similarly, in the mood disorders literature which often utilizes diathesis–stress models, both genetically based vulnerabilities (e.g., shy temperament) and environmentally based vulnerabilities (e.g., learned helplessness) have been the focus of research. In contrast, research on conduct disorders has primarily focused on vulnerability processes acquired through socialization processes in early development. This is not surprising given that the predominate theories guiding this research are rooted in behavioral (e.g., Patterson, 1993) and cognitive–social learning theories (e.g., Dodge, 1993).

Third, in general, vulnerability processes are viewed as being relatively stable and enduring. However, the extent to which a factor is seen as enduring depends on whether the factor is seen as a biological process that has its roots in hereditary processes, is the result of some sort of environmentally based trauma or injury, or has been acquired through learning processes (e.g., a negative self-schema). Whereas vulnerability processes rooted in hereditary processes or some sort of environmentally based injury are perceived as stable and enduring, vulnerability processes resulting from learning are seen as more malleable. Yet, even learning-based vulnerability processes are often viewed as being relatively stable and even enduring, especially if the environmental context in which the individual is developing consists of features that maintain the learning-based vulnerability process (e.g., persistent parental rejection).

HISTORY OF THEORY AND RESEARCH ON VULNERABILITY FACTORS RELATED TO CHILD AND ADOLESCENT PSYCHOPATHOLOGY

Theoretical Models

Prior to the 20th century, there was a glaring absence of knowledge about child psychopathology and professional specialties that focused on child psychopathology (Rie, 1971). This was due, in part, to the general social philosophy that permeated mainstream culture that children were not valued persons but, rather, family possessions (Aries, 1962). During this period, child behavioral disorders were believed to be the result of either organic imbalances, inherent evil, or possession by supernatural forces.

During the latter half of the 19th century the philosophies of Locke (1690/1913), Rousseau (1762/1955) and others began to have an influence on societal conceptualizations of childhood. These philosophers asserted that the direction of children's lives were not necessarily biologically determined and could be influenced by moral guidance and support. Consequently, concern for the needs of children in general began to increase across Europe and North America. By the turn of the century, specific concern for the welfare of children with mental and behavioral disorders was also increasing. However, due to the heavy influence of the medical sciences and the organic disease model, mental disorders among children were viewed as being biologically based. Although not discussed in terms of vulnerability processes, the causal mechanisms in the development of child disorders were seen as being rooted in the child's physiological makeup. This perspective continued to dominate during the early part of this century. However, during the middle part of the 20th century, the role of the environment in the development of childhood disorders became more widely recognized and accepted as psychoanalytic and behavioral theories increased in influence.

By 1962, Meehl introduced the diathesis–stress model of schizophrenia, which formally introduced the concept of vulnerability, along with the notion that psychopathology was a result of the interplay between both biological vulnerability processes and environmental stressors and influences. Meehl's model helped to integrate the biological and environmental models of psychopathology. Since that time, the diathesis–stress model has been used to understand myriad childhood disorders including childhood schizophrenia (e.g., Asarnow & Asarnow, 1996), anxiety (e.g., Barlow, 1988), and depression (e.g., Blatt & Homann, 1992). The diathesis–stress model was also instrumental in launching the research on risk for psychopathology, which has expanded from an earlier focus on identifying risk factors associated with schizophrenia to the identification of risk factors associated with a wide range of child and adolescent disorders.

Recently, with the advent of the field of developmental psychopathology, there has been a trend toward moving beyond diathesis–stress models to multidimensional models that reflect more of the dynamic nature of the interactions or "transactions" between the child and his or her environment, with particular importance given to developmental processes (e.g., Cicchetti & Cohen, 1995; Hammen & Rudolph, 1996; Sroufe, 1997). Most of these developmental theories integrate the basic components of the general diathesis–stress model with developmental principles. The general characteristics of developmental models of psychopathology include several elements.

First, vulnerability processes are viewed as being either hereditarily or environmentally based. Hereditary factors include such biological processes as neurological functioning and temperament. Environmental vulnerability factors include both environmentally based trauma or injury (e.g., obstetrical complications) or socialization processes (e.g., cognitions of self that emerge from parent–child interactions).

Second, the developmental psychopathology perspective asserts that vulnerability factors can exist within any of the physiological, affective, cognitive, or social/behavioral systems. Table 2.1 lists several vulnerability factors that have been found to be related to several different forms of psychopathology among children and adolescents. We have attempted to categorize each of these factors according to the type of developmental system it represents. As is evident from this table, for each of the forms of psychopathology listed, a number of vulnerability factors have been found within each of the major domains or systems of development. According to the developmental psychopathology perspective, with age these systems become more integrated, thus enabling various vulnerability processes, as well as protective processes, to act in a synergistic fashion to influence the development of disorder.

TABLE 2.1. Vulnerability Factors Related to Child Psychopathology

	Cognitive	Affective	Social/behavioral	Biological
Anxiety	• Cognitions of diminished control over events or situations	• Difficulty regulating and monitoring emotional expression	• Insecure attachment • Social avoidance and withdrawal	• Heritability • Behavioral inhibition • Dysregulation in neurological subsystems
Depression	• Dysfunctional cognitive appraisal style of self and others • Internal, global, stable attributions for negative events • Negative models of self and others	• Difficulty controlling depressive affect • Increased use of lower-quality, mal-adaptive emotional regulation strategies	• Anxious, insecure attachment • Social impairments such as withdrawal	• Heritability • Dysfunctional HPA axis regulation • Increased sensitivity to stressful events
Conduct disorder	• Memory structures that the world is a hostile place • Automatic processing that includes aggressive, hostile attributions	• Higher levels of depressed and angry affect • High variability and intensity of emotional responses	• Insecure relationships and attachments • Poor social competence, such as negative problem solving skills • Social rejection	• Neurological • Heritability • Deficits in the brain's noradrenergic and serotonergic systems

TABLE 2.1. (cont.)

	Cognitive	Affective	Social/behavioral	Biological
Attention-deficit/hyperactivity disorder	• Deficits in information processing • Deficits in processing and encoding information • Allocation of attention to fewer stimuli • Fewer response access from memory	• Variability in negative mood and variability in arousal • Difficulty processing emotional cues	• Poor social competence, such as poor problem solving skills • Difficulty modulating social communication • Deficits in self-control such as impulsivity	• Irregular metabolism of monoamines • Diminished brain dopamine • Underarousal of the reticular activation system • Difficulty in selective attention, distractibility, and sustained attention
Schizo-phrenia	• Deficits in informational/attentional processing • Difficulty processing information under controlled circumstances	• Blunted affect • Emotional withdrawal	• Deficits in social competence, such as interpersonal problem soling skills and communication	• Heritability • Dopaminergic hyperactivity • Central integrative dysfunction

Take, for example, the vulnerability processes associated with conduct disorders (CD). *Biological* vulnerability appears in the following areas: (1) neurological (i.e., from disruption in the ontogenesis of the fetal brain such as exposure to toxic agents or child abuse and neglect; Craig & Pepler, 1997; Moffitt, 1993); (2) heritability (i.e., increased risk for CD in families); and (3) biochemical (i.e., deficits in efficiency of the brain's noradrenergic and serotonergic system, especially lower levels of serotonin; Kruesi et al., 1990; Richters & Cicchetti, 1993). Individuals with CD also tend to manifest certain *social/behavioral* vulnerabilities, including a lack of positive social schema and poor attachment relationships (Greenberg, Speltz, & DeKlyen, 1993; Kagan, 1984). These social vulnerabilities interact with *cognitive* vulnerabilities so these individuals negatively approach and perceive the environment to be consistent with their negative experiences with others. These memory structures and expectations negatively affect the ability to form positive relationships and perpetuate the likelihood of negative social interactions (Cicchetti, 1990; Richters & Cicchetti, 1993). These individuals display a variety of cognitive, perceptual, and attributional biases related to their CD problems (Dodge et al., 1990) which are difficult to monitor and control. Individuals develop memory structures of the world as a hostile place that requires coercive behavior to achieve desired goals. *Affective* vulnerability to CD can be expressed in difficulty controlling their emotional responses. This is marked by high activity and intensity of emotional response (Malhotra, 1989) as well as negative mood (Weinberger & Gomes, 1996) including both angry and depressed affect (Sanders, Dadds, Johnston, & Cash, 1992). Thus, individuals who are most vulnerable to CD are those who have a biological vulnerability for aggressive behavior as well as difficulty controlling and managing hostile and negative affect. Further, they also tend to view the world and others as negative and hostile and demonstrate a variety of deficits in social competence. Conduct disorders then can be viewed as developing as a result of an interactional process among vulnerability processes from various developmental systems.

Third, vulnerability processes within the individual are viewed as being in a dynamic interaction with environmental systems throughout the lifespan. This dynamic interaction, or transaction, is reciprocal in nature, allowing vulnerability processes both to influence and be influenced by environmental conditions.

Fourth, the degree to which an individual successfully negotiates the important developmental tasks at one phase of development (e.g., development of language skills in infancy and integration in the peer group in childhood) will have an impact on the degree to which developmental tasks are negotiated at subsequent phases of development (Sroufe, 1997). The development of various cognitive, affective, and social competencies acquired as a consequence of successful negotiation of developmental tasks will contribute to successful negotiation of the developmental requirements at the next phase of development and help to maintain a normative developmental trajectory. These competencies, in turn, can make the individual more resilient to the development of disorder, even in the presence of a vulnerability factor (Sameroff & Seifer, 1990). Conversely, failure to develop necessary competencies becomes an obstacle to the negotiation of subsequent developmental tasks, thus contributing to the individual's vulnerability to psychopathology later in development and increasing the possibility of an atypical developmental trajectory.

Fifth, as might well be expected, developmental models emphasize the importance of understanding the particular pathway an individual takes in the development of a disorder. Even though two individuals may develop the same form of psychopathology (e.g., depression), the specific vulnerability factors and the dynamics of the interaction between these factors and the environment in route to the development of the disorder can differ (Cicchetti & Rogosch, 1996). Thus, a specific disorder may be reached from a variety of different initial conditions and through a variety of different processes. This phenomenon represents the construct referred to in general systems theory as *epifinality*. It is also recognized that the same vulnerability processes (e.g., inaccurate interpretations of other's intentions) may lead to different types of disorders across different individuals, due to each person's unique genotype and developmental history. This represents the complementary construct of *multifinality*. Thus, a particular vulnerability factor is not necessarily seen as leading to the same psychopathological outcome in every individual.

Finally, unlike traditional disease models, developmental models do not assume discontinuity between dysfunctional behavior and normal behavior, where the former is viewed as being different in kind from normal behavior. Rather, developmental models of psychopathology make no prior assumptions about continuity or discontinuity between normal and pathological behavior (Cicchetti & Cohen, 1995; Sameroff & Seifer, 1990). Furthermore, there is also no assumption as to whether vulnerabilities should be conceptualized as dichotomous or continuous variables.

What clearly distinguishes the models emerging from the field of developmental psychopathology from the earlier diathesis–stress models are emphases on developmental processes and change and on the dynamic interactions between the individual and his or her experiences throughout the lifespan. From all appearances, current theory and research on vulnerability to child and adolescent psychopathology is becoming increasingly dominated by a developmental psychopathology perspective. As Garmezy (1991) notes: "Developmental psychopathology and risk research have now become inextricably linked in their common focus on those ontogenetic and environmental processes that influence the longitudinal evolution of adaptive and maladaptive behavior patterns extending from infancy to adulthood" (p. 32).

As the developmental psychopathology perspective has become more influential in the study of vulnerability, changes have also occurred in both the methods used to study vulnerability and in the direction of the research on vulnerability. These changes are reviewed briefly in the following section.

Research Methodology and Research Trends

The 1960s saw the birth of a research tradition that focused on identifying the factors that put individuals at risk for psychopathology, which thus became the formal beginning of research on vulnerability processes. Initially those efforts used cross-sectional designs that focused almost exclusively on the characteristics of adults manifesting a disorder (e.g., schizophrenia). However, as Mednick and McNeil (1968) pointed out in reference to research on schizophrenia, there were serious weaknesses in studying etiological factors in individuals who had already been diagnosed with the disorder. Among the weaknesses cited were inaccurate and distorted retrospective reports, effects of psychiatric care, and, most serious, the inability to separate the causes from the consequences of the disorder. In response to these shortcomings, Mednick and McNeil (1968) began advocating the use of prospective, longitudinal designs to the study of the etiology of psychopathology. They argued that by studying a group of children, many of whom would later develop the disorder, the methodological shortcomings of cross-sectional designs could be avoided. One of the clear advantages of prospective designs is that because the individuals in the study do not possess symptoms of the disorder, their responses on various measures taken during the course of the investigation, particularly early on, are unlikely to be influenced by features of the disorder or by any treatment. Likewise, the assessments provided by others during the course of development are also less likely to be influenced by manifested features of the disorder, or by any expectations that might result from a prior diagnosis of a disorder. Another real advantage of the prospective design is that because of the temporal sequencing of the assessment of risk factors and the emergence of the disorder, the causes, symptoms, and consequences of the disorder can be more easily separated and identified.

Based on these considerations, researchers interested in understanding the etiology of schizophrenia began to examine the children of individuals diagnosed with schizophrenia. Given that children with one diagnosed parent are 10 to 15 times more likely to develop schizophrenia than the offspring of nondiagnosed parents, this represented a particularly high-risk group of individuals to study. Over the past 30 years, many researchers have studied samples of these high-risk children to examine the etiology of schizophrenia (e.g., Garmezy, 1974; Mednick & Schulsinger, 1968). To date, a fairly wide range of personal and environmental characteristics of the children of parents diagnosed with schizophrenia have been assessed, resulting in an extensive literature on risk factors for schizophrenia (see Gooding & Iacono, 1995, for a review). Having proven useful for the study of the origins of schizophrenia, prospective longitudinal designs have been used to understand the etiology of child and adolescent disorders as well. For example, prospective longitudinal designs have been used extensively to understand the etiology of both mood disorders (e.g., Nolen-Hoeksema, Girgu, & Seligman, 1986, 1992) and conduct disorders (see Dodge et al., 1990; Patterson, 1993).

Although the more formal and focused study of risk and vulnerability factors emerged from the study of schizophrenia during the 1960s, the use of longitudinal research to study developmental outcomes in children and adolescents actually has its roots in the 1920s. During this time, a number of "growth studies" of children were initiated. Perhaps the most well-known of these studies were conducted at the Institute of Human Development at the University of California, Berkeley (Jones, Bayley, MacFarlane, & Honzik, 1971). The first of these studies, the Guidance Study, was designed to reveal the frequency of behavior and personality problems displayed by a sample of children in therapeutic preschool clinics. As a precursor to the more formal study of risk that emerged several decades later, the aims of this study were to identify the 'bioenvironmental' and family factors associated with the presence or absence of specific presenting problems. What began as a 5-year study, eventually turned into a series of follow-up studies of the original cohort when they were 30 and 40 years of age.

The second study to have its genesis at the Institute was the Berkeley Growth Study (Jones et al., 1971), which began the same year as the Guidance Study. The major goal of this study was to examine the physical, mental, physiological, and motor development in the first 15 months of life among a homogeneous sample of healthy Caucasian infants. However, as with the Guidance Study, a short-term longitudinal study turned into a follow-up investigation of the original cohort from ages 3 to 18 and again at 21, 26, and 36 years of age. What began as a study of the growth and development of infants became a study of the linkages between child and adult personality patterns, predictors of adult relationships, and an evaluation of the offspring born to the members of the original cohort. Both of these investigations made early contributions to our understanding of risk for psychopathology and of the methodology that could be used to examine risk and vulnerability.

So as not to leave the impression that longitudinal research should always be viewed as the "best" design for studying vulnerability processes, studies using cross-sectional designs still have an important place in vulnerability research, especially in the process of identifying potential vulnerability factors. For example, Garber and Flynn (Chapter 8, this volume) point out how cross-sectional methodology has been fruitful to the identification of vulnerability factors in depression. Using this methodology, groups of individuals who are currently depressed are compared to those who have never been depressed and those who were formerly depressed. A stable vulnerability factor would be expected to be present in both the currently depressed individuals and the formerly depressed individuals. However, if this factor indeed represents some sort of vulnerability to depression, it would be less likely to be evident among the individuals who were never depressed.

Over the course of the three decades since the formal study of risk research emerged, a number of changes have also occurred in the focus of risk research. Reflecting the transition from disease models to models based on a developmental psychopathology perspective, research on vulnerability to psychopathology in children and adolescents has shifted from the *identification* of single vulnerability processes to a more comprehensive *analysis of the interaction* between multiple vulnerability and protective processes, environmental stressors, and developmental change. Because the disease models guiding earlier research focused on identifying a single endogenous pathogen within the individual, initial vulnerability research was set up to determine linkages between a single endogenous factor (e.g., attentional deficits) and a specific type of disorder (e.g., schizophrenia). With the emergence of diathesis–stress models, the focus of research began to shift toward attempting to understand the interaction between the diathesis (the vulnerability factor) and stressful life experiences that might trigger the disorder.

More recently, another shift has occurred in the research on vulnerability to child and adolescent disorders as a result of the influence of developmental models of vulnerability. As mentioned earlier, these models emphasize that the development of psychopathology is a consequence of the unfolding of the complex interaction between characteristics of the child and his or her social environment. Following from this model, many recent studies of risk have sought to identify sets of vulnerability and protective factors involved in the development of specific disorders. For example, Cicchetti and his colleagues have examined the roles of vulnerability processes, such as a negative self and other representations (Lynch & Cicchetti, 1991), and dysfunctional emotional regulation (Cicchetti, Ganihan, & Barnett, 1991) and protective factors, including social competencies and perceived self-efficacy (e.g., Toth & Cicchetti, 1996) in the development of psychopathology in a sample of maltreated children. Finally, there is also a recent trend toward understanding vulnerability *processes* and *mechanisms* rather than simply identifying a vulnerability factor via a correlational connection between the vulnerability factor and a specific form of psychopathology.

As a consequence of the research on vulnerability factors over the past three decades, a wide range of biological and psychological processes has been identified as being vulnerability factors that contribute to the development of child and adolescent psychopathology. Although the specifics on how these vulnerability factors are translated into a specific form of psychopathology is still relatively unknown, we at least have a starting point for understanding better the vulnerability processes that underlie child and adolescent psychopathology.

CONCLUSIONS

After three decades, the research on vulnerability to child and adolescent disorders has clearly come into its own. New models for conceptualizing vulnerability have emerged, along with methodological approaches used to examine the processes described in these models. Also, as is evident from the chapters in this volume, a wide range of biologically and environmentally based vulnerability processes have been found to be linked to the development of psychopathology in children and adolescents. Whereas some vulnerability factors have been linked to specific types of psychopathology (e.g., dopaminergic hyperactivity in schizophrenia), other vulnerability factors have been linked to more than one type of disorder (e.g., attentional deficits).

One of the challenges that remains is uncovering the reasons why certain vulnerability factors may be associated with more than one form of psychopathology. One possibility is that during childhood, particularly early on in development, there may be a lack of differentiation between developmental systems, such that vulnerability processes would naturally have an effect on a number of different domains of functioning. Another possibility is that even though developmental systems will eventually differentiate, these systems are so well integrated that a single vulnerability process within one developmental system, such as deficits in sustained attention, could indeed be related to a variety of forms of psychopathology (attention-deficit/hyperactivity disorder and conduct disorders). Yet another possibility is that our measurement of vulnerability constructs still lacks the precision to detect subtle distinctions between vulnerability factors. For instance, although attention deficits have been found to be associated with several forms of psychopathology, it is possible that more subtle distinguishing forms of attention deficits are associated with different disorders. Relatedly, it is possible that a closer examination of the operational definitions of the same vulnerability process across studies will reveal subtle differences in measurements that reflect differences in the vulnerability processes. Finally, it is possible that the association between a particular vulnerability process with several types of disorders reflects overlap between the nature of the disorders. For example, in the model of anxiety proposed by Chorpita and Barlow (1998), anxiety and depression are hypothesized to lie on the same continuum in terms of perceived personal control. Thus it should be no surprise to find that the two disorders share some of the same vulnerability processes.

These and other challenges remain for those interested in understanding better the vulnerability processes associated with psychopathology during childhood and adolescence. If the progress that has been made over the last three decades is any indication of what can be accomplished in the future, then we enter the new millennium with a renewed optimism for increasing our understanding of vulnerability to psychopathology during childhood and adolescence.

REFERENCES

Albano, A. M., Chorpita, B. F., & Barlow, D. H. (1996). Childhood anxiety disorders. In E. J. Mash & R. A. Barkley (Eds.), *Child psychopathology* (pp. 196–241). New York: Guilford Press.

American Psychiatric Association. (1994). *Diagnostic and statistical manual of mental disorders* (4th ed.). Washington, DC: Author.

Aries, P. (1962). *Centuries of childhood*. New York: Knopf.

Asarnow, J. R., & Asarnow, R. F. (1996). Childhood-onset schizophrenia. In E. J. Mash & R. A. Barkley (Eds.), *Child psychopathology* (pp. 340–361). New York: Guilford Press.

Barlow, D. H. (1988). *Anxiety and its disorders: The nature and treatment of anxiety and panic*. New York: Guilford Press.

Blatt, S. J., & Homann, E. (1992). Parent–child interaction in the etiology of dependent and self-critical depression. *Clinical Psychology Review, 12,* 47–91.

& S. Weintraub (Eds.) *Risk and protective factors in the development of psychopathology* (pp. 67–96). New York: Cambridge University Press.

Rie, H. E. (1971). Historical perspective of concepts of child psychopathology. In H. E. Rie (Ed.), *Perspectives in child psychopathology* (pp. 3–50). Chicago: Aldine-Atherton.

Rousseau, J. J. (1955). *Emile*. New York: Dutton. (Original work published 1762)

Sameroff, A. J., & Seifer, R. (1990). Early contributors to developmental risk. In J. Rolf, A. S. Masten, D. Cicchetti, K. H. Nuechterlein, & S. Weintraub (Eds.), *Risk and protective factors in the development of psychopathology* (pp. 52–66). New York: Cambridge University Press.

Sanders, M. R., Dadds, M. R., Johnston, B. M., & Cash, R. (1992). Childhood depression and conduct disorder: I. Behavioral, affective, and cognitive aspects of family problem-solving interactions. *Journal of Abnormal Psychology, 101,* 495–504.

Schwab-Stone, M. E., & Briggs-Gowan, M. J. (1998). The scope and prevalence of psychiatric disorders in childhood and adolescence. In J. G. Young & P. Ferrari (Eds.), *Designing mental health services and systems for children and adolescents: A shrewd investment* (pp. 2–25). Philadelphia: Brunner/Mazel.

Sroufe, L. A. (1997). Psychopathology as an outcome of development. *Development and Psychopathology, 9,* 251–268.

Toth, S. L., & Cicchetti, D. (1996). Patterns of relatedness, depressive symptomatology, and perceived competence in maltreated children. *Journal of Consulting and Clinical Psychology, 64,* 32–41.

Weinberger, D. A., & Gomes, M. E. (1996). Changes in daily mood and self-restraint among undercontrolled preadolescents: A time-series analysis of "acting out." *Journal of the American Academy of Child & Adolescent Psychiatry, 34,* 1473–1482.

World Health Organization. (1992). *The ICD-10 classification of mental and behavioral disorders: Clinical descriptions and diagnostic guidelines.* Geneva, Switzerland: Author.

3

The Nature of Adult Vulnerability
History and Definitions

RICK E. INGRAM
MICHELLE FORTIER

As is evident from the organization of this volume, vulnerability theory and research can, at least for the sake of discussion, be partitioned into vulnerability to psychopathology in childhood and adolescence and vulnerability to psychopathology in adulthood. As previously noted (Ingram & Price, Chapter 1, this volume), such a distinction is in many respects artificial, but it nevertheless serves some important purposes. Perhaps most important, differentiating between child/adolescence and adult psychopathology renders more manageable the task of understanding vulnerability. Indeed, for all but the most extraordinary theorists and researchers, it is difficult to have a firm grasp on the most important vulnerability factors for both adults and children, let alone for both. Moreover, the sheer range and diversity of different forms of psychopathology in both adulthood and childhood/adolescence present formidable challenges for any attempt to adequately understand the factors that predispose to disorders. Partitioning theory and research on child and adult factors thus helps to make theory and research more manageable for both the producers and the consumers of this information.

In pursuing this partition, Price and Lento (Chapter 2, this volume) discuss a number of important issues that must be considered in understanding theory and research on childhood vulnerability. The current chapter explores some of the issues that surround conceptualizations of adult vulnerability. A variety of issues dictate that we confine our discussion to a limited number of psychological problems, and we thus start this exploration by briefly noting the disorders that are classified as adult psychopathology. We next address why we believe it is important to study vulnerability to disorders in adulthood and suggest three broad reasons that justify this approach. Next we trace the history of the vulnerability approach to adult psychopathology.

THE DISORDERS OF ADULTHOOD: A BRIEF SUMMARY

The number of disorders that exist in various classification schemes, and that are proposed by various schools of thought, is enormous. Deciding which disorders to examine therefore requires making some choices. Although some psychologists concentrate on extremely rare disorders (e.g., Franzini & Grossberg, 1995), the fact that they are so rare suggests that they affect few people, thus rendering discussion of them an inappropriate subject for serious psychology. On the other hand, some relatively rare disorders are quite serious (e.g., dissociative identity disorder), but because systematic empirical research on them is also rare, it is difficult to examine vulnerability factors with any degree of confidence. We will thus limit our discussion in this chapter to the major disorders of adulthood as recognized by the fourth edition of the *Diagnostic and Statistical Manual of Mental Disorders* (DSM-IV; American Psychiatric Association, 1994), and which have been the subject of empirical research. Although the classification scheme offered by DSM-IV is far from perfect (Ingram, Miranda, & Segal, 1998), it does tend to represent a consensus among researchers on a reasonable way to understand at least the descriptive features of psychopathology. We thus summarize here the descriptive features of several DSM-IV Axis I (clinical syndrome) disorders that (1) are not extremely uncommon, (2) have been the subject of vulnerability theorizing and research, and (3) are not the clear result of organic causes (e.g., Alzheimer's disease). Axis II disorders (personality disorders), of course, can also be disorders of adulthood, but we will leave an examination of these disorders to Geiger and Crick (Chapter 4, this volume). The disorders we examine make up the vast majority of psychopathological conditions experienced by adults (see Robins & Regier, 1991) and, correspondingly, are the disorders that are examined in more depth in the chapters throughout this volume.

Substance-Related Disorders

Substance-related disorders may be the most detailed compilation of disorders that are included in DSM-IV. They include the abuse of numerous substances as well as intoxication resulting from these substances. *Intoxicated states* are diagnosed as a disorder when they are associated with maladaptive functioning (e.g., cognitive impairment and interpersonal difficulty) that is the result of the ingestion of a psychoactive substance and occur in circumstances associated with significant risk (driving while intoxicated, behaviors that lead to legal problems, etc.). Although a convenient diagnostic category in some instances, substance intoxication generally falls outside the scope of our interest in psychopathology.[1]

A category that does fall within our view of psychopathology is that of *substance abuse* disorders. According to DSM-IV, substance abuse disorders are defined as "a maladaptive pattern of substance use manifested by recurrent adverse consequences related to the repeated use of substances" (p. 182). DSM-IV lists several criteria for an overall diagnosis of substance abuse, including (1) chronic use of a substance that results in the failure to fulfill one's major life obligations; (2) recurrent use in situations that can be hazardous, such as driving; (3) legal problems that result from repeated substance use; and (4) recurrent use that occurs despite the problems caused by the abuse. Any one of these criteria can be sufficient for a diagnosis of substance abuse if it occurs within a period of 12 months.

DSM-IV also lists numerous substances whose chronic use can result in a diagnosis. A notable but not exhaustive list includes alcohol, amphetamines, cannabis, cocaine, hallucinogens, opioids, and phencyclidines (PCP). Also included in this list of substances that can form the basis of a disorder is caffeine, a legal and popular drug. For example, according to DSM-IV, for those who ingest caffeine in the form of coffee, tea, soda, cold remedies, or chocolate, the average caffeine intake in the United States is around 200 mg per day (the equivalent of about two brewed cups of coffee, or about 50 oz. of soda). Excessive use of even these legal substances can result in a DSM-IV diagnosis, although this is extremely rare.

Each of these have criteria that are specific to the particular substance. Criteria for a diagnosis of alcohol intoxication, for example, include features such as slurred speech, lack of coordination, faulty memory and attention impairment. On the other hand, cannabis intoxication includes primary features such as motor impairment, euphoria, and impaired judgment and peripheral features such as increased appetite and dry mouth. Continual use of such substances may be associated with a substance abuse diagnosis if this use results in the impairment noted in the general DSM-IV criteria for substance abuse.

Eating Disorders

Eating disorders, characterized by a significant disturbance in eating habits, are divided into two more specific disorders: anorexia nervosa and bulimia nervosa. Each of these disorders also has a specific subtype.

---

[1]DSM-IV also includes a category for substance withdrawal, but inasmuch as this also falls outside the scope of our interest in psychological disorders, it is not discussed here.

Anorexia Nervosa

DSM-IV criteria suggest that this eating disorder is characterized by the refusal to maintain a minimally normal body weight for the individual's age and height (i.e., less than 85% of the expected weight). The disorder is also characterized by a significant fear of becoming fat, unrelated to actual weight. Correspondingly, anorexia nervosa features a distorted body image in which individuals do not acknowledge the weight deficit. Prevalence rates for this disorder range from 0.5% to 1.0%. Onset typically occurs in late adolescence or early adulthood, with a mean onset of approximately 17 years of age. An enormous gender difference is widely acknowledged, with more than 90% of anorexia diagnoses being assigned to women (American Psychiatric Association, 1994). The disorder carries significant risk for illness and premature death through starvation or electrolyte imbalance. Suicide rates are also high for this disorder.

Two specific subtypes of anorexia nervosa are recognized: the *binge eating/purging type* and the *restricted type*. The binge eating/purging subtype regularly engages in binge eating and then purges through the use of methods such as induced vomiting or laxative use. In contrast to this subtype, the restricted subtype *does not* binge eat and purge but, rather, severely restricts food intake (e.g., excessive dieting).

Bulimia Nervosa

While anorexia nervosa is characterized by the refusal to maintain a normal weight, the primary features of bulimia nervosa are binge eating a large amount of food, relative to what most individuals would eat within a relatively limited amount of time, and feelings of a lack of control about eating. As with those with anorexia, the individual with bulimia uses an inappropriate way to compensate for the binge eating (e.g., vomiting). Also as with anorexia, the onset of this disorder occurs in late adolescence or early adulthood and is far often more assigned to women than to men (by about the same 90% figure). This disorder is somewhat more commonly diagnosed than anorexia, with estimates ranging from 1% to 3%. The key difference between bulimia nervosa and anorexia is that individuals with bulimia are able to maintain a body weight at a normal level, or at a minimally normal level.

Bulimia nervosa has two subtypes: the purging subtype and the nonpurging subtype. The purging subtype chronically uses inappropriate ways to avoid weight gain such as laxative overuse or self-induced vomiting. The nonpurging subtype compensates for bingeing by methods such as fasting or excessive physical exercise rather than through inappropriate use of laxatives, self-induced vomiting, and so on.

Mood/Affective Disorders

The key feature of mood or affective disorders is a disturbance in, naturally enough, mood. Beyond this central feature, mood disorders generally fall into two broad categories: bipolar disorders and unipolar disorder.[2] The key unipolar disorder is major depressive episode while the key bipolar disorder can be either a depressive episode and a manic episode or the occurrence of a manic episode only. Mood disturbances of a less severe magnitude occur relatively frequently in the general population, and at present there is no consensus whether these states represent downward extensions of clinically severe states or fundamentally different phenomena (Ingram & Hamilton, 1999; Tennen, Hall, & Affleck, 1995).

Unipolar Disorder: Major Depressive Episode

The core feature of a depressive episode is a minimum 2-week period in which the individual experiences either a significantly depressed mood or, alternatively, a loss of interest or pleasure in virtually all activities. Beyond these core symptoms, DSM-IV specifies that at least four additional symptoms must be experienced. Although a minimum of 2 weeks is specified, untreated major depressive episode can last for up to 2 years (Goodwin & Jamison, 1990)

Among the DSM-IV criteria from which these four additional symptoms must be experienced are (1) a significant weight change (either loss or gain), (2) insomnia or hypersomnia, (3) motor retardation or agitation, (4) a continual sense of exhaustion or fatigue, (5) feelings of worthlessness or guilt, (6) cognitive impairment such as concentration difficulties or indecisiveness, and (7) suicidal ideation, a plan for committing suicide, or a suicide attempt. Other features, such as hopeless and negative or distorted information processing, are not included in DSM-IV as specific criteria but are nonetheless widely recognized as characterizing many cases of depression.

A first onset of depression can occur at any age but typically occurs in young adulthood. Because many individuals experience numerous depressive episodes over the course of their lifetime, depression is also widely recognized as a chronic disorder (Hammen, 1991; Lavori, Kessler, & Klerman, 1984). Prevalence estimates vary widely and can range from lifetime estimate of 20% to 5% (Ingram et al., 1998). Suicide rates are high in individuals with a depressive disorder; DSM-IV reports that approximately 15% of

---

[2]Within each of these major catagories are a number of subcatagories such as dysthymia and cyclothymia. Although these are important, because our focus is on the major disorders, we do not address them here.

individuals with a major depressive disorder commit suicide, and, exclusive of suicide, overall mortality rates in depressed individuals are higher than average. There is a widely recognized gender difference in depression, with approximately twice as many women as men being diagnosed with the disorder. Such gender differences are observed worldwide and are unlikely to be accounted for by artifacts such as diagnostic bias (Ingram et al., 1998).

Bipolar Disorder

In DSM-IV, bipolar disorders are separated into bipolar I and bipolar II. Bipolar I is characterized by the occurrence of at least one manic episode. The occurrence of a major depressive episode at some point in the person's life is not required for this diagnosis, but such episodes are nevertheless frequent, and when they have occurred, the disorder is classified as a mixed episode. Bipolar II is defined as the occurrence of at least one major depressive episode, and the occurrence of at least one hypomanic (but not manic) episode.

Like unipolar mood disorder, bipolar disorder usually first occurs in young adulthood, and in many cases is quite chronic. For example, DSM-IV reports that more than 90% of people who have experienced a manic episode will experience another episode in the future. Prevalence rates are lower for bipolar disorder than for unipolar disorder. For bipolar I disorder, lifetime prevalence rates range from 0.04% to 1.6%, with the large-scale Epidemiologic Catchment Area (ECA) study (Robins & Regier, 1991) finding a rate of 0.8%. Prevalence rates for bipolar II tend to hover around 0.5% (Robins & Regier, 1991). Unlike major depression, there do not appear to be gender differences in the incidence of bipolar disorder, although there are some differences in the timing and onset of the disorder between genders. For example, women are more likely to experience the onset of depression first while men are more likely to experience a manic episode first (American Psychiatric Association, 1994).

Anxiety Disorders

The category of anxiety disorders encompasses a number of specific anxiety states that are considered clinically problematic. For example, panic attacks, panic disorder, agoraphobia with and without panic, social phobia, specific phobia, obsessive–compulsive disorder, posttraumatic stress disorder, acute stress disorder, and generalized anxiety disorder all fall under the more general rubric of anxiety disorders. These specific disorders do not include the residual problems included in virtually all the DSM-IV categories—anxiety disorder not otherwise specified.

Rather than discuss each of these specific disorders here, we instead note the central features that characterize, and thus define, a condition as an anxiety disorder. Quite obviously, the core feature of anxiety disorders is anxiety or fear or apprehensiveness. Although in some cases anxiety manifests itself only in certain situations (e.g., in social situations for social phobia), in other cases the anxiety is quite generalized and seems to pervade most of the individual's functioning (e.g., generalized anxiety disorder). Although fear and apprehensiveness are the key emotional states involved in anxiety disorders, these disorders are also characterized by cognitive, behavioral, and somatic symptom patterns.

Cognitive characteristics of many anxiety states include problems with effective task performance when the person is experiencing anxiety and the possible misinterpretation of situations as dangerous or threatening when the actual danger or threat is either limited or nonexistent. Behaviorally, many anxiety states are characterized by avoidance of perceived threatening situations (e.g., social situations). Somatic features involve physiological changes that occur in anxiety-provoking situations, such as dry mouth, shallow breathing, increased perspiration, and heart palpitations. The various characteristics that occur in the cognitive, behavioral, and somatic domains vary not only across individuals but also across the more specific anxiety disorders. Likewise, course, prevalence, and gender differences also vary considerably across the different disorders.

Schizophrenia

Like anxiety and depression, the category of schizophrenia includes a number of different conditions and specific schizophrenic states. Unlike anxiety and depression, the defining feature of schizophrenia is psychosis—a condition that is typically defined as involving hallucinations, delusions, and psychological and behavioral disorganization (although not all these symptoms need be present in any given case of schizophrenia). Schizophrenia falls under the DSM-IV category of schizophrenia and other psychotic disorders. Some of these other psychotic disorders include delusional disorder (previously labeled paranoia), brief psychotic disorder, shared psychotic disorder, and schizoaffective disorder, the latter of which is defined as a combination of psychotic and affective features, making it difficult to diagnose as either schizophrenia or an affective (or mood) disorder.

Clearly, schizophrenia is the most prevalent of the various psychotic disorders, although its overall prevalence in the general population is quite low in comparison to other psychiatric conditions. DSM-IV estimates lifetime prevalence rates between 0.5% and 1%, whereas the ECA study estimates rates at 1.3% (Keith, Regier, & Rae, 1991). Estimates also vary concerning gender differences with some studies indicating higher rates for males, others suggesting higher rates for females (possibly due to overlap between schizophrenia and mood disorders), and others suggesting no gender differences at all. Although it is still unclear whether there are gender differences in schizophrenia, if these differences do exist they are clearly much less pronounced than those seen in other disorders. Despite the lack of a consensus regarding gender differences in the *incidence* of schizophrenia, there is more of a consensus that gender differences exist in the *course* of the disorder. For example, the average age of onset of schizophrenia in men is earlier (typically in the early to mid 20s) than it is for women (in the late 20s).

The symptom pattern for schizophrenia is quite varied but generally reflects the presentation of negative and positive symptoms. Positive symptoms refer to those reflected in the presence of abnormal behaviors such as hallucinations and delusions; negative symptoms are those that refer to the absence of normal behaviors (e.g., deficits in the expression of affect and speech deficits). Schizophrenia is also characterized by significant interpersonal and occupational dysfunction and, like other disorders, can be a quite chronic condition, although accurate data tend not to be available because of differences in definitions and assessment of schizophrenia (American Psychiatric Association, 1994). Nevertheless, it is commonly acknowledged that the majority of individuals who are diagnosed with schizophrenia will, if they do not remain continuously afflicted, experience chronic relapses and recurrences.

WHY STUDY VULNERABILITY TO DISORDERS IN ADULTHOOD?

It is unlikely that most of the precursors to psychopathology in adulthood arise solely with the onset of adulthood. Rather, most researchers acknowledge that in many if not most cases, these precursors are rooted in experiences encountered early in life. The range of such early experiences is quite diverse. For example, such experiences can include a variety of prenatal insults, as has been suggested by some schizophrenia researchers (e.g., Zubin & Spring, 1977). Postnatal insults, such as those arising from obstetrical complications, can also occur and may produce vulnerability. And in many cases, especially those in which dysfunctional learning is involved, the development of vulnerability factors can occur throughout the childhood years. Why then focus on vulnerability in adulthood? We believe that there are several reasons why such a focus is both warranted and important.

Some Vulnerability Factors May Develop in Adulthood

Although most vulnerability factors arise before adulthood, some of these processes do in fact occur during adulthood. For example, if we posit (from a psychopathological standpoint) that learning experiences can serve as the basis for vulnerability to psychopathology, then we cannot rule out that some of these learning experiences take place in adulthood. Take the example of anxiety states. Even though the root of many of these disorders is found in childhood or adolescent experiences, sufficient exposure to inescapable aversive circumstances as an adult should, in principle, also elicit the development of anxiety. In the case of posttraumatic stress disorder (PTSD), for instance, although it is known that some processes that appear in childhood (e.g., neuroticism) are linked to vulnerability to this disorder in adulthood (see McNally, Chapter 12, this volume), repeated exposure to traumatic events as an adult (e.g., repeated prison or wartime rape) may be sufficient to create lasting vulnerability to a variety of disorders that differ from the adulthood onset of PTSD (e.g., phobic states and depression may also develop). Hence, vulnerability to several disorders may be created by horrific experiences encountered as an adult. Although it is undoubtedly true that vulnerability to many psychopathological states arise prior to adulthood, in some cases vulnerability processes may indeed first appear in adulthood and thus justify both theoretical and empirical attention.

Factors That Actualize Vulnerability Occur in Adulthood

Although the vulnerability roots of adult psychopathology may not develop in adulthood, an extremely important reason to examine vulnerability factors in adulthood is the *activation* or *actualization* of vulnerability factors that initiate the onset of adult psychopathology. As noted by Ingram et al. (1998) and Ingram and Price (Chapter 1, this volume), vulnerability variables are typically seen as stable traits. Psychological disorders, on the other hand, are considered to be states—that is, conditions that occur and then, in most cases either disappear or enter at least some state of remission. These trait and state distinctions underscore the fact that most vulnerability models are explicitly *diathesis–stress models*—models that locate the genesis of psychopathology in the combination of vulnerability traits and life stress. Thus, even though the vulnerability factors for a given disorder may have developed prior to adulthood, the variables that initiate the realization of these vulnerability traits into a psychopathological state (typically aversive life events) occur during adulthood. Indeed, the onset of all adult disorders is arguably a function of these triggering events, certainly according to those models that embrace a diathesis–stress approach.[3] Understanding when, how, and why stress interacts with latent vulnerability factors to produce an active psychopathological state in adulthood is thus an extremely important goal for researchers.

---

[3]A clear exception would be seen in personality disorders that do not represent the kinds of clinical syndromes that are coded on Axix I of the DSM.

Modification of Vulnerability Factors Can Occur in Adulthood

It is possible to view vulnerability factors as static, unchanging, and unchangeable, and in some cases of vulnerability this may be an accurate conceptualization. For example, Zubin and Spring (1977), are clear about the unyielding nature of vulnerability: "we regard [vulnerability] as a relatively permanent, enduring trait" (p. 109). Such assumptions of permanence are likely rooted in the genetic level of analysis employed by researchers who examine disorders such as schizophrenia (e.g., McGue & Gottesman, 1989; Nicholson & Neufeld, 1992) and clearly argue for a relatively static view of vulnerability mechanisms.

Although these perspectives suggest that vulnerability mechanisms may not be modifiable, they do not necessarily argue that *functional* vulnerability levels cannot be attenuated by processes that affect neurochemistry. For instance, pharmacological agents such as lithium carbonate may alter the likelihood of developing the symptoms of a bipolar episode by presumably controlling the underlying neurochemistry of the vulnerability. Similar diminishment of functional vulnerability may be seen in the actions of psychopharmacological treatments for depression with medications such as selective serotonin reuptake inhibitors or the various generations of tricyclic agents. However, even though functional vulnerability may be altered and individuals are less likely to develop the disorder while on medication, the vulnerability persists; in the case of all the pharmacological agents we have noted, increased risk returns once the medication is discontinued (Hollon, 1999). Thus, even though the emergent vulnerability may be controlled, the vulnerability process itself remains.

In other cases, vulnerability processes that arise before adulthood may in fact become modified during adulthood. For instance, changes may reflect variables that *intensify* the vulnerability. To illustrate, in the area of mood disorders, Post (1992) proposed a process that he labeled *kindling*. Kindling is thought to be a neuronal process that intensifies vulnerability to affective disorders. In brief, Post suggests that each episode of an affective disorder leaves a residual neuronal trace. As these neurobiological traces become more distinct, they lead to the development of pathways by which increasingly minimal stress becomes sufficient to activate the affective mechanisms that result in the onset of a disorder. In the most extreme cases, disorder onsets become autonomous from the external triggering mechanisms that are acknowledged to occur in most disorders. From a somewhat different level of analysis, Segal, Williams, Teasdale, and Gemar (1996) argue that kindling may be associated with the likelihood that dysfunctional cognitive patterns are activated with increasingly minimal stimulation (e.g., aversive life events). Regardless of whether this process is viewed from a neurobiological level of analysis or a cognitive level of analysis, kindling intensifies the adult vulnerability processes that may have developed at an earlier time in life and thus serves to alter vulnerability levels.

Changes in vulnerability processes do not always have to be in a negative direction; a lessening of vulnerability may also be possible. Whether or not a model specifies that decreases in vulnerability are possible depends on the disorder in question (e.g., schizophrenia as conceptualized by Zubin & Spring, 1977) and the level of vulnerability analysis (e.g., learning-based vs. neurobiological). For instance, psychological approaches typically rely on assumptions of maladaptive learning as the basis of vulnerability (Ingram et al., 1998). Given these learning assumptions, vulnerability may be affected by new learning experiences. The most obvious example of a new learning experience is that of psychotherapy, which in most cases is intended not only to treat the symptoms of a disorder but also to alter the underlying vulnerability. In addition, naturally occurring "corrective" learning experiences may also affect vulnerability. Although it is unlikely that new learning experiences will totally ameliorate vulnerability (see Mahoney, 2000), these conceptualizations nevertheless suggest that some modification of vulnerability is possible and, by extension, suggest that vulnerability having its genesis in childhood or adolescence may be altered in adulthood.

In sum, even though vulnerability to adulthood disorders may arise before adulthood, several circumstances suggest the importance of studying vulnerability in adulthood. These circumstances reflect the fact that some vulnerability processes do arise in adulthood, that the factors that actualize vulnerability to psychopathology occur in adulthood, and that vulnerability processes may be modified (both functionally and dysfunctionally) in adulthood. To fully appreciate the implications of these circumstances, it is helpful to understand the historical context for the study of vulnerability, a topic to which we now turn.

A BRIEF HISTORY OF VULNERABILITY THEORY AND RESEARCH

Virtually all theories of psychopathology at least implicitly encompass notions of vulnerability. The history of vulnerability perspectives on adult psychopathology therefore depends to a large extent on the time frame one wants to cover. For example, as any abnormal psychology textbook tells us, many historical conceptualizations of psychopathology evidence the belief that individuals were possessed by demons and were presumably vulnerable to such possession by virtue of living immoral, or nonreligious, lifestyles. Somewhat more recent, and scientifically credible, origins of adult vulnerability theory can be seen in the work of the earliest psychiatrists. We refer most centrally to Freud, whose theory of trauma and fixation is every bit a vulnerability theory. Likewise, neo-Freudians such as Alder, who located vulnerability to psychopathology in fears of inferiority, also propose what can be considered to be theories of vulnerability. Our focus, however, is on the more contemporary origins of current vulnerability perspectives.

The Advent of Contemporary Approaches to Vulnerability

Despite the various theories that imply vulnerability processes, explicit (and somewhat more contemporary) ideas of vulnerability as an explanatory concept for adult psychopathology most likely have their conceptual origins in theorizing about schizophrenia. In a classic paper, Meehl (1962) was probably the first to allude to a psychogenic vulnerability to schizophrenia when he proposed that the disorder is the result of a neural deficit ("schizotaxia") that is combined with the individual's learning history. Meehl (1962) referred to this as schizotypia and suggested that the confluence of these variables conferred vulnerability to schizophrenia. Meehl also hypothesized, however, that schizotypia, although necessary for the development of schizophrenia, was not sufficient in and of itself for the development of schizophrenia. Rather, Meehl suggested that only some schizotypic individuals would eventually develop clinical schizophrenia. Specifically, these were the individuals who were reared by a schizophrenogenic mother who would provide a developmental climate of ambivalent, unpredictable, and aversive mother–child interactions: "it seems likely that the most important causal influence pushing the schizotype toward schizophrenic decompensation is the schizophrenogenic mother" (p. 830). Meehl's (1962) theory therefore argued that the onset of schizophrenia was a joint function of both biological (genetically determined schizotaxia) and psychological factors (e.g., the individual's learning history and disturbed mother–child interactions). Despite the focus on childhood factors, which as we have noted underlie many approaches to adult psychopathology, Meehl's theory represents, we believe, the inauguration of the vulnerability approach to understanding psychopathology in adults.

The empirical origins of the vulnerability approach are again linked to schizophrenia and appear traceable to work reported by Kety, Rosenthal, Wender, and Schulsinger (1968), Mednick and Schulsinger (1968), and Rosenthal et al. (1968). Although interested in schizophrenia in adulthood, this work examined a variety of variables in the children of a parent (or parents) with a diagnosis of schizophrenia, with the idea that these variables may predict the eventual onset of schizophrenia in these children. To examine such individuals, these researchers used extensive registers in Denmark known as the National Psychiatric Register and the Folkeregister. The National Psychiatric Register documents all psychiatric hospitalizations in Denmark while the Folkeregister contains the addresses of virtually all Danish residents. Using these databases, Mednick and Schulsinger (1968) located a sample of 207 children of schizophrenic mothers and a control group of more than 100 children whose mothers did not show evidence of psychopathology. These offspring were then tested on a number of variables and were followed longitudinally over time.

The historical antecedents for disorders other than schizophrenia vary according to a number of factors. In the area of depression, for example, Beck (1967) was undoubtedly the first to articulate a cognitive theory of affective disorder and suggested that vulnerability to adult depression developed in childhood. In particular, he argued that problematic situations in childhood serve as the basis for the development of cognitive structures that place individuals at later risk.

> In childhood and adolescence, the depression-prone individual becomes sensitized to certain types of life situations. The traumatic situations initially responsible for embedding or reinforcing the negative attitudes that comprise the depressive constellation are the prototypes of the specific stresses that may later activate these constellations. When a person is subjected to situations reminiscent of the original situations, he may then become depressed. (p. 278)

Beck's ideas clearly represent a vulnerability hypothesis that focuses on both vulnerability mechanisms and on how and under what circumstances these mechanisms developed and were later activated. Although the vulnerability approach had its earliest origins in schizophrenia, Beck's theory appears to have developed independently of this vulnerability theory and research, as most likely did most of the vulnerability ideas discussed in the various chapters in this volume.

As this brief review demonstrates, the history of vulnerability theory and research in adult psychopathology is fairly recent. Discounting the notion of possession by evil spirits, contemporary perspectives on vulnerability can probably be traced to Meehl's pioneering work on schizophrenia and to some extent to Zubin and Spring's suggestions that the only way to truly understand the development of schizophrenia itself is through understanding the processes that lead to the development of vulnerability factors. Although these perspectives originated with the study of schizophrenia, they nevertheless represent important influences on the study of vulnerability to a variety of disorders.

CONCLUSIONS: WHAT DOES THE FUTURE HOLD FOR ADULT VULNERABILITY PERSPECTIVES?

Despite the reality that most vulnerability factors develop in childhood or adolescence, children and adolescents grow up to be adults. Hence, the examination of vulnerability in adult psychopathology indicates few signs of slowing down. This is due in large part to the three reasons we noted earlier. First, because some vulnerability factors may in fact develop in adulthood, it is important to continue to examine when and how these factors develop. Second, vulnerability to adult psychopathology will continue to be important because vulnerability factors for disorders that occur in adulthood, even if developed in childhood or adolescence, are actualized in adulthood. This perspective is captured the most clearly in diathesis–stress models that focus on the interactive effects of stressful events and endogenous mechanisms (whether psychological or physiological), which together produce vulnerability. And third, vulnerability factors may be modified in adulthood. As we noted, sometimes vulnerability increases in adulthood, while in other cases, and depending on the origins of the vulnerability, these factors may decrease in adulthood.

Although there are numerous possible future directions for adult vulnerability theorizing and research, we end this chapter with a comment about one possible future direction. Ingram and Price (Chapter 1, this volume) suggested that the line between childhood/adolescence and adulthood can be difficult to find. From a conceptual standpoint it would be helpful if the line did not exist at all. That is, to truly understand vulnerability, theorists and researchers need to adopt a lifespan perspective. For childhood and adolescence researchers this means realizing that children and adolescents eventually become adults and, thus, vulnerability factors, although developed in childhood or adolescence, may nevertheless affect individuals for a lifetime. Understanding the long-term trajectory of these vulnerability factors and their consequences is thus an extremely important quest.

From the adult psychopathologist's perspective this means recognizing that adults were once children. Adult researchers tend to confine their investigations to variables that occur after childhood and adolescence, but it is becoming increasingly clear that in order to understand adult vulnerability, we must begin with understanding children and adolescents. This dual recognition—that functioning continues after childhood and that adult processes must be understood in terms of earlier processes—suggests that vulnerability must be understood across the lifespan. With rare exceptions, this situation does not currently exist, as can be seen in the division of chapters in this volume. Nevertheless, only a lifespan perspective will move us closer to understanding the vulnerability processes that are linked to the devastating consequences of psychopathology in both children and adults.

REFERENCES

American Psychiatric Association. (1994). *Diagnostic and statistical manual of mental disorders* (4th ed.). Washington, DC: Author.

Beck, A. T. (1967). *Depression: Causes and treatment.* Philadelphia: University of Pennsylvania Press.

Franzini, L., & Grossberg, J. (1995). *Eccentric and bizarre behaviors.* New York: Wiley.

Goodwin, F. K., & Jamison, K. R. (1990). *Manic–depressive illness.* New York: Oxford University Press.

Hammen, C. (1991). *Depression runs in families: The social context of risk and resilience in children of depressed mothers.* New York: Springer-Verlag.

Hollon, S. D. (1999). Psychotherapy and pharmacotherapy: Efficacy, generalizability, and cost-effectiveness. In N. E. Miller & K. M. Magruder, (Eds.), *Cost-effectiveness of psychotherapy: A guide for practitioners, researchers, and policymakers* (pp. 14–26). New York: Oxford University Press.

Ingram, R. E., & Hamilton, N. A. (1999). Evaluating precision in the social psychological assessment of depression: Methodological considerations, issues, and recommendations. *Journal of Social and Clinical Psychology, 18,* 160–180.

Ingram, R. E., Miranda, J., & Segal, Z. V. (1998). *Cognitive vulnerability to depression.* New York: Guilford Press.

Keith, S. J., Regier, D. A., & Rae, D. S. (1991). Schizophrenia disorders. In L. N. Robins & D. A. Regier (Eds.), *Psychiatric disorders in America: The Epidemiologic Catchment Area study* (pp. 33–52). New York: Free Press.

Kety, S. S., Rosenthal, D., Wender, P. H., & Schulsinger, F. (1968). The types and prevalence of mental illness in the biological and adoptive families of adopted schizophrenics. In D. Rosenthal & S. S. Kety (Eds.), *Transmission of schizophrenia* (pp. 14–23). Oxford: Pergamon Press.

Lavori, P. E., Kessler, M. B., & Klerman, G. L. (1984). Relapse in affective disorder: A reanalysis of the literature using life table methods. *Journal of Psychiatric Research, 18,* 13–25.

Mahoney, M. J. (2000). A changing history of efforts to understand and control change: The case of psychotherapy. In C. R. Snyder & R. E. Ingram (Eds.), *Handbook of psychological change: Psychotherapy processes and practices for the 21st century* (pp. 2–18). New York: Wiley.

McGue, M., & Gottesman, I. I. (1989). Genetic linkage in schizophrenia: Perspectives from genetic epidemiology. *Schizophrenia Bulletin, 15,* 453–464.

Mednick, S. A., & Schulsinger, F. (1968). Some premorbid characteristics related to breakdown in children of with schizophrenic mothers. In D. Rosenthal & S. S. Kety (Eds.), *Transmission of schizophrenia* (pp. 41–57). Oxford: Pergamon Press.

Meehl, P. E. (1962). Schizotaxia, schizotypy, schizophrenia. *American Psychologist, 17,* 827–838.

Nicholson, I. R., & Neufeld, R. W. J. (1992). A dynamic vulnerability perspective on stress and schizophrenia. *American Journal of Orthopsychiatry, 62,* 117–130.

Post, R. M. (1992). Transduction of psychosocial stress into the neurobiology of affective disorder. *American Journal of Psychiatry, 149,* 999–1010.

Robins, L. N., & Regier, D. A. (Eds.). (1991). *Psychiatric disorders in America: The Epidemiologic Catchment Area study.* New York: Free Press.

Rosenthal, D., Wender, P. H., Kety, S. S., Schulsinger, F., Welner, J., & Ostergaard, L. (1968). Schizophrenics' offspring reared in adoptive homes. In D. Rosenthal & S. S. Kety (Eds.), *Transmission of schizophrenia* (pp. 97–113). Oxford: Pergamon Press.

Segal, Z. V., Williams, J. M., Teasdale, J. D., & Gemar, M. (1996). A cognitive science perspective on kindling and episode sensitization in recurrent affective disorder. *Psychological Medicine, 26,* 371–380.

Tennen, H., Hall, J. A., & Affleck, G. (1995). Depression research methodologies in the *Journal of Personality and Social Psychology:* A review and critique. *Journal of Personality and Social Psychology, 68,* 870–884.

Zubin, J., & Spring, B. (1977). Vulnerability: A new view of schizophrenia. *Journal of Abnormal Psychology, 86,* 103–126.

Part II
PERSONALITY DISORDERS

4

A Developmental Psychopathology Perspective on Vulnerability to Personality Disorders

TASHA C. GEIGER
NICKI R. CRICK

Numerous authors have noted the lack of empirical evidence for the reliability of personality disorder assessment and the existence of clearly distinguishable types of personality disorders as they are described in the current diagnostic system (e.g., Skodol, 1997; Westen, 1997). The difficulty in locating empirical research on the developmental precursors of such pathology may be one consequence of these systemic problems. Millon and Davis (1995) state that "although a generative theoretical basis and much clinical lore exists from which the developmental antecedents of these disorders can be extrapolated, longitudinal studies are sorely lacking" (p. 673). Despite these difficulties, the personality disorders especially lend themselves to examination according to developmental theory because personality is hypothesized to begin forming early in life—substrates of which are thought to be present at birth (Hartup & van Lieshout, 1995).

Our goal for this chapter is to examine possible childhood precursors to adult personality disorders. Although sparse, longitudinal research has indicated that behavioral characteristics associated with adult personality disorders can be observed in childhood (Bernstein, Cohen, Skodol, Bezirganian, & Brook, 1996; Rey, Morris-Yates, Singh, Andrews, & Stewart, 1995). These studies are limited, however, by the fact that the diagnoses were obtained during adolescence, a developmental period often marked by deviant behavior (Moffitt, 1993), increased stress, and emotional lability

(Arnett, 1999). Such a pattern of adolescent behavior may result in a false inflation in the prevalence rate of personality disorders for that population. For example, one study found that of the adolescents who were diagnosed with a personality disorder according to the the revised third edition of the *Diagnostic and Statistical Manual of Mental Disorders* (DSM-III-R; American Psychiatric Association, 1987), less than half of them retained the diagnosis at a 2-year follow-up (Bernstein et al., 1993). Although some authors have methodologically addressed the instability of diagnoses during this transition period (e.g., Bernstein et al., 1996), it is not clear whether these youths would go on to obtain a personality disorder diagnosis during adulthood. The relative instability of personality disorder diagnoses from early adolescence to late adolescence or young adulthood has been acknowledged in both clinical (Mattanah, Becker, Levy, Edell, & McGlashan, 1995) and nonclinical samples (Korenblum, Marton, Golombek, & Stein, 1990).

Given the limitations of the current personality disorder diagnostic system as delineated in the fourth edition of the DSM (DSM-IV; American Psychiatric Association, 1994), and given the limited research on childhood precursors of personality pathology, we are approaching the examination of childhood vulnerability to personality disorder in two ways. First, we have chosen to address common themes that cut across diagnostic categories. For example, rather than focusing on precursors to borderline personality disorder, we identify possible antecedents to core aspects of the disorder such as "overly close relationships," a broader concept descriptive of not only borderline personality disorder but histrionic and dependent personality disorder as well. A similar approach has been used by Costello (1996) to describe personality characteristics of personality-disordered adults. Second, we have selected to explore childhood vulnerability to personality disorder by adopting a developmental psychopathology perspective.

This two-pronged approach was taken for three reasons. First, this framework represents an attempt to address the inadequacy of the current diagnostic system (i.e., lack of discriminant validity). Although not explicitly acknowledging the difficulties of conducting research with the current personality disorder taxonomy, a review of the literature seems to indicate that researchers use methods or data reduction techniques that compensate for the inadequacy of this classification system. For example, researchers have chosen to assess dimensions of personality pathology instead of, or in addition to, using the categorical approach of the DSM (e.g., Daley et al., 1999; Lewinsohn, Rohde, Seeley, & Klein, 1997). Other researchers find it necessary to combine the personality disorders into clusters, groupings based on the personality clusters in the DSM (e.g., Bernstein et al., 1996) or newly created groupings (e.g., Korenblum et al., 1990). Still others have resorted to combining all the personality disorder symptoms into one summary variable in order to locate predictors of personality pathology (e.g., Cohen, 1996). Thus, the approach taken in this chapter is an attempt to take into account the difficulties encountered in research concerned with the distinctiveness of the individual personality disorders and their precursors.

Second, by not relying on the relatively nondevelopmental criteria of the DSM categories, but rather by describing behavior relevant to a particular age group, this approach may help to address some of the difficulties of assessing features of personality disorders during adolescence. Third, these common themes more readily map themselves onto skills and competencies addressed in the developmental psychology literature. When the diagnostic system is "abandoned" and common themes are considered, the result is often a dimensional system (van Praag, 1996, p. 131). Therefore, many of the themes listed here describe dimensions or continua of behaviors and characteristics with an excess of one quality as one end point and a lack of that quality as the other end point (e.g., "overly close relationships" to "distant/avoidant relationships"; see Table 4.1 for a list of the core behavioral areas to be discussed and the DSM-IV diagnostic criteria hypothesized to compose each area).

Thus, we adopt a developmental psychopathology model to examine how empirically based concepts in developmental psychology may evolve over time, laying the foundation for features of maladaptive personality functioning in adulthood. It is important, therefore, to start with a description of some of the fundamental principles of developmental psychopathology. One guiding principle maintains that the study of normative behavior is essential to the understanding of deviant development (Cicchetti & Cohen, 1995). Therefore, we often describe normal developmental processes before presenting deviations from this typical pattern that may be implicated as precursors to pathology. The developmental psychopathology model also embraces an organizational perspective such that attention is paid to cognitive, biological, social, and emotional processes and how these systems become integrated over time. Therefore, we include a discussion of vulnerability processes that may be implicated within each of these domains.

Another important feature of the developmental psychopathology perspective is a focus on a pattern of adaptation to significant tasks or requirements appropriate for a particular age group (Cicchetti & Cohen, 1995). For example, during infancy, an important task is the formation of an appropriate attachment relationship with the caregiver (Sroufe & Waters, 1977), whereas during middle childhood important accomplishments may include successful negotiation of peer relationships, academic endeavors, and appropriate behavior and conduct (Masten & Coatsworth, 1998). Throughout this chapter, we examine different developmental periods, and failure to deal effectively with pertinent developmental tasks is discussed as a possible indicator of future psychopathology.

An additional aspect of the developmental psychopathology model is that pathways of development are emphasized such that the pattern of adaptation (both successful and maladaptive) to developmental tasks is exam-

TABLE 4.1. A Developmental Approach to the Identification of Child and Adolescent Features of Personality Disorders

Personality feature	Personality disorder	Example DSM-IV symptom
1. Hostile, paranoid world view	PPD	Suspects, without sufficient basis, that others are exploiting, harming, or deceiving him or her
	SPPD	Suspiciousness or paranoid ideation
	BPD	Transient, stress-related paranoid ideation or severe dissociative symptoms
2a. Intense unstable, inappropriate emotion	BPD	Affective instability due to a marked reactivity of mood
	HPD	Displays rapidly shifting and shallow expression of emotions
2b. Restricted, flat affect	SZPD	Shows emotional coldness, detachment, or flattened affectivity
	SPPD	Inappropriate or constricted affect
3a. Impulsivity	APD	Impulsivity or failure to plan ahead
	BPD	Impulsivity in at least two areas that are potentially self-damaging (e.g., spending, sex, substance abuse)
3b. Rigidity	OCPD	Shows perfectionism that interferes with task completion
	AVPD	Is unusually reluctant to take personal risks or to engage in any new activities because they may prove embarrassing
4a. Overly close relationships	BPD	A pattern of unstable or intense interpersonal relationships characterized by alternating between extremes of idealization and devaluation
	HPD	Considers relationships to be more intimate than they actually are
	DPD	Goes to excessive lengths to obtain nurturance and support from others, to the point of volunteering to do things that are unpleasant
4b. Distant/ avoidant relationships	OCPD	Is excessively devoted to work and productivity to the exclusion of leisure activities and friendships (not accounted for by obvious economic necessity)
	PPD	Is reluctant to confide in others because of unwarranted fear that the information will be used maliciously against him or her
	SZPD	Neither desires or enjoys close relationships, including being part of a family
	SPPD	Lack of close friends or confidants other than first-degree relatives
	AVPD	Avoids occupational activities that involve significant interpersonal contact, because of fears of criticism, disapproval, or rejection

TABLE 4.1. (cont.)

Personality feature	Personality disorder	Example DSM-IV Symptom
5a. Negative sense of self	NPD	Is often envious of others or believes that others are envious of him or her
	AVPD	Views self as socially inept, personally unappealing, or inferior to others
	DPD	Has difficulty initiating projects or doing things on his or her own (because of a lack of self-confidence in judgment or abilities rather than a lack of motivation or energy)
5b. Lack of sense of self	BPD	Identity disturbance: Markedly and persistently unstable self-image or sense of self
5c. Exaggerated sense of self	HPD	Is uncomfortable in situations in which he or she is not the center of attention
	NPD	Has a grandiose sense of self-importance
6. Peculiar thought processes and behaviors	SPPD	Behavior or appearance that is odd, eccentric, or peculiar
7. Lack of concern for social norms and needs of others	APD	Lack of remorse, as indicated by being indifferent to or rationalizing having hurt, mistreated, or stolen from another
	NPD	Lacks empathy: is unwilling to recognize or identify with the feelings and needs of others

Note. From American Psychiatric Association (1994). Copyright 1994 by the American Psychiatric Association. Reprinted by permission. PPD, paranoid personality disorder; SZPD, schizoid personality disorder; SPPD, schizotypal personality disorder; APD, antisocial personality disorder; BPD, borderline personality disorder; HPD, histrionic personality disorder; NPD, narcissistic personality disorder; AVPD, avoidant personality disorder; DPD, dependent personality disorder; OCPD, obsessive–compulsive personality disorder.

ined over time. Thus, individuals are thought to take into future situations and challenges the cognitive, social, biological, and emotional resources, skills, and knowledge they gained in early negotiations with important tasks. For example, an individual who was not successful at maintaining adequate relationships with peers during childhood may lack a solid foundation for the development of later positive, fulfilling adult friendships and romantic relationships. Failure at these important developmental tasks does not necessarily signify pathology but, rather, serves as an indicator that an individual may be on a deviant pathway, and perhaps at an increased risk for further maladaptive behavior. The longer an individual remains on this deviant pathway, the more difficult it may be to return to a normal, typical developmental progression. Change, however, is still possible, but given the organizational structure of development, this change is constrained by the individual's previous history (Sroufe, 1997).

Within this focus on the organizational structure of development, such that the cognitive, emotional, biological, and social systems become integrated over time as the individual adapts to the environment and various experiences, it is possible to study the coherence of development. Coherence implies that there is a logical progression to this development. Emphasis, therefore, is not necessarily on the particular form of a behavior but, rather, on the function or meaning of a behavior and how it may change over time. Therefore, behaviors that are similar in appearance may have different meanings at different ages (Sroufe, 1997; Sroufe & Rutter, 1984). Coherence has two implications for this chapter. First, behaviors are examined for their appropriateness for a particular age group. Second, childhood behaviors are examined that are meaningfully related (but not necessarily phenotypically similar) to adult symptoms of personality disorder.

In sum, this chapter illustrates how common concepts in developmental psychology that have functional or symptomatic similarity to features of personality disorders may represent vulnerabilities or liabilities that predispose children to developing a personality disorder in adulthood. However, given the paucity of empirical research on the antecedents of personality disorders, the developmental processes we select for discussion are not meant to provide a comprehensive review of the potential precursors of personality disorders. Rather, the concepts are chosen because a wide research base supports their validity in developmental psychology, and because these concepts possess a conceptual or functional similarity linking them with the symptomatic picture of respective personality disorders of adulthood. We attempt to address vulnerability in several domains including cognition, behavior, biology, emotion, and social interaction and also to discuss vulnerability processes that may be occurring during infancy, childhood, and adolescence. Currently, the link between these processes and the development of a personality disorder is only speculative, but we hope they will serve as a springboard for future research endeavors. In keeping with the aims for this volume, we provide an overview of research on the assessment and stability of personality disorders before discussing childhood precursors of these disorders.

ASSESSMENT AND STABILITY
OF PERSONALITY DISORDERS

"A Personality Disorder is an enduring pattern of inner experience and behavior that deviates markedly from the expectations of the individual's culture, is pervasive and inflexible, has an onset in adolescence or early adulthood, is stable over time, and leads to distress or impairment" (American Psychiatric Association, 1994, p. 629). Assessment of these disorders, however, can be complicated. First, the Axis II diagnostic system, the one used to assess personality disorders, appears to lack adequate coverage of clinically significant character pathology. In a survey of a random sample of psychiatrists and psychologists, Westen and Arkowitz-Westen (1998) found that almost 60% of the clients being treated for personality pathology did not fit into a personality disorder category and therefore remained undiagnosed on Axis II. A second concern regarding this diagnostic system is its relatively low discriminant validity (Westen, 1997). Comorbidity rates are very high among the personality disorders (for a review, see Widiger & Rogers, 1989) such that in some samples, 80% of clients with a personality disorder qualified for another Axis II diagnosis (Oldham et al., 1992).

Several measures exist for assessing normal and pathological personality functioning for adults (for a review, see Butcher & Rouse, 1996). The features vary among the instruments and thus the goals of the researcher or clinician should be considered in choosing the appropriate measure. In selecting an appropriate instrument, several factors should be considered including reliability, degree of structure, false-positive rates, correspondence to DSM criteria, coverage, administration procedures, content, and interviewer qualifications (for a review, see Zimmerman, 1994). Existing measures vary considerably with respect to these features. For example, the Personality Disorders Examination (PDE; Loranger, 1988) is structured to cover domains of functioning (e.g., work, interpersonal relationships), whereas the Structured Clinical Interview for the DSM-IV Axis II Disorders (SCID-II; First, Spitzer, Gibbon, & Williams, 1995) includes questions relating directly to each criteria for each personality disorder. Another commonly used instrument is the Millon Clinical Multiaxial Inventory (MCMI; Millon, 1994); however, the correspondence between the MCMI and the DSM-III or III-R has been questioned (Zimmerman, 1994). Further, the MCMI tends to overdiagnose personality disorders. This has also been shown to be true of another widely used instrument, the Personality Diagnostic Questionnaire (PDQ; Hyler et al., 1988), but to a lesser degree (Zimmerman, 1994).

In comparison to adult measures, relatively few instruments have been developed to assess personality disorders during childhood or adolescence. Currently, little agreement or consistent discussion exists in the literature concerning the conceptualization of personality development in children (Shiner, 1998). Therefore, it may be difficult to determine not only which constructs assess normal personality but also which constructs measure deviant personality processes. The available instruments seem to represent two approaches: (1) standardizing versions of adult personality disorder measures with younger samples or (2) designing new instruments specifically for use with children but based on adult criteria.

Concerning the former approach, the validity of the PDE for assessing personality disorders in a sample of psychiatric adolescents has been examined. Unfortunately, the internal consistency was lower and the overlap among the criteria for different disorders was greater for adolescents than for adults (Becker et al., 1999). In another example of this approach, an early version of the SCID, the Structured Interview for the DSM-III, was examined for a sample of adolescents, and convergent validity was demonstrated for the DSM-III Cluster B disorders (borderline, histrionic, and narcissistic personality disorder; Brent, Zelenak, Bukstein, & Brown, 1990).

Corresponding to the second approach, instruments designed specifically for children (for reviews, see Knoff, 1986; Martin, 1988), three measures assessing personality pathology in children show promise. The Kid's Coolidge Axis II Inventory (KCATI; Coolidge et al., 1990) is a parent report instrument thought to assess personality disorders and related characteristics in children ages 5 to 11. The Personality Inventory for Children (PIC; Lachar & Wirt, 1981) is a parent report measure of personality dimensions such as self-control and anxiety, with normative data available for children ages 6 through 16. Based on the PIC, the Personality Inventory for Children Preschool Version (PPIC; Heindselman, Wingenfeld, & Smith, 1999) was recently developed for the assessment of younger children, ages 2 to 6. To date, research supporting the validity and psychometric properties of these three instruments is in its infancy.

Research concerning the stability of personality disorder diagnoses in adults has numerous methodological limitations including follow-back designs, nonblind diagnoses, and unreliable diagnoses (for a review, see McDavid & Pilkonis, 1996). Little research has addressed the stability of these diagnoses in children or adolescents. One study has demonstrated that of the adolescents (age range 9–19) who were diagnosed with a DSM-III-R personality disorder, less than half of them retained the diagnosis at a 2-year follow-up (Bernstein et al., 1993). These authors also found that of their random community sample, approximately half of the adolescents were diagnosed with a personality disorder, a prevalence rate much higher than that for adults (American Psychiatric Association, 1994). In addition, the older the adolescents, the less likely they were to receive a personality disorder diagnosis, another finding at odds with the DSM conceptualization of personality disorders (i.e., the chance of obtaining a personality disorder diagnosis should increase with age). Taken together, these findings suggest that the measures of personality disorders used to assess adolescents may not be tapping the same constructs as those designed for adults but may, rather, be measuring more normal behaviors of adolescence including an increase in antisocial behaviors (Moffitt, 1993), narcissistic tendencies, and an immature sense of self (Harter, 1998).

Accepting the limited discriminant validity of the personality disorders, it may be possible to demonstrate the stability of *general* personality disturbance from childhood through adulthood. For example, two separate studies using different criteria and different ages of assessment both demonstrated that a borderline-related diagnosis during childhood is associated with the development of any personality disorder 10 to 15 years later (Lofgren, Bemporad, King, Lindem, & O'Driscoll, 1991; Thomsen, 1996).

Neither study addressed, however, whether particular symptoms were associated with the later development of a specific personality disorder.

CHILDHOOD AND ADOLESCENT PRECURSORS TO ADULT PERSONALITY DISORDERS

To identify themes that cut across the personality disorders and have potential for increasing our understanding of the childhood precursors of adult personality disorders, we conducted a content analysis of the 79 personality disorder symptoms described in DSM-IV. The authors separately examined a list of the symptoms and divided them into categories based on their conceptual similarities. The content of the items within each category was then examined and themes were created that seemed to encompass the variety of symptoms within each grouping. The authors then compared their categories and the symptoms that constituted those categories. Any differences were discussed and the discrepancies were resolved by discussion and consultation of the literature. This analysis yielded seven themes, each of which is discussed here. As described previously, most themes describe continua of behaviors or characteristics with an excess of a particular quality as one end point and a lack of that quality as the second end point. The seven themes are (1) hostile, paranoid world view; (2) intense, unstable, and inappropriate emotion to restricted, flat affect; (3) impulsivity to rigidity; (4) overly close relationships to distant/avoidant relationships; (5) negative sense of self or lack of self to exaggerated sense of self; (6) peculiar thought processes and behaviors; (7) lack of concern for social norms and needs of others. Table 4.1 (see pp. 60–61) lists these themes, the personality disorders that are encompassed by each theme, and example DSM-IV symptoms for each theme–disorder pairing.

Hostile, Paranoid World View

Individuals with paranoid, schizotypal, or borderline personality disorder tend to view the world in a hostile or paranoid manner. Persons with paranoid personality disorder believe that others are inherently persecutory, disloyal, and dishonest. Although these individuals lack sufficient proof of the malfeasance of others, they maintain that others are intentionally trying to harm them. These individuals may prematurely respond to social situations with aggressive outbursts. Persons with schizotypal or borderline personality disorder may also be suspicious and paranoid of others (American Psychiatric Association, 1994).

The development of a hostile view of the world has been examined in childhood through a social information-processing model that describes the social and cognitive mechanisms related to children's maladjustment (Dodge & Crick, 1990). According to this model, the cognitive steps of making sense of one's environment and reacting to it include the following: (1) encoding important cues, (2) interpreting the information, (3) generating a set of possible responses, (4) choosing a response, and (5) performing the selected response. Dodge and Crick (1990) posit that "Skillful processing at each step will lead to competent performance within the situation, whereas biased or deficient processing will lead to deviant, possibly aggressive, social behavior" (p. 13). For example, aggressive children are more likely to encode negative stimuli and to interpret ambiguous situations as hostile. This initiates a process where a bias toward attributing hostile intent to an ambiguous situation may lead to an aggressive response, which, in turn, may cause retaliation, an event that reinforces the child's initially incorrect interpretation. Such a pattern may underlie the suspiciousness and the tendency to be "quick to react angrily or to counterattack" (American Psychiatric Association, 1994, p. 638) characteristic of persons with paranoid personality disorder.

Poor social information-processing skills may serve as a risk factor for the development of later personality pathology that involves a paranoid or hostile view of others, but how might this pattern of interpreting the world develop, and what is the process by which this risk factor might play a role in making an individual vulnerable to the development of a personality disorder in adulthood? Cognitive deficits and biases have been associated with temperamental variables such as impulsivity (Dodge & Newman, 1981) and environmental factors such as harsh parenting (Weiss, Dodge, Bates, & Pettit, 1992), and "early temperamental characteristics in combination with early social experiences can set up anticipatory attitudes that lead the individual to project particular interpretations onto new social relationships and situations" (Caspi, 1998, p. 356).

An example of the processes involved in vulnerability may begin with a hyperactive and impulsive child who may be more likely to jump to conclusions without sufficient information. The difficulties for a child with such a tendency may be compounded if he or she lives in a chaotic household with harsh parenting or is exposed to aggressive peers. In such an antagonistic or unfriendly environment, a hostile attribution may be accurate in most cases, only becoming a "bias" when this tendency is carried into new contexts in which more positive social relationships may be available.

At this point, there is no opposing end point such as "overly positive views" on a continuum with hostile views of the world. Although some research has been conducted on children who demonstrate a benign attributional bias, this behavior has not been considered pathological but, rather, has been associated with prosocial tendencies in a normative sample of children (Nelson & Crick, 1999). It is possible, however, that a pervasive and extreme benign attribution may lead to an inappropriate tolerance of negative behaviors, possibly making the child vulnerable to victimization by peers.

Intense, Unstable, and Inappropriate Emotion to Restricted, Flat Affect

Intense, Unstable, and Inappropriate Emotion

Intense, unstable, and inappropriate emotional expression is characteristic of both borderline and histrionic personality disorder. Symptoms of borderline personality disorder include "affective instability due to a marked reactivity of mood" and "inappropriate, intense anger," whereas "exaggerated expression of emotion" and emotional lability are descriptive of histrionic personality disorder (American Psychiatric Association, 1994, pp. 654, 658). Such behavior may implicate difficulty with emotion regulation as a risk factor underlying the development of these particular disorders.

Emotion regulation concerns individuals' ability to control their arousal, and the foundation for such a skill begins forming in infancy. During infancy, a secure attachment style is one mechanism or process through which children learn to regulate their emotions. A secure attachment is one in which the caregiver has demonstrated that he or she is consistently available for the infant, even in times of stress. Within a secure relationship, negative emotions such as anger or fear are more easily managed by infants because such arousal has been associated with a soothing, effective response by the caregiver (Sroufe, 1996).

Initially, the caregiver is responsible for regulating the emotional arousal of the infant by recognizing the infant's distress and relieving the infant's state of disorganization. The infant gradually plays a larger role in regulating his or her own arousal by, for example, seeking contact with the caregiver or displaying wariness at separation. Having success at returning to a settled state after high arousal teaches the infant that expressing intense emotion need not be an extremely disorganizing experience. Therefore, he or she becomes able to experience more intense emotions and withstand greater arousal, at first with the assistance of the caregiver and gradually on his or her own (Sroufe, 1996).

When this process is aberrant, for example, when the caregiver is not effective at providing responsive and consistent care, the infant may experience arousal as confusing and unsettling. The infant who has not experienced a pattern of intense arousal coupled with attentive care and soothing may not learn that emotion can be experienced and then quelled. As a result, a smooth transition from parent-guided regulation in infancy to self-regulation during childhood may not occur, laying the groundwork for an inability to cope with intense arousal and emotions experienced later in life (Sroufe, 1996).

An adequate parent–child relationship also appears to be involved in the development of important biological systems involved in emotion regulation. For example, Schore (1994) describes how the development of the central nervous system is implicated in emotion regulation. Specifically, the development of the inhibitory processes of the limbic system can influence control over the earlier maturing excitatory processes of the limbic system. Importantly, however, it is the caregiver's assistance in regulating the infant's arousal that may influence the relative power of inhibitory/excitatory functions of the limbic system.

Research on patterns of brain activity in infancy has also implicated the importance of brain development for emotion regulation. Davidson (1991) has studied the frontal and anterior temporal regions, two cortical zones associated with the limbic system that are involved in controlling emotion expression. By examining electroencephalographic (EEG) measures of brain activation, it has been found that activation in the left hemisphere is associated with approach behavior and positive emotion, whereas right-sided activation is associated with withdrawal and negative emotions. The relative balance of this activation pattern has been associated with stable, trait-like tendencies toward negative (relatively stronger left activation) and positive (relatively stronger right activation) emotional responses to eliciting situations. Thus, having a trait-like tendency toward negative emotional responding may make it more difficult to regulate that response.

Dawson, Hessl, and Frey (1994) have studied the effects of maternal depression on infants and have described how depressed mothers may not provide responsive care or be effective at soothing their infants' distress. It has been hypothesized, therefore, that these infants develop a lower threshold for the elicitation of negative emotion and have not learned how to regulate this negative arousal. The researchers suggest that "the infants of depressed mothers are experiencing negative emotions more frequently and intensely and that this results in selective amplification of those neural circuits involved in such emotion" (Dawson et al., 1994, p. 774).

This work on biological systems underlying emotion may be related to research on temperament. Temperament styles consist of early emerging emotional and behavioral tendencies such as activity level, irascibility, ability to regulate arousal ("soothability"), inhibition, and sociability (Goldsmith et al., 1987), and these styles are often considered a foundation for personality (Hartup & van Lieshout, 1995). Temperament researchers often maintain that individual differences in biological dispositions may underlie differences in emotional and behavioral responsivity among children. Kagan, Reznick, and Snidman (1988), for example, argue that inhibited infants, who are fearful of novel situations, may have a central nervous system that has a low threshold for arousal. Thus, stimuli that may cause no response or a positive response for some infants may elicit fear or anxiety in others. This hypersensitivity is important. For example, maltreatment or other chaotic family life experiences may have devastating consequences for the development of any child; however, the combination of a child physiologically predisposed to be overly sensitive to aversive stimuli and an extremely negative environment may be disastrous. Such a process may be implicated in the proneness to unprovoked episodes of extreme anxiety characteristic of individuals with borderline personality disorder (American Psychiatric Association, 1994; Cicchetti & Olsen, 1990). This research on temperament and the work of Schore (1994) and Davidson (1991) highlight the interdependence of the social, emotional, and biological systems.

Poor emotion regulation skills begin forming during infancy, but consistent with the organizational nature of development, this foundation is carried into the early childhood years where it can have significant implications for behavior. Having an insecure attachment history may place a child at risk for problematic behaviors associated with a lack of emotional control. There are important links between how an individual feels and how he or she acts. Emotions not only require regulation themselves but also serve as regulators of behavior. Coping behaviors are one example of how emotions regulate behavior. In a study of 4- to 6-year-olds, intense emotionality was related to ineffective coping, and this was hypothesized to be due to the high intensity of the children's negative emotions making them more "distractible" and less able to focus on the situation (Eisenberg et al., 1993; see section on "Impulsivity" for behavioral manifestations of dysregulated emotion during childhood and adolescence).

Poor emotion regulation skills in the context of chaotic, negative home environments have been specifically implicated in the etiology of borderline personality disorder (Cicchetti & Olsen, 1990). One process that may be involved in the etiology of this disorder includes the impact of intense emotional arousal on cognitive processes. Although the social information-processing model described previously has most typically been applied to the study of aggression (Dodge & Crick, 1990), this model offers a broad framework for understanding cognitive processing that has proven useful in describing other types of maladjustment, including depression (Dodge, 1993). Therefore, this model may also be helpful in outlining a cognitive vulnerability toward developing borderline personality disorder.

Individuals who come from families marked with violence, disorganization, or abuse are likely to become overly sensitive to negative stimuli. They may interpret potentially benign situations as particularly hostile because such an interpretation is consistent with their past experiences. They may react with anger, a hostile outburst, or anxiety, which may lead to a negative response from other family members. This negative response by others likely works to reinforce the individual's misinterpretation of the benign event and may play a role in furthering inappropriate emotional arousal to events. Because children with borderline characteristics may view some events as traumatic that would not usually be experienced in such a manner by other children (Cicchetti & Olsen, 1990), the development of these types of biological, emotional, and cognitive systems may make particular individuals more sensitive to negative events and may explain this phenomenon. Further, these vulnerabilities may be linked to another defining feature of borderline personality disorder—that of being "prone to outbursts of anger and bouts of paralyzing anxiety, both of which happen seemingly without provocation" (American Psychiatric Association, 1994, p. 364).

In sum, emotion regulation skills may serve as one avenue for developmental research targeting personality disorders characterized by intense, unstable, and inappropriate affect. It appears as if the development of particular biological systems, patterns of cognitive processing, and an inability to regulate emotion not only set the stage for intense emotional reactivity but may also play a role in the impulsive behaviors (see section on "Impulsivity") and in the tendency to overreact to personally important situations (see section on "Overly Close Relationships") characteristic of particular personality disorders.

Restricted, Flat Affect

On the other end of our emotion continuum is restricted or flat affect, a characteristic typical of individuals with schizoid or schizotypal personality disorder. Schizoid personality disorder involves "a restricted range of expression of emotions in interpersonal settings," and schizotypal personality disorder is characterized by "inappropriate or constricted affect" (American Psychiatric Association, 1994, pp. 638, 642). Behavioral precursors of these two disorders have been identified; for example, children who were later diagnosed with schizotypal personality disorder were described as high on such characteristics as "seldom laughs or smiles with others," "quiet and unengaged," "passive," and "shy, reserved, and silent" (Olin et al., 1997, p. 96). Depressive symptoms in childhood have also been predictive of the later development of Cluster A personality disorders (which include schizotypal and schizoid personality disorder), especially for boys (Bernstein et al., 1996).

Schizoid and schizotypal personality disorders are considered schizophrenia spectrum disorders, and because of this link with schizophrenia (Grove et al., 1991; Wolff & Chick, 1980), research on the development of schizophrenia may also be useful for identifying vulnerability processes. Infants with a genetic risk for the development of schizophrenia have been found to be atypically quiet and underactive (Fish, 1977). Further, by examining home movies, children who later developed schizophrenia were found to demonstrate more negative affect than their healthy siblings, and pre-schizophrenic girls were found to exhibit fewer expressions of joy (Walker, Grimes, Davis, & Smith, 1993). From infancy through age 5, pre-schizophrenic children were found to be less responsive than their nonaffected siblings (Walker & Lewine, 1990).

It has been hypothesized that individuals with schizoid personality disorder may present with a physiological dysfunction present in infancy "favoring the cholinergic or parasympathetic system" which is thought to underlie a temperamental "emotional unresponsiveness" (Millon & Davis, 1995, p. 666). This lack of emotional expression may also have its roots in the attachment process of infancy. Some infants who have been exposed to a rejecting caregiver may learn to restrain the healthy proximity-seeking behavior toward a caregiver, as discussed earlier. Having met with rejection when approaching the caregiver for comfort, these infants may instead avoid and ignore the caregiver when distressed. In contrast to infants with secure attachments, arousal for these infants is associated with increased avoidance, because to exhibit intense emotions and approach a rejecting caregiver would likely exacerbate the distress rather than calm the infant. Thus, the infant may learn to inhibit the expression of distressing emotions (Sroufe, 1996).

In keeping with the principles of developmental psychopathology, the formation of an attachment relationship is considered an ongoing process involving the behavior of both the caregiver and the infant mutually influencing each other. From one perspective, the infant–caregiver attachment relationship may play a role in the young child's learning to suppress emotion and engage in avoidance of social partners. From a complementary perspective, however, an especially emotionally unresponsive infant may elicit particular reactions from the environment (e.g., less involvement from a caregiver). Evidence indicates that an infant's behavior may influence the type of caregiving that is received. For example, the mothers of "irritable" babies have been shown to engage in less face-to-face contact, physical contact, appropriate stimulation, soothing, and responsiveness as compared to the behavior of mothers of "nonirritable" babies (van den Boom & Hoeksma, 1994). Thus, the behavioral characteristics of children who later developed a schizophrenia spectrum disorder may be both the result of important processes (e.g., the development of an insecure attachment) and the instigators or facilitators of an aberrant process.

Although a particular attachment style does not indicate that a disorder will develop, it does suggest that an individual may be on a deviant pathway and may therefore reflect a vulnerability to later psychopathology. An insecure attachment may influence how an individual relates to others, resulting in a maladaptive pattern of social interacting that accumulates over time. The pattern of emotional unresponsiveness of the infant and toddler may play a role in the formation of detached relationships later in life, a fundamental characteristic of persons diagnosed with schizoid or schizotypal personality disorders (see section on "Distant/Avoidant Relationships").

Impulsivity to Rigidity

Impulsivity

Impulsivity appears to be manifested in two related behavior patterns in adult personality pathology: an inability to inhibit excesses in behavior and behaviors related to aggressive outbursts. The former pattern of impulsivity may include behaviors such as excessive spending or substance use characteristic of individuals with borderline personality disorder, the inability to delay gratification characteristic of individuals with histrionic personality disorder, and the lack of planning associated with antisocial personality disorder. The latter pattern of impulsivity associated with personality pathology is related to aggression and includes the "reckless disregard for safety of self or others" characteristic of individuals with antisocial personality disorder and the "physical fights" commonly exhibited by persons with either antisocial or borderline personality disorder (American Psychiatric Association, 1994, pp. 650, 654).

The display of intense, unstable, and inappropriate emotion characteristic of individuals with borderline or histrionic personality disorder described in the above section may be considered an emotional component of impulsivity. For example, it has been found that relatively low levels of negative emotionality and high levels of emotion regulation predict competent and appropriate social behavior (Eisenberg et al., 1995). Because an inability to regulate emotional arousal may interfere with the ability to inhibit behavior (Eisenberg & Fabes, 1998), emotion regulation difficulties may be predictive of later personality pathology involving impulsivity.

The individual with antisocial personality disorder demonstrates behavioral impulsivity and repeated aggressive outbursts. In childhood, aggressive behavior and impulsivity often present together. One example concerns reactive aggression, a form of aggression in which anger and/or negative affect due to the perceived thwarting of a goal or other provocation plays a role in children's hurting others (Dodge & Coie, 1987). The display of aggression, therefore, is linked with an inability to regulate emotional arousal. Second, emotional arousal can interfere with the information-processing steps of encoding and interpreting events and also with selecting, evaluating, and enacting possible responses. When children experience negative emotions, adequate regulation can often result in inhibiting impulses to behave inappropriately (Eisenberg & Fabes, 1998). Thus, emotion regulation is an important component of an individual's ability to regulate his or her behavior.

Self-regulatory skills may offer another avenue for research on the development of impulsivity in adult character pathology. An inability to inhibit behavior, hyperactivity, and attention problems form the syndrome of attention-deficit/hyperactivity disorder (ADHD; American Psychiatric Association, 1994). Conduct disorder during childhood, a necessary precursor to diagnosing antisocial personality disorder in adulthood, is often found to co-occur with ADHD (Hinshaw, 1987). In addition, individuals with borderline personality disorder also exhibit marked impulsivity, anger-control problems, and the recurrent expression of "inappropriate, intense anger" (American Psychiatric Association, 1994, p. 651), and these individuals may have a history of ADHD (Rey et al., 1995).

The relation between ADHD and aggressive behavior is unclear (for a review, see Lahey & Loeber, 1997). Early attention problems may make an individual vulnerable to the later development of aggressive behavior. Moffitt (1993) has posited that early attention problems may be related to delinquent behavior during adolescence. Consistent with the developmental psychopathology model, attention problems may be a risk factor that interacts with other variables, placing a child on the pathway toward aggressive behavior. For example, parents may use more harsh discipline with an impulsive child (Hinshaw & Simmel, 1994), and harsh discipline has been associated with later aggressive behavior (Weiss et al., 1992). It has also been demonstrated that children's ability to exhibit self-restraint mediates the relation between parenting measures and later antisocial behavior (Feldman & Weinberger, 1994). Another pathway toward aggressive behavior may include ADHD and academic failure. Attention problems may cause academic difficulties, which can increase the risk for aggressive behavior (Maughan, Gray, & Rutter, 1985). It is not clear, however, whether attention and impulsivity difficulties precede or antecede academic problems (Coie & Dodge, 1998; Dishion, French, & Patterson, 1995). Attention difficulties and academic problems likely serve as risk factors that may interact with other biological, social, or cognitive systems to increase the child's tendency to engage in aggressive behavior.

Several processes have been implicated in the development of antisocial behavior (for reviews, see Coie & Dodge, 1998; Dishion et al., 1995), and future research will need to determine which of these processes is linked with impulsivity in adult personality pathology. For example, lack of empathy for others is a defining feature of antisocial personality disorder (see section on "Lack of Concern for Social Norms and Needs of Others") that may be associated with biological or cognitive processes not implicated in other impulse-control disorders such as intermittent explosive disorder, in which the individual may feel regretful after an aggressive episode.

Rigidity

On the other end of the continuum from impulsivity, lack of planning, and lack of emotion-regulation and self-regulation is the inflexibility and rigidity characteristic of individuals with obsessive–compulsive personality disorder or avoidant personality disorder. The rigidity observed in individuals with avoidant personality disorder refers to their excessive unwillingness "to take personal risks or to engage in any new activities because they may prove embarrassing" (American Psychiatric Association, 1994, p. 665). One potential vulnerability to this extreme inhibition has been identified by Kagan (Kagan, 1992; Kagan & Snidman, 1991). As described previously, infants exhibiting behavioral inhibition are fearful of novel situations, and this behavior has been argued to reflect a physiological sensitivity to stimuli (i.e., a low threshold for arousal; Kagan et al., 1988). Similarly, Gray (1982) has posited a behavioral inhibition system (BIS) which is thought to underlie temperamental differences. An overly active BIS may be associated with feelings of anxiety leading to the inhibition of behavior. Over time, an overly active BIS might predispose an individual to experience generalized feelings of anxiety leading to extreme inhibition in both negative circumstances and potentially positive situations.

On the other hand, individuals with obsessive–compulsive personality disorder demonstrate rigidity in that they exhibit "perfectionism that interferes with task completion," "stubborness," and "inflexib[ility] about matters of morality, ethics, or values" (American Psychiatric Association, 1994, pp. 672–673). Although an abundance of research exists concerning childhood obsessive–compulsive disorder (OCD), and some research points toward a linkage between OCD and obsessive–compulsive personality disorder (e.g., Pollak, 1987), current studies have shown that these two disorders are not necessarily related (Thomsen & Mikkelsen, 1993). Therefore, it may not be fruitful to draw on the extensive childhood OCD literature to examine precursors to obsessive–compulsive personality disorder.

Because individuals with obsessive–compulsive personality disorder are excessively perfectionist, organized, detail oriented, and concerned about making errors, the study of perfectionism in children and adolescents may provide a viable research avenue for understanding the development of a rigid personality style. Perfectionism has been found to predict obsessive–compulsive features such as excessive checking in a nonclinical sample of adolescents and adults (Wade, Kyrios, & Henry, 1998). Further, it has been found that a negative form of perfectionism, "maladaptive evaluation concerns" rather than "positive striving," is associated with obsessive–compulsive features in a psychiatric sample of adolescents and adults (Norman, Davies, Nicholson, Cortese, & Malla, 1998).

Interestingly, perfectionism has also been considered an important component of anorexia nervosa in female adolescents and young adults (Attie & Brooks-Gunn, 1995), and an association between anorexia nervosa and obsessive–compulsive personality disorder has been observed in adolescents (Gillberg & Rastam, 1992). These findings point toward excessive perfectionism as a risk factor that may place a child on a deviant pathway for psychopathological outcomes. How this risk factor interacts with other biological and social systems may determine whether it manifests itself in obsessive–compulsive personality traits, disordered eating, or related disorders.

Future research could examine the processes that may be involved in an association between childhood strivings for perfection and obsessive–compulsive features during adulthood. Individuals with obsessive–compulsive personality disorder are also preoccupied with control, and many of their problematic behaviors, including excessive organization and unwillingness to trust others to complete tasks satisfactorily, reflect attempts to "maintain a sense of control" (American Psychiatric Association, 1994,

p. 669). Thus, the strivings for perfection that may be associated with later personality pathology may be related to an excessive need to maintain control.

Overly Close Relationships to Distant/Avoidant Relationships

Overly Close Relationships

Overly close relationships as typified by excessive dependency, a preoccupation with relationship concerns, and heightened emotionality about relationship concerns are characteristic of individuals with borderline, histrionic, or dependent personality disorder. For example, persons with borderline personality disorder demonstrate "a pattern of unstable or intense interpersonal relationships" and are preoccupied with fears of abandonment, individuals with histrionic personality disorder may engage in "inappropriate sexually seductive . . . behavior," and those with dependent personality disorder may rely on others to the point that they feel helpless to function on their own (American Psychiatric Association, 1994, pp. 654, 657). These adults appear to demonstrate a pattern of overvaluing relationships while using these same relationships to manipulate or control others.

One possible precursor to the development of disorders characterized by overly close relationships may be found in children who engage in a similar pattern of overvaluing and manipulating relationships. This pattern of behavior has been observed in children who engage in relatively high rates of relationally aggressive behavior (Crick, Werner, Casas, et al., 1999). Evidence has demonstrated an association between relationally aggressive behaviors and borderline personality features in both children's (Crick, Werner, & Rockhill, 1999) and adolescents' peer relationships (Werner & Crick, 1999) and adolescents' romantic relationships (Morales & Cullerton-Sen, 2000). Relational aggression has at its core a focus on relationships such that these children harm others by manipulating or damaging social relationships (e.g., spreading rumors in retaliation to damage a child's reputation and withdrawing friendship in order to control a peer; Crick & Grotpeter, 1995).

Similar to adults with borderline, histrionic, or dependent personality disorder, despite their manipulative behaviors within relationships, relationally aggressive children also engage in "enmeshed" relationships and demonstrate heightened sensitivity to relational events. For example, relationally aggressive children tend to maintain friendships that are overly intimate, exclusive, and marked with jealousy. These children also manipulate their friends in order to obtain control within the friendship (Grotpeter & Crick, 1996). Further, adolescents who are relationally aggressive have been found to exhibit this relational event sensitivity and an elevated level of desire for exclusivity in their close relationships (Morales & Crick, 1999).

Relationally aggressive children also report feeling more anger than do nonrelationally aggressive children when faced with relational conflicts (Crick, 1995; Crick, Grotpeter, & Bigbee, 1998). Thus, the intense emotionality discussed in the section, "Intense, Unstable, and Inappropriate Emotion" may be activated in situations that threaten the integrity of important relationships. Given their preoccupation with maintaining close relationships and their sensitivity to relational slights, children who are successful at obtaining their goals and controlling others through this form of social manipulation may continue this pattern in adult relationships.

The social information-processing model described previously may also highlight social and cognitive aspects of the oversensitivity to relationship events. For example, individuals with borderline personality disorder worry about abandonment, and these individuals may be more alert to cues signaling potential loss, or may misinterpret temporary separation as possible abandonment. Their intense reaction may ultimately push others away, beginning a process that reinforces the initial incorrect interpretation of the event. This sensitivity to interpersonal events may be compounded by the intense, uncontrolled emotion often experienced by these individuals. Such a cognitive pattern may explain why neutral events, such as a friend being a few minutes late, is so easily misinterpreted and related to feelings of "panic or fury" (American Psychiatric Association, 1994, p. 650).

As discussed previously, these cognitive processes likely interact with environmental events to produce vulnerability to the development of disorders characterized by overly close relationships. For example, a chaotic family life may be related to a heightened sensitivity to negative stimuli. Further, these individuals may misinterpret situations and react with an angry outburst which may lead to a negative response from other family members, thereby reinforcing the initial misinterpretation. Whereas chaotic home environments may be a risk factor for the development of borderline personality disorder, the possible contribution of overinvolved parenting in children's low self-esteem may be more relevant for the individual who later goes on to develop dependent personality disorder (see section on "Negative Sense of Self").

Distant/Avoidant Relationships

A pathological absence of adequate, nurturing, and fulfilling social relationships is a shared feature of obsessive–compulsive, paranoid, schizoid, schizotypal, and avoidant personality disorders. The emotional unresponsiveness discussed in the previous section, "Restricted, Flat Affect," may play an important role in the inability to maintain adequate social relationships. Children with schizoid features have been described as having "an acutely constricted and underdeveloped affective life, with emotional distance in human relations" (Cicchetti & Olsen, 1990, p. 359). As mentioned earlier, the relation between schizoid and schizotypal personality disorders and schizophrenia, a disorder associated with several neurological impairments, may indicate a biological risk factor that is involved in the emotional unresponsiveness and social withdrawal observed in children who later develop these disorders.

An important risk factor therefore may be a biological predisposition toward emotional unresponsiveness, and the processes involved in creating a vulnerability to the development of a personality disorder marked by distant relationships may begin as early as infancy. If the infant–caregiver bond is characterized by a secure attachment, the infant can learn to trust the caregiver, and this first relationship serves as a model for future relationships. As mentioned previously, it is plausible that an emotionally unresponsive infant may elicit less involvement from a caregiver and may make appropriate caregiving more difficult. A history marked by a series of insecure attachments may instill an inability to trust others, and this inherent distrust is a primary feature of paranoid personality disorder. On the other hand, a series of insecure attachments and a tendency to distrust others may develop instead into the ambivalence toward maintaining close, interpersonal relationships that is characteristic of the individual with schizoid or schizotypal personality disorder. Thus, an insecure attachment may influence how an individual interacts with others, resulting in a deviant pattern of social interacting that worsens over time.

For example, an insecure attachment during infancy has been associated with "passive withdrawal" for boys during middle childhood (Renken, Egeland, Marvinney, Mangelsdorf, & Sroufe, 1989), suggesting that the study of this behavior during childhood may provide important information about precursors to social detachment. Although each of the personality disorders addressed in this section is characterized by a lack of fulfilling social relationships, the reasons underlying this social withdrawal differ among the disorders. The individual with paranoid personality disorder avoids relationships because of pervasive feelings of distrust and suspicion toward others. Individuals with schizoid or schizotypal personality disorder have no interest in maintaining social relationships, whereas individuals with avoidant personality disorder are distressed by their lack of close relationships with others. Although persons with avoidant personality disorder long to form lasting relationships with others, they are plagued by feelings of inadequacy and fear of rejection (American Psychiatric Association, 1994). Recent research on social withdrawal in children has identified three subtypes of withdrawn children, those who are characterized as passive–anxious, unsociable, or active–isolates (Harrist, Zaia, Bates, Dodge, & Pettit, 1997), and it is interesting to speculate whether these subtypes parallel the different types of social detachment descriptive of adult personality disorders.

Passive–anxious children are those who refrain from playing with other children because they are afraid of the social interchange (Rubin & Mills,

1988). These children tend to be easily aroused by unfamiliar situations (Harrist et al., 1997). This type of withdrawn behavior may be similar to the behavior of adults with avoidant personality disorder because these children would like to play with others but are too inhibited to engage in social activities. The second subtype of withdrawn children is referred to as unsociable. In contrast to passive–anxious children, unsociable children prefer playing by themselves (Harrist et al., 1997). These withdrawn children may demonstrate behaviors similar in function and appearance to adults with schizoid or schizotypal personality disorder who exhibit little desire to engage in social activities. This hypothesis is consistent with the finding that children who later developed schizophrenia were described by their kindergarten through 12th-grade teachers as being low in interpersonal competence (e.g., maturity level, group participation, popularity, and sociability; Lewine, Watt, Prentky, & Fryer, 1980).

The third subtype of withdrawn children, active–isolates, includes those who want to play with others but are rejected as play partners because of their aggressive behavior and/or lack of social skills (Harrist et al., 1997). In accordance with the social information-processing model described earlier, aggressive children may exhibit poor social skills, including the maintenance of a hostile attribution bias. For some individuals, it is possible that these negative peer interactions accumulate over time and contribute to the negative and hostile view of others that is prominent in individuals with paranoid personality disorder. Thus, the risk factor may be poor social skills and/or aggressive behavior; however the mechanisms by which the individual becomes vulnerable to the development of paranoid personality disorder may involve the process by which this risk factor influences the child's social system (e.g., peer rejection) and cognitive system (e.g., an intensification of a hostile attribution bias).

Recall that within a developmental psychopathology model, pathways of development are emphasized such that knowledge, resources, and skills gained in early negotiations with important tasks assist in the completion of future accomplishments. Children who are rejected by their peers do not have a setting in which to learn appropriate social skills and relationship-building skills such as sharing, trusting, cooperating, and generating intimacy. In fact, children who are not accepted by their peers have been found to be at an increased risk for future maladjustment (Parker & Asher, 1987). Early social withdrawal may begin a process by which children become increasingly incapable of maintaining successful relationships with peers and ultimately with romantic partners.

The vulnerability process may continue with increasing age because with better cognitive skills, the manner in which individuals perceive the environment may play a larger role in the preference for social detachment. Whereas the interaction between the environment and neurological impairments pertaining to emotional unresponsiveness may be an especially important factor in the development of schizoid personality disorder, the formation of self-defeating cognitive schemes may be particularly significant for the development of avoidant personality disorder. Early experience such as overly critical parenting and experiences of humiliation or rejection, in combination with a hypersensitivity to aversive stimuli, may cause these children to learn that they are ineffectual, impotent, and inconsequential (Millon & Davis, 1995). These individuals may develop cognitive schemes concerning their ineffectiveness to maintain relationships, which, in turn, might lead to biased encoding of the unfavorable aspects of relationships and negative misinterpretations of benign interpersonal events.

For example, it is likely that individuals with avoidant personality disorder develop social–cognitive biases, selectively encoding negative information and interpreting ambiguous information in a self-defeating manner. They may interpret an acquaintance's failure to show up at a meeting as a direct indication that the acquaintance does not accept or approve of them. Further, biased comparisons of personal qualities and accomplishments with those of others may reinforce low self-esteem and feelings of worthlessness. With increasing age and independence, individuals also have more control over their environment such that persons uncomfortable with social situations may choose to remain in settings that suit their fear or ambivalence toward personal relationships (e.g., an isolated occupational setting). Such personal choices may exacerbate the lack of interpersonal skills of these individuals.

Negative Sense of Self or Lack of Self to Exaggerated Sense of Self

A core symptom of several of the personality disorders is a disturbed sense of self. A negative self-view is a key aspect of both avoidant and dependent personality disorder, an unstable self-image or lack of self is characteristic of borderline personality disorder (American Psychiatric Association, 1994), and an inflated self-image is an element of both narcissistic and histrionic personality disorders (American Psychiatric Association, 1994; Kernberg, 1989). Whereas an exaggerated sense of self represents one end of the continuum, the other end may be conceptualized as either a negative sense of self or a lack of a coherent sense of self. In congruence with a developmental psychopathology model, an exploration of the normative development of self-representations may offer clues to aberrant processes underlying the distorted view of the self that is inherent in certain types of maladaptive personality functioning in adulthood.

In a recent review, Harter (1998) describes the typical pattern of the developing self. Due to increasing cognitive skills that allow children to perceive the distinction between what they hope to achieve and what they actually can achieve (Crain, 1996), it is normal for children's self-concepts to become more negative (less unrealistically positive) during middle childhood (Harter, 1982). In early adolescence, there may be a second decrease in self-esteem, followed by a slow increase over the later adolescent years (Marsh, 1989). Deviations in this normal pattern may be indicative of an increased potential for the development of one of the patterns of distorted self-concept characteristic of an adult personality disorder. For example, during the middle childhood years, a child who maintains the unrealistically high self-view characteristic of early childhood may be on a pathway toward developing narcissistic personality features. Similarly, an adolescent who maintains the typically low self-esteem characteristic of early adolescence without undergoing the gradual increase in self-concept generally experienced by older adolescents may be on a pathway toward developing the chronic, negative self-concept characteristic of persons with avoidant or dependent personality disorder.

Thus, the question arises as to what mechanisms might be responsible for these deviations in the development of self-representations. Many normal processes in children appear to mirror symptoms of personality disorders in adults, suggesting that personality-disordered adults have adopted immature ways of dealing with the environment. This theory is consistent with the notion that some features of personality disorder represent immature patterns of behavior (Ryglewicz & Pepper, 1996). It is possible that overlearned behavioral patterns of childhood were maintained because they were effective, reinforced, or because the learning of new, more effective behavior was somehow hindered. Thus, the following are possible processes in the development of the self that may serve as markers or liabilities for the development of the distorted self-representations characteristic of particular personality disorders.

Negative Sense of Self

Beginning in infancy, the development of a negative self-view may be fostered by the internalization of the experience of the caregivers' responsiveness. A consistent and responsive caregiver teaches the infant that he or she can elicit desirable events in the environment and more generally that the infant is effective, worthy of care, and lovable. A caregiver who is rejecting or a caregiver who is inconsistent in responding to an infant's bids for attention, however, may set the stage for the child to learn that he or she is ineffective and not worthy of attention. Sroufe (1990) has demonstrated that children with an insecure attachment history are rated as lower on self-esteem than those with secure attachment histories.

With increasing age, cognitive processes may play an important role in creating a vulnerability toward personality disorders characterized by low self-esteem. Specifically, the child may be more sensitive to social cues that undermine his or her confidence or ability to be successful. The child may misinterpret ambiguous social information as indicative of his or her inferiority. This tendency to interpret an ambiguous situation negatively may lead to feelings of inadequacy, which, in turn, could result in a failure to complete a task. This failure may serve to reinforce the child's initially incorrect interpretation of his or her ability.

The above processes involve the development and maintenance of a general sense of negative self-worth, characterized by inferiority and fear of negative evaluation, that may make the child vulnerable to a personality disorder such as avoidant personality disorder. The following processes involved in negative self-concept, however, may be more associated with dependent personality disorder because of their relation to helplessness and overreliance on others. Because it is generally during middle childhood that children more clearly realize the kind of individual that others might want them to become (Higgins, 1991), this period may be where the foundation is laid for excessive concern with the desires of others. It is in adolescence, however, that the opinions of others appear to have an overwhelming influence on an individual's sense of self (Elkind, 1967; Lapsley & Rice, 1988).

To deal with the perceived demands or opinions of others, many adolescents have reported engaging in "false-self behavior," which includes "not saying what you think," "expressing things you don't really believe or feel," and "changing yourself to be something that someone *else* wants you to be" (Harter, 1998, p. 581). Harter has suggested that some adolescents believe that they receive little support from important others and that they will only be able to obtain this limited support by meeting exceptionally high demands. These adolescents may "feel hopeless about pleasing others, which in turn causes them to suppress their true self as a potential means of garnering the desired support" (Harter, 1998, p. 581). Given the similarity between examples of "false-self behavior" and the symptoms of dependent personality disorder such as "has difficulty expressing disagreement with others because of fear of loss of support or approval" (American Psychiatric Association, 1994, p. 668), it makes sense that such behaviors may function as precursors to the development of this disorder. In addition, the proposed link between negative self-concept and the "fear of loss of support" typical of individuals with dependent personality disorder (American Psychiatric Association, 1994, p. 668) is mirrored in Gilligan's (1982) argument that false-self behavior may be related to an individual's notion that to reveal his or her particular opinions may damage close relationships.

Individuals with dependent personality disorder also have "difficulty initiating projects or doing things on their own (because of a lack of self-confidence in judgment or abilities rather than a lack of motivation or energy)" (American Psychiatric Association, 1994, p. 668). Another possible source of the negative self-concept related to an overreliance on others may involve the type of parenting a child receives. Child maltreatment has often been associated with the development of a personality disorder, especially with the development of borderline personality disorder. Although maltreatment is likely to have a direct, negative impact on several domains of a child's development, it has been specifically linked with the formation of a negative self-view. Fischer and Ayoub (1994) posit that maltreatment can lead children to believe that they are unimportant and useless, instilling within them the notion that they are generally "bad."

Maltreatment is an extreme example of negative parenting; however, more normative types of parenting may also influence a child's sense of self. Caregivers who are sensitive to and helpful with their child's efforts at achievement generally aid in the development of a positive self-image. For children with a negative sense of self, however, such involvement may indicate to the child that he or she is not capable of independent success (Harter, 1998). For example, Shell and Eisenberg (1992) have found that children who have already developed a notion that they are not smart, tend to perceive assistance as a sign that they are incapable of accomplishing tasks on their own. This perception may lead to negative views of the self and to feelings of inadequacy. This example also highlights the role of interpretation of social events in the maintenance of a negative self-image, as discussed previously.

Lack of Sense of Self

The characteristics of borderline personality disorder such as "identity disturbance," "unstable self-image or sense of self," and "chronic feelings of emptiness" (American Psychiatric Association, 1994, p. 654) suggest that the individual with this disorder suffers from a lack of an integrated, coherent sense of self. This state is to be distinguished from a negative self-image because individuals with borderline personality disorder "at times have feelings that they do not exist at all" (American Psychiatric Association, 1994, p. 651).

The changing self-image of individuals with borderline personality disorder involves shifting between viewing the self as all good or all bad (Ryglewicz & Pepper, 1996). This inability to integrate different facets of individuals, particularly characteristics that are opposites, is common in normally developing children (Fischer, 1980). During early and middle childhood, children often separate these opposing qualities to such an extent that the idea that individuals may have aspects of both characteristics is difficult to comprehend.

As mentioned earlier, it is normal for children to view themselves in an overly positive manner. Because children have difficulty integrating opposite characteristics, this overdistinction between "good" and "bad" tends to result in a "unidimensional or all-or-none thinking that typically leads to self-descriptions that remain laden with virtuosity" (Harter, 1998, p. 570). Under adverse circumstances, however, this "all-or-none thinking" may have the opposite effect: leading a child to think that he or she is all bad (Harter, 1986). Thus, it seems logical that if individuals with borderline personality disorder partially maintain this earlier "unidimensional" thinking such that they view the self as all positive or all negative, it may result in both an unstable switching between positive and negative self-views and a general lack of a cohesive self-representation.

Further, for most children, it is normal for the "all good" or "all bad" view of the self to be associated with specific external events. For example, if a teacher scolds a child, he may think that he is a "bad" child. Between 7 and 8 years of age, children undergo a cognitive shift marked by moving away from associating negative feelings with absolute events that can change from situation to situation and also by an increasing tendency to compare oneself to peers. This process can affect self-evaluation by the formation of global attributions rather than event-related attributions (Cicchetti & Toth, 1995). The individual with borderline personality disorder, for example, may demonstrate an inability to make these global attributions but instead will rely on the more immature view of the self—that which is tied to absolute events and therefore fluctuates depending on the nature of the eliciting occurrence. For instance, events of perceived abandonment common in persons with borderline personality disorder may imply for these individuals that they are generally "bad." Those individuals who continue to attribute their self-image to external events during adolescence may be especially at risk for identity problems. Damon and Hart (cited in Harter, 1998) argue that "adolescents who do not move to the stage of internalized standards but continue to rely on external social standards and feedback will be at risk because they will not have developed an internalized, relatively stable sense of self that will form the basis for subsequent identity development" (p. 586).

Adolescents are capable of thinking of themselves in a more abstract manner, for example by combining similar concepts into broader categories. An example might include conceptualizing oneself as "trustworthy," a category that encompasses other notions of the self such as "responsible" and "honest" (Fischer, 1980; Harter, 1998). Adolescents, however, are still cognitively limited in their ability to integrate the abstract concepts that are opposite in nature (Harter & Monsour, 1992). In fact, self-constructs in middle adolescence are characterized by "an immature form of relating . . . abstract concepts to one another because one cannot yet integrate such self-representations in a manner that would resolve the apparent contradiction" (Harter, 1998, p. 573). This inability to meaningfully integrate abstract traits that are opposite in nature during adolescence has been linked directly with an unstable self-image that fluctuates between the two extremes (e.g., viewing oneself as extremely productive and creative at times, but feeling inadequate and like a complete failure another time; Harter, 1990).

As stated previously, one experiential factor that may influence the continuation of this less well-developed conceptualization of the self, and therefore may make an individual vulnerable to the development of borderline personality disorder, is child maltreatment. Physical and sexual abuse have often been identified as risk factors associated with the development of this disorder (American Psychiatric Association, 1994; Cicchetti & Olsen, 1990). This maltreatment may encourage an immature conceptualization of the self. For example, Harter (1998) argues that in an abusive home "family members typically offer and continue to reinforce negative evaluations of the child that are then incorporated into the self-portrait. As a result, there may be little scaffolding for the kind of self structure that would allow the child to develop as well as integrate both positive and negative self-evaluations" (p. 571). This maltreatment at the hands of a caregiver is especially confusing for the child's developing sense of self because the child's abuser at times also fulfills the role of nurturer. It has been hypothesized that exposure to these opposing roles may result in the child receiving conflicting messages about his or her self-worth. Given the conflicting notions about the self, a disorganized form of behavior, characterized by a disorganized attachment style, may result in interactions with the parent (Liotti, 1992; Main & Hesse, 1990).

Child maltreatment (Briere & Runtz, 1988; Chu & Dill, 1990), and other trauma in general (Irwin, 1994), has been found to be related to dissociation, a symptom of borderline personality disorder that is associated with a lack of sense of self. Dissociation refers to the inability to integrate aspects of the self including "consciousness," "memory," and "identity" (American Psychiatric Association, 1994, p. 766) and can include amnesic or depersonalization experiences (Waller, Putnam, & Carlson, 1996). Dissociation is thought to be a defense mechanism enacted in response to trauma in order to protect the self (Putnam, 1994). "Self, in fact, refers to the integration and organization of diverse aspects of experience, and dissociation can be defined as the failure to integrate experience" (Ogawa, Sroufe, Weinfield, Carlson, & Egeland, 1997, p. 855).

There are several ways in which dissociation, a lack of sense of self, trauma, and insecure attachment may be related. Ogawa et al. (1997) have demonstrated that having a weak sense of self during infancy and toddlerhood predicts dissociation during adolescence, suggesting that a less well-developed sense of self may serve as a vulnerability factor for later dissociation. Further, insecure attachment during infancy was associated with increased adolescent dissociative behaviors for individuals who had undergone substantial trauma. Thus, an insecure attachment may serve as a vulnerability factor for later dissociation in the context of traumatic experiences. Ogawa et al. (1997) speculated that "the vulnerable self will be more likely to adopt dissociation as a coping mechanism because it does not have either the belief in worthiness gained from a loving and responsive early relationship or the normal level of defenses and integration that such a belief affords" (p. 15).

This incoherent sense of self appears to be a highly important component of borderline personality disorder. A poor self-concept emerged among a host of other cognitive and affective variables (e.g., anger, depression, and locus of control) as the only variable that distinguished female adolescents who were comorbid for depression and borderline personality disorder from those suffering from depression only (Pinto, Grapentine, Francis, & Picariello, 1996). Thus, disturbances in self-concept during childhood and adolescence and how this risk factor may interfere with social, emotional, and cognitive processes may indicate vulnerability processes associated with the later development of borderline personality disorder.

Exaggerated Sense of Self

On the other end of the continuum from negative sense of self or lack of self is an inflated self-view, another distorted view of the self that characterizes aspects of both narcissistic and histrionic personality disorders. Childhood precursors of such a self-concept are difficult to identify because most children typically boast excessively about their accomplishments, indulge in grandiose fantasies (Kernberg, 1989), and maintain an unrealistically positive view of the self (Harter, 1998). It is possible that individuals with narcissistic or histrionic personality disorder have carried this early pattern of grandiose self-appraisal into adulthood. This pattern of behavior may have been reinforced, or the child may have failed to develop appropriate skills that might have later served as a foundation for a more mature and realistic assessment of the self. In addition, although children generally describe themselves positively, many of them do not endorse purely virtuous attributes, but also acknowledge that they are less than perfect (Cassidy, 1988). Thus, it may be that those children who do not acknowledge even minor faults may be on an early pathway toward developing a maladaptive overevaluation of their attributes and accomplishments.

This grandiose view of the self may function to mask a negative self-concept. For example, individuals with narcissistic personality disorder demonstrate "a grandiose sense of self-importance," "a sense of entitlement," and arrogance (American Psychiatric Association, 1994, p. 661). Despite this aggrandizement, the inflated self-esteem and boasting behavior appears to belie an "invariably very fragile" self-esteem such that these individuals may become excessively distressed by criticism (American Psychiatric Association, 1994, p. 658). One process that may have predisposed the individual to adopt this pattern of masking feelings of inferiority with grandiosity may have been the early attachment process with the primary caregiver discussed previously. It appears that children with a history of an insecure/avoidant attachment may present with a pattern of self-representation that strikingly resembles that of the narcissistic personality. Specifically, despite observer, teacher, or counselor ratings of low self-esteem (Sroufe, 1990), some children with insecure attachment histories have been reported to describe themselves rather positively, suggesting that these children report high self-esteem to hide their feelings of worthlessness (Cassidy, 1988).

Peculiar Thought Processes and Behaviors

In general, individuals with a personality disorder maintain thoughts and beliefs about events, people, or behaviors that most would consider maladaptive and are often unsubstantiated. For example, individuals with borderline, histrionic, or dependent personality disorder exhibit distorted beliefs concerning relationships, whereas persons with paranoid personality disorder may demonstrate untenable beliefs about the hostility of others. These individuals may behave in a manner that seems to perpetuate and reinforce these maladaptive thoughts, such that these beliefs appear to be understandable given the particular circumstances of the individual. Another category of eccentric thought processes—psychotic thoughts—includes those that are extremely unusual and not likely to be justified given most circumstances. These thoughts and their associated behaviors include the "ideas of reference," "unusual perceptual experiences," "odd beliefs or magical thinking," "belief[s] in clairvoyance, [or] telepathy," and "odd thinking and speech" that characterize the individual with schizotypal personality disorder (American Psychiatric Association, 1994, p. 645). Persons with borderline personality disorder may also exhibit hallucinations, ideas of reference, and hypnagogic episodes (American Psychiatric Association, 1994).

Psychotic processes include hallucinations, delusions, and formal thought disorder. Research on the development of these phenomena is limited (for a review, see Volkmar, Becker, King, & McGlashan, 1995). Hallucinations are perceptual experiences that lack an appropriate stimulus (American Psychiatric Association, 1994). Individual differences in vulnerability to hallucinations have been identified such that persons more vulnerable to hallucinatory experiences tend to be highly suggestible. Also, vulnerability to hallucinating has been associated with individuals who are overconfident in judging the source of experimentally produced perceptual events (e.g., determining the location of a sound; Bentall, 1990). Further, the experience of hallucinations has been related to difficulties distinguishing reality from imagination (Slade & Bentall, 1988).

Delusions are beliefs that cannot possibly be true given an individual's social and cultural context. Delusions are not symptomatic of the personality disorders; however, a related phenomenon, ideas of reference, is characteristic of schizotypal personality disorder. Ideas of reference are notions that everyday occurrences, such as newspaper articles or television programs, have special importance, usually negative, for the individual (American Psychiatric Association, 1994). The individual does not exhibit the delusional intensity of such phenomenon but, rather, maintains some insight that the occurrence may not be real. In children and adolescents, symptoms of schizotypal personality disorder may include "bizarre fantasies or preoccupations" (American Psychiatric Association, 1994, p. 645). Possible precursors of ideas of reference and related unusual behavior may be identified during childhood. Children who later developed schizotypal personality disorder were rated by a psychiatrist interviewer as more "peculiar" (e.g., eccentric, queer, and awkward) than psychiatric and nonpsychiatric controls (Parnas & Jorgensen, 1989).

Patterns of "odd thinking and speech" have also been detected in a high-risk sample of children (mean age 15) who later developed schizotypal personality disorder. In this longitudinal, prospective study, evidence of formal thought disorder was observed in these children (Parnas, Schulsinger, Schulsinger, Mednick, & Teasdale, 1982). Formal thought disorder refers to deviance in the form of thinking as demonstrated by vague, tangential, or incoherent speech as opposed to deviance in thought content (e.g., delusions or hallucinations).

Assessing psychotic processes in children can be a daunting task which makes research in this area difficult. Knowledge of normal development and abilities for particular age groups may be beneficial. For example, it may be difficult to determine the presence of psychotic processes in young children because of their limited language ability. Children may not be able to articulate their hallucinatory experiences (Volkmar et al., 1995). Also, it is normal for young children to have difficulty distinguishing real from fantasy (e.g., Ceci & Huffman, 1997), and this normative behavior must not be confused with hallucinatory experiences. Further, hallucinations have been observed to occur in normal, but anxious, children of preschool age (Volkmar et al., 1995). Behavior resembling loose associations and irrational thinking, two examples of formal thought disorder, are observed in normal children before the age of 7 (Caplan, Foy, Asarnow, & Sherman, 1990). Further, psychosis must be distinguished from normal behaviors that are similar in appearance (e.g., imaginary friends; Volkmar et al., 1995).

For all of these reasons, identifying and researching antecedents to peculiar thought processes and behaviors may be difficult and the ideas posited here should be considered speculative. It seems likely however, that given the numerous biological correlates of the schizophrenia spectrum disorders, physiological risk factors may also play an important role in psychotic thought processes. Perhaps the combination of psychological vulnerability such as an increased tendency to withdraw into fantasy and a family history significant for a schizophrenia spectrum disorder is characteristic of children who later display personality pathology marked by eccentric thoughts and behavior.

Lack of Concern for Social Norms and Needs of Others

A lack of concern for the needs of others, as demonstrated by an inability to experience remorse or empathy, is characteristic of individuals with antisocial or narcissistic personality disorder. For individuals with antisocial personality disorder, this lack of concern for others may also be manifested in lying, cheating, and criminal behavior (American Psychiatric Association,

1994). Research on the cognitive, emotional, biological, and social interaction processes associated with empathy and the development of a conscience may offer insight into vulnerability to these disorders.

A social–cognitive perspective on the development of empathy-related behaviors has implicated the role of intelligence. A moderate correlation has been found between prosocial behavior and intelligence, and this relation may be due to children's ability to take the perspective of others, their ability to articulate their motivation for helping others, and their skills in reasoning about moral issues (Eisenberg & Fabes, 1998). Other evidence indicates that children's understanding of a peer's need for help, along with the knowledge of their own ability to be helpful, influences children's decision of whether to provide assistance to others. Older children tend to rely on this information more than do younger children, suggesting that with increasing cognitive skills, children are better at evaluating situations requiring prosocial, helping behaviors (Ladd, Lange, & Stremmel, 1983). Thus, relatively lower cognitive functioning, especially related to understanding social interaction and moral reasoning, may provide a vulnerability to a pathological unconcern for the needs of others.

A lack of concern for others also has an emotional component. Research on adult psychopathy, a behavioral syndrome related to antisocial personality disorder that is also characterized by a lack of remorse, has demonstrated diminished autonomic and reflex responses to fearful and startling stimuli (Patrick, Bradley, & Lang, 1993; Patrick, Cuthbert, & Lang, 1994). This research suggests that individual differences in emotional reactivity may be one risk factor for the development of a lack of concern for others.

As mentioned earlier in the discussion of impulsivity, emotions can regulate behavior in that varying intensities of different emotional responses are often associated with different actions. In general, children who display emotional indicators of sympathy often behave in a prosocial manner (Eisenberg & Fabes, 1998). Eisenberg and Fabes (1998) describe a series of studies conducted with their colleagues in which children were exposed to videos designed to bring about an empathic response. Children's demonstration of physiological indicators of empathy (e.g., measures of heart rate, facial expressions, and skin conductance) was associated with their tendency to engage in prosocial behavior toward the individuals portrayed in the video. When discussing rigidity, an overactive BIS was implicated in the expression of anxiety or negative affect (Gray, 1982). An *underactive* BIS, however, has been hypothesized to predispose an individual to remain relatively unaffected by punishment, setting the stage for later antisocial behavior (Quay, 1993). Thus, individuals with a reduced emotional response to empathy-inducing events may be at risk for the development of antisocial or narcissistic personality disorder.

These cognitive and emotional risk factors must be examined within a social context to understand the processes relevant to the development of impaired empathy-related behaviors. Parents often assume initial responsibility for instructing their children about appropriate emotional and behavioral responses to events that children should "internalize" into standards for behavior. In her review on the development of conscience, Kochanska (1993) states that "the gradual developmental shift from external to internal regulation that results in a child's ability to conform to societal standards of conduct and to restrain antisocial or destructive impulses, even in the absence of surveillance, is the essence and hallmark of successful socialization" (pp. 325–326).

Harsh parenting may interact with cognitive and emotional risk factors in predisposing a child to developing an impaired sense of empathy. One example is offered by Dienstbier (1984), who argues that when children break a rule, they become distressed and attempt to understand the cause of this discomfort. If parents are excessively negative, angry, and punishing, the child may attribute his or her negative feelings to external reasons (i.e., being discovered misbehaving by the parents). In contrast, parents who use a calm approach to discipline may be more effective in teaching the child to internalize standards of behavior because the child may be more likely to attribute the negative emotion to internal reasons. In another example of the role of parenting on empathy-related behavior, Kochanska (1993) proposes that the development of conscience involves meaningful interactions between the individual characteristics of the child and the parenting style used. Kochanska (1995) found that compliance in children is most likely to occur when the parent's disciplinary style matches the child's individual characteristics. Gentle discipline was effective in obtaining compliance in children who tend to be fearful; however, the subtlety of this parenting style did not elicit compliance in fearless children. For fearless children, compliance was instead related to maternal sensitivity and mutual engagement between the child and caregiver.

CONCLUSION

Individual Differences

The previous discussion of vulnerability factors offers an account of meaningful individual differences in children that may be related to the future development of personality disorders. For example, it is hypothesized that individuals with a negative sense of self may be at an increased risk for avoidant or dependent personality disorder compared to individuals with a positive self-concept. Nonspecific individual differences including age or gender also may be related to the previously discussed vulnerability factors and processes. First, vulnerability processes are related to the age of the child; for example, the development of an aberrant attachment relationship begins during infancy, whereas cognitive processes are not likely primary vulnerabilities until later in childhood. Further, it has been found that in general, behavioral excess tends to decline whereas solitary, isolated behavior tends to increase with age. With respect to gender, research has found that during childhood and adolescence, males are more likely to exhibit impulsivity problems, physical aggression, and avoidant behaviors (McDermott, 1996).

Nonspecific individual differences may also be related to personality disorders directly. In a sample of psychiatric adolescents, gender differences were generally not related to personality disorder diagnosis (assessed by DSM-III-R criteria), with the exceptions that females were more often diagnosed with borderline personality disorder whereas narcissistic personality disorder was found only among the males (Grilo et al., 1996). Age effects have also been noted in a separate clinical sample that included both adolescents and adults such that individuals with a diagnosis of dependent personality disorder tended to be older compared with individuals with other personality disorders. In addition, females constituted approximately 70% of individuals diagnosed with this disorder in contrast with the approximately 60% female prevalence in other personality disorder categories (Loranger, 1996).

Nonspecific individual differences have also been found to be associated with the measurement of personality disorders. In a prospective study of childhood risk factors associated with later personality pathology, Cohen (1996) has found that prediction was more precise among girls, particularly younger girls.

Implications for Intervention

In this chapter, we have attempted to identify possible vulnerabilities to the development of personality disorders by conceptualizing the process within a developmental psychopathology framework. This perspective also has implications for intervention research and treatment. Proponents of the diagnostic system adopted in the DSM attempt to identify therapeutic interventions that benefit most individuals with the same diagnosis. A developmental perspective, however, suggests that treatment should not necessarily be dictated by how an individual's behavior patterns are classified but, rather, by attention to the developmental pathway of each individual. Thus, persons who manifest similar behaviors (e.g., borderline features) may have arrived at this outcome from very different histories and patterns of success and failure throughout childhood and adolescence (Sroufe, 1997). Addressing the processes involved in particular outcomes may assist clinicians in creating treatment plans that take into account the development of a disorder rather than primarily addressing the similar behavioral outcome among a group of possibly heterogeneous individuals.

Further, by identifying well-researched, broad areas of functioning that may be antecedents or important components of adult personality disorders, it may be possible to direct preventive efforts at these personality dimensions. Such an approach would prevent the delay of treatment until maladaptive patterns of behavior become deeply ingrained and interact with each other to produce a full-blown psychiatric disorder. For example, whereas individuals with antisocial personality disorder may be highly resistant to psychotherapy, research on the developmental manifestations of empathy may be informative for interventionists and preventionists interested in targeting children who demonstrate a lack of empathy. In their review of empathic responding, Eisenberg, Wentzel, and Harris (1998) identify two processes, emotionality and regulation, that may be involved in children's empathy, describe how to measure empathic feelings and behavior, and review several intervention programs designed to enhance empathy. By focusing on the processes of emotionality and regulation rather than on a similar behavioral manifestation (i.e., empathic responding), these researchers concluded that different types of interventions would be indicated for children who differ on these characteristics. Whereas children who become too emotionally distressed to be helpful to others might need assistance in regulation, those children who are generally less emotional may need help identifying and understanding the emotions of others.

Another treatment implication of the dimensional model used in this chapter involves a search for therapeutic intervention beyond the individual child. Traditionally, researchers develop treatment programs that are thought to benefit individuals who "have" a psychiatric disorder. General maladaptation during childhood, as described by extremes on the above dimensions, does not necessarily reflect a disorder that a child has or does not have but, rather, implies problematic functioning within a particular domain. Thus, difficulties such as impulsivity or behaviors related to low self-esteem may be addressed by examining the context in which these negative behaviors are exhibited. For example, some researchers intervene to reduce aggressive behavior in children by altering family interaction patterns of negative reinforcement and coercion (Patterson, DeBaryshe, & Ramsey, 1989). Rather than emphasizing treatment research that conceptualizes these problems as a disorder endogenous to the child, a child's treatment needs could be considered within his or her context (Sroufe, 1997).

A developmental model allows researchers and clinicians to identify maladaptive behaviors that are not necessarily pathological in themselves but increase an individual's risk for serious psychopathology. Using normal developmental accomplishments as a guide, it is possible to identify children who fail at important developmental milestones. Such an approach may bring more success to the commonly pessimistic prognosis of therapeutic intervention for personality-disordered individuals.

Future Directions

Throughout the chapter, we have attempted to describe how several risk factors and vulnerability processes within different domains of developmental psychology might serve as fruitful avenues for the study of the antecedents of personality disorders. Longitudinal studies are necessary to test whether these processes in childhood predispose an individual to the later development of a personality disorder and whether these hypothesized precursors differentially predict the personality disorders as conceptualized in DSM. In addition to pointing toward the benefits of longitudinal research, the developmental psychopathology perspective adopted in this chapter has implications for the type of research that is conducted. A developmental approach would call for research that begins before the onset of a disorder. Despite similar symptom expression (and similar diagnostic label), two individuals may have arrived at the disorder from different pathways. This information may shed light on heterogeneity within a particular disorder. For example, these individuals may have different prognoses or may be amenable to different types of treatment given their developmental history (Sroufe, 1997).

Future researchers should also consider normal developmental processes in their hypotheses and models of psychopathology. By studying the development of normal emotion regulation, strivings for perfection, sense of self, and other processes, researchers will better be able to identify when these processes are aberrant and indicative of increased risk for pathology. Throughout the chapter we examined childhood behaviors that were functionally or conceptually similar to symptoms of adult personality disorders. The developmental psychopathology perspective, however, reminds researchers that childhood symptoms need not be phenotypically similar to adult behaviors; rather, the hypothesized links between childhood and adult problems should appear logical given what is known about normal development. For example, aggressive behavior in a preschool boy may not predict adult aggression because such behavior is more typical at this age. Similarly, apparently dependent behavior during toddlerhood is considered a healthy, developmentally appropriate behavior associated with future *in*dependence rather than pathological dependency. Thus, researchers should not limit their search for vulnerability factors by searching for childhood symptoms that are identical to adult symptoms of disorder. Rather, researchers should strive to examine general patterns of adaptation in important developmental periods in order to identify childhood predictors of adult disorders that may appear, on the surface, to be quite distinct patterns of behavior (Sroufe & Rutter, 1984).

Further, attention should be paid to normative personality processes during childhood. The difficulty in finding empirical research on childhood antecedents of personality disorders is understandable given the lack of agreement concerning what constitutes normal personality development in children and how it should be measured. Grove and Tellegen (1991) suggest that the classification problems of the personality disorders may be partially addressed by considering the research on normal personality. They draw parallels between factor models of normal personality and personality disorder clusters in DSM. Further, by examining normal personality dimensions, they speculate that it would be possible to determine to what extent personality disorders represent problematic interactions among normal personality traits.

In addition, research should address how various risk and protective factors influence each other to produce an outcome rather than studying any hypothesized variable in isolation (Masten, 1999). As mentioned earlier, not only do the social, cognitive, biological, and emotional systems influence each other, but each of these systems is developing within an environmental context that plays an important role in the vulnerability process. Perhaps this attention to vulnerability processes within a particular context, as opposed to an emphasis on isolated risk factors, might pave the way for answering questions of specificity, for example, how a pattern of distant/avoidant relationships during childhood may play a role in the development of schizoid personality disorder for one individual and avoidant personality disorder for another. The answer may lie in how a particular risk factor interacts with other risk and protective factors within a given context. Although such a comprehensive approach to identifying the numerous variables and processes playing a role in the development of a particular disorder may appear daunting, by examining basic patterns of maladaptation within essential developmental tasks, patterns may appear that reliably predict psychopathology (Sroufe & Rutter, 1984). Further, new data-analytic techniques have been developed to examine pathways of individuals by identifying both common and infrequent patterns in complex data sets (Bergman & Magnusson, 1997).

Researchers, however, may be called on to address another challenging issue. Perhaps reliable antecedent processes will not be predictive of one particular personality disorder versus another because these disorders do not represent coherent syndromes. As discussed previously, the current personality disorder taxonomy is problematic as demonstrated by its low discriminant validity, the high rates of comorbidity, and insufficient coverage of general personality pathology. Sroufe (1997) challenges researchers to consider "classification schemes centered on patterns of adaptation and developmental trajectories" (p. 257) rather than using diagnoses as a "starting point for studying problem behaviors over time" (p. 255).

ACKNOWLEDGMENTS

Preparation of this chapter was supported by an Eva O. Miller Graduate Fellowship to Tasha C. Geiger and a FIRST award from the National Institute of Mental Health (No. MH53524) and a Faculty Scholars Award from the William T. Grant Foundation to Nicki R. Crick.

REFERENCES

American Psychiatric Association. (1987). *Diagnostic and statistical manual of mental disorders* (3rd ed., rev.). Washington, DC: Author.

American Psychiatric Association. (1994). *Diagnostic and statistical manual of mental disorders* (4th ed.). Washington, DC: Author.

Arnett, J. J. (1999). Adolescent storm and stress, reconsidered. *American Psychologist, 54,* 317–326.

Attie, I., & Brooks-Gunn, J. (1995). The development of eating regulation across the life span. In D. Cicchetti & D. J. Cohen (Eds.), *Developmental psychopathology: Risk, disorder, and adaptation* (Vol. 2, pp. 332–368). New York: Wiley.

Becker, D. F., Grilo, C. M., Morey, L. C., Walker, M. L., Edell, W. S., & McGlashan, T. H. (1999). Applicability of personality disorder criteria to hospitalized adolescents: Evaluation of internal consistency and criterion overlap. *Journal of the American Academy of Child and Adolescent Psychiatry, 38,* 200–205.

Bentall, R. P. (1990). The illusion of reality: A review and integration of psychological research on hallucinations. *Psychological Bulletin, 107,* 82–95.

Bergman, L. A., & Magnusson, D. (1997). A person-oriented approach in research on developmental psychopathology. *Development and Psychopathology, 9,* 291–319.

Bernstein, D. P., Cohen, P., Skodol, A., Bezirganian, S., & Brook, J. S. (1996). Childhood antecedents of adolescent personality disorders. *American Journal of Psychiatry, 153,* 907–913.

Bernstein, D. P., Cohen, P., Velez, C. N., Schwab-Stone, M., Siever, L. J., & Shinsato, L. (1993). Prevalence and stability of the DSM-III-R personality disorders in a community-based survey of adolescents. *American Journal of Psychiatry, 150,* 1237–1243.

Brent, D. A., Zelenak, J. P., Bukstein, O., & Brown, R. V. (1990). Reliability and validity of the structured interview for personality disorders in adolescents. *Journal of the American Academy of Child and Adolescent Psychiatry, 29,* 349–354.

Briere, J., & Runtz, M. (1988). Symptomatology associated with childhood sexual victimization in a non-clinical adult sample. *Child Abuse and Neglect, 12,* 51–59.

Butcher, J. N., & Rouse, S. V. (1996). Personality: Individual differences and clinical assessment. *Annual Review of Psychology, 47,* 87–111.

Caplan, R., Foy, J. G., Asarnow, R. F., & Sherman, T. (1990). Information-processing deficits of schizophrenic children with formal thought disorder. *Psychiatry Research, 31,* 169–177.

Caspi, A. (1998). Personality development across the life course. In W. Damon (Series Ed.) & N. Eisenberg (Vol. Ed.), *Handbook of child psychology: Vol. 3. Social, emotional, and personality development* (5th ed., pp. 311–388). New York: Wiley.

Cassidy, J. (1988). Child–mother attachment and the self at age six. *Child Development, 57,* 331–337.

Ceci, S. J., & Huffman, M. L. C. (1997). How suggestible are preschool children?

Cognitive and social factors. *Journal of the American Academy of Child and Adolescent Psychology, 36,* 948–958.

Chu, J. A., & Dill, D. L. (1990). Dissociative symptoms in relation to childhood physical and sexual abuse. *American Journal of Psychiatry, 147,* 887–892.

Cicchetti, D., & Cohen, D. J. (1995). Perspectives on developmental psychopathology. In D. Cicchetti & D. J. Cohen (Eds.), *Developmental psychopathology: Theory and methods* (Vol. 1, pp. 3–20). New York: Wiley.

Cicchetti, D., & Olsen, K. (1990). Borderline disorders in childhood. In M. Lewis & S. M. Miller (Eds.), *Handbook of developmental psychopathology* (pp. 355–370). New York: Plenum.

Cicchetti, D., & Toth, S. L. (1995). Developmental psychopathology and disorders of affect. In D. Cicchetti & D. J. Cohen (Eds.), *Developmental psychopathology: Risk, disorder, and adaptation* (Vol. 2, pp. 369–420). New York: Wiley.

Cohen, P. (1996). Childhood risks for young adult symptoms of personality disorder: Method and substance. *Multivariate Behavioral Research, 31,* 121–148.

Coie, J. D., & Dodge, K. A. (1998). Aggression and antisocial behavior. In W. Damon (Series Ed.) & N. Eisenberg (Vol. Ed.), *Handbook of child psychology: Vol. 3. Social, emotional, and personality development* (5th ed., pp. 779–862). New York: Wiley.

Coolidge, F. L., Philbrick, P. B., Wooley, M. J., Bunting, E., Hyman, J. N., & Stager, M. A. (1990). The KCATI: Development of an inventory for the assessment of personality disorders in children. *Journal of Personality and Clinical Studies, 6,* 225–232.

Costello, C. G. (Ed.). (1996). *Personality characteristics of the personality disordered.* New York: Wiley.

Crain, R. M. (1996). The influences of age, race, and gender on child and adolescent multidimensional self-concept. In B.A. Bracken (Ed.), *Handbook of self-concept* (pp. 395–420). New York: Wiley.

Crick, N. R. (1995). Relational aggression: The role of intent attributions, feelings of distress, and provocation type. *Development and Psychopathology, 7,* 313–322.

Crick, N. R., & Grotpeter, J. K. (1995). Relational aggression, physical aggression, and social-psychological aggression. *Child Development, 66,* 710–722.

Crick, N. R., Grotpeter, J. K., & Bigbee, M. A. (1998). *Relationally and physically aggressive children's intent attributions and feelings of distress for relational and instrumental peer provocations.* Manuscript submitted for publication.

Crick, N. R., Werner, N. E., Casas, J. F., O'Brien, K. M., Nelson, D. A., Grotpeter, J. K., & Markon, K. (1999). Childhood aggression and gender: A new look at an old problem. In R. A. Dienstbier (Series Ed.) & D. Bernstein (Vol. Ed.), *Nebraska Symposium on Motivation: Vol. 45. Gender and motivation* (pp. 75–141). Lincoln: University of Nebraska Press.

Crick, N. R., Werner, N. E., & Rockhill, C. M. (1999). *Childhood aggression and borderline personality features.* Manuscript submitted for publication.

Daley, S. E., Hammen, C., Burge, D., Davila, J., Paley, B., Lindberg, N., & Herzberg, M. A. (1999). Depression and axis II symptomatology in an adolescent community sample: Concurrent and longitudinal associations. *Journal of Personality Disorders, 13,* 47–59.

Davidson, R. J. (1991). Cerebral asymmetry and affective disorders: A developmental perspective. In D. Cicchetti & S. Toth (Eds.), *Internalizing and externalizing expressions of dysfunction* (pp. 123–154). Hillsdale, NJ: Erlbaum.

Dawson, G., Hessl, D., & Frey, K. (1994). Social influences on early developing biological and behavioral systems related to risk for affective disorder. *Development and Psychopathology, 6,* 759–779.

Dienstbier, R. A. (1984). The role of emotion in moral socialization. In C. Izard, J. Kagan, & R. B. Zajonc (Eds.), *Emotions, cognitions, and behaviors* (pp. 484–513). New York: Cambridge University Press.

Dishion, T. J., French, D. C., & Patterson, G. R. (1995). The development and ecology of antisocial behavior. In D. Cicchetti & D. J. Cohen (Eds.), *Developmental psychopathology: Risk, disorder, and adaptation* (Vol. 2, pp. 421–471). New York: Wiley.

Dodge, K. A. (1993). Social–cognitive mechanisms in the development of conduct disorder and depression. *Annual Review of Psychology, 44,* 559–584.

Dodge, K. A., & Coie, J. D. (1987). Social information-processing factors in reactive and proactive aggression in children's peer groups. *Journal of Personality and Social Psychology, 53,* 1146–1158.

Dodge, K. A., & Crick, N. R. (1990). Social information-processing bases of aggressive behavior in children. *Personality and Social Psychology Bulletin, 16,* 8–22.

Dodge, K. A., & Newman, J. P. (1981). Biased decision-making processes in aggressive boys. *Journal of Abnormal Psychology, 90,* 375–379.

Eisenberg, N., & Fabes, R. A. (1998). Prosocial development. In W. Damon (Series Ed.), & N. Eisenberg (Vol. Ed.), *Handbook of child psychology: Vol. 3. Social, emotional, and personality development* (5th ed., pp. 701–778). New York: Wiley.

Eisenberg, N., Fabes, R. A., Bernzweig, J., Karbon, M., Poulin, R., & Hanish, L. (1993). The relations of emotionality and regulation to preschoolers' social skills and sociometric status. *Child Development, 64,* 1418–1438.

Eisenberg, N., Fabes, R. A., Murphy, B., Maszk, P., Smith, M., & Karbon, M. (1995). The role of emotionality and regulation in children's social functioning: A longitudinal study. *Child Development, 66,* 1360–1384.

Eisenberg, N., Wentzel, M., & Harris, J. D. (1998). The role of emotionality and regulation in empathy-related responding. *School Psychology Review, 27,* 506–521.

Elkind, D. (1967). Egocentrism in adolescence. *Child Development, 38,* 1025–1034.

Feldman, S. S., & Weinberger, D. A. (1994). Self-restraint as a mediator of family influences on boys' delinquent behavior: A longitudinal study. *Child Development, 65,* 195–211.

First, M. B., Spitzer, R. L., Gibbon, M., & Williams, J. B. W. (1995). The Structured Clinical Interview for DSM-III-R personality disorders (SCID-II): Part I. Description. *Journal of Personality Disorders, 9,* 83–91.

Fischer, K. W. (1980). A theory of cognitive development: The control and construction of hierarchies of skills. *Psychological Review, 87,* 477–531.

Fischer, K. W., & Ayoub, C. (1994). Affective splitting and dissociation in normal and maltreated children: Developmental pathways for self in relationships. In D. Cicchetti, S. L. Toth, (Eds.), *Rochester Symposium on Developmental*

Psychopathology: Vol. 5. Disorders and dysfunctions of the self. (pp. 149–222). Rochester, NY: University of Rochester Press.

Fish, B. (1977). Neurobiologic antecedents of schizophrenia in children. Evidence for an inherited, congenital neurointegrative defect. *Archives of General Psychiatry, 34,* 1297–1313.

Gillberg, C., & Rastam, M. (1992). Do some cases of anorexia nervosa reflect underlying autistic-like conditions? *Behavioural Neurology, 5,* 27–32.

Gilligan, C. (1982). *In a different voice: Psychological theory and women's development.* Cambridge, MA: Harvard University Press.

Goldsmith, H. G., Buss, A. H., Plomin, R., Rothbart, M. K., Thomas, A., Chess, S., Hinde, R. A., & McCall, R. B. (1987). What is temperament? Four approaches. *Child Development, 58,* 505–529.

Gray, J. A. (1982). *The neuropsychology of anxiety: An inquiry into the functions of the septo-hypocampal system.* New York: Clarendon Press.

Grilo, C. M., Becker, D. F., Fehon, D. C., Walker, M. L., Edell, W. S., & McGlashan, T. H. (1996). Gender differences in personality disorders in psychiatrically hospitalized adolescents. *American Journal of Psychiatry, 153,* 1089–1091.

Grotpeter, J. K., & Crick, N. R. (1996). Relational aggression, physical aggression, and friendship. *Child Development, 67,* 2328–2338.

Grove, W. M., Lebow, B. S., Clementz, B. A., Cerri, A., Medus, C., & Iaocono, W. G. (1991). Familial prevalence and coaggregation of schizotypy indicators: A multitrait family study. *Journal of Abnormal Psychology, 100,* 115–121.

Grove, W. M., & Tellegen, A. (1991). Problems in the classification of personality disorders. *Journal of Personality Disorders, 5,* 31–41.

Harrist, A. W., Zaia, A. F., Bates, J. E., Dodge, K. A., & Pettit, G. S. (1997). Subtypes of social withdrawal in early childhood: Sociometric status and social–cognitive differences across four years. *Child Development, 68,* 278–294.

Harter, S. (1982). The perceived competence scale for children. *Child Development, 53,* 87–97.

Harter, S. (1986). Cognitive–developmental processes in the integration of concepts about emotions and the self. *Social Cognition, 4*(2), 119–151.

Harter, S. (1990). Self and identity development. In S. S. Feldman & G. R. Elliot (Eds.), *At the threshold: The developing adolescent* (pp. 352–387). Cambridge, MA: Harvard University Press.

Harter, S. (1998). The development of self-representations. In W. Damon (Series Ed.) & N. Eisenberg (Vol. Ed.), *Handbook of child psychology: Vol. 3. Social, emotional, and personality development* (5th ed., pp. 553–617). New York: Wiley.

Harter, S., & Monsour, A. (1992). Developmental analysis of conflict caused by opposing attributes in the adolescent self-portrait. *Developmental Psychology, 28,* 251–260.

Hartup, W. W., & van Lieshout, C. F. M. (1995). Personality development in social context. *Annual Review of Psychology, 46,* 655–687.

Heindselman, T. L., Wingenfeld, S. A., & Smith, D. W. (1999, April). *A preliminary examination of the reliability and validity of the Personality Inventory for Children Preschool Version (PICP).* Poster session presented at the biennial meeting of the Society for Research in Child Development, Albuquerque, NM.

Higgins, E.T. (1991). Development of self-regulatory and self-evaluative processes: Costs, benefits, and tradeoffs. In M. R. Gunnar & L. A. Sroufe (Eds.), *Minnesota Symposia on Child Development: Vol. 23. Self processes and development* (pp. 125–166). Hillsdale, NJ: Erlbaum.

Hinshaw, S. P. (1987). On the distinction between attentional deficits/hyperactivity and conduct problems/aggression in child psychopathology. *Psychological Bulletin, 101,* 443–463.

Hinshaw, S. P., & Simmel, C. (1994). Attention-deficit hyperactivity disorder. In M. Hersen, R.T. Ammerman, & L.A. Sisson (Eds.), *Handbook of aggressive and destructive behavior in psychiatric patients* (pp. 339–354). New York: Plenum.

Hyler, S. E., Rieder, R. D., Williams, J. B. W., Spitzer, R. L., Hendler, J., & Lyons, M. (1988). The Personality Diagnostic Questionnaire: Development and preliminary results. *Journal of Personality Disorders, 2,* 229–237.

Irwin, H. J. (1994). Proneness to dissociation and traumatic childhood events. *Journal of Nervous and Mental Disease, 182,* 456–460.

Kagan, J. (1992). Behavior, biology, and the meaning of temperamental constructs. *Pediatrics, 90,* 510–513.

Kagan, J., Reznick, J. S., & Snidman, N. (1988). Biological bases of childhood shyness. *Science, 240,* 167–171.

Kagan, J., & Snidman, N. (1991). Temperamental factors in human development. *American Psychologist, 46,* 856–862.

Kernberg, P. F. (1989). Narcissistic personality disorder in childhood. *Psychiatric Clinics of North America, 12,* 671–694.

Knoff, H. M. (Ed.). (1986). *The assessment of child and adolescent personality.* New York: Guilford Press.

Kochanska, G. (1993). Toward a synthesis of parental socialization and child temperament in early development of conscience. *Child Development, 64,* 325–347.

Kochanska, G. (1995). Children's temperament, mother's discipline, and security of attachment; Multiple pathways to emerging internalization. *Child Development, 66,* 597–615.

Korenblum, M., Marton, P., Golombek, H., & Stein, B. (1990). Personality status: Changes through adolescence. *Psychiatric Clinics of North America, 13,* 389–399.

Lachar, D., & Wirt, R.D. (1981). A data-based analysis of the psychometric performance of the Personality Inventory for Children (PIC): An alternative to the Achenbach review. *Journal of Personality Assessment, 45,* 614–616.

Ladd, G.W., Lange, G., & Stremmel, A. (1983). Personal and situational influences on children's helping behavior: Factors that mediate compliant helping. *Child Development, 54,* 488–501.

Lahey, B.B., & Loeber, R. (1997). Attention-deficit/hyperactivity disorder, oppositional defiant disorder, conduct disorder, and adult antisocial behavior: A life span perspective. In D. M. Stoff, J. Breiling, & J. D. Maser (Eds.), *Handbook of antisocial behavior* (pp. 51–59). New York: Wiley.

Lapsley, D. K., & Rice, K. (1988). The "New Look" at the imaginary audience and personal fable: Toward a general model of adolescent ego development. In D. K. Lapsley & F. C. Power (Eds.), *Self, ego, and identity: Integrative approaches* (pp. 109–129). New York: Springer-Verlag.

Lewine, R. R. J., Watt, N. F., Prentky, R. A., & Fryer, J. H. (1980). Childhood social competence in functionally disordered psychiatric patients and in normals. *Journal of Abnormal Psychology, 89,* 132–138.

Lewinsohn, P. M., Rohde, P., Seeley, J. R., & Klein, D. N. (1997). Axis II psychopathology as a function of Axis I disorders in childhood and adolescence. *Journal of the American Academy of Child and Adolescent Psychiatry, 36,* 1752–1759.

Liotti, G. (1992). Disorganized/disoriented attachment in the etiology of the dissociative disorders. *Dissociation, 4,* 196–204.

Lofgren, D. P., Bemporad, J., King, J., Lindem, K., & O'Driscoll, G. (1991). A prospective follow-up study of so-called borderline children. *American Journal of Psychiatry, 148,* 1541–1547.

Loranger, A. W. (1988). *Personality Disorder Examination (PDE) manual.* Yonkers, NY: DV Communications.

Loranger, A. W. (1996). Dependent personality disorder: Age, sex, and Axis I comorbidity. *Journal of Nervous and Mental Disease, 184,* 17–21.

Main, M., & Hesse, E. (1990). Parents' unresolved traumatic experiences are related to infant disorganized attachment status: Is frightened and/or frightening behavior the linking mechanism? In M. T. Greenberg, D. Cicchetti, & E. M. Cummings (Eds.), *Attachment in the preschool years: Theory, research, and intervention* (pp. 161–182). Chicago: University of Chicago Press.

Marsh, H. W. (1989). Age and sex effects in multiple dimensions of self-concept: Preadolescence to early adulthood. *Journal of Educational Psychology, 81,* 417–430.

Martin, R. P. (1988). *Assessment of personality and behavior problems: Infancy through adolescence.* New York: Guilford Press.

Masten, A. S. (1999). Resilience comes of age: Reflections on the past and outlook for the next generation of research. In M. D. Glantz, J. Johnson, & L. Huffman (Eds.), *Resilience and development: Positive life adaptations* (pp. 282–296). New York: Plenum.

Masten, A. S., & Coatsworth, J. D. (1998). The development of competence in favorable and unfavorable environments: Lessons from research on successful children. *American Psychologist, 53,* 205–220.

Mattanah, J. J. F., Becker, D. F., Levy, K. N., Edell, W. S., & McGlashan, T. H. (1995). Diagnostic stability in adolescents followed up two years after hospitalization. *American Journal of Psychiatry, 152,* 889–894.

Maughan, B., Gray, G., & Rutter, M. (1985). Reading retardation and antisocial behavior: A follow-up in employment. *Journal of Child Psychology and Psychiatry, 26,* 741–758.

McDavid, J. D., & Pilkonis, P. A. (1996). The stability of personality disorder diagnoses. *Journal of Personality Disorders, 10,* 1–15.

McDermott, P. A. (1996). A nationwide study of developmental and gender prevalence for psychopathology in childhood and adolescence. *Journal of Abnormal Child Psychology, 24,* 53–66.

Millon, T. (1994). *Manual for the Millon Clinical Multiaxial Inventory—III.* Minneapolis, MN: National Computer Systems.

Millon, T., & Davis, R. D. (1995). The development of personality disorders. In D. Cicchetti & D. J. Cohen (Eds.), *Developmental psychopathology: Risk, disorder, and adaptation* (Vol. 2, pp. 633–676). New York: Wiley.

Moffitt, T. E. (1993). Adolescence-limited and life-course persistent antisocial behavior: A developmental taxonomy. *Psychological Review, 100,* 674–701.

Morales, J. R., & Crick, N. R. (1999). *Hostile attribution and aggression in adolescents' peer and romantic relationships.* Poster session presented at the biennial meeting of the Society for Research in Child Development, Albuquerque, NM.

Morales, J. R., & Cullerton-Sen, C. (2000, March). *Relational and physical aggression and psychological adjustment in adolescent peer and romantic relationships.* Poster presented at the biennial meeting of the Society for Research in Adolescence, Chicago.

Nelson, D. A., & Crick, N. R. (1999). Rose-colored glasses: Examining the social information-processing of prosocial young adolescents. *Journal of Early Adolescence, 19,* 17–38.

Norman, R. M. G., Davies, F., Nicholson, I. R., Cortese, L., & Malla, A. K. (1998). The relationship of two aspects of perfectionism with symptoms in a psychiatric outpatient population. *Journal of Social and Clinical Psychology, 17,* 50–68.

Ogawa, J. R., Sroufe, L. A., Weinfield, N. S., Carlson, E. B., & Egeland, B. (1997). Development and the fragmented self: Longitudinal study of dissociative symptomatology in a nonclinical sample. *Development and Psychopathology, 4,* 855–879.

Oldham, J. M., Skodol, A. E., Kellman, H. D., Hyler, S. E., Rosnick, L., & Davies, M. (1992). Diagnosis of DSM-III-R personality disorders by two structured interviews: Patterns of comorbidity. *American Journal of Psychiatry, 149,* 213–220.

Olin, S. S., Raine, A., Cannon, T. D., Parnas, J., Schulsinger, F., & Mednick, S. A. (1997). Childhood behavior precursors of schizotypal personality disorder. *Schizophrenia Bulletin, 23,* 93–103.

Parker, J. & Asher, S. R. (1987). Peer acceptance and later personal adjustment: Are low-accepted children at risk? *Psychological Bulletin, 102,* 357–389.

Parnas, J., & Jorgensen, A. (1989). Pre-morbid psychopathology in schizophrenia spectrum. *British Journal of Psychiatry, 155,* 623–627.

Parnas, J., Schulsinger, F., Schulsinger, H., Mednick, S., & Teasdale, T. (1982). Behavioral precursors of schizophrenia spectrum. *Archives of General Psychiatry, 39,* 658–664.

Patrick, C. J., Bradley, M., & Lang, P. J. (1993). Emotion in the criminal psychopath: Startle reflex modulation. *Journal of Abnormal Psychology, 102,* 82–92.

Patrick, C. J., Cuthbert, B. N., & Lang, P. J. (1994). Emotion in the criminal psychopath: Fear imagery processing. *Journal of Abnormal Psychology, 103,* 523–534.

Patterson, G., DeBaryshe, B., & Ramsey, E. (1989). A developmental perspective on antisocial behavior. *American Psychologist, 44,* 329–335.

Pinto, A., Grapentine, W. L., Francis, G., & Picariello, C. M. (1996). Borderline personality disorder in adolescents: Affective and cognitive features. *Journal of the American Academy of Child and Adolescent Psychiatry, 35,* 1338–1343.

Pollak, J. (1987). Relationship of obsessive–compulsive personality to obsessive–compulsive disorder: A review of the literature. *Journal of Psychology, 121,* 137–148.

Putnam, F. W. (1994). Dissociation and disturbances of the self. In D. Cicchetti & S. L. Toth (Eds.), *Rochester Symposium on Developmental Psychopathology: Vol. 5. Disorders and dysfunctions of the self.* (pp. 251–265). Rochester, NY: University of Rochester Press.

Quay, H. C. (1993). The psychobiology of undersocialized aggressive conduct disorder: A theoretical perspective. *Development and Psychopathology, 5,* 165–180.

Renken, B., Egeland, B., Marvinney, D., Sroufe, L. A., & Mangelsdorf, S. (1989). Early childhood antecedents of aggression and passive withdrawal in early elementary school. *Journal of Personality, 57,* 257–281.

Rey, J. M., Morris-Yates, A., Singh, M., Andrews, G., & Stewart, G. W. (1995). Continuities between psychiatric disorders in adolescents and personality disorders in young adults. *American Journal of Psychiatry, 152,* 895–900.

Rubin, K. H., & Mills, R. S. L. (1988). The many faces of social isolation in childhood. *Journal of Consulting and Clinical Psychology, 56,* 916–924.

Ryglewicz, H. & Pepper, B. (1996). *Lives at risk: Understanding and treating young people with dual disorders.* New York: Free Press.

Schore, A. (1994). *Affect regulation and the origin of the self: The neurobiology of emotional development.* Hillsdale, NJ: Erlbaum.

Shell, R. M., & Eisenberg, N. (1992). A developmental model of recipients' reaction to aid. *Psychological Bulletin, 111,* 413–433.

Shiner, R. L. (1998). How shall we speak of children's personalities in middle childhood? A preliminary taxonomy. *Psychological Bulletin, 124,* 308–332.

Skodol, A. E. (1997). Classification, assessment, and differential diagnosis of personality disorders. *Journal of Practical Psychiatry and Behavioral Health, 3,* 261–274.

Slade, P. D., & Bentall, R. P. (1988). *Sensory deception: A scientific analysis of hallucination.* Baltimore: Johns Hopkins University Press.

Sroufe, L. A. (1990). An organizational perspective on the self. In D. Cicchetti & M. Beeghly (Eds.), *The self in transition: Infancy to childhood* (pp. 281–307). Chicago: University of Chicago Press.

Sroufe, L. A. (1996). *Emotional development: The organization of emotional life in the early years.* New York: Cambridge University Press.

Sroufe, L. A. (1997). Psychopathology as an outcome of development. *Development and Psychopathology, 9,* 251–268.

Sroufe, L. A., & Rutter, M. (1984). The domain of developmental psychopathology. *Child Development, 55,* 17–29.

Sroufe, L. A., & Waters, E. (1977). Attachment as an organizational construct. *Child Development, 48,* 1184–1199.

Thomsen, P. H. (1996). Borderline conditions in childhood: A register-based follow-up study over a 22-year period. *Psychopathology, 29,* 357–362.

Thomsen, P. H., & Mikkelsen, H. U. (1993). Development of personality disorders in children and adolescents with obsessive–compulsive disorder: A 6- to 22-year follow-up study. *Acta Psychiatrica Scandinavica, 87,* 456–462.

van den Boom, D. C., & Hoeksma, J. B. (1994). The effect of infant irritability on mother–infant interaction: A growth-curve analysis. *Developmental Psychology, 30,* 581–590.

van Praag, H. M. (1996). Comorbidity (psycho) analysed. *British Journal of Psychiatry, 168,* 129–134.

Volkmar, F. R., Becker, D. F., King, R. A., & McGlashan, T. H. (1995). Psychotic processes. In D. Cicchetti & D. J. Cohen (Eds.), *Developmental psychopathology: Risk, disorder, and adaptation* (Vol. 2, pp. 512–534). New York: Wiley.

Wade, D., Kyrios, M., & Henry, J. (1998). A model of obsessive–compulsive phenomena in a nonclinical sample. *Australian Journal of Psychology, 50,* 11–17.

Walker, E. F., Grimes, K. E., Davis, D. M., & Smith, A. J. (1993). Childhood precursors of schizophrenia: Facial expressions of emotion. *American Journal of Psychiatry, 150,* 1654–1660.

Walker, E. F., & Lewine, R J. (1990). Prediction of adult-onset schizophrenia from childhood home movies of the patients. *American Journal of Psychiatry, 147,* 1052–1056.

Waller, N., Putnam, F. W., & Carlson, E. B. (1996). Types of dissociation and dissociative types: A taxometric analysis of dissociative experiences. *Psychological Methods, 1,* 300–321.

Weiss, B., Dodge, K. A., Bates, J. E., & Pettit, G. S. (1992). Some consequences of early harsh discipline: Child aggression and a maladaptive social information processing style. *Child Development, 63,* 1321–1335.

Werner, N. E., & Crick, N. R. (1999). Relational aggression and social–psychological adjustment in a college sample. *Journal of Abnormal Psychology, 108,* 615–623.

Westen, D. (1997). Divergence between clinical and research methods for assessing personality disorders: Implications for research and the evolution of Axis II. *American Journal of Psychiatry, 154,* 895–903.

Westen, D., & Arkowitz-Westen, L. (1998). Limitations of Axis II in diagnosing personality pathology in clinical practice. *American Journal of Psychiatry, 155,* 1767–1771.

Widiger, T. A., & Rogers, J. H. (1989). Prevalence and comorbidity of personality disorders. *Psychiatric Annuals, 19,* 132–136.

Wolff, S., & Chick, J. (1980). Schizoid personality in childhood: A controlled follow-up study. *Psychological Medicine, 10,* 85–100.

Zimmerman, M. (1994). Diagnosing personality disorders: A review of issues and research methods. *Archives of General Psychiatry, 51,* 225–245.

Part III

CLINICAL SYNDROMES

SUBSTANCE USE
DISORDERS

5

Vulnerability to Substance Use Disorders in Childhood and Adolescence

LAURIE CHASSIN
JENNIFER RITTER

Although substance use disorders are not typically diagnosed until late adolescence or early adulthood, they have been referred to as "developmental" disorders because of their predictable antecedents in childhood and early adolescence (Tarter & Vanyukov, 1994). The category of substance use disorders includes both substance abuse (a maladaptive pattern of use involving negative consequences to the individual) and substance dependence (a maladaptive pattern of use marked by psychological or physical dependence such as tolerance to drug effects and withdrawal symptoms when drug use is discontinued; American Psychiatric Association, 1994). However, such actual clinical diagnoses are rarely studied in childhood or early adolescence because they are rarely seen in these young populations. Instead, most research in childhood and early adolescence focuses on the initiation of substance use, with some studies examining the development of heavy substance use and substance use–related problems in older adolescents.

Developmentally, substance use initiation occurs in early adolescence. Substance use typically begins with use of the so-called gateway drugs such as alcohol and cigarettes (Kandel, 1975). Both alcohol and cigarette use show peak initiation rates in sixth to ninth grades (Johnston, O'Malley, & Bachman, 1998). The use of illegal drugs begins somewhat later, with peak initiation rates for marijuana use reported in grades 9–11 and for other illegal drugs in grades 10–12 (Johnston et al., 1998). By the end of the high school years, substantial numbers of adolescents report some experience with substance use. For example, national data for 1998 show illegal drug use in the past month by 12% of 8th graders, 22% of 10th graders, and 26% of 12th graders. Alcohol use in the past month was reported by 23% of 8th graders, 39% of 10th graders, and 52% of 12th graders (Johnston, O'Malley, & Bachman, 1999).

Although some adolescent experimentation may be statistically normative, an early onset of alcohol and drug use itself has been reported as a risk factor for later substance abuse and dependence. Alcohol use before age 14 is associated with a greater likelihood of later alcohol diagnoses (Grant & Dawson, 1997) and illegal drug use before age 15 is associated with later drug abuse or dependence (Robins & Pryzbeck, 1985). Thus, although some experimentation with substance use in adolescence is a normative phenomenon, early onset is one risk factor for the development of clinical substance use disorders. Moreover, the quantity and frequency of substance use during adolescence may also be a risk factor. In the middle school and high school years, subgroups of adolescents escalate the extent of their use (Chassin, Curran, Hussong, & Colder, 1996; Wills, McNamara, Vaccaro, & Hirky, 1996). At least for alcohol use, escalation to high levels of consumption during adolescence is a risk factor for later alcohol-related problems (Hawkins et al., 1997; Schulenberg et al., 1996).

Late adolescence and early adulthood are marked by increases in alcohol, cigarette, and other drug use, and these years represent both the peak periods of substance use (Chen & Kandel, 1995) and the peak ages for the development of substance abuse and dependence (Anthony & Helzer, 1991). Increases in substance use in this period appear to be related to departures from the parental home, as well as the fact that individuals' living situations and social environments become less restrictive and more tolerant of substance use (Bachman, O'Malley, & Johnston, 1984; Bachman, Wadsworth, O'Malley, Johnston, & Schulenberg, 1997; Cashin, Presley, & Meilman, 1998). With the lessening of these environmental restrictions, use rates for alcohol and drug use peak in the early 20s (Bachman et al., 1997; Chen & Kandel, 1995).

However, with the assumption of adult role responsibilities associated with marriage, work, and parenthood come normative declines in the prevalence of substance use, and by the mid 20s substance use typically begins to decline (Bachman et al., 1997; Gotham, Sher, & Wood, 1997). A similar role-related decline has been reported for symptoms of alcohol abuse and dependence (Chilcoat & Breslau, 1996). Given this age-related pattern, it has been suggested that a subgroup of alcohol and drug disorders are "developmentally limited" (Zucker, Fitzgerald, & Moses, 1995) and that these individuals "mature out" of their problems with the assumption of adult roles and responsibilities.

To this point, we have emphasized patterns of alcohol and drug use rather than clinical disorders because this is the focus of most research on young populations. However, there has been some attempt to examine substance use disorders in adolescence and young adulthood as well. Available evidence suggests that patterns of alcohol and drug abuse symptoms in adolescents differ somewhat from symptom patterns found in adult substance abusers, and that criteria for substance dependence, according to the fourth edition of the *Diagnostic and Statistical Manual of Mental Disorders* (DSM-IV; American Psychiatric Association, 1994), may not adequately reflect the unique features of adolescent substance involvement. For example, Vik, Brown, and Myers (1997) argue that relative to adults, it may be difficult to detect withdrawal symptoms among adolescent substance abusers because of their limited duration of substance involvement. Indeed, evidence from adolescents hospitalized for substance abuse problems indicates that affective symptoms are the most common withdrawal symptom (Stewart & Brown, 1995). Other studies indicate that symptoms of withdrawal, tolerance, and medical complications occur infrequently among adolescent substance abusers and, instead, that alcohol-related blackouts, cravings, and risky sexual behavior are common among adolescents with substance abuse disorders (Martin, Kaczynski, Maisto, Bukstein, & Moss, 1995). Frequent polydrug use poses an additional complication in assessing symptom patterns of adolescent substance abusers. Recent evidence indicates that as many as 72% of adolescents with an alcohol dependence diagnosis use multiple substances, with the most common combinations of polydrug use being alcohol and marijuana, followed by alcohol and hallucinogens (Martin, Kaczynski, Maisto, & Tarter, 1996). Finally, the developmental status of adolescents decreases the likelihood of impairment in occupational or romantic functioning that forms part of the typical definitions of substance use disorders (Vik et al., 1997). Thus, given the nature of adolescent substance abuse disorders, DSM-IV diagnostic criteria may have some limitations when used with adolescent populations.

RESEARCH APPROACHES AND METHODOLOGICAL ISSUES

Most empirical studies of child and adolescent populations have been focused on describing drug use and its developmental trajectories, identifying correlates of drug use, and identifying prospective predictors of drug use. Most of these studies have been carried out in the general population, using longitudinal studies of school-based samples (e.g., Bentler, 1992; Chassin, Presson, Sherman, Corty, & Olshavsky, 1984; Jessor & Jessor, 1977; Kandel, Yamaguchi, & Chen, 1992; Johnston et al., 1998), although some have used community samples (see, e.g., Brook, Whiteman, Cohen, Shapiro, & Balka, 1995; Bates & Labouvie, 1997). Some of these studies have followed samples that have received preventive interventions aimed at deterring drug use (e.g., Botvin, Baker, Dusenbery, Botvin, & Diaz, 1995; Ellickson, Bell, & McGuigan, 1993; MacKinnon et al., 1991). These studies have made important contributions because they follow large samples of participants for long periods. This allows them to describe the natural history of substance use and its vulnerability factors. However, these studies also have limitations. Because they focus on drug use in the general population, their results may not always generalize to predicting clinical substance abuse/dependence outcomes. Also, because of the large samples that are involved, the assessments in these studies (particularly the school-based studies) have typically been restricted to paper-and-pencil surveys.

Another research approach has been to focus on high-risk samples, most typically on offspring of alcoholic or drug-abusing parents (Chassin et al., 1996; Chassin, Pitts, & DeLucia, 1999; Harden & Pihl, 1995; Sher, Walitzer, Wood, & Brent, 1991; Tarter, Kirisci, & Clark, 1997; Zucker, Ellis, Bingham, & Fitzgerald, 1996). These high-risk studies have been able to use more intensive methods including psychophysiological assessment (e.g., Harden & Pihl, 1995) and neuropsychological assessment (Ozkaragoz & Noble, 1995; Tarter, Jacob, & Bremer, 1989) but have been restricted to smaller samples than the school-based studies.

Finally, a smaller number of studies have focused on clinical populations of adolescents with substance use disorders (Brown, 1993a; Brown, Myers, Mott, & Vik, 1994; Martin et al., 1996). Although these are the most clinically relevant approaches, they cannot separate the antecedents of substance use disorders from the effects of those disorders. Thus, it is difficult to draw inferences about vulnerability from these studies.

For the current chapter, summarizing and interpreting the rather large body of literature on vulnerability to substance use disorders presents several problems. First, much of the child and adolescent literature is restricted to drug use rather than problem use or clinical substance use disorders. Thus, our review of vulnerability factors includes vulnerability to substance use as well as abuse/dependence. Second, vulnerability for substance use disorders includes both factors that are common across multiple drugs and factors that are drug specific. For example, children who are prone to conduct problems are at heightened risk for a range of substance use and substance use disorders. Thus, conduct problems are a common vulnerability factor for the use and abuse of different types of drugs. In contrast, other risk factors are drug specific. For example, the influence of advertising may raise risk for alcohol or cigarette use but is not a factor for illegal drugs. A single chapter cannot do justice to the complexity of substance-specific pathways of vulnerability. Accordingly, we will focus more on common vulnerabilities than on drug-specific vulnerabilities (see Sher, 1991, for an extended discussion of vulnerability to alcoholism, and Glantz & Pickens, 1992, for a discussion more specific to illegal drug use vulnerability). Finally, it is necessary to choose some operational definition of childhood and adolescence in order to focus our discussion. Given the age-related epidemiological patterns of substance use and substance use disorders, the current chapter focuses on populations from childhood up to the early 20s. This age range covers the period from normative initiation of substance use behavior to early-onset forms of substance use disorders.

PATHWAYS OF VULNERABILITY TO SUBSTANCE USE DISORDERS

Identifying pathways of vulnerability to substance use disorders is a complex undertaking. Evidence to date suggests that no single model can explain vulnerability but, rather, that multiple pathways underlie the development of substance use disorders (Cloninger, Sigvardsson, & Bohman, 1996; Institute of Medicine, 1996; Sher et al., 1991; Zucker, Boyd & Howard, 1994). One basic starting place for vulnerability research is the common observation that alcohol and drug problems "run in families." Empirical studies have shown that parental alcoholism raises risk for offspring alcoholism, although the magnitude of the risk varies from risk ratios of 2–3 in community samples to a risk ratio of 9 for severely alcohol-dependent and antisocial samples (McGue, 1994; Russell, 1990). Similarly, there is an elevated risk (as high as eight-fold) for drug disorders among relatives of probands with drug disorders (Merikangas et al., 1998).

A major challenge for vulnerability research has been to understand how this family history risk is mediated. To date, results suggest that these risk processes are biopsychosocial in nature. Both twin studies (Heath et al., 1993; Kendler & Prescott, 1998; Tsuang et al., 1996) and adoptee studies (see McGue, 1994, for a review) have concluded that there are significant genetic components to the intergenerational transmission of risk. Theorizing has suggested that this genetic risk may be mediated through personality characteristics (e.g., propensities for negative affectivity, poor self-regulation, and sensation seeking, see Sher, 1991, 1996) and/or individual differences in the pharmacological effects of substances (see, e.g., Schuckit, 1998). Evidence for environmental components of family history risk has also been produced (through either shared or nonshared environment depending on the sample and the specific drug that is studied). Moreover, effects of prenatal environments have also been demonstrated. For example, prenatal exposure to alcohol has recently been shown to raise risk for adolescent alcohol use and use-related negative consequences above and beyond a family history of alcoholism (Baer, Barr, Bookstein, Sampson, & Streissguth, 1998).

Given the complexity of these processes that consist of both genetic and environmental components, most theories of vulnerability for substance use disorders hypothesize that there are multiple pathways underlying risk, that these pathways are interrelated and interacting rather than mutually exclusive, and that these pathways are biopsychosocial in nature rather than either "genetic" or "environmental." A heuristic model of such pathways has been offered by Sher (1991) and will provide the guiding framework for the current review. Sher (1991) hypothesizes that vulnerability to substance use disorders can be described by three pathways: a deviance proneness pathway, a stress and negative affect pathway, and a pathway that focuses on substance use effects. Although Sher's model was proposed to explain the effects of familial alcoholism on vulnerability to alcoholism, the same pathways can be examined with respect to substance use disorders more broadly.

Vulnerability to Substance Use Disorders through "Deviance Proneness" and Conduct Problems

The deviance-proneness model of substance abuse (Sher, 1991) focuses on deficits in self-regulation and socialization. Ineffective parenting is hypothesized to interact with difficult temperamental, personality, and cognitive characteristics in offspring, setting off a process of school failure and emotional distress. This, in turn, increases risk for affiliation with a deviant peer network whose norms promote substance use and other forms of problem behavior. Heavy substance use is thus considered a specific manifestation of more broad-based conduct problems (Donovan & Jessor, 1985). Consistent with this conceptualization, many studies indicate that externalizing behavior and conduct problems in childhood and early adolescence are powerful predictors of substance abuse later in adolescence and in young adulthood (Chassin et al., 1999; Hawkins, Catalano, & Miller, 1992; Henry et al., 1993; Robins & Pryzbeck, 1985).

Much cross-sectional evidence indicates that temperamental and personality traits reflecting behavioral disregulation and undercontrol are associated with adolescent substance use. In two recent reviews, the adolescent temperament and personality characteristics most consistently associated with adolescent substance abuse were unconventionality, low ego control, novelty/sensation seeking, aggression, impulsivity, and an inability to delay gratification (Bates, 1993; Hawkins et al., 1992). Others have found that adolescent substance abuse is associated with greater behavioral activity and negative emotionality (Colder & Chassin, 1997; Wills, DuHamel, & Vaccaro, 1995).

Similar temperamental characteristics are longitudinally predictive of risk for substance use from childhood to adolescence and young adulthood. Longitudinal research by Block (Block, Block, & Keyes, 1988; Shedler & Block, 1990) found that adolescents who used marijuana weekly were emotionally distressed as children and characterized by impulsivity, difficulty in concentrating, difficulty in forming close relationships, and poor ego control. Caspi, Moffitt, Newman, and Silva (1996) found that 3-year-old boys described by observers as impulsive, restless, and distractible were at increased risk to be diagnosed with alcohol dependence by age 21. Lerner and Vicary (1984) found that 5-year-old children with a "difficult temperamental profile," characterized by withdrawal from novel stimulation, slow adaptability, high intensity of reactions, negative mood, and biological irregularity, were more likely than non-"difficult" children to use substances in adolescence and young adulthood. Interestingly, these temperamental and behavioral characteristics are also found more frequently among offspring of alcoholics (themselves a group at risk for substance-related problems) compared to controls (Carbonneau et al., 1998; Fitzgerald et al., 1993; Martin et al., 1994; Tarter, Alterman, & Edwards, 1985). Offspring of alcoholics who do not possess these characteristics are less likely to develop substance abuse problems (Vitaro, Dobkin, Carbonneau, & Tremblay, 1996). This suggests that one component of intergenerational transmission of substance abuse involves a temperamental style characterized by behavioral undercontrol and disregulation.

Additional evidence for deficient self-regulation among adolescents at risk for substance abuse may be found in the neuropsychology literature, particularly in studies of executive functioning. Executive functioning is defined as a higher-order cognitive construct encompassing a diverse set of abilities, including sustained attention, concentration, abstract reasoning, formulating goals, anticipating and planning, initiating purposive behavior, self-monitoring, inhibiting inappropriate behaviors and interrupting ongoing behavior to engage in more adaptive behaviors (Moffitt, 1993). Deficits in various aspects of executive functioning have been found in youth at high-risk for alcoholism as well as in conduct-disordered and substance-abusing samples. Harden and Pihl (1995) found that 12-year-old boys with multigenerational histories of paternal alcoholism performed more poorly than did controls on a battery of neuropsychological tests measuring executive functioning. Other investigators have found that sons of substance-abusing fathers show specific deficits on tasks tapping sustained attention, motor restraint, abstract reasoning, and problem solving (e.g., Atyaclar, Tarter, Kirisci, & Lu, 1999; Giancola, Moss, Martin, Kirisci, & Tarter, 1996). Overall level of executive functioning has also been found to prospectively predict increases in alcohol consumption among young adult offspring of alcoholics (Atyaclar et al., 1999; Deckel & Hesselbrock, 1996).

As indicated earlier, ineffective parenting is hypothesized to moderate the relation between deficits in self-regulation and the development of substance use problems by exacerbating the likelihood for undercontrolled children to experience school failure and affiliate with a deviant peer network. Sher (1991) did not originally specify which, if any, aspects of parenting moderated the relationship between temperament, school failure, and the development of adolescent substance use and other problem behaviors. However, other models of parenting and substance abuse have focused on aspects of parenting that include monitoring, consistency of discipline, and social support (e.g., Hawkins et al., 1992; Jacob & Leonard, 1994).

Many cross-sectional studies have found that low levels of parental monitoring, inconsistent discipline, and poor social support are associated with adolescent substance use and other externalizing behaviors (Dobkin, Charlebois, & Tremblay, 1997; Foxcroft & Lowe, 1991; Jacob & Leonard, 1994; Stice & Barrera, 1995; Wills et al., 1996). These parenting deficits are also found in alcoholic and drug-abusing families (Chassin et al., 1996; Curran & Chassin, 1996; Dishion, Patterson, & Reid, 1988; Jacob & Leonard, 1994; Moos & Billings, 1982; Zucker et al., 1996). Although these findings suggest that poor parenting may play a causal role in the development of "deviance proneness" in adolescents, it is also important to recognize that children with poor self-regulatory capacities may elicit poor parenting. Dobkin et al. (1997) found that disruptive sons of male alcoholics had poorer mother–son dyadic interactions relative to nondisruptive sons of alcoholics and controls. Other researchers (Ge et al., 1996) have found that poor parenting may be provoked by a conduct-disordered child, and that children with high-risk temperaments remain at high-risk for conduct problems despite optimal parenting (Wootton, Frick, Shelton, & Silverthorn, 1997). Parental socialization may thus be an effect, as well as a cause, of deficits in self-regulation.

Few mediational tests have been conducted to examine how offspring temperament and parenting characteristics each influence later offspring academic adjustment, peer networks, and development of substance use/abuse. However, several studies have tested particular components of the deviance-proneness model. Dishion (1990) found that the effect of parent discipline practices on male children was mediated by academic performance and antisocial behavior. Another study by Dishion and his colleagues, which also used a sample of male children, found that poor parental socialization (poor discipline and monitoring), peer rejection, and academic failure at age 10 was predictive of involvement with antisocial peers at age 12 (Dishion, Patterson, Stoolmiller, & Skinner, 1991). The effect of parental monitoring remained significant after controlling for previous levels of antisocial behavior. In our own research, we have found significant cross-sectional associations between decreased levels of parental monitoring and membership in drug-using peer groups, which in turn are proximal pathways for the initiation of drug use (Chassin, Pillow, Curran, Molina, & Barrera, 1993). A follow-up study with the same sample revealed that growth in substance use over time was related to paternal alcoholism and decreased paternal monitoring, which in turn predicted associations with drug-using peers (Chassin et al., 1996). We have also found that adolescent externalizing behavior mediates the effects of parent alcoholism on later young adult substance abuse and dependence diagnoses (Chassin et al., 1999).

Despite these findings, there are several components of the deviance-proneness pathway that are in need of future investigation. One issue concerns possible moderating effects of gender. Many of the studies cited previously are restricted to samples of male children (e.g., Dishion, 1990; Dishion et al., 1991), and those studies that include both male and female participants have found increased evidence for deviance-proneness effects in males relative to females (e.g., Caspi et al., 1996; Chassin et al, 1993, 1996; Windle, 1990). However, Crick (1996; Crick, Bigbee, & Howes, 1996) has suggested that a reliance on overt measures of antisocial behavior and aggression may underestimate the effects of conduct problems in girls, because girls may be more likely to express aggression covertly (e.g., by undermining relationships and social reputation). Accordingly, additional research concerning deviance-proneness effects in females should incorporate measures of this more covert or "relational" form of aggression.

A related issue concerns possible moderating effects of ethnicity. The concept of a "general deviance" syndrome has not been tested in different ethnic groups, and it is uncertain whether factors that influence substance abuse and delinquent behavior are equally salient across cultures (Newcomb, 1995). In addition, the development of substance abuse problems among ethnic adolescents may be influenced by culturally unique factors. For instance, Castro, Harmon, Coe, and Tafoya-Barraza (1994) hypothesize that peer influence, disrupted family systems, and level of acculturation exert unique cultural effects on the development of substance abuse problems among Hispanic adolescents. However, their theoretical model has not been empirically tested.

Several studies suggest that certain components of the deviance-proneness model may differ across ethnic groups. In a comparison of Caucasian, Hispanic, African American, and Asian American adolescents, Maddahian, Newcomb, and Bentler (1988) found that deviant behaviors posed a higher-risk for substance abuse among Hispanic youth. Sensation seeking posed less of a risk for African Americans than it did for others, whereas parental and peer substance use posed less of a risk for Asian Americans than it did for others. A similar study which compared deviance-proneness effects in Caucasian, Cuban, other Hispanic, and African American youth found that low family pride was a more prevalent risk factor for Caucasian youth than for others, and that African American youth perceived the greatest peer approval for using drugs (Vega, Zimmerman, Warheit, Apospori, & Gil, 1993). More recently, Swaim, Bates, and Chavez (1998) used structural equation modeling to examine the effects of peer influence, family sanctions, and school adjustment on polydrug use among a sample of Hispanic and Caucasian school dropouts. They found that peer influence exerted direct effects on substance abuse for both ethnic groups. However, school adjustment exerted a buffering effect against association with drug-using peers for Caucasian but not Hispanic youth, suggesting that the interrelatedness between various forms of deviance may be stronger for Hispanic youth than for Caucasian youth. Additional work that tests mediational models of deviance proneness in different ethnic groups is needed.

Another issue concerns the developmental significance of deviance-proneness effects. As we have previously noted, externalizing behaviors in childhood are powerful predictors of early-onset substance use (e.g., Hawkins et al., 1992), thus suggesting that certain symptoms of deviance proneness may be observed before the onset of alcohol use. Other studies have found cross-sectional associations between adolescent substance use and other problem behaviors beginning as early as seventh grade (Donovan & Jessor, 1985). Rates of substance use as well as symptoms of alcohol abuse and dependence peak in late adolescence and then decline with the assumption of adult role responsibilities (Bachman et al., 1997; Chilcoat & Breslau, 1996). This same pattern has also been found for conduct problems (Moffitt, 1993). These findings suggest that some of the deviance-proneness effects may be developmentally limited. Indeed, Newcomb and McGee (1991) found that covariation among a diverse range of adolescent problem behaviors (e.g., licit and illicit drug use, precocious sexual behavior, criminal behavior, low religiosity, and negative attitudes toward law abidance) decreased over time, suggesting that the concept of general deviance may not hold from adolescence into young adulthood. However, longitudinal studies that examine risk for substance abuse and conduct-related problems from adolescence to adulthood are needed to more fully illuminate this issue.

Vulnerability to Substance Use Disorders through Negative Affect Pathways

Negative affect regulation pathways of vulnerability hypothesize that substance use/abuse is caused by a motive to regulate negative affect. Individuals who are at risk for substance use/abuse are those who are either temperamentally prone to experience negative affectivity (e.g., high in neuroticism, and/or low in stress resilience) and/or those who experience high levels of environmental stress that produce a negative affective state (Cooper, Frone, Russell, & Muldar, 1995; Sher, 1991). Interestingly, children of alcoholics, who are at high risk for substance abuse/dependence, are also reported to experience high levels of environmental stress and negative affectivity (Chassin et al., 1993; Roosa, Beals, Sandler, & Pillow, 1990). Thus, the stress and negative affect pathway hypothesizes that substance use serves a self-medicating function, helping individuals cope with negative affective states.

There is substantial cross-sectional evidence that negative affectivity is related to substance use and substance use–related problems in adolescence. A cluster of adolescent alcoholics who are high in negative affectivity has been identified in clinical samples (Mezzich et al., 1993), and depression is comorbid with adolescent drug abuse (Deykin, Buka, & Zeena, 1992), with heavy alcohol use in adolescence (Rohde, Lewinsohn, & Seeley, 1996), and with nicotine dependence in adolescence (Fergusson, Lynskey, & Horwood, 1996). Negative life stress events have also been repeatedly found to correlate with higher levels of adolescent substance use (Castro, Mahaddian, Newcomb, & Bentler, 1987; Newcomb & Harlow, 1986; Wills, Vaccaro, & McNamara, 1992). Moreover, consistent with a negative affect pathway,

Cooper et al. (1995) found that negative emotion was significantly related to a motive to drink in order to cope, which in turn was related to drinking problems among a sample of adolescents (see also Laurent, Catanzaro, & Callan, 1997, for a replication). Similarly, Colder and Chassin (1993) found that negative affect partially mediated the relation between stress and adolescent alcohol use.

Despite these cross-sectional data, the relation of negative affectivity to adolescent substance use problems remains controversial for several reasons. First, researchers have argued that negative affectivity has only weak relations to adolescent substance use compared to factors such as peer affiliations, and that the effects of emotional distress are only small and indirect (Swaim, Oetting, & Beauvais, 1989). Second, studies linking negative affect with adolescent substance use have often failed to consider the effects of externalizing symptoms or conduct problems. Because there is considerable covariation between conduct problems and negative affect, it has not been clearly established that negative affectivity has a unique relation to adolescent substance use (above and beyond conduct problems). Third, cross-sectional studies cannot establish the directionality of the relation between negative affect and adolescent substance use, and negative affect might be the result rather than a cause of adolescent substance use.

Prospective studies have shown weaker support for negative affect pathways of vulnerability to adolescent substance use problems. Henry et al. (1993) found that depression was a unique prospective predictor of adolescent substance use (above and beyond conduct problems) but only for boys. Hansell and White (1991) failed to find a prospective effect of psychological distress on later adolescent drug use. Our own data showed that negative affect had a direct relation to adolescent substance use cross-sectionally, but this direct relation was not found for prospective prediction (Chassin et al., 1993, 1996). Moreover, in a follow-up of the same sample, we found that externalizing symptoms but not internalizing symptoms mediated parental alcoholism effects on substance use diagnoses in young adulthood (Chassin et al., 1999). In contrast, Caspi et al. (1996) found that boys who were inhibited at age 3 were at elevated risk for alcohol problems at age 21 (but not more frequent alcoholism diagnoses), and Shedler and Block (1990) found that childhood emotional distress predicted heavy marijuana use at age 18.

Thus, there are conflicting findings concerning prospective effects of negative affect on child and adolescent substance use. This pattern may have several interpretations. First, it may be that the negative affect pathway does not represent a major vulnerability process for substance use problems in adolescence. Some theorists suggest that early-onset substance use problems are more determined by conduct problems and deviance proneness, whereas later adult-onset problems are more likely to be driven by self-medication and negative affect regulation motives (Zucker, Fitzgerald, et al., 1995). Second, conflicting findings may reflect the fact that only some

forms of negative affect raise risk for adolescent substance use and substance use–related problems. Many studies fail to distinguish among different forms of negative affect (Hussong & Chassin, 1994). Support has been
stronger for depression, irritability, and anger as predictors of adolescent
substance use than for anxiety (Block et al., 1988; Forgays, Forgays,
Wrzesniewski, & Bonaiuto, 1992). For example, Hussong and Chassin
(1994) found that depression but not anxiety mediated the relation between
stress and adolescent alcohol use. Swaim et al. (1989) found that among
different forms of emotional distress, only anger had a unique direct effect
on adolescent substance use (above and beyond the effects of peer influences).
Clark, Kirisci, and Moss (1998) found that *lower* levels of anxiety predicted
the onset of adolescent tobacco use in a sample of high-risk adolescents.

   Thus, conflicting findings may be due to variation in the types of negative affect that are assessed. One way to explain the different effects for
different types of negative affect is to consider the unique characteristics of
substance use during the adolescent age period. Namely, adolescent substance use is strongly embedded in a peer social context (Kaplan, 1980;
Swaim et al., 1989). Kaplan (1980) proposed a related model of adolescent
vulnerability that linked negative affectivity to adolescent substance use
through deviant peer affiliations. Kaplan proposed that early and middle
adolescents whose self-esteem was threatened by rejection from mainstream
peer networks would seek out deviant peers as a way of receiving more
positive feedback and increasing self-esteem. These deviant peer affiliations
would then increase the likelihood of substance use. Indeed, such indirect
effects of negative affect through peer affiliations have been supported in
both cross-sectional and prospective studies (Swaim et al., 1989; Chassin et
al., 1996). Thus, negative affect may influence adolescent substance use
indirectly by affecting peer relationships rather than through a self-medication
mechanism. However, to the extent that highly anxious adolescents are more
likely to withdraw from the kinds of peer networks that support substance
use behaviors, anxiety would be associated with less adolescent substance
use. This would explain why anger and irritability would be better predictors of adolescent substance use than is anxiety.

   It is also possible that conflicting findings concerning the relation of
stress and negative affect to adolescent substance use are due to the presence of moderator variables. Not all adolescents who experience negative
affective states will cope with this negative affect by using alcohol or other
drugs. Thus, only adolescents who both experience negative affect and have
deficient coping strategies, or who believe substance use will help to cope
with negative affect, will be at risk for substance use because of this pathway (Cooper et al., 1995; Wills & Filer, 1996).

   Broader temperament theories of vulnerability have also proposed
moderator variables. Eisenberg and Fabes (1992) suggest that children who
are both highly reactive (and thus likely to experience intense negative affect states) and also deficient in self-regulation will be most vulnerable to

stress-related conduct problems. These adolescents will be most likely to act impulsively under stress. Such stress-related impulsive behavior might be hypothesized to include substance use. That is, adolescents who experience negative affect but who are poorly self-regulated will be more likely to cope with their negative affect by engaging in substance use because they are less likely to be restrained from engaging in socially disapproved or illegal behaviors. In addition, these adolescents are more likely to be embedded in peer social contexts that tolerate or encourage these behaviors. Combinations of high levels of negative affectivity and poor self-regulation (e.g., impulsivity and disinhibition) have been found to predict adolescent substance use and substance use problems (Colder & Chassin, 1997; Pandina, Johnson & Labouvie, 1992). Similarly, in Shedler and Block's (1990) study, childhood characteristics of those who used marijuana frequently at age 18 included both high levels of emotional distress and low levels of ego control, and Miller, Lochman, Coie, Terry, and Hyman (1998) found that comorbid conduct and depression problems prospectively predicted adolescent substance use. Thus, inconsistent findings for the negative affect pathway of vulnerability may reflect the moderating role of self-regulation such that negative affect is particularly predictive for those who are poorly self-regulated.

Finally, it has been suggested that females will be more likely to use alcohol and drugs to cope with negative affect (Hoffman & Su, 1998). Rohde et al. (1996) found that anxiety was marginally related to alcohol use for females but not for males, and similar findings were noted by Chassin et al. (1999). However, Laurent et al. (1997) found few gender effects in testing stress and negative affect regulation models of alcohol use for adolescents, and both Henry et al. (1993) and Caspi et al. (1996) found prospective effects of negative affect (depression and behavioral inhibition respectively in the two studies) for males but not for females. Thus, there are conflicting data concerning gender differences in the importance of negative affectivity for adolescent substance use/abuse.

Vulnerability to Substance Use Disorders through Sensitivity to Reinforcing Effects

The enhanced-reinforcement model focuses on individual differences in the pharmacological effects of substances. Certain individuals are hypothesized to be more sensitive to the reinforcing effects of alcohol and other substances while being less sensitive to their adverse effects. These individuals would be more likely to use substances frequently and in larger amounts, consequently placing them at increased risk for substance abuse and dependence.

Studies that administer substances to participants provide the most direct test of this hypothesis. However, given the ethical and legal constraints of administering substances to research participants, studies have been largely limited to alcohol challenge studies with participants who are of legal drinking age. Consistent with the enhanced reinforcement hypothesis, several studies have found that a moderate dose of alcohol (e.g., 1 gram per kilogram of body weight) dampens psychophysiological response to laboratory stressors in nonalcoholic Caucasian college-age subjects, particularly those whose personality profiles and/or family histories place them at high-risk for alcoholism (Finn & Pihl, 1987, 1988; Finn, Zeitouni, & Pihl, 1990; Levenson, Oyama, & Meek, 1987; Sher & Levenson, 1982). Moreover, other studies have found that sons of male alcoholics are less sensitive to the negative effects of alcohol (i.e., depressive and anxiogenic effects as blood-alcohol levels drop; Newlin & Thomson, 1990). However, few data exist to link such alcohol effects with actual diagnosis in the natural environment. In one exception, Schuckit (1994; Schuckit & Smith, 1996) found that sons of male alcoholics who had particularly low levels of negative responses to an alcohol challenge (measured subjectively by feelings of intoxication and objectively by degree of body sway) were more likely to receive diagnoses of alcohol abuse or dependence over the subsequent decade.

These findings support the notion that certain subgroups of individuals may be at heightened risk for alcoholism because they derive more pleasurable effects and fewer adverse effects from alcohol. However, there are several limitations to these findings. First, it is unknown whether stress-response dampening and enhanced excitatory effects are unique to alcohol or whether they may be induced by ingestion of other substances. Second, few studies have examined whether enhanced-reinforcement effects are moderated by offspring gender, gender of the alcoholic parent, or ethnicity (in one exception, Levenson et al., 1987, found that stress-response dampening effects did not differ as a function of gender). Also, because ethnic minority groups (e.g., African Americans and Asian Americans) have been found to metabolize alcohol at a different rate than do Caucasians (Naranjo & Bremner, 1993), most alcohol-challenge studies restrict their samples to Caucasian participants. As such, it is uncertain whether the enhanced-reinforcement model is applicable to populations of high-risk individuals other than Caucasian sons of male alcoholics. Third, because of ethical concerns, participants with alcohol problems are eliminated from alcohol-challenge studies. However, those high-risk individuals who reach early adulthood without any indications of alcohol problems may represent a particularly resilient subgroup (rather than actually a group at risk). Finally, because most alcohol-challenge studies are cross-sectional investigations (with the exception of Schuckit's work), the developmental antecedents and consequences of observed enhanced-reinforcement effects remain unknown.

Although alcohol-challenge studies are not conducted using children and adolescents, studies can be conducted that focus on the perceptions of substance use effects in this age group. For instance, Zucker, Kincaid, Fitzgerald, and Bingham (1995) found that preschool age children of alcoholics possessed more knowledge about and were better able to identify alcoholic beverages relative to controls, suggesting that alcohol-related cognitive schemas are detectable early in development and prior to the ingestion of alcohol. Because these subjects were too young to drink, it is unclear whether these early schemas truly reflect vulnerability for alcohol use. However, other longitudinal studies with older (adolescent) subjects have found that adolescents who have positive expectancies about the pharmacological effects of alcohol (e.g., social facilitation, increased arousal, and improvement of cognitive/motor functioning) are more likely to initiate drinking (Christiansen, Smith, Roehling, & Goldman, 1989) and to continue their use of alcohol over time (Smith, Goldman, Greenbaum, & Christiansen, 1995). Continued affirmation of positive alcohol expectancies in late adolescence may be prognostic for the development of alcohol abuse and/or dependence in adulthood (Brown, Creamer, & Stetson, 1987; Christiansen, Goldman, & Brown, 1985). Similar findings have emerged with respect to perceptions of drug use effects. Specifically, affirmation of drug-specific expectancies for marijuana and cocaine distinguishes between college students who actually use each of these respective drugs and influences the maintenance of this behavior (Brown, 1993b; Schafer & Brown, 1991).

Some experimental studies suggest that cognitions and perceptions about the pharmacological effects of alcohol and drugs are implicitly represented in semantic memory networks whose activation influences the decision to use. Stacy and his colleagues (Stacy, Ames, Sussman, & Dent, 1996) have found that substance-specific measures of memory association (i.e., including memory associations for alcohol and marijuana effects) are powerful and direct predictors of concurrent alcohol and drug use in adolescents and may thus mediate the relationship between previous and future substance use by fostering drug-consistent decisions and behaviors. Longitudinal research with college students supports this contention. Stacy (1997) found that previous marijuana use and memory activation for marijuana cues significantly predicted subsequent marijuana use, whereas previous alcohol use, sensation seeking, alcohol memory activation, and alcohol expectancies each exerted unique predictive effects on subsequent alcohol use.

In summary, a growing body of evidence suggests that at least some subgroups of youth are predisposed to substance abuse disorders due to positive expectancies of alcohol and drug effects, which perhaps reflect actual enhanced reinforcement. However, longitudinal studies that test the potential associations between positive alcohol expectancies and the pharmacological effects of alcohol are needed.

IMPLICATIONS OF THESE MODELS FOR DRUG PREVENTION

The prevention of substance abuse/dependence has been the focus of considerable research and public health effort in the last decades. Most of these programs have been school-based, focused on social influences, and attempting to reduce the incidence and prevalence of drug use among adolescents

(Institute of Medicine, 1996). These programs are "universal" in that they address drug use in the general population rather than in high-risk subgroups. By changing norms about substance use, recasting the social image associated with use, and teaching skills to resist peer pressure, these programs have shown short-term reductions in substance use prevalence (Institute of Medicine, 1996). Two programs that have demonstrated long-term success have both used such social influence approaches and also added techniques for coping with life stress (Botvin et al., 1995) or added community and family components (Pentz et al., 1989).

In addition to these universal approaches, the vulnerability research reviewed previously suggests further directions for the prevention of substance use disorders. Universal interventions alone may not be powerful enough to combat the family and intrapersonal factors that are associated with risk for substance abuse and dependence. For example, factors such as parental drug abuse, childhood conduct problems, aggression, difficulties in regulating emotional arousal, impulsivity, poor school achievement, and difficulty coping are not easily amenable to modification within typical school-based drug prevention programs. Thus, interventions targeted at high-risk subgroups may be a useful addition.

First, the fact that children of addicted parents are at heightened risk suggests that interventions aimed at changing parental substance abuse might function as a form of targeted prevention for the next generation. Successful treatment of alcoholic parents has been associated with better mental health outcomes for their children (Moos & Billings, 1982), although our data from a sample of recovered alcoholic parents who were not in formal treatment had less optimistic findings (DeLucia & Belz, 1999). Even if targeting parental recovery alone is insufficient, treatment settings could prove to be important contexts for delivering preventive services. These services might include parent training (to reduce the risk of deviance proneness), education about the personalized risk of addiction (suggested by the enhanced-reinforcement model), and stress-management techniques (suggested by the negative affect model) as well as the prevention of fetal alcohol effects. Because of the stigma of addiction, children of addicted parents are difficult to target in typical school settings, but they could be reached through treatment settings. Although these interventions may have greater intensity than do school-based programs, they unfortunately will reach a smaller subgroup of children because the majority of addicted parents do not receive formal treatment.

Another approach has been suggested by the deviance-proneness model. Namely, interventions might seek to reduce aggression and conduct problems and to increase academic achievement (to increase chances of bonding to conventional institutions and peer groups). Methods such as parent training programs, academic strengthening programs, and cognitive-behavioral programs to reduce aggressive behavior may have long-term potential to reduce substance abuse and dependence outcomes (Institute of Medicine, 1996). Thus, programs that are currently being evaluated for their ability to reduce or prevent conduct disorder should also be evaluated for their effects on substance abuse and dependence.

TREATMENT IMPLICATIONS

Despite increasing concern about the risk for substance abuse problems among youth, relatively few investigations have tested factors associated with successful treatment for this population. Indeed, most treatment models for adolescents with substance abuse problems are derived from studies of adult treatment for substance abuse which may not generalize to some of the unique treatment concerns of adolescents, including high rates of concomitant psychopathology, peer pressure, and familial influences (Brown, Mott, & Myers, 1990).

Longitudinal work with clinical samples suggests that peer factors are important to address in treating adolescent substance abusers. Brown has reported that the most common precipitant of adolescent substance abuse relapse is social peer pressure (Brown, Vik, & Creamer, 1989). Other research has found that adolescents who remain abstinent following treatment are characterized by supportive social networks and affiliations with new, non-substance-using peers (Brown et al., 1990). Thus, one treatment component for adolescent substance abusers should focus on promoting friendships with peers who are emotionally supportive but who do not themselves use drugs or encourage drug use.

Family factors are also important targets for modification. Many comparative studies have found that family-based approaches provide the most success in treating adolescents with substance abuse problems (see Liddle & Dakof, 1995, for a review). The importance of working with family systems is further underscored when considering the unique treatment needs of ethnically diverse populations. In their extensive research on the treatment of substance abuse in Hispanic youth, Kurtines and Szapocznik (1995) stress the importance of identifying culturally relevant family dynamics that influence the development of adolescent substance abuse and conduct problems. For instance, they have found that differences in acculturation exacerbate parent–adolescent conflict, consequently leading to decreased behavioral management on the part of parents and increases in delinquent behavior on the part of their offspring. Kurtines and Szapocznik (1995) have found that family-oriented treatment promoting bicultural understanding is most successful in treating such problems.

CONCLUSIONS AND FUTURE RESEARCH DIRECTIONS

As the earlier discussion illustrates, vulnerability for substance abuse and dependence is likely to consist of multiple pathways that exert their influence at different developmental stages. Current theorizing focuses on deviance-proneness pathways, which conceptualize substance abuse and dependence as part of a broader pattern of adolescent problem behavior; negative affect pathways, which conceptualize substance abuse and dependence as the end result of using substances to regulate negative affect; and enhanced-reinforcement pathways, which focus on individual differences in the pharmacological effects of alcohol and drug consumption. In terms of early-onset substance abuse and dependence (i.e., onset in adolescence and early adulthood), there is clear evidence in support of the deviance-proneness pathways, more controversy about negative affect regulation models, and indirect evidence for enhanced-reinforcement pathways (because studies of children and adolescents rely on perceptions of substance use effects rather than observation of actual effects).

Although a substantial data base has been generated on child and adolescent vulnerability to substance abuse and dependence, many directions for future research also remain. For the deviance-proneness pathway, studies need to be done that test relevant measures for adolescent girls (e.g., relational aggression; Crick, 1996) as well as studies of variation across ethnic groups. Moreover, more research needs to be done on the psychological underpinnings of "problem behaviors" to identify ways in which temperamental and personality characteristics contribute to substance abuse and dependence. Finally, longitudinal studies are needed to examine the extent to which deviance-proneness pathways are related to developmentally limited substance abuse and dependence.

For the negative affect pathway, research is needed to understand the role of negative affect regulation in adolescent and young adult substance abuse and dependence and to determine whether these factors are more appropriately viewed as causes of late onset disorders. To do this, research must consider the comorbidity between internalizing and externalizing symptoms in childhood and adolescence and must differentiate between different forms of negative affect. Finally, research should examine the potential moderators of the relation between negative affect and substance use in adolescence, including gender, coping, and temperamental self-regulation.

For the enhanced-reinforcement model, research should better integrate laboratory and field data to relate pharmacological effects of ingestion with the extent of consumption in the natural environment. These studies should also relate pharmacological effects to individuals' perceptions and expectations about consumption and should follow subjects over time to study the relation between these perceptions and actual consumption. For studies of pharmacological effects, more studies of women and ethnic minority participants are also needed.

Finally, for all the pathways, future research needs to take more seriously the biopsychosocial nature of these hypothesized mechanisms. Studies should test the ways in which genetic predispositions, biologically based individual differences, and temperamental and personality characteristics relate to the kinds of family, peer, and community environments within which children and adolescents are embedded. Studies should also examine ways in which these individual level factors moderate the effects of broader social environments. Similarly, ways in which the pharmacological effects of substances may mediate genetic risk and also be related to sociocultural norms and expectations should be evaluated. To accomplish this, researchers must take advantage of recent advances in quantitative methods for testing mediating and moderating relations within longitudinal designs (Rose, Chassin, Presson, & Sherman, 2000). From these studies will emerge a better understanding both of vulnerability processes and of factors that promote resilience to substance abuse and dependence.

ACKNOWLEDGMENT

Preparation of this chapter was supported by Grant No. DA 05227 from the National Institute on Drug Abuse.

REFERENCES

American Psychiatric Association. (1994). *Diagnostic and statistical manual of mental disorders* (4th ed.). Washington, DC: Author.

Anthony, J., & Helzer, J. (1991). Syndromes of drug abuse and dependence. In L. Robins & D. Reiger (Eds.), *Psychiatric disorders in America: The Epidemiologic Catchment Area study* (pp. 116–154). New York: Free Press.

Atyaclar, S., Tarter, R .E., Kirisci, L., & Lu, S. (1999). Association between hyperactivity and executive cognitive functioning in childhood and substance use in early adolescence. *Journal of the American Academy of Child and Adolescent Psychiatry, 38,* 172–178.

Bachman, J., O'Malley, P., & Johnston, L. (1984). Drug use among young adults: The impact of role status and social environments. *Journal of Personality and Social Psychology, 47,* 629–645.

Bachman, J., Wadsworth, K., O'Malley, P., Johnston, L., & Schulenberg, J. (1997). *Smoking, drinking, and drug use in young adulthood: The impact of new freedoms and responsibilities.* Mahwah, NJ: Erlbaum.

Baer, J. S., Barr, H. M., Bookstein, F. L., Sampson, P. D., & Streissguth, A. P. (1998). Prenatal alcohol exposure and family history of alcoholism in the etiology of adolescent alcohol problems. *Journal of Studies on Alcohol, 59,* 533–543.

Bates, M. E. (1993). Psychology. In Marc Galanter (Ed.), *Recent developments in alcoholism: Vol. 11. Ten years of progress* (pp. 45–72). New York: Plenum.

Bates, M., & Labouvie, E. (1997). Adolescent risk factors and the prediction of persistent alcohol and drug use into adulthood. *Alcoholism: Clinical and Experimental Research, 21,* 944–950.

Bentler, P. M. (1992). Etiologies and consequences of adolescent drug use: Implications for prevention. *Journal of Addictive Disorders, 11,* 47–61.

Society for Research in Child Development Biennial Meeting, Albuquerque, NM.

Deykin, E. Y., Buka, S. L. & Zeena, T. H. (1992). Depressive illness among chemically dependent adolescents. *American Journal of Psychiatry, 149,* 1341–1347.

Dishion, T. (1990). The family ecology of boys' peer relations in middle childhood. *Child Development, 61,* 874–892.

Dishion, T., Patterson, G. R., & Reid, J. R. (1988). Parent and peer factors associated with drug sampling in early adolescence. In E.R. Rahdert & J. Graboswski (Eds.), *Adolescent drug abuse: Analyses of treatment research* (NIDA Research Monograph 77, pp. 69–93). Rockville, MD: National Institute on Drug Abuse.

Dishion, T. J., Patterson, G. R., Stoolmiller, M., & Skinner, M. L. (1991). Family, school, and behavioral antecedents to early adolescent involvement with antisocial peers. *Developmental Psychology, 27,* 127–180.

Dobkin, P. L., Charlebois, P., & Tremblay, R. E. (1997). Mother–son interactions in disruptive and non-disruptive adolescent sons of male alcoholics and controls. *Journal of Studies on Alcohol, 58,* 546–553.

Donovan, J. E., & Jessor, R. (1985). Structure of problem behavior in adolescence and young adulthood. *Journal of Consulting and Clinical Psychology, 53,* 890–904.

Eisenberg, N., & Fabes, R. (1992). Emotion, regulation, and the development of social competence. In M. Clark (Ed.) *Review of personality and social psychology: Vol. 14. Emotion and social behavior* (pp. 119–150). Newbury Park, CA: Sage.

Ellickson, P., Bell, R., & McGuigan, K. (1993). Preventing adolescent drug use: Long-term results of a junior high program. *American Journal of Public Health, 83,* 856–861.

Fergusson, D., Lynskey, M., & Horwood, L. (1996). Comorbidity between depressive disorders and nicotine dependence in a cohort of 16 year olds. *Archives of General Psychiatry, 53,* 1043–1047.

Finn, P. R., & Pihl, R. O. (1987). Men at high risk for alcoholism: The effect of alcohol on cardiovascular response to unavoidable shock. *Journal of Abnormal Psychology, 96,* 230–236.

Finn, P. R., & Pihl, R. O. (1988). Risk for alcoholism: A comparison between two different groups of sons of alcoholics on cardiovascular reactivity and sensitivity to alcohol. *Alcoholism: Clinical and Experimental Research, 12,* 742–747.

Finn, P. R., Zeitouni, N., & Pihl, R. O. (1990). Effects of alcohol on psychophysiological hyperreactivity to nonaversive and aversive stimuli in men at high risk for alcoholism. *Journal of Abnormal Psychology, 99,* 79–85.

Fitzgerald, H. E., Sullivan, L. A., Ham, H. P., Zucker, R. A., Bruckel, S., Schneider, A. M., & Noll, R. B. (1993). Predictors of behavior problems in three-year-old sons of alcoholics: Early evidence for the onset of risk. *Child Development, 64,* 110–123.

Forgays, D., Forgays, D. G., Wrzesniewski, K., & Bonaiuto, P. (1992). Alcohol use and personality: relationships in U.S. and Polish adolescents. *Journal of Substance Abuse, 4,* 393–402.

Foxcroft, D. R., & Lowe, G. (1991). Adolescent drinking behavior and family socialization factors: A meta-analysis. *Journal of Adolescence, 14,* 255–273.

Ge, X., Conger, R., Cadoret, R., Neiderhiser, J., Yates, W., Troughton, E., & Stewart, M. (1996). The developmental interface between nature and nurture: A mutual influence model of child antisocial behavior and parent behaviors. *Developmental Psychology, 32,* 574–589.

Giancola, P. R., Moss, H. B., Martin, C. S., Kirisci, L., & Tarter, R. E. (1996). Executive cognitive functioning predicts reactive aggression in boys at high risk for substance abuse. *Alcoholism: Clinical and Experimental Research, 20,* 740–744.

Glantz, M., & Pickens, R. (1992). *Vulnerability to drug abuse.* Washington, DC: American Psychological Association.

Gotham, H., Sher, K., & Wood, P. (1997). Predicting stability and change in frequency of intoxication from the college years to beyond: Individual difference and role transition variables. *Journal of Abnormal Psychology, 106,* 619–629.

Grant, B. F., & Dawson, D. (1997). Age of onset of alcohol use and its association with DSM-IV alcohol abuse and dependence: Results from the National Longitudinal Alcohol Epidemiological Survey. *Journal of Substance Abuse, 9,* 103–110.

Hansell, S., & White, H. R. (1991). Adolescent drug use, psychological distress, and physical symptoms. *Journal of Health and Social Behavior, 32,* 288–301.

Harden, P., & Pihl, R. (1995). Cognitive function, cardiovascular reactivity, and behavior in boys at high risk for alcoholism. *Journal of Abnormal Psychology, 104,* 94–103.

Hawkins, J. D., Catalano, R. F., & Miller, J. Y. (1992). Risk and protective factors for alcohol and other drug problems in adolescence and early adulthood: Implications for substance abuse prevention. *Psychological Bulletin, 112,* 64–105.

Hawkins, J., Graham, J., Maguin, E., Abbott, R., Hill, K., & Catalano, R. (1997). Exploring the effects of age of alcohol use initiation and psychosocial risk factors on subsequent alcohol misuse. *Journal of Studies on Alcohol, 58,* 280–290.

Heath, A., Cates, R., Martin, N., Meyer, J., Hewitt, J., Neale, M., & Eaves, L. (1993). Genetic contribution to risk of smoking initiation: Comparisons across birth cohorts and across cultures. *Journal of Substance Abuse, 5,* 221–246.

Henry, B., Feehan, M., McGee, R., Stanton, W., Moffitt, T., & Silva, P. (1993). The importance of conduct problems and depressive symptoms in predicting adolescent substance use. *Journal of Abnormal Child Psychology, 21,* 469–480.

Hoffman, J., & Su, S. (1998). Stressful life events and adolescent substance use and depression: Conditional and gender-differentiated effects. *Substance Use and Misuse, 33,* 2219–2262.

Hussong, A., & Chassin, L. (1994). The stress–negative affect model of adolescent alcohol use: Disaggregating negative affect. *Journal of Studies on Alcohol, 55,* 707–719.

Institute of Medicine. (1996). *Pathways of addiction: Opportunities in drug abuse research.* Washington, DC: National Academy Press.

Jacob, T., & Leonard, K. E. (1994). Family and peer influences in the development of adolescent alcohol abuse. In R. Zucker, G. Boyd, & J. Howard (Eds.), *The development of alcohol problems: Exploring the biopsychosocial ma-*

trix of risk (NIAAA Research Monograph 26, NIH Pub. No. 64-3495, pp. 123–156). Washington, DC: U.S. Government Printing Office.

Jessor, R., & Jessor, S. L. (1977). *Problem behavior and psychosocial development: A longitudinal study of youth*. New York: Academic Press.

Johnston, L., O'Malley, P., & Bachman, G. (1998). *National survey results on drug use from The Monitoring the Future Study, 1975–1997*. Washington, DC: National Institute on Drug Abuse, U.S. Government Printing Office.

Johnston, L., O'Malley, P., & Bachman, G. (1999). *National survey results on drug use from the Monitoring the Future Survey, 1975–1998, Vol. I: Secondary school students*. (NIH Pub. No. 99-4660, p. 70). Rockville, MD: National Institute on Drug Abuse.

Kandel, D. B. (1975). Stages in involvement in adolescent drug use. *Science, 190,* 912–914.

Kandel, D. B., Yamaguchi, K., & Chen, K. (1992). Stages of progression in drug involvement from adolescence to adulthood: Further evidence for the gateway theory. *Journal of Studies on Alcohol, 53,* 447–457.

Kaplan, H. B. (1980). *Deviant behavior in defense of self*. New York: Academic Press.

Kendler, K., & Prescott, C. (1998). Cannabis use, abuse, and dependence in a population-based sample of female twins. *American Journal of Psychiatry, 155,* 1016–1022.

Kurtines, W. M., & Szapocznik, J. (1995). Cultural competence in assessing Hispanic youth and families: Challenges in the assessment of treatment needs and treatment evaluation for Hispanic drug-abusing adolescents. In E. Rahdert & D. Czechowitz (Eds.), *Adolescent drug abuse: Clinical assessment and therapeutic interventions* (NIDA Research Monograph 156, pp. 172–189). Rockville, MD: National Institute on Drug Abuse.

Laurent, J., Catanzaro, S., & Callan, M. (1997). Stress, alcohol-related expectancies and coping preferences: A replication with adolescents of the Cooper et al. (1992) model. *Journal of Studies on Alcohol, 58,* 644–651.

Lerner, J. V., & Vicary, J. R. (1984). Difficult temperament and drug use: Analyses from the New York Longitudinal Study. *Journal of Drug Education, 14,* 1–8.

Levenson, R. W., Oyama, O. N., & Meek, P. S. (1987). Greater reinforcement from alcohol for those at risk: Parental risk, personality risk, and sex. *Journal of Abnormal Psychology, 96,* 242–253.

Liddle, H. A., & Dakof, G. A. (1995). Family-based treatment for adolescent drug use: State of the science. In E. Rahdert & D. Czechowitz (Eds.), *Adolescent drug abuse: Clinical assessment and therapeutic interventions* (NIDA Research Monograph 156, pp. 218–255). Rockville, MD: National Institute on Drug Abuse.

MacKinnon, D. P., Johnson, C. A., Pentz, M. A., Dwyer, J. H., Jansen, W. B., Flay, B. R., & Wang, E. (1991). Mediating mechanisms in a school-based drug prevention program: First year effects. *Health Psychology, 10,* 164–172.

Mahaddian, E., Newcomb, M. D., & Bentler, P. M. (1988). Risk factors for substance use: Ethnic differences among adolescents. *Journal of Substance Abuse, 1,* 11–23.

Martin, C. S., Earleywine, M., Blackson, T. C., Vanyukov, M. M., Moss, H. B., & Tarter, R. E. (1994). Aggressivity, inattention, hyperactivity, and impulsivity in boys at high and low risk for substance abuse. *Journal of Abnormal Child Psychology, 22,* 177–203.

Martin, C. S., Kaczynski, N. A., Maisto, S. A., Bukstein, O. M., & Moss, H. B. (1995). Patterns of DSM-IV alcohol abuse and dependence symptoms in adolescent drinkers. *Journal of Studies on Alcohol, 56,* 672–680.

Martin, C. S., Kaczynski, N. A., Maisto, S. A., & Tarter, R. E. (1996). Polydrug use in adolescent drinkers with and without DSM-IV alcohol abuse and dependence. *Alcoholism: Clinical and Experimental Research, 20,* 1099–1108.

McGue, M. (1994). Genes, environment, and the etiology of alcoholism. In R. Zucker, G. Boyd, & J. Howard (Eds.), *The development of alcohol problems: Exploring the biopsychosocial matrix of risk* (NIAAA Research Monograph 26, pp. 1–40). Washington, DC: U.S. Government Printing Office.

Merikangas, K., Stolar, M., Stevens, D., Goulet, J. Preisig, M., Fenton, B., Zhang, J., O'Malley, S., & Rounsaville, B. (1998). Familial transmission of substance use disorders. *Archives of General Psychiatry, 55,* 973–979.

Mezzich, A., Tarter, R., Kirisci, L., Clark, D., Bukstein, O., & Martin, C. (1993). Subtypes of early age onset alcoholism. *Alcoholism: Clinical and Experimental Research, 17,* 767–770.

Miller, S., Lochman, J., Coie, J., Terry, R., & Hyman, C. (1998). Comorbidity of conduct and depressive problems at sixth grade: Substance use outcomes across adolescence. *Journal of Abnormal Child Psychology, 26,* 221–232.

Moffitt, T. E. (1993). The neuropsychology of conduct disorder. *Development and Psychopathology, 5,* 135–151.

Moos, R., & Billings, A. G. (1982). Children of alcoholics during the recovery process: Alcoholic and matched control families. *Addictive Behavior, 7,* 155–163.

Naranjo, C. A., & Bremner, K. E. (1993). Behavioral correlates of alcohol intoxication. *Addiction, 88,* 25–35.

Newcomb, M. D. (1995). Drug use etiology among ethnic minority adolescents: Risk and protective factors. In G. J. Botvin, S. P. Schinke, & M. A. Orlandi (Eds.), *Drug abuse prevention with multiethnic youth* (pp. 105–129). Thousand Oaks, CA: Sage.

Newcomb, M., & Harlow, L. (1986). Life events and substance use among adolescents: Mediating effects of perceived loss of control and meaninglessness in life. *Journal of Personality and Social Psychology, 51,* 564–577.

Newcomb, M. D., & McGee, L. (1991). Influence of sensation seeking on general deviance and specific problem behaviors from adolescence to young adulthood. *Journal of Personality and Social Psychology, 61,* 614–628.

Newlin, D. B., & Thomson, J. B. (1990). Alcohol challenge with sons of alcoholics: A critical review and analysis. *Psychological Bulletin, 108,* 383–402.

Ozkaragoz, T. Z., & Noble, E. P. (1995). Neuropsychological differences between sons of active alcoholic and non-alcoholic fathers. *Alcohol and Alcoholism, 30,* 115–123.

Pandina, R., Johnson, V., & Labouvie, E. (1992). Affectivity: A central mechanism in the development of drug dependence. In M. Glantz & R. Pickens (Eds.), *Vulnerability to drug abuse* (pp. 179–209). Washington, DC: American Psychological Association.

Pentz, M. A., Dwyer, J., MacKinnon, D., Flay, B., Hansen, W., Wang, E., & Johnson, C. A,. (1989). A multicommunity trial for primary prevention of adolescent drug abuse. *Journal of the American Medical Association, 261,* 3259–3266.

Robins, L., & Pryzbeck, T. (1985). Age of onset of drug use as a factor in drug and other disorders. In C. R. Jones & R. J. Battjes (Eds.), *Etiology of drug abuse: Implications for prevention* (pp. 178–192). Washington, DC: U.S. Government Printing Office.

Rohde, P., Lewinsohn, P. M., & Seeley, J. R. (1996). Psychiatric comorbidity with problematic alcohol use in high school students. *Journal of the American Academy of Child and Adolescent Psychiatry, 35,* 101–109.

Roosa, M., Beals, J., Sandler, I., & Pillow, D. (1990). The role of risk and protective factors in predicting symptomatology in adolescent self-identified children of alcoholic parents. *American Journal of Community Psychology, 18,* 725–741.

Rose, J., Chassin, L., Presson, C., & Sherman, S. J. (2000). *Multivariate applications in substance abuse research: New methods for new questions.* Mahwah, NJ: Erlbaum.

Russell, M. (1990). Prevalence of alcoholism among children of alcoholics. In M. Windle & J. S. Searles (Eds.), *Children of alcoholics: Critical perspectives* (pp. 9–38). New York: Guilford Press.

Schafer, J., & Brown, S.A. (1991). Marijuana and cocaine effect expectancies and drug use pattern. *Journal of Consulting and Clinical Psychology, 59,* 558–565.

Schuckit, M. A. (1994). Low level of response to alcohol as a predictor of future alcoholism. *American Journal of Psychiatry, 151,* 184–189.

Schuckit, M. A. (1998). Biological, psychological, and environmental predictors of the alcoholism risk: A longitudinal study. *Journal of Studies on Alcohol, 59,* 485–494.

Schuckit, M. A., & Smith, T. L. (1996). An 8-year follow-up of 450 sons of alcoholic and control subjects. *Archives of General Psychiatry, 53,* 202–210.

Schulenberg, J., Wadsworth, K., O'Malley, P., Bachman, G., & Johnston, L. (1996). Adolescent risk factors for binge drinking during the transition to adulthood: Variable and pattern-centered approaches to change. *Developmental Psychology, 32,* 659–674.

Shedler, J., & Block, J. (1990). Adolescent drug use and psychological health: A longitudinal inquiry. *American Psychologist, 45,* 612–630.

Sher, K. J. (1991). *Children of alcoholics: A critical appraisal of theory and research.* Chicago: University of Chicago Press.

Sher, K. J. (1996). Psychological characteristics of children of alcoholics. *Alcohol Health and Research World, 21,* 247–254.

Sher, K. J., & Levenson, R.W. (1982). Risk for alcoholism and individual differences in the stress-response dampening effect of alcohol. *Journal of Abnormal Psychology, 91,* 350–367.

Sher, K. J., Walitzer, K., Wood, P., & Brent, E. (1991). Characteristics of children of alcoholics: Putative risk factors, substance use and abuse, and psychopathology. *Journal of Abnormal Psychology, 100,* 427–448.

Smith, G. T., Goldman, M. S., Greenbaum, P. E., & Christiansen, B. A. (1995). Expectancy for social facilitation for drinking: The divergent paths of high-expectancy and low-expectancy adolescents. *Journal of Abnormal Psychology, 104,* 32–40.

Stacy, A. W. (1997). Memory activation and expectancy as prospective predictors of alcohol and marijuana use. *Journal of Abnormal Psychology, 106,* 61–73.

Stacy, A. W., Ames, S. L., Sussman, S., & Dent, C. W. (1996). Implicit cognition in adolescent drug use. *Psychology of Addictive Behavior, 10,* 190–203.

Stewart, D. G., & Brown, S. A. (1995). Withdrawal and dependency symptoms among adolescent alcohol and drug abusers. *Addiction, 90,* 627–635.

Stice, E., & Barrera, M. (1995). A longitudinal examination of the reciprocal relations between perceived parenting and adolescents' substance use and externalizing behaviors. *Developmental Psychology, 31,* 322–334.

Swaim, R. C., Bates, S. C., & Chavez, E. L. (1998). Structural equation socialization model of substance use among Mexican-American and white non-Hispanic school dropouts. *Journal of Adolescent Health, 23,* 128–138.

Swaim, R., Oetting, R., & Beauvais, F. (1989). Links from emotional distress to adolescent drug use: A path model. *Journal of Consulting and Clinical Psychology, 57,* 227–231.

Tarter, R. E., Alterman, A. I., & Edwards, K. L. (1985). Vulnerability to alcoholism in men: A behavior–genetic perspective. *Journal of Studies on Alcohol, 46,* 329–356.

Tarter, R. E., Jacob, T., & Bremer, D. A. (1989). Cognitive status of sons of alcoholic men. *Alcoholism: Clinical and Experimental Research, 13,* 232–235.

Tarter, R. E., Kirisci, L., & Clark, D. B. (1997). Alcohol use disorder among adolescents: Impact of paternal alcoholism on drinking behavior, drinking motivation, and consequences. *Alcoholism: Clinical and Experimental Research, 21,* 171–178.

Tarter, R. E., & Vanyukov, M. (1994). Alcoholism: A developmental disorder. *Journal of Consulting and Clinical Psychology, 62,* 1096–1107.

Tsuang, M., Lyons, M. Eisen, S., Goldberg, J., True, W., Lin, N., Meyer, J., Toomey, R., Faraone, S., & Eaves, L. (1996). Genetic influences on DSM-III-R drug abuse and dependence: A study of 3,372 twin pairs. *American Journal of Medical Genetics, 67,* 473–477.

Vega, W. A., Zimmerman, R. S., Warheit, G. J., Apospori, E., & Gil, A. (1993). Risk factors for early adolescent drug use in four ethnic and racial groups. *American Journal of Public Health, 83,* 185–189.

Vik, P. W., Brown, S. A., & Myers, M. G. (1997). Adolescent substance use problems. In E. J. Mash & L. G. Terdal (Eds.), *Assessment of childhood disorders* (3rd ed., pp. 717–748). New York: Guilford Press.

Vitaro, F., Dobkin, P., Carbonneau, R., & Tremblay, R. E. (1996). Personal and familial characteristics of resilient sons of male alcoholics. *Addiction, 91,* 1161–1177.

Wills, T. A., DuHamel, K., & Vaccaro, D. (1995). Activity and mood temperament as predictors of adolescent substance use: Test of a self-regulation mediational model. *Journal of Personality and Social Psychology, 68,* 901–916.

Wills, T. A., & Filer, M. (1996). Stress-coping model of adolescent substance use. In T. Ollendick & R. Prinz (Eds.). *Advances in clinical child psychology* (Vol. 18, pp. 91–132). New York: Plenum.

Wills, T. A., McNamara, G., Vaccaro, D., & Hirky, E. (1996). Escalated substance use: Longitudinal grouping analysis from early to middle adolescence. *Journal of Abnormal Psychology, 105,* 166–180.

Wills, T. A., Vaccaro, D., & McNamara, G. (1992). The role of life events, family support, and competence in adolescent substance use: A test of vulnerability and protective factors. *American Journal of Community Psychology, 20,* 349–374.

Windle, M. (1990). Temperament and personality attributes of children of alcoholics. In M. Windle & J. S. Searles (Eds.), *Children of alcoholics: Critical perspectives* (pp. 129–167). New York: Guilford Press.

Wootton, J., Frick, P., Shelton, K., & Silverthorn, P. (1997). Ineffective parenting and childhood conduct problems: The moderating role of callous–unemotional traits. *Journal of Consulting and Clinical Psychology, 65*, 301–308.

Zucker, R. A., Boyd, G., & Howard, J. (Eds.). (1994). *The development of alcohol problems: Exploring the biopsychosocial matrix of risk* (NIAAA Research Monograph 26, NIH Pub. No. 64-3495). Washington, DC: U.S. Government Printing Office.

Zucker, R. A., Ellis, D. A., Bingham, C. R., & Fitzgerald, H. E. (1996). The development of alcoholic subtypes: Risk variation among alcoholic families during the childhood years. *Alcohol Health and Research World, 20*, 46–54.

Zucker, R. A., Fitzgerald, H. E., & Moses, H. D. (1995). Emergence of alcohol problems and the several alcoholisms: A developmental perspective on etiological theory and life course trajectory. In D. Cicchetti & D. Cohen (Eds.), *Manual of developmental psychopathology* (Vol. 2, pp. 677–711). New York: Wiley.

Zucker, R. A., Kincaid, S. B., Fitzgerald, J. E., & Bingham, C. R. (1995). Alcohol schema acquisition in preschoolers: Differences between children of alcoholics and children of nonalcoholics. *Alcoholism: Clinical and Experimental Research, 19*, 1011–1017.

6

Vulnerability to Substance Use Disorders in Adulthood

R. LORRAINE COLLINS
MARIELA C. SHIRLEY

Many factors related to vulnerability to alcohol/substance abuse occur during adolescence, but adulthood is the time when more stable patterns of use are established and problems become apparent. In this chapter, we describe issues related to vulnerability to substance use during adulthood. As we try to understand the roles that different vulnerability factors play, our focus is on alcohol abuse research, with reference to other substances when appropriate. We begin with a definition of substance use/abuse and prevalence data then move to a brief historical overview of different approaches to alcohol and substance abuse. Using a biopsychosocial framework, we discuss current theory and empirical evidence on vulnerability to substance abuse during adulthood. We end with a discussion of the implications for prevention and treatment, as well as future directions for research.

DEFINITION AND PREVALENCE
OF SUBSTANCE USE DISORDERS

Substance abuse is generally defined as unsafe psychoactive substance use to alter psychological or physiological functioning in a manner that is socially unacceptable (Jaffe, 1985). Dependence has been more difficult to define (e.g., Edwards, Arif, & Hodgson, 1981; Nathan, 1991) but is usually equated with physical dependence and a withdrawal syndrome that varies with the substance of abuse (Kalant, 1989). In the United States, the most commonly used diagnostic system is the *Diagnostic and Statistical Manual of Mental Disorders* (DSM) published by the American Psychiatric Association. The current version, DSM-IV (American Psychiatric Association, 1994), divides substance-related disorders into two groups: substance use disorders (e.g., substance dependence and substance abuse) and substance-induced disorders (e.g., substance intoxication, substance withdrawal, and substance-induced mood disorder). Substance use disorders are further classified by 11 drug types (e.g., alcohol, stimulants, cocaine, and opioids). Substance-induced disorders presuppose that the substance use predates the development of other coexisting disorders. For example, abuse of alcohol precedes and causes mood disorders.

Substance dependence is defined as a "pattern of repeated self-administration of alcohol or other drug use which results in tolerance, withdrawal, and compulsive drug-taking behavior" (American Psychiatric Association, 1994, p. 176). The continued use of the substance leads to behavioral, physiological, and cognitive symptoms and impairments. There are seven criteria related to the diagnosis of dependence. They include tolerance (either the need to increase amounts to achieve intoxication or reduced effects derived from continued use of the substance), withdrawal (cognitive and physiological changes due to drug discontinuation), and impairment in life areas (e.g., social, occupational, and recreational). In contrast, substance abuse is a "maladaptive pattern of substance use" associated with negative consequences related to recurrent use. Such consequences include the failure to meet major obligations and continued use despite social, legal, or interpersonal problems.

Classification systems such as DSM are developed to promote communication among researchers and clinicians to further explain, predict, and control the problem behavior. However, difficulties often arise in the classification of problem behavior. They include (1) a lack of clearcut operational definitions of the behavior, (2) the use of disjunctive or overlapping categories, (3) a failure to consider base rates of disorders in the general population, (4) the influence of empirical findings versus clinical impressions in influencing diagnostic practices, (5) reliability in the application of diagnostic criteria, and (6) the failure to subject diagnostic criteria to concurrent and predictive validity testing (Adams & Cassidy, 1993; Nathan, 1991). These problems and more can result in poor validity and reliability of classification schemes and inflated prevalence estimates.

Prevalence rates are determined from surveys of the general population. Two such surveys are the Epidemiologic Catchment Area (ECA) study (Regier et al., 1990) and the National Longitudinal Alcohol Epidemiologic Survey (NLAES). The ECA study (Regier et al., 1990) is a general population study of 20,291 individuals. The results indicated lifetime prevalence rates of 13.5% for alcohol dependence and abuse and 6.1% for other drug dependence or abuse. Lifetime prevalence rates for other (nonsubstance use) psychiatric disorders was 22.5% of the population. Approximately 29% of those with a mental disorder had an overlapping addictive disorder (22%

alcohol use disorder, 15% other drug use disorder). The highest comorbidity observed was for alcohol and other drug use disorders (i.e., those with an alcohol disorder were seven times more likely to also have another drug use disorder; those with another drug use disorder were seven times more likely to have an alcohol use disorder). Of those with an alcohol disorder, 37% had a coexisting mental disorder and of those with another drug use disorder, 53% had an overlapping mental disorder. The ECA study found, of the mental disorders examined, that those with the highest degree of overlap with substance use disorders included antisocial personality disorder, mood and anxiety disorders, and schizophrenia. Results also suggested that coexisting mental disorders are more prevalent in individuals with other (nonalcohol) drug use disorders, and that mental disorders may precede the development of substance use disorders. Although the ECA is the largest general population study conducted to date, it has some limitations. The ECA is based on DSM-III diagnostic criteria where lifetime diagnoses for substance abuse/dependence disorders were based on non–time-clustered criteria. In addition, the only personality disorder assessed in this study was antisocial personality disorder.

Other studies have found that demographic characteristics are related to comorbidity of substance abuse and mental disorders. The National Comorbidity Study (NCS; Kessler et al., 1994) found that women were at a greater risk for mood and anxiety disorders and nonaffective psychosis, whereas men were at greater risk for substance use and antisocial personality disorders. Men were more likely to be diagnosed as drug dependent than women (Warner, Kessler, Hughes, Anthony, & Nelson, 1995). Furthermore, this study showed that the rates of psychiatric disorders declined with age, that ethnic differences in prevalence rates could be identified (e.g., African Americans had lower prevalence of mood, substance use, and lifetime comorbidity than European Americans; Hispanic Americans had a higher prevalence rate of mood disorders than European Americans); and socioeconomic status was inversely related to rates of psychiatric disorders.

Grant (1997) examined the prevalence and demographic correlates of alcohol use and DSM-IV alcohol dependence in a national sample of 42,862. Unlike earlier studies, the NLAES employed a much larger sample representative of the U.S. adult population, used a more sensitive measure to assess alcohol dependence, and included older adults. The results showed a lifetime prevalence rate of 66% for alcohol use and a current use prevalence rate of 44%. Alcohol use, dependence diagnoses, and long-term histories of dependence were more prominent among men than among women. Younger drinkers (age range 18–44) appeared to account for the largest portion of alcohol consumed and had a greater frequency of dependence diagnoses than did older drinkers (a finding consistent with consumption patterns reported by Greenfield & Rogers, 1999). Regardless of generational effects, alcohol use peaked during adolescence (ages 14–19) with greater stabilization around age 29. The youngest members of the sample showed the greatest probability of dependence after adolescence, even though lifetime consumption rates were lower in this age group. Grant (1997) suggests that younger members of this sample "may be more vulnerable to dependence as the result of a history of other psychopathology" (p. 472). Similar to the NCS, alcohol use was more prevalent among European Americans than African Americans or Hispanic Americans as well as among those who were more educated and affluent. European Americans and Hispanic Americans were more likely to be dependent on alcohol than were African Americans but were less likely to remain dependent than the other two ethnic groups.

HISTORY OF APPROACHES USED TO EXAMINE THE VULNERABILITY TO THE DISORDER

Vulnerability to substance abuse has been conceptualized in a variety of ways and research methods have matched the different conceptualizations. Much of the initial research on vulnerability to alcohol and substance abuse focused on adults. Historical accounts typically described alcohol abuse and the use of illicit substances as signs of depravity and moral weakness and, for the most part, not worthy of study. For adult alcohol abusers, a breakthrough in notions of vulnerability and treatment occurred when research introduced disease-oriented notions. Jellinek (1960) helped to popularize the disease model of alcohol when he described different types of alcohol abusers, based on his review of research and his clinical experience. Alcoholism came to be seen as a medical disorder for which a formal system of diagnosis and medical treatment was appropriate. Research on alcoholism often focused on persons with an identified problem and on the medical and biological consequences of alcohol abuse. There also was some interest in the course of the disorder, exemplified in a 40-year, longitudinal study of young men, which provided information on the natural course of alcoholism (Vaillant, 1983). Interestingly, most such research focused on men and on persons of European ancestry.

Successful challenges to the basic tenets of the disease model came from behaviorally trained clinicians and researchers who sought to apply learning theory to the conceptualization and treatment of alcohol and substance abuse. For example, the disease model assumed that certain types of alcoholics, characterized by Jellinek as "gamma alcoholics," would lose control over drinking if exposed to any alcohol; therefore abstinence was the only viable option for alcohol treatment. Experiments designed to test this notion indicated that after one drink alcoholics did not lose control of their drinking (e.g., Merry, 1966), thus undermining a basic tenet of the model and paving the way for other approaches.

Behavioral psychologists who challenged disease notions tended to characterize drinking as occurring on a continuum, ranging from abstinence to problematic heavy drinking. They assumed that the laws of learning pertained to all aspects of the drinking continuum and so saw the study of processes in social drinking as having relevance to the conceptualization and treatment of problem drinking (Bandura, 1969; Maisto, Carey, & Bradizza, 1999). The laws of learning are universal; thus they were seen as being applicable to women and to persons from various ethnic backgrounds. Methods used in learning-based studies of vulnerability to substance abuse among adults ranged from survey studies of the general population described earlier to experiments and analog studies involving college students and clinical populations. Studies of adults have employed cross-sectional and longitudinal designs. However, given their complexity and cost, longitudinal designs are much less common. As the complexity of substance use disorders came to be understood, the need for a broader conceptual framework became apparent. Such a framework is provided by a biopsychosocial perspective on vulnerability, which encompasses a variety of concepts, disciplines, and related research methods (Zucker & Gomberg, 1986). This perspective serves as the framework for our upcoming discussion of theory and research on vulnerability to substance abuse during adulthood.

CLASSIFICATION AND ASSESSMENT
OF SUBSTANCE USE DISORDERS

Models of vulnerability have been linked to classification of alcohol and substance use disorders into typologies. Such typologies have been based on clinical observations, systems of diagnosis, and a variety of other factors that connote risk for alcohol and/or substance abuse. Jellinek's (1960) description of types of alcoholics was based on clinical observation. Other researchers have attempted to develop more empirically based typologies of alcoholics based on patterns of drinking and impairment (e.g., Cloninger, Bohman, & Sigvardsson, 1981; Morey & Skinner, 1986), age of onset and motivation for use (e.g., Babor et al., 1992), and developmental/emotional factors contributing to risk (e.g., Schuckit, 1985; Zucker, 1994). Cloninger and colleagues (Cloninger, 1987; Cloniger et al., 1987) distinguished two types of alcoholics based on heritability and environmental factors. According to this typology, Type I alcoholics have a later age of onset of problematic use, are more likely to binge drink, are not antisocial, are prone to be more neurotic and anxious, often develop health problems related to use, and are of both genders. Thus, Type I alcoholism seems to involve a diathesis–stress model in which both genetic and environmental factors are required for the expression of alcoholism. In contrast, Type II alcoholics have an earlier onset of problematic drinking (usually adolescence) and a more severe course of alcoholism. They are unable to abstain, antisocial and highly aggressive, more impulsive and sensation seeking, predominantly male, and have greater disruption in levels of social and occupational functioning. For Type II alcoholism, genetic/biological factors may predominate.

Babor and colleagues extended Cloninger's classification to alcohol and cocaine abusers. Using cluster analyses of premorbid risk and vulnerability, severity of dependence, chronicity, consequences of use, and comorbid psychopathology (Babor et al., 1992; Ball, Carroll, Babor, & Rounseville, 1995; Brown, Babor, Litt, & Kranzler, 1994), they designated two types of substance abusers. Type A was found to have a later onset of use, less premorbid vulnerability, less severe dependence, fewer alcohol/drug-related problems, less chronic course of the substance use disorder, and less concurrent psychopathology. Type B had greater premorbid risk, family history of substance abuse, earlier onset of use, more severe dependence and chronic course, and more consequences as a result of substance use and were more aggressive, more impulsive and less conventional, and had more concurrent psychopathology (Brown et al., 1994). Babor et al. (1992) showed that the Type A/B typology had predictive validity at 12 and 36 months after treatment cessation in that Type Bs displayed more alcohol-related impairment, distress, and pathological use patterns. Ball et al. (1995) suggested that family history, childhood conduct problems, and sensation seeking may contribute to a more severe form of cocaine dependence (Type Bs), whereas Type As' cocaine dependence is more strongly influenced by environmental variables, thereby validating Cloninger's Type I/II typology. They also suggested that antisocial personality and alcoholism severity may best distinguish Type A from Type B cocaine-dependent individuals but that psychiatric and substance use severity are better predictors for use in treatment matching studies.

Morey and Skinner (1986) proposed a classification system based on types of drinkers related to severity and contextual aspects of use. The three types of drinkers are early-stage problem drinkers (alcohol-related problems without symptoms of dependence), affiliative drinkers (socially motivated frequent or daily use, moderate dependence), and schizoid drinkers (socially isolated binge drinkers, severely dependent). Although this model describes the drinking patterns of alcoholics, it does not address causal variables involved in the etiology of alcoholism. That is, these patterns may be subsequent to the development of alcoholism.

Zucker (1994) proposed a developmental model of alcoholism based on four subtypes including (1) antisocial alcoholism (high genetic loading, early onset, antisocial behavior, greater substance use severity, greater likelihood of other substance use/abuse, history of childhood aggression); (2) developmentally limited alcoholism (greater severity of alcohol symptoms, externalizing deviant behaviors, frequent heavy drinking, lower risk load in adolescence, maturation out of problematic use with the assumption of adult roles); (3) negative affect alcoholism (primarily seen in women, use of alcohol to manage depressive and anxiety symptoms or deal with interpersonal conflict); and (4) primary alcoholism (a diagnosis of exclusion where the alcohol dependence is unrelated to and precedes the development of other psychiatric disorders). According to Zucker, a developmental perspective allows for an evaluation of alcoholism based on multiple etiologies, which suggest different courses of the disorder.

Schuckit (1985) proposed two types of alcoholics based on the order of onset of the alcoholism relative to the onset of depression. In primary alcoholics, the alcoholism preceded the development of depression. Primary alcoholics have a later onset and lower intensity of substance use, and a slower progression to alcohol abuse. Whether depressive symptoms are due to substance use (central nervous system depressant effects) or to an underlying depressive disorder has been questioned as depressive symptoms remit following a period of abstinence (Brown & Schuckit, 1988). In secondary alcoholics, the depression preceded the development of alcoholism with alcohol used to "medicate" depressive symptoms (Schuckit & Monteiro, 1988). Secondary alcoholism is associated with more family histories positive for mood disorders, suicide attempts, psychopathology, treatment utilization, less substance use; it is more frequently observed in women, and is associated with poorer treatment outcomes in men (Rounsaville, Dolinsky, Babor, & Meyer, 1987).

THEORY AND RESEARCH ON VULNERABILITY

Substance abuse is a highly complex behavior that has multiple causes. Recognition of this complexity has led to the propagation of a biopsychosocial model of vulnerability. This model incorporates research from a variety of disciplines including genetic, neurobiological, psychological, and personality factors, as well as social factors as contributing to risk for substance use disorders (Zucker & Gomberg, 1986). We examine vulnerability to substance abuse in adulthood by highlighting the evidence from the various components of this multidisciplinary perspective. Much of this research has largely been conducted on males (particularly regarding genetic and neurobiological markers), making firm conclusions about vulnerability processes in females tenuous at best.

Biological Aspects of Vulnerability

Genetics has been the basis of the biological approach to alcohol and substance abuse. Genetic evidence has been gathered from a variety of methods that focus on biological family linkages as a basis for transmitting alcoholism. Studies of alcoholics show that individuals with a family history of alcoholism in a first-degree relative have a sevenfold increased risk of developing alcoholism (Merikangas, 1990). Genetic studies suggest that gender (genetic link predominantly found in males) and severity of dependence (greater severity of dependence) may influence concordance rates (e.g., Cloninger, 1987; Cloninger et al., 1981; Goodwin, Schulsinger, Knopf,

Mednick, & Guze, 1977; McGue, Pickins, & Svikis, 1992) . The most powerful evidence comes from studies of monozygotic (MZ; identical) and dizygotic (DZ; fraternal) twins. Identical twins share 100% of genetic material whereas fraternal twins share on average 50% of genetic material. If we assume that twins share similar environments, we could simplistically conclude that similarities between MZ twins are a function of their shared genes. Generally, the evidence shows the highest concordance for alcoholism as occurring between male MZ twins (68–76%), with lower rates for female MZ twins (32–47%). The rates for male DZ twins range from 46 to 61% and for female DZ twins from 24 to 42% (Zuckerman, 1999).

A variation on the twin studies method involves MZ twins that have been separated and raised in different environments. Adoption studies are the most powerful design in which to separate genetic from environmental influences (McGue, 1994). The evidence from adoption studies typically has been seen as providing support for a genetic explanation of alcoholism. Cloninger's (1981) study of Swedish adoptees led to the designation of two types of alcoholics described earlier. Each type varied in heritability and psychosocial correlates, with Type I alcoholism having both a genetic and an environmental component and Type II alcoholism being limited to males, highly heritable, and not related to environmental factors. Searles (1988) has raised a number of conceptual and methodological issues related to this body of research. He cites problems such as the criteria used for diagnosis and the high rates of psychopathology in the foster parents of adoptees as reasons for caution in interpreting the results of these adoption studies. He suggests the use of more complex models that treat genes and environments as dynamic systems as a way to enhance our understanding of the role of biological factors in the abuse of alcohol and other substances.

Researchers also are trying to identify the specific genes or combination of genes that are implicated in alcohol disorders. Genetic marker studies have focused on allelic variation in two specific genes (at the aldehyde dehydrogenase or ALDH locus, and the D_2 dopamine receptor or DRD2 locus) (McGue, 1994; National Institute on Alcohol Abuse and Alcoholism, 1997). The ALDH locus gene is responsible for the inability of some ethnic groups to metabolize alcohol (e.g., Asians), thereby protecting them from alcoholism (Zuckerman, 1999). However, as only 2% of Japanese alcoholics have this gene, this theory does not explain why most Asian drinkers fail to develop alcoholism. Cultural differences may contribute to the relationship between ALDH deficiency and risk for alcoholism (National Institute on Alcohol Abuse and Alcoholism, 1997).

The A1 form of the DRD_2 gene found on chromosome 11 was believed to mediate the reward effects of alcohol use (McBride, Murphy, Lumeng, & Li, 1990). However, some studies reported inconsistent findings on whether this gene was more prevalent in alcoholics (Blum et al., 1990; Turner et al., 1992), and more recent research has suggested no association between DRD_2 locus and alcoholism. Genetic vulnerability may be more related to (1) personality variables (Zuckerman, 1999) supporting a diathesis–stress vulnerability model of environmental influences relative to genetic loading (McGue, 1994); (2) failure to include appropriate control groups matched for ethnicity (National Institute on Alcohol Abuse and Alcoholism, 1997); (3) lack of awareness of the heterogeneity of alcoholism (Cloninger, 1991); and (4) utilization of inappropriate sampling and statistical methodologies (National Institute on Alcohol Abuse and Alcoholism, 1997).

Studies of biological markers for alcohol and drug abuse target comparisons of biological processes between substance abusers versus nonsubstance abusers or the children of substance abusers, and have focused on neurophysiological, biochemical, and alcohol sensitivity measures. The idea is that the identification of global markers of a predisposition to alcohol and other drugs or to specific drugs (e.g., alcohol, opiates) would allow for risk prediction. Alcohol and opiate reinforcement is perhaps mediated by the endogenous opioid system with these drugs producing an increase in beta-endorphins in individuals with positive family histories (Zuckerman, 1999). Thus, alcoholics, for example, may be underaroused and use alcohol to stimulate reward centers. Electroencephalographic (EEG) brain wave activity has been evaluated as sons of alcoholics have lower alpha wave activity (National Institute on Alcohol Abuse and Alcoholism, 1997) and beta brain wave activity and show fewer changes in brain wave activity following alcohol challenge (Newlin, 1994). However, changes in brain wave activity may be due to overlapping diagnoses of antisocial personality disorder or to rising and falling blood alcohol concentration levels (National Institute on Alcohol Abuse and Alcoholism, 1997).

Brain-evoked potentials have been linked to alcoholism risk (Begleiter, Porjesz, Bihari, & Kissin, 1984) and are suggestive of trait variables involved in its etiology. The P300 has been more systematically evaluated because it happens about 300 milliseconds after the presentation of a stimulus and may be a good measure of attention. Studies evaluating P300 amplitudes show that alcoholics have reduced amplitudes or are unable to even attend to unpredictable or infrequent stimuli (Begleiter et al., 1984; Begleiter & Porjesz, 1988). These studies suggest that some individuals are at a greater risk for alcoholism simply because they are unable to detect the behavioral effects of alcohol, even at moderate doses. A drawback to the P300 amplitude is that it is not specific to alcohol (Polich & Bloom, 1988), and its effects are demonstrated under visual stimuli only (Polich, Pollock, & Bloom, 1994). Low P300 amplitudes also have been found in individuals with other mental disorders and may be more indicative of cognitive (vs. specific vulnerability to substance abuse) and neurological developmental differences among individuals (National Institute on Alcohol Abuse and Alcoholism, 1997).

Enzymes have been evaluated because they are genetic by-products and are involved in the breakdown of neurotransmitters. The monoamine oxidase activity (MAO) enzyme has been implicated in antisocial personality disorder, borderline personality disorder, and alcoholism. Low MAO levels have been linked to alcoholism, particularly among Type II alcoholics (Sher, 1991; Tabakoff, Whelan, & Hoffman, 1990; von Knorring, Hallman, von Knorring, & Oreland, 1991). MAO is involved in the metabolism of dopamine (in addition to serotonin and norepinephrine), a neurotransmitter implicated in alcohol reward. However, MAO levels can be the result of alcohol consumption and have been found to be low in other personality disorders characterized by low impulse control. The neurotransmitter serotonin also may contribute to alcoholism risk as low levels of serotonin may relate to antisocial behaviors, poor impulse control, and aggression (Zuckerman, 1999). In addition, low serotonin levels are observed in nonalcoholics with a positive family history of alcoholism, suggesting implications for order of onset in substance use disorders (National Institute on Alcohol Abuse and Alcoholism, 1997). As low serotonin levels may be found in some depressed individuals, it is likely that substance abuse is not the result of a single neurotransmitter, but an interaction among several neurotransmitters.

Sensitivity to the effects of alcohol and/or drugs has been evaluated in several studies (Finn, Zeitouni, & Pihl, 1990; Newlin & Thomson, 1990; Schuckit & Gold, 1988). Finn et al. (1990) found that increased heart rate responsivity was common in multigenerational relatives of alcoholics, suggesting a greater sensitivity to the effects of alcohol and greater reward from alcohol stimulation. More frequent heavy drinking also occurs in individuals who show greater heart rate responsivity (Pihl & Peterson, 1991). Schuckit and Gold (1988) have shown that sons of alcoholics are less sensitive (measured by body sway and subjective intoxication) to the effects of alcohol on behavior and thus report less intoxicating effects from alcohol use. Newlin and Thomson (1990) suggest that sensitivity to alcohol effects is based on rising and falling blood alcohol levels (i.e., a "differentiator model") with increased sensitivity to the rewarding effects when blood alcohol levels are rising and reduced sensitivity to intoxication when these levels are falling. Although all the alcohol sensitivity markers have been identified, they fail to show consistent results as indicators of vulnerability. It is highly likely that these biological markers interact with psychological, personality, and sociocultural variables to increase vulnerability and risk for substance use disorders.

Psychological Aspects of Vulnerability

Personality is one of the more compelling psychological variables that has been related to alcohol and substance abuse, and as with all components of biopsychosocial models, it is a complex phenomenon. Contributing to the complexity is the heterogeneity of alcohol and substance abuse, including the existence of different typologies within substance abuse and the comorbidity of these disorders with other forms of psychopathology. Methodological issues include the nature of the design (cross-sectional vs. longitudinal), the sample (diagnosed/treated vs. general population) and the psychometric properties of the vast number of personality measures that exist.

Personality has long been linked to substance use (the notion of the "alcoholic" or "addictive personality" comes to mind). Over the years, the number of personality dimensions studied has been great, some measures and study designs have been flawed, findings have been inconsistent, and popular notions often have gone without empirical substantiation (Cox, 1987; Lang, 1983). Much of the research has been conducted using measures derived from clinical samples, such as the Minnesota Multiphasic Personality Inventory, which presupposes psychopathology (Sutker & Allain, 1988). Critics of this literature have questioned the utility of personality constructs in differentiating substance abusers from non-substance abusers, and suggested that behavior, rather than personality, is the more compelling indicator of the potential for substance abuse (e.g., Nathan, 1988). More recent research has featured methodologically sound designs and psychometrically sound measures and has examined the role of personality in substance use in a variety of samples ranging from college students to drug abusers in treatment. The results of various studies suggest that adult personality dimensions relate to substance use in a relatively consistent fashion, regardless of the nature of the sample.

One useful development in the area of personality research is the rising prominence of the five-factor model of personality as a useful conceptual framework for the variety of trait names that have served as descriptors of normal personality. As described by Costa and McCrae (1989) in their development of the NEO Personality Inventory (NEO-PI), the five factors are Neuroticism (e.g., anxiety, depression, and impulsiveness); Extraversion (e.g., warmth, assertiveness, and sociability); Openness (e.g., aesthetics and intellectual curiosity); Agreeableness (e.g., altruistic and sympathetic); and Conscientiousness (e.g., persistent, reliable, and task oriented). Martin and Sher (1994) used the NEO-FFI, a short form of the NEO-PI, to examine the links among personality, family history of alcoholism, and alcohol problems in a sample (mainly college students) of young adults. They found relationships between alcohol use disorders and personality such that subjects with alcohol disorders scored higher on neuroticism and lower on conscientiousness and agreeableness than did subjects without alcohol use disorders. Relationships between these personality dimensions and alcohol use also were found in analyses involving subtypes of alcohol disorders (e.g., mood disorders, other drug use, and antisocial personality disorder). Interestingly, within the subtype analyses, neither antisocial personality disorder nor family history of alcoholism was associated with the NEO-FFI scales.

Studies of personality as an indicator of vulnerability also have been conducted in samples in which problems of alcohol and substance abuse have already developed. For example, in a sample of male and female drug abusers on methadone maintenance, those who reported the highest drug use were high on Neuroticism, and low on Extraversion and Conscientiousness. Clients with the lowest drug use were low on Neuroticism and high on the other four factors of the NEO (Gollnisch, 1997; Gollnisch, 1999a). Community-based drug users also showed patterns in which high Neuroticism, and low Agreeableness and Conscientiousness were associated with more drug use and poorer psychosocial functioning (Gollnisch, 1999b). McCormick, Dowd, Quirk, and Zegarra (1998) used the NEO-PI to assess the relationships among personality, coping, and substance use among a large sample of male VA patients. Results indicated that substance abusers scored higher on Neuroticism and lower on Agreeableness and Conscientiousness than did the NEO's normative male sample. There were differences based on primary substance of abuse; when compared to alcohol abusers, polysubstance users had significantly higher scores on Neuroticism and lower scores on Agreeableness and Conscientiousness. Cocaine-only users had higher scores on Extraversion and Openness. The consistency of findings across samples that include college students, community drug users, and substance abusers in treatment suggests that some aspects of personality play an important role in vulnerability to substance use and abuse.

In considering the relationship between personality and alcohol/substance abuse, it is useful to consider broad dimensions of personality rather than specific traits. Sher and Trull (1994) identified three dimensions commonly seen in the literature on alcoholism: neuroticism/emotionality; impulsivity/disinhibition; and extraversion/sociability. They concluded that whereas neuroticism is often correlated with alcohol/substance abuse, its etiological significance has varied based on the nature of the sample and the research design. Generally, neuroticism is not seen as predictive of alcohol abuse for men, but it may have some relevance for women. Most recently, McGue, Slutske, and Iacono (1999) reported that alcoholism is associated with negative affectivity, of the sort included in the neuroticism/emotionality dimension. They controlled for comorbid drug use disorders and found that the behavioral disinhibition identified with alcoholism was present in the subset of alcoholics who also abused drugs. This study highlights the heterogeneity among substance abusers and the need for careful controls in research on personality and substance use.

Impulsivity/disinhibition encompasses sensation seeking, aggressiveness, impulsivity, and other traits that are said to characterize behavioral undercontrol or deviance proneness (Sher, 1991). Individuals with these characteristics are likely to have an earlier age of onset of alcohol and other drug use (see Chassin & Ritter, Chapter 5, this volume), score higher on sensation-seeking measures (Ball et al., 1995; Zuckerman, 1999), be consistent with Cloninger's Type II alcoholics (Cloninger, 1987), and be more likely to meet DSM criteria for childhood conduct disorders and adult antisocial personality disorders (National Institute on Alcohol Abuse and Alcoholism, 1997). Whether behavioral undercontrol is specific to the development of alcoholism (vs. conduct or antisocial personality disorder) is a matter of contention. Nathan (1988) has questioned the distinction between antisocial behavior and antisocial personality suggesting that it is behavior that is key in predicting problems such as alcohol/substance abuse. The issue then becomes the extent to which antisocial personality is uniquely predictive of alcohol and substance abuse. Again, gender differences may exist such that for men, a history of conduct problems, impulsivity, and aggression is linked to alcohol/substance use. Finally, substance abuse is one of the criteria required for the diagnosis of antisocial personality disorder; thus, externalizing behaviors may simply lead to greater exposure to alcohol/drugs (Sher, Walitzer, Wood, & Brent, 1991).

Antisocial personality disorder is the Axis II disorder more strongly associated with vulnerability for substance use disorders (Hesselbrock, 1986; von Knorring, von Knorring, Smigan, Lindberg, & Edholm, 1987; Zuckerman, 1999). Both the ECA (Regier et al., 1990) and NCS (Kessler et al., 1994) show a high prevalence of alcohol and other drug use disorders in individuals with antisocial personality disorders. Morgenstern, Langenbucher, Labouvie, and Miller (1997) examined the relationship between alcohol typologies and the presence of Axis II disorders. Results from this study indicated that antisocial and borderline personality disorders were associated with more severe alcohol dependence. Comorbid antisocial personality disordered individuals displayed characteristics similar to Cloninger's Type II alcoholics and were predominantly male. In contrast, subjects with overlapping borderline personality disorders were more likely female with significant interpersonal, affect regulation, and coping difficulties (Morganstern et al., 1997). Hesselbrock (1986) indicated that antisocial personality disorder usually preceded the development of alcoholism and was associated with a more severe course of alcoholism, an earlier age of onset of substance use, greater impairment, and greater severity of dependence. This pattern also is seen when antisocial personality disorder occurs in individuals with severe mental illness (Hodgins, Toupin, & Cote, 1996; Robins, Tipp, & Przybeck, 1991) and mood disorders (Epstein, Ginsburg, Hesselbrock, & Schwarz, 1994). Often, a childhood diagnosis of conduct disorder and/or hyperactivity is present in antisocial alcoholics (Hesselbrock, 1986; Mueser, Drake, & Wallach, 1998). Zuckerman (1999) has suggested that antisocial personality disorder may be a mediator of the relationship between family history and subsequent vulnerability for alcoholism and drug abuse in offspring. However, Mueser et al. (1998) question the role of antisocial personality disorder as a risk factor in the development of substance use disorders as it may instead be a "by-product" (p. 720) in light of the developmental process from childhood conduct disorder to adult antisocial personality disorder. Alterman and Cacciola (1991) suggest that antisocial personality disorder in substance abusers represents a heterogeneous population that may not lend itself to subtyping based on single dimensions; more complex models of antisociality are needed than those presented in DSM classification systems. Other research suggests that personality characteristics such as sensation seeking (Ball, Carroll, & Rounsaville, 1994; Ball et al., 1995; Sher & Trull, 1994; Zuckerman, 1999) or temperament (Windle, 1994) may comprise the pathway linking antisocial personality disorder and substance abuse disorders. Sher and Trull (1994) have suggested that more sophisticated prospective models, which include consideration of third variables that are related to both impulsivity and substance use, might enhance our understanding of the role of personality in vulnerability.

The role of extraversion/sociability in vulnerability to alcohol/substance abuse is uncertain. Some studies have indicated that sociability is related to frequency of intoxication. However, a key unresolved issue is whether the sociability that is seen as predictive of alcohol problems is sociability per se or a manifestation of disinhibition. Much of the research reviewed here suggests that Extraversion does not play an important role in alcohol or substance abuse (Gollnisch, 1997; Martin & Sher, 1994; McCormick et al., 1998).

Among other psychological factors, psychopathology (Meyer, 1986), stress (Greeley & Oei, 1999), expectancies (Goldman, Del Boca, & Darkes, 1999), and drinking restraint (Collins, 1993) have been examined as predictors of risk for alcoholism and/or other substance abuse. Research on the role of psychopathology has been interwoven into our earlier discussion of research on the prevalence and the types of alcohol and substance abuse and so will not be repeated here. Research on stress, expectancies, and drinking restraint are briefly discussed in turn.

Measures of stressful life events (e.g., Perceived Stress Scale, Daily Hassles Questionnaire, Social Readjustment Rating Scale) have been administered to evaluate the relationship of real-life stressors to the onset of substance abuse or use patterns with results showing no clear links (Cappell & Greeley, 1987). Laboratory studies in which subjects have been subjected to a stressor (e.g., physical, social, or cognitive) also have produced inconsistent results. The same is true for naturalistic studies of stress in which the failure to show a direct link between stress and alcohol use may be due to the heterogeneity of alcohol/drug use disorders, reasons for use, the nature of the stressor, and amounts being consumed (Zuckerman, 1999). Greeley and Oei (1999) suggest that individual differences such as family history of alcoholism (Sher et al., 1991) and positive expectancies (Cooper, Russell, Skinner, Frone, & Mudar, 1992) influence whether individuals drink to reduce stress.

Initiation of substance use has been explained by expectancy theories, which suggest that individuals who develop positive beliefs about the effects of alcohol/drug use are more likely to use substances. Studies using measures such as the Alcohol Expectancy Questionnaire (Brown, Goldman, Inn, & Anderson, 1980) show that substance abusers tend to score higher on positive expectancies, and these scores predict future use even in current nonusers (Christiansen, Roehling, Smith, & Goldman, 1989; Smith, Goldman, Greenbaum, & Christiansen, 1995; Stacy, Widaman, & Marlatt,

1990). Sher et al. (1991) suggest that as expectancies occur prior to actual substance use, they may mediate the relationship between family history of substance abuse and vulnerability. Other researchers (e.g., Goldman & Rather, 1993) suggest that expectancies mediate not only biological aspects but also psychological and social aspects of vulnerability for substance abuse. Further, expectations for positive outcomes may be more frequently observed in heavy versus light drinkers (Stacy, Leigh, & Weingardt, 1994). Theorizing and research on the role of expectancy in alcohol use and abuse continues to grow. What started out as a largely correlational approach to understand drinking is now being broadened to include a variety of research designs as well as consideration of the causal processes involved in substance use (Goldman et al., 1999).

Drinking restraint is a relatively new construct, which research suggests may enhance risk for alcohol and substance abuse. The restraint model posits that the preoccupation with controlling the intake of a substance can paradoxically increase the risk for excessive use of that substance. Collins and Lapp (1991) modified Marlatt and Gordon's (1980, 1985) abstinence violation effect to propose a limit violation effect (LVE) in which the failure to regulate alcohol intake leads to negative reactions that may include negative affect and self-blaming attributions. The drinker consumes more alcohol as a way of repairing the negative mood, thereby drinking to excess. Over time, restrained drinkers experience a cycle in which limit setting leads to failures to regulate intake. Negative reactions to the failures contributes to excessive drinking, which in turn accentuates the need to set limits. Research has provided support for aspects to the model including the occurrence of negative affective reactions following the failure to regulate drinking (Collins & Lapp, 1991; Collins, Lapp, & Izzo, 1994). In studies with social drinkers, drinking restraint has been associated with heavy drinking, binge drinking, and alcohol problems (Bensley, 1991; Collins, 1993). Alcohol and substance abusers have confirmed the factor structure of a measure of drinking restraint (Connors, Collins, Dermen, & Koutsky, 1998), and restraint has predicted treatment outcome for a sample of heavy-drinking women (Walitzer & Connors, 1994).

Social Aspects of Vulnerability

Social aspects of vulnerability include the social environment (family, peers) as well as the physical environment (access to substances, poor neighborhood) in which the individual lives. A key component of the social environment is the family. The family environment, including the substance use behavior of family members, can increase vulnerability to substance abuse. Family members can serve as models of maladaptive drinking, thereby contributing to the development of drinking problems in adults. For example, husbands' heavy drinking has been found to influence the drinking behavior of their wives, some of which may be related to companionable drinking (Hammer & Vaglum, 1989; Leonard & Eiden, 1999; Wilsnack et al., 1984) or the desire to maintain relationships (Covington & Surrey, 1997). In one of the few examinations of the reciprocal influences of husbands' and wives' drinking, Leonard and Eiden (1999) examined drinking behavior of newlyweds through the first year of marriage. They found similarity in the drinking behavior of the couple in the year prior to marriage. In the year following marriage, husbands' drinking predicted wives' drinking, such that a heavy-drinking husband served as a risk factor for his wife. Interestingly, wives' drinking did not influence husbands' drinking, so a light-drinking wife would not be protective for a heavy-drinking husband.

Heavy-drinking peers also can influence the drinking behavior of adults. Evidence from experiments involving adult drinking dyads suggest that the alcohol intake of moderate to heavy drinkers is fairly malleable. When exposed to models of heavy drinking, they increase their alcohol intake. When exposed to models of light drinking, they decrease their alcohol intake (Quigley & Collins, 1999). Interestingly, light drinkers seem to have a "ceiling" on their alcohol intake and thus will not drink to match the alcohol intake of a heavy-drinking model.

Drinking peers often are part of the individual's social network. Social network analyses of drinking have typically focused on the drinking behavior of adolescents and have failed to examine the social networks of adults. However, there is evidence to suggest that adult social networks influence drinking behavior. The density, closeness, and companionship of social networks of male college students have been related to the quantity and frequency of drinking (Fondacaro & Heller, 1983). The number of males in the social network has been related to alcohol consumption; however, the number of females did not influence drinking (Burda & Vaux, 1987). Compared to light drinkers, heavier drinkers were more likely to report alcohol use while socializing in a variety of contexts including with people from work, people from church, neighbors, and close friends (Hilton, 1991).

The social network also can define norms for drinking. To the extent that these norms are perceived to be permissive of drinking, they can provide a context for excessive drinking and alcohol abuse. For example, college students often overestimate the extent to which their friends drink as well as the amount they consume. This misperception can provide an excuse and/or a context for heavy drinking (Baer & Carney, 1993; Baer, Stacy & Larimer, 1991). Rothbard and Leonard (1998) examined social network factors in the alcohol consumption of newly married couples. Analyses indicated that the drinking of friends and spouses accounted for variance in individual drinking, over and above the effects of sociodemographic (e.g., education and ethnicity) and individual difference (e.g., antisocial behavior and expectancies) variables. Interestingly, their results suggested that friends had the most influence on drinking. There were no associations between individual intake and family drinking patterns.

For adults with alcohol problems, the direct and indirect social influences of other drinkers is often cited as a reason for relapse following treatment. Research using Marlatt and Gordon's (1980, 1985) relapse taxonomy has identified direct (e.g., being offered a drink) and indirect (e.g., seeing others drink) social influences as being involved in 12 to 24% of alcohol relapses, dependent on the clinical sample and the phase of treatment during which data were collected (Lowman, Allen, Stout, & Relapse Research Group, 1996). Thus, the sum of the evidence suggests that the individual's social network, particularly peers, influences drinking behavior. Drinkers who spend time with heavy drinkers are at risk for developing and/or maintaining heavy-drinking patterns.

The socioeconomic environment (neighborhood characteristics, crime) also may play a role in vulnerability to alcohol and substance abuse. There is evidence to suggest that although higher socioeconomic status (SES) is related to a greater likelihood of being a drinker, a lower SES is related to a greater likelihood of having problems with alcohol or other drugs (Abbey, Scott, Oliansky, Quinn, & Andreski, 1990). Whether poverty is a cause or a consequence of alcohol or substance use can be a difficult issue. Evidence indicates a downward drift as a function of developing problems of alcohol or substance abuse. As the individual becomes more preoccupied with substance use, the ability to earn money may be compromised. In addition, the individual's limited financial and personal resources are focused on maintaining drug use and are not available for non-drug-related activities that enhance the quality of life for the individual, family, or neighborhood. Evidence also suggests that poverty and related living conditions can increase the propensity to use substances. Neighborhood characteristics that enhance access to alcohol and other drugs, including a high density of alcohol outlets and sellers of illicit drugs, often are cited as reasons for relatively higher rates of alcohol and substance use in poor communities. For example, Abbey et al. (1990) suggested that density of alcohol outlets is related to drinking not through physical availability but, rather, through the drinker's perception that alcohol is readily available. This notion of ready availability also may support norms concerning heavier drinking.

In the United States, poverty and low SES often are related to race/ethnicity. Thus, examination of alcohol problems as related to poverty and/or race/ethnicity can provide useful information on social aspects of vulnerability for abuse of alcohol and other substances. Jones-Webb, Snowden, Herd, Short, & Hannen (1997) examined the role of poverty and race in alcohol problems of male adults. They made the important contribution of considering location-based indicators of SES, such as neighborhood poverty, which had not been considered in previous research; the notion being that environmental (lack of jobs, social instability, antisocial behavior) as well as individual level factors can affect alcohol use. Consistent with earlier individually based studies of SES and alcohol (e.g., Herd, 1994; Jones-Webb, Hsiao, & Hannen, 1995), they found that African American men living in poor neighborhoods reported more alcohol problems than did their European American counterparts. Analyses indicated that even among men of lower SES, neighborhood poverty in African American neighborhoods included more areas with low family incomes and higher unemployment. Interestingly, neighborhood poverty did not have an effect on the alcohol problems of Hispanic men, who, among other things, were more likely to be married and employed as compared to African American men. The studies reviewed here indicate that aspects of the social and physical environment play an important role in adult vulnerability to alcohol and substance abuse. As such, they provide support for consideration of social variables in a biopsychosocial approach to conceptualizing vulnerability to the abuse of alcohol and other substances.

IMPLICATIONS FOR PREVENTION AND TREATMENT

The initiation to alcohol use and many illicit substances typically begins in adolescence. Therefore, prevention efforts during adulthood usually focus on secondary prevention. That is preventing the development of problems related to substance use rather than preventing or delaying the initiation of use, as is the case in primary prevention. The biopsychosocial framework provides a host of possibilities for secondary prevention and/or intervention. Substance abuse is complex and heterogeneous with regard to drugs of choice, the level and nature of biological contributions, and the interplay among the various contributors to enhanced risk. Even if specific biological markers or genes for alcohol or drug use are identified, a direct correspondence between possession of those particular genes or biological markers and the development of a substance abuse disorder is unlikely. It is always possible that some individuals with such markers will not develop a substance use disorder or that individuals who do not possess these biological risk factors will develop a disorder. These truths raise ethical issues related to biological testing and present challenges to secondary prevention efforts at the individual and societal levels. The most obvious point of prevention/ intervention based on biological vulnerability is to educate and counsel those identified as being at risk for problems with alcohol and other drugs so that they can take appropriate action to develop patterns of moderate (nonproblematic) substance use. For example, family-based prevention and treatment programs, which integrate knowledge of biological and social vulnerability factors, could serve as effective points of intervention for high-risk families. Secondary prevention programs to bring problem drinkers into treatment before they develop dependence (e.g., Yates 1988) also might be helpful to persons at high risk.

Similar recommendations can be made with regard to the variety of psychological factors (e.g., personality, expectancies, and restraint) that enhance vulnerability to substance abuse. A major issue is the extent to which we can identify those factors that determine, moderate, or mediate risk. The identification of individual characteristics or constellation of factors that place individuals at risk and implementation of interventions before problems develop could enhance prevention of substance abuse during adulthood. For example, interventions to reduce positive expectancies for alcohol while also enhancing negative expectancies have been suggested as a way to reduce alcohol intake (Jones & McMahon, 1998). Darkes and Goldman (1993, 1998) challenged positive expectancies and produced significant reductions in social/sexual expectancies as well as short-term (up to 6 weeks) reductions in alcohol intake among male college students. Marlatt (1985) has described a "programmed relapse" to disconfirm positive expectancies in problem drinkers. His anecdotal evidence suggests that such disconfirmation of beliefs about the specific effects of alcohol lead to reductions in alcohol intake. Collins's (1993) restraint model suggests a number of strategies for secondary prevention. They include interventions to reduce preoccupation with alcohol, training in behavioral skills to regulate alcohol intake, and training in cognitive and behavioral strategies to cope with negative attributions and affect.

The myriad factors that increase vulnerability may require approaches that go beyond individual risk. Holder (1998) has proposed the adoption of a broader community systems perspective on the prevention of alcohol problems. The approach involves acknowledgment of the complexity of the system that maintains access to alcohol (alcohol makers, distributors and retailers, taxes generated by alcohol sales) as well as the part that alcohol problems play in the broader society (e.g., alcohol-related injuries stimulate the medical sector). This perspective involves a focus on the entire population rather than individuals at highest risk or those who already have been identified as having a problem. Policies that affect the entire community (e.g., policies that lessen the availability of alcohol or reflect community values against risky drinking) can reduce adult vulnerability and related alcohol problems. Successful alcohol policies to date include raising the minimum drinking age to 21 years and passing tax legislation to increase the price of alcohol.

Aspects of a broader community and policy-oriented approach are compatible with harm reduction. As described by Larimer et al. (1998), a harm reduction approach acknowledges the continuum of drinking/substance use and the variable course of the development of problems. This results in a broader set of options for intervention, ranging from approaches linked to the individual (e.g., more detox and treatment for substance abusers) to those that require changes in the physical or social environment and/or changes in policy (e.g., decriminalize use of illicit drugs). They suggest that the best outcomes may result from a combination of methods. Thus, "to reduce the harm of drunk driving, it is possible to combine programs mandated for drunk drivers (e.g., programs designed to modify drinking and prevent intoxicated driving) with physical and social environmental changes (e.g., use of car ignition systems that are designed to foil intoxicated drivers) and policy changes (e.g., reductions in the blood alcohol level used to define driver intoxication)." (Larimer et al., 1998, p. 109).

Evidence suggests that a poor socioeconomic environment contributes to substance abuse (e.g., Jones-Webb et al., 1997). Thus, efforts to improve the socioeconomic environment may be effective for secondary prevention of substance abuse. Such efforts are likely to involve political and social agents at levels ranging from the neighborhood to the federal government. Community action to lessen alcohol and tobacco advertising, such as painting over billboards or complaining about advertising that targets minority populations, has served the purposes of both primary and secondary prevention (Hacker, Collins, & Jacobson, 1987; Maxwell & Jacobson, 1989). Policy changes to lessen alcohol intake and support light to moderate drinking can be implemented in settings varying from primary health care clinics to workplaces. Such policies have been successfully used to control the use of tobacco. Similarly, policies to reduce the availability of alcohol and tobacco using local zoning and licensing laws and other strategies for decreasing the density of outlets in poorer neighborhoods can help to change norms as well as behavior (Abbey et al., 1990; Holder, 1998). At the broadest level, federal and state policies and interventions to alleviate poverty and improve the quality of life for vast numbers of persons in poorer urban and rural areas (e.g., improve education, provide decent housing, and provide job training and meaningful opportunities to work) are interventions that are likely to lessen substance use linked to socioeconomic conditions. Such programs and policies represent the ideal. Reality suggests that changes in public policy and/or funding for social programs to reduce poverty vary with the political climate and that such change is typically slow. Thus, substance abuse linked to socioeconomic conditions is likely to be an ongoing challenge. The other examples of secondary prevention that we have outlined suggest that broadening the base for prevention and treatment will enhance our ability to intervene on many of the factors that contribute to adult vulnerability to alcohol and substance abuse.

FUTURE DIRECTIONS FOR RESEARCH

Research to enhance our understanding of biological contributions to vulnerability to substance abuse is occurring at levels ranging from the molecular genetic to the entire organism. This research is taking place in the context of developments in biological technology and in our understanding and mapping of the human genome. Future research should focus on resolving controversies in the biological research to date, including various methodological issues, and on improving our understanding of the processes involved in various biological markers. Many studies use single-typology frameworks (e.g., familial alcoholics and antisocial personality disorder), yet research suggests that there is much heterogeneity in the nature of substance abuse problems and the factors that contribute to vulnerability to alcohol and substance abuse. Babor (1994) has suggested that the use of multidimensional typologies may be a better approach to addressing the complexities involved in the etiology of substance use disorders.

Even within typologies, consideration of biopsychosocial characteristics such as gender (biological), negative affect and stress (psychological), and socioeconomic status (social) is necessary for a better understanding of vulnerability. For example, research on biological factors is beginning to clarify alcoholism in men, but findings for women remain inconsistent. Studies on women are limited due to sample size and the tendency to compare genders on only one dimension (e.g., psychopathology). Variables such as age and sociocultural factors affecting use patterns (Del Boca, 1994), victimization (Miller, Downs, Gondoli, & Keil, 1987; Wilsnack, Vogeltanz, Klassen, & Harris, 1997), or the phenotypic expression of disorders (Hesselbrock & Hesselbrock, 1997) may better account for gender differences. Gender effects also may be due to sociocultural variables related to the initiation of use and certain patterns of use (e.g., companion drinking). All these topics are likely to be fruitful areas for future research.

Among psychological factors, more research on the role of personality is clearly needed. The etiological significance of the high level of association between certain personality characteristics (e.g., antisocial personality) and substance use needs to be clarified. Neuroticism and negative affect may (see McGue et al., 1999) or may not be a causal variable in substance abuse. The fact that negative affect plays an important role in women's substance abuse is of interest, although the higher rates of depression and anxiety in female alcoholics may simply reflect the high base rates in the general population of women (Regier et al., 1990; Ross, 1995; Ross & Shirley, 1997) or gender-based biases in the diagnosis of certain disorders. Cunningham, Sobell, Gavin, and Annis's (1995) suggestion that negative affect may represent a shift in drinking patterns, from abuse to dependence, can serve as a useful point of departure for new research. The pharmacological properties of specific drugs (e.g., alcohol is a central nervous system depressant) also influences affect. The role of stress is unclear as stress is both positive and negative in valence. It is more likely that perceived predictability and controllability of stress are related to vulnerability, a pattern clearly documented in the development of certain chronic illnesses (Taylor & Brown, 1988).

Individual difference variables such as expectancies and restrained drinking may mediate vulnerability to substance abuse. In a review of the expectancy literature, Smith (1994) suggests that expectancies play a variety of roles. They precede the onset of teenage alcohol use, predict future drinking onset and problematic use, contribute to further progression of abusive use patterns via more positive expectancies, mediate the effects of family drinking history, and interact with personality variables to predict risk for problem drinking. Collins (1993) has suggested that drinking restraint can enhance the move from moderate social drinking to excessive drinking and alcohol problems. Future research on the causal role of expectancies and the processes through which cognitive factors such as restraint and expectancies influence vulnerability and/or interact with other components of a biopsychosocial model could enhance our knowledge of substance abuse (Collins, 1993; Goldman et al., 1999).

The role of social factors in vulnerability for alcohol and substance abuse is understudied and thus offers many opportunities for new research. A particularly difficult question is whether poverty is a cause or consequence of alcohol and substance abuse. The influence of stereotypical gender roles, as in the case of companionable drinking, in women's drinking also is worthy of further study. Regardless of the specific issue being studied, a multidisciplinary biopsychosocial perspective is likely to increase our understanding of adult vulnerability to substance abuse.

Research on almost any topic related to substance abuse policy, particularly as it pertains to secondary prevention, is very much needed. Policy change can occur at many levels ranging from restrictions on smoking to increases in taxes on licit drugs; thus researchers have a wide range of areas in which they can make a contribution. One important concern across all areas of research is the dissemination of findings. As we develop knowledge about policies and strategies that influence substance use behavior, it is incumbent that researchers make this knowledge available to the lay public, persons in positions of influence, and policymakers. Dissemination of research findings may not produce hoped for changes. For example, there is a body of research suggesting that treatment can be effective in lessening substance abuse and related social problems, yet current drug control policy focuses on criminal sanctions and interdiction (Massing, 1998). Research on effective strategies for disseminating research findings as well as the development and implementation of policies also seem important topics for the future.

REFERENCES

Abbey, A., Scott, R. O., Oliansky, D. M., Quinn, B., & Andreski, P. M. (1990). Subjective, social, and physical availability: II. Their simultaneous effects on alcohol consumption. *International Journal of the Addictions, 25*, 1011–1023.

Adams, H. E., & Cassidy, J. F. (1993). The classification of abnormal behavior: An overview. In P. B. Sutker & H. E. Adams (Eds.), *Comprehensive handbook of psychopathology* (2nd ed., pp. 3–25). New York: Plenum.

Alterman, A. I., & Cacciola, J. S. (1991). The antisocial personality disorder diagnosis in substance abusers: Problems and issues. *Journal of Nervous and Mental Disease, 179*, 401–409.

American Psychiatric Association. (1994). *Diagnostic and statistical manual of mental disorders* (4th ed.). Washington, DC: Author.

Babor, T. F. (1994). Introduction: Method and theory in the classification of alcoholics. In T. F. Babor, V. Hesselbrock, R. E. Meyer, & W. Shoemaker (Eds.), *Types of alcoholics: Evidence from clinical, experimental, and genetic research* (pp. 1–6). New York: New York Academy of Sciences.

Babor, T. F., Dolinsky, Z. S., Meyer, R. E., Hesselbrock, M., Hofmann, M., & Tennen, H. (1992). Types of alcoholics: Concurrent and predictive validity of some common classification schemes. *British Journal of Addictions, 87,* 1415–1431.

Baer, J. S., & Carney, M. M. (1993). Biases in the perceptions of the consequences of alcohol use among college students. *Journal of Studies on Alcohol, 54,* 54–60.

Baer, J. S., Stacy, A.W., & Larimer, M. (1991). Biases in the perception of drinking norms among college students. *Journal of Studies on Alcohol, 52,* 540–586.

Ball, S. A., Carroll, K. M., Babor, T. F., & Rounsaville, B. J. (1995). Subtypes of cocaine abusers: Support for a Type A–Type B distinction. *Journal of Consulting and Clinical Psychology, 63,* 115–124.

Ball, S. A., Carroll, K. M., & Rounsaville, B. J. (1994). Sensation seeking, substance abuse, and psychopathology in treatment-seeking and community cocaine abusers. *Journal of Consulting and Clinical Psychology, 62,* 1053–1057.

Bandura, A. (1969). *Principles of behavior modification.* New York: Holt, Rinehart & Winston.

Begleiter, H., & Porjesz, B. (1988). Neurophysiological dysfunction in alcoholism. In R. M. Rose & J. E. Barrett (Eds.), *Alcoholism: Origins and outcome* (pp. 157–172). New York: Raven Press.

Begleiter, H., Porjesz, B., Bihari, B., & Kissin, G. (1984). Event-related brain potentials in boys at risk for alcoholism. *Science, 225,* 1493–1496.

Bensley, L. S. (1991). Construct validity evidence for the interpretation of drinking restraint as a response conflict. *Addictive Behaviors, 16,* 139–150.

Blum, K., Nobel, E. P., Sheridan, P. J., Montgomery, A., Ritchie, T., Jagadeeswaran, P., Nogami, H., Briggs, A. H., & Cohn, J. B. (1990). Allelic association of human dopamine D2 receptor gene in alcoholism. *Journal of the American Medical Association, 263,* 2055–2060.

Brown, J., Babor, T. F., Litt, M. D., & Kranzler, H. R. (1994). The Type A/Type B distinction: Subtyping alcoholics according to indicators of vulnerability and severity. In T. F. Babor, V. Hesselbrock, R. E. Meyer, & W. Shoemaker (Eds.), *Types of alcoholics: Evidence from clinical, experimental, and genetic research* (pp. 23–33). New York: New York Academy of Sciences.

Brown, S. A., Goldman, M. S., Inn, A., & Anderson, L. R. (1980). Expectations of reinforcement from alcohol: Their domain and relation to drinking patterns. *Journal of Consulting and Clinical Psychology, 48,* 419–426.

Brown, S. A., & Schuckit, M. A. (1988). Changes in depression among abstinent alcoholics. *Journal of Studies on Alcohol, 49,* 412–417.

Burda, P.C., & Vaux, A.C. (1987). The social support process in men: Overcoming sex-role obstacles. *Human Relations, 40,* 31–44.

Cappell, H., & Greeley, J. (1987). Alcohol and tension reduction: An update on research and theory. In H. T. Blane & K. E. Leonard (Eds.), *Psychological theories of drinking and alcoholism* (pp. 15–54). New York: Guilford Press.

Christiansen, B. A., Roehling, P. V., Smith, G. T., & Goldman, M .S. (1989). Using alcohol expectancies to predict adolescent drinking behavior after one year. *Journal of Consulting and Clinical Psychology, 57,* 93–99.

Cloninger, R. (1987). Neurogenetic adaptive mechanisms in alcoholism. *Science, 236,* 410–416.

Cloninger, R., Bohman, M., & Sigvardsson, S. (1981). Inheritance of alcohol abuse. *Archives of General Psychiatry, 38,* 861–868.

Collins, R. L. (1993). Drinking restraint and risk for alcohol abuse. *Experimental and Clinical Psychopharmacology, 1,* 44–54.

Collins, R. L, & Lapp, W. M. (1991). Restraint and attributions: Evidence of the abstinence violation effect in alcohol consumption. *Cognitive Therapy and Research, 15,* 69–84.

Collins, R. L., Lapp, W. M., & Izzo, C. V. (1994). Affective and behavioral reactions to the violation of limits on alcohol consumption. *Journal of Studies on Alcohol, 55,* 475–486.

Connors, G. J., Collins, L. R., Dermen, K. H., & Koutsky, J. R. (1998). Substance use restraint: An extension of the construct to a clinical population. *Cognitive Therapy and Research, 22,* 75–87.

Cooper, M. L., Russell, M., Skinner, J. B., Frone, M. R., & Mudar, P. (1992). Stress and alcohol use: Moderating effects of gender, coping and alcohol expectancies. *Journal of Abnormal Psychology, 101,* 139–152.

Costa, P. T., & McCrae, R. R. (1989). *NEO-PI/FFI Manual Supplement.* Odessa, FL: Psychological Assessment Resources.

Covington, S. S., & Surrey, J. L. (1997). The relational model of women's psychological development: Implications for substance abuse. In R. W. Wilsnack & S. C. Wilsnack (Eds.), *Gender and alcohol: Individual and social perspectives* (pp. 335–351). New Brunswick, NJ: Rutgers Center of Alcohol Studies.

Cox, W. M. (1987). Personality theory and research. In H. T. Blane & K. E. Leonard (Eds.), *Psychological theories of drinking and alcoholism* (pp. 55–89). New York: Guilford Press.

Cunningham, J. A., Sobell, M. B., Gavin, D. R., & Annis, H. M. (1995). Heavy drinking and negative affective situations in a general population and a treatment sample: Alternative explanations. *Psychology of Addictive Behaviors, 9,* 123–127.

Darkes, J., & Goldman, M. S. (1993). Expectancy challenge and drinking reduction: Experimental evidence for a mediational process. *Journal of Consulting and Clinical Psychology, 61,* 344–353.

Darkes, J., & Goldman, M. S. (1998). Expectancy challenge and drinking reduction: Process and structure in the alcohol expectancy network. *Experimental and Clinical Psychopharmacology, 6,* 64–76.

Del Boca, F. K. (1994). Sex, gender, and alcoholic typologies. In T. F. Babor, V. Hesselbrock, R. E. Meyer, & W. Shoemaker (Eds.), *Types of alcoholics: Evidence from clinical, experimental,and genetic research* (pp. 34–48). New York: New York Academy of Sciences.

Edwards, G., Arif, A., & Hodgson, R . J. (1981). Nomenclature and classification of drug and alcohol related problems. *Bulletin of WHO, 59,* 225–242.

Epstein, E. E., Ginsburg, B., Hesselbrock, V. M., & Schwarz, J. C. (1994). Alcohol and drug abusers subtyped by antisocial personality and primary or secondary depression disorder. In T. F. Babor, V. Hesselbrock, R. E. Meyer, & W. Shoemaker (Eds.), *Types of alcoholics: Evidence from clinical, experimental, and genetic research* (pp. 187–201). New York: New York Academy of Sciences.

Finn, P. R., Zeitouni, N. C., & Pihl, R. O. (1990). Effects of alcohol on psycho-physiological hyperreactivity to nonaversive and aversive stimuli in men at high risk for alcoholism. *Journal of Abnormal Psychology, 99,* 79–85.

Fondacaro, M. R., & Heller, K. (1983). Social support factors and drinking among college student males. *Journal of Youth and Adolescence, 10,* 363–383.

Goldman, M.S., Del Boca, F. K., & Darkes, J. (1999). Alcohol expectancy theory: The application of cognitive neuroscience. In K. E. Leonard & H. T. Blane (Eds.), *Psychological theories of drinking and alcoholism* (2nd ed. pp. 203–246). New York: Guilford Press.

Goldman, M. S., & Rather, B. C. (1993). Substance use disorders: Cognitive models and architecture. In K. Dobson & P. C. Kendall (Eds.), *Psychopathology and cognition* (pp. 245–292). San Diego: Academic Press.

Gollnisch, G. (1997). Multiple predictors of illicit drug use in methadone maintenance clients. *Addictive Behaviors, 22,* 353–366.

Gollnisch, G. (1999a) *Cluster-analytic profiles on methadone maintenance clients.* Unpublished manuscript. Buffalo, NY: Research Institute on Addictions.

Gollnisch, G. (1999b) *The validity of the five-factor model of personality with community-based drug users.* Unpublished manuscript. Buffalo, NY: Research Institute on Addictions.

Goodwin, D. W., Schulsinger, F., Knopf, J., Mednick, S., & Guze, S. B. (1977). Alcoholism and depression in adopted daughters of alcoholics. *Archives of General Psychiatry, 34,* 1005–1009.

Grant, B. F. (1997). Prevalence and correlates of alcohol use and DSM-IV alcohol dependence in the United States: Results of the National Longitudinal Alcohol Epidemiologic Survey. *Journal of Studies on Alcohol, 58,* 464–473.

Greeley, J., & Oei, T. (1999). Alcohol and tension reduction. In K. E. Leonard & H. T. Blane (Eds.), *Psychological theories of drinking and alcoholism* (2nd ed., pp. 14–53). New York: Guilford Press.

Greenfield, T. K., & Rogers, J. D. (1999). Who drinks most of the alcohol in the U.S.?: The policy implications. *Journal of Studies on Alcohol, 60,* 78–89.

Hacker, G. A., Collins, R., & Jacobson, M. (1987). *Marketing booze to Blacks.* Washington, DC: Center for Science in the Public Interest.

Hammer, T., & Vaglum, P. (1989). The increase in alcohol consumption among women: A phenomenon related to accessibility or stress? A general population study. *British Journal of Addiction, 84,* 767–775.

Herd, D. (1994). Predicting drinking problems among black and white men: Results from a national survey. *Journal of Studies on Alcohol, 55,* 61–71.

Hesselbrock, M. (1986). Alcoholic typologies: A review of empirical evaluations of common classification schemes. In M. Galanter (Ed.), *Recent developments in alcoholism* (4th ed., pp. 191–206). New York: Plenum.

Hesselbrock, M., & Hesselbrock, V. (1997). Gender, alcoholism, and psychiatric comorbidity. In R. W. Wilsnack & S. C. Wilsnack (Eds.), *Gender and alcohol: Individual and social perspectives* (pp. 49–71). New Brunswick, NJ: Rutgers Center of Alcohol Studies.

Hilton, M. E. (1991). Regional diversity in U.S. drinking practices. In W. B. Clark & M. E. Hilton (Eds.), *Alcohol in America: Drinking practices and problems* (pp. 256–279). Albany: State University of New York Press.

Hodgins, S., Toupin, J., & Cote, G. (1996). Schizophrenia and antisocial personality disorder: A criminal combination. In L. B. Schlesinger (Ed.), *Explora-*

tions in criminal psychopathology: Clinical syndromes with forensic implications (pp. 217–237). Springfield, IL: Charles C Thomas.

Holder, H. D. (1998). *Alcohol and the community.* Cambridge, UK: Cambridge University Press.

Jaffe, J. (1985). Drug addiction and drug abuse. In A. Gilman, L. Goodman, T. Rall, & F. Murad (Eds.), *The pharmacological basis of therapeutics* (7th ed., pp. 532–581). New York: Macmillan.

Jellinek, E. M. (1960). *The disease concept of alcoholism.* New Haven, CT: College and University Press.

Jones, B. T., & McMahon, J. (1998). Alcohol motivation as outcome expectancies. In W. R. Miller & N. Heather (Eds.), *Treating addictive behaviors* (2nd ed., pp. 75–91). New York: Plenum.

Jones-Webb, R J., Hsiao, C. Y., & Hannan, P. (1995). Relationships between socio-economic status and drinking problems among black and white men. *Alcoholism: Clinical and Experimental Research, 19,* 623–627.

Jones-Webb, R. J., Snowden, L., Herd, D., Short, B., & Hannan, P. (1997). Alcohol-related problems among black, Hispanic and white men: The contribution of neighborhood poverty. *Journal of Studies on Alcohol, 58,* 539–545.

Kalant, H. (1989). The nature of addiction: An analysis of the problem. In A. Goldstein (Ed.), *Molecular and cellular aspects of the drug addictions* (pp. 1–28). New York: Springer-Verlag.

Kessler, R. C., McGonagh, K. A., Zhao, S., Nelson, C. B., Hughes, M., Eshleman, S., Wittchen, U., & Kendler, K. S. (1994). Lifetime and 12-month prevalence of DMI-III-R psychiatric disorders in the United States. *Archives of General Psychiatry, 51,* 8–19.

Lang, A. R. (1983). Addictive personality: A viable construct? In P. K. Levison, D. R. Gerstein, & D. R. Maloff (Eds.), *Commonalities in substance abuse and habitual behavior* (pp. 157–235). Lexington, MA: Lexington Books.

Larimer, M. E., Marlatt, G. A., Baer, J. S., Quigley, L. A., Blume, A. W., & Hawkins, E. H. (1998). Harm reduction for alcohol problems: Expanding access to and acceptability of prevention and treatment services. In G. A. Marlatt (Ed.), *Harm reduction* (pp. 69–121). New York: Guilford Press.

Leonard, K. E., & Eiden, R. D. (1999). Husband's and wife's drinking: Unilateral or bilateral influences among newlyweds in a general population sample. *Journal of Studies on Alcohol, 13,* 130–138.

Lowman, C., Allen, J. P., Stout, R. L., & Relapse Research Group. (1996). Replication and extension of Marlatt's taxonomy of relapse precipitants: Overview of procedures and results. *Addiction, 91,* S51–S71.

Maisto, S. A., Carey, K. B., & Bradizza, C. M. (1999). Social learning theory. In K. E. Leonard & H. T. Blane (Eds.), *Psychological theories of drinking and alcoholism* (2nd ed., pp. 106–163). New York: Guilford Press.

Marlatt, G. A. (1985). Cognitive assessment and intervention procedures for relapse prevention. In G. A. Marlatt & J. R. Gordon (Eds.), *Relapse prevention: Maintenance strategies in the treatment of addictive behaviors* (pp. 201–279). New York: Guilford Press.

Marlatt, G. A., & Gordon, J. R. (1980). Determinants of relapse: Implications for the maintenance of behavior change. In P. O. Davidson & S. M. Davidson (Eds.), *Behavioral medicine: Changing health lifestyles* (pp. 410–452). New York: Brunner/Mazel.

Marlatt, G. A. & Gordon, J. R. (1985). *Relapse prevention: Maintenance strategies in the treatment of addictive behaviors.* New York: Guilford Press.

Martin, E. D., & Sher, K. J. (1994). Family history of alcoholism, alcohol use disorders and the five-factor model of personality. *Journal of Studies on Alcohol, 55,* 81–90.

Massing, M. (1998). The fix: Under the Nixon Administration, America had an effective drug policy. We should restore it (Nixon was right). New York: Simon & Schuster.

Maxwell, B., & Jacobson, M. (1989). *Marketing disease to Hispanics.* Washington, DC: Center for Science in the Public Interest.

McBride, W. J., Murphy, J. M., Lumeng, L., & Li, T. K. (1990). Serotonin, dopamine, and GABA involvement in alcohol drinking of selectively bred rats. *Alcohol, 7,* 199–205.

McCormick, R. A., Dowd, E. T., Quirk, S., & Zegarra, J. H. (1998). The relationship of the NEO-PI performance to coping styles, patterns of use, and triggers for use among substance abusers. *Addictive Behaviors, 23,* 497–507.

McGue, M. K. (1994). Genes, environment, and the etiology of alcoholism. In R. A. Zucker, G. Boyd, & J. Howard (Eds.), *The development of alcohol problems: Exploring the biopsychosocial matrix of risk* (NIAAA Research Monograph 26, NIH Pub. No. 94-3495, pp. 1–40). Rockville, MD: National Institute on Alcohol Abuse and Alcoholism.

McGue, M. K., Pickens, R. W., & Svikis, D. S. (1992). Sex and age effects on the inheritance of alcohol problems: A twin study. *Journal of Abnormal Psychology, 101,* 3–17.

McGue, M. K., Slutske, W., & Iacono, W. G. (1999). Personality and substance use disorders: II. Alcoholism versus drug use disorders. *Journal of Consulting and Clinical Psychology, 67,* 394–404.

Merikangas, K. R. (1990). The genetic epidemiology of alcoholism. *Psychological Medicine, 20,* 11–22.

Merry, J. (1966). The "loss of control" myth. *Lancet, 1,* 1257–1258.

Meyer, R. E. (1986). How to understand the relationship between psychopathology and addictive disorders: Another example of the chicken and the egg. In R. E. Meyer (Ed.), *Psychopathology and addictive disorders* (pp. 3–16). New York: Guilford Press.

Miller, B. A., Downs, W. R., Gondoli, D. M., & Keil, A. (1987). The role of childhood sexual abuse in the development of alcoholism in women. *Violence and Victims, 2,* 157–172.

Morey, L. C., & Skinner, H. A. (1986). Empirically derived classifications of alcohol-related problems. In M. Galanter (Ed.), *Recent developments in alcoholism* (5th ed., pp. 45–168). New York: Plenum.

Morgenstern, J., Langenbucher, J., Labouvie, E., & Miller, K. J. (1997). The comorbidity of alcoholism and personality disorders in a clinical population: Prevalence rates and relation to alcohol typology variables. *Journal of Abnormal Psychology, 106,* 74–84.

Mueser, K. T., Drake, R. E., & Wallach, M. A. (1998). Dual diagnosis: A review of etiological theories. *Addictive Behaviors, 23,* 717–734.

Nathan, P. E. (1988). The addictive personality is the behavior of the addict. *Journal of Consulting and Clinical Psychology, 56,* 183–188.

Nathan, P. E. (1991). Substance use disorders in the DSM-IV. *Journal of Abnormal Psychology, 100*, 356–361.

National Institute on Alcohol Abuse and Alcoholism. (1997). *Ninth special report to the U.S. Congress on alcohol and health* (97-4017). Washington, DC: U.S. Department of Health & Human Services.

Newlin, D. B. (1994). Alcohol challenge in high-risk individuals. In R. Zucker, G. Boyd, & J. Howard (Eds.), *The development of alcohol problems: Exploring the biopsychosocial matrix of risk* (NIAAA Research Monograph 26, NIH Pub. No. 94-3495, pp. 47–68). Rockville, MD: National Institute on Alcohol Abuse and Alcoholism.

Newlin, D. B., & Thomson, J. B. (1990). Alcohol challenge with sons of alcoholics: A critical review and analysis. *Psychological Bulletin, 108*, 383–402.

Pihl, R. O., & Peterson, J. B. (1991). Attention-deficit hyperactivity disorder, childhood conduct disorder, and alcoholism: Is there an association? *Alcohol Health and Research World, 15*, 25–31.

Polich, J., & Bloom, F. E. (1988). Event-related brain potentials in individuals at high and low risk for developing alcoholism: Failure to replicate. *Alcoholism: Clinical and Experimental Research, 12*, 368–373.

Polich, J., Pollock, V. E., & Bloom, F. E. (1994). Meta-analysis of P300 amplitude from males at risk for alcoholism. *Psychological Bulletin, 115*, 55–73.

Quigley, B. M., & Collins, L. R. (1999). The modeling of alcohol consumption: A meta-analytic review. *Journal of Studies on Alcohol, 60*, 90–98.

Regier, D. A., Farmer, M. E., Rae, D. S., Locke, B. Z., Keith, S. J., Judd, L. L., & Goodwin, F. K. (1990). Comorbidity of mental disorders with alcohol and other drug abuse: Results from the Epidemiologic Catchment Area (ECA) Study. *Journal of the American Medical Association, 264*, 2511–2518.

Robins, L., Tipp, J., & Przybeck, T. R. (1991). Antisocial personality. In L. Robins & D. A. Regier (Eds.), *Psychiatric disorders in America: The Epidemiologic Catchment Area Study* (pp. 285–290). New York: Free Press.

Ross, H. E. (1995). DSM-III-R alcohol abuse and dependence and psychiatric comorbidity in Ontario: Results from the Mental Health Supplement to the Ontario Health Survey. *Drug and Alcohol Dependence, 39*, 111–128.

Ross, H. E., & Shirley, M. (1997). Life-time problem drinking and psychiatric comorbidity among Ontario women. *Addiction, 92*, 183–196.

Rothbard, J. C., & Leonard, K. E. (1998, November). *Alcohol use in adulthood: Peer and family influences.* Paper presented at the meeting of the Association for Advancement of Behavior Therapy, Washington, DC.

Rounsaville, B .J., Dolinsky, Z. S., Babor, T. F., & Meyer, R. E. (1987). Psychopathology as a predictor of treatment outcome in alcoholics. *Archives of General Psychiatry, 44*, 505–513.

Schuckit, M. A. (1985). The clinical implications of primary diagnostic groups among alcoholics. *Archives of General Psychiatry, 42*, 1043–1049.

Schuckit, M. A., & Gold, E. O. (1988). A simultaneous evaluation of multiple markers of ethanol/placebo challenges in sons of alcoholics and controls. *Archives of General Psychiatry, 45*, 211–216.

Schuckit, M. A., & Monteiro, M. G. (1988). Alcoholism, anxiety and depression. *British Journal of Addiction, 83*, 1373–1380.

Searles, J. S. (1988). The role of genetics in the pathogenesis of alcoholism. *Journal of Abnormal Psychology, 97*, 153–167.

Sher, K. J. (1991). *Children of alcoholics: A critical appraisal of theory and research.* Chicago: University of Chicago Press.

Sher, K. J., & Trull, T. J. (1994). Personality and disinhibitory psychopathology: Alcoholism and antisocial personality disorder. *Journal of Abnormal Psychology, 103,* 92–102.

Sher, K. J., Walitzer, K. S., Wood, P. K., & Brent, E. E. (1991). Characteristics of children of alcoholics: Putative risk factors, substance use and abuse, and psychopathology. *Journal of Abnormal Psychology, 100,* 427–448.

Smith, G. T. (1994). Psychological expectancy as mediator of vulnerability to alcoholism. In T. F. Babor, V. Hesselbrock, R. E. Meyer, & W. Shoemaker (Eds.), *Types of alcoholics: Evidence from clinical, experimental, and genetic research* (pp. 165–171). New York: New York Academy of Sciences.

Smith, G. T., Goldman, M. S., Greenbaum, P. E., & Christiansen, B. A. (1995). Expectancy for social facilitation from drinking: The divergent paths of high-expectancy and low-expectancy adolescents. *Journal of Abnormal Psychology, 104,* 32–40.

Stacy, A. W., Leigh, B. C., & Weingardt, K. R. (1994). Memory accessibility and association of alcohol use and its positive outcomes. *Experimental and Clinical Psychopharmacology, 2,* 269–282.

Stacy, A. W., Widaman, K. F., & Marlatt, A. G. (1990). Expectancy models of alcohol use. *Journal of Personality and Social Psychology, 58,* 918–928.

Sutker, P. B., & Allain, A. N., Jr. (1988). Issues in personality conceptualizations of addictive behaviors. *Journal of Consulting and Clinical Psychology, 56,* 172–182.

Tabakoff, B., Whelan, J. P., & Hoffman, P. L. (1990). Two biological markers of alcoholism. In R. Cloninger & H. Begleiter (Eds.), *Genetics and biology of alcoholism* (pp. 195–204). Cold Spring Harbor, NY: Cold Spring Harbor Laboratory Press.

Taylor, S. E., & Brown, J. (1988). Illusion and well-being: A social psychological perspective on mental health. *Psychological Bulletin, 103,* 193–210.

Turner, E., Ewing, J., Shilling, P., Smith, T. L., Irwin, M., Schuckit, M. A., & Kelsoe, J. R. (1992). Lack of association between an RFLP near the D2 dopamine receptor gene and severe alcoholism. *Biological Psychiatry, 31,* 285–290.

Vaillant, G. E. (1983). *The natural history of alcoholism: Causes, patterns, and paths to recovery.* Cambridge, MA: Harvard University Press.

von Knorring, A. L., Hallman, J., von Knorring, L., & Oreland, L. (1991). Platelet monoamine oxidase activity in type 1 and type 2 alcoholism. *Alcohol, 26,* 409–416.

von Knorring, L., von Knorring, A. L., Smigan, L., Lindberg, U., & Edholm, M. (1987). Personality traits in subtypes of alcoholics. *Journal of Studies on Alcohol, 48,* 523–527.

Walitzer, K. S., & Connors, G. J. (1994, June). *Drinking restraint and mediation of changes in heavy drinking.* Poster presented at the meeting of the Research Society on Alcoholism, Maui, HI.

Warner, L. A., Kessler, R. C., Hughes, M., Anthony, J. C., & Nelson, C. B. (1995). Prevalence and correlates of drug use and dependence in the United States: Results from the National Comorbidity Survey. *Archives of General Psychiatry, 52,* 219–229.

Wilsnack, S. C., Vogeltanz, N. D., Klassen, A. D., & Harris, T. R. (1997). Childhood sexual abuse and women's substance abuse: National survey findings. *Journal of Studies on Alcohol, 58,* 264–271.

Wilsnack, S. C., Wilsnack, R. W., & Klassen, A. D. (1984). Drinking and drinking problems among women in a U.S. national survey. *Alcohol, Health, and Research World, 9,* 3–13.

Windle, M. (1994). Temperamental inhibition and activation: Hormonal and psychosocial correlates and associated psychiatric disorders. *Personality and Individual Differences, 17,* 61–70.

Yates, F. E. (1988). The evaluation of a "Co-operative Counseling" alcohol service which uses family and affected others to reach and influence problem drinkers. *British Journal of Addiction, 83,* 1309–1319.

Zucker, R. A. (1994). Pathways to alcohol problems and alcoholism: A developmental account of the evidence for multiple alcoholisms and for contextual contributions to risk. In R. Zucker, G. Boyd, & J. Howard (Eds.), *The development of alcohol problems: Exploring biopsychosocial matrix of risk* (NIAAA Research Monograph 26, NIH Pub. 94-3495, pp. 255–290). Rockville, MD: National Institute on Alcohol Abuse and Alcoholism.

Zucker, R. A., & Gomberg, E. S. L. (1986). Etiology of alcoholism reconsidered: The case for a biopsychosocial process. *American Psychologist, 41,* 783–793.

Zuckerman, M. (1999). *Vulnerability to psychopathology: A biosocial model.* Washington, DC: American Psychological Association.

7

Vulnerability to Substance Use Disorders across the Lifespan

LAURIE CHASSIN
R. LORRIANE COLLINS
JENNIFER RITTER
MARIELA C. SHIRLEY

ESTABLISHING COMMON GROUND: SIMILAR THEMES AND ISSUES ACROSS THE LIFESPAN

Models of vulnerability to substance use and abuse in adolescence and adulthood suggest several areas of overlap and continuity. We highlight four common areas of vulnerability across the lifespan: genetic and biological factors, temperament and personality factors, social environmental influences, and cognitive influences, particularly expectancies about the effects of alcohol and drugs.

A number of different genetic and biological factors have been postulated for explaining familial transmission of risk for substance abuse, particularly alcohol abuse. Theoretically, several of these factors might be expected to operate in similar ways across the lifespan. For example, it has been hypothesized that children of alcoholics obtain different psychopharmacological effects of alcohol, and these effects might be expected to be present in both childhood, adolescence, and adulthood. However, the effects of these heritable individual differences would be expressed only when the individual has access to abusable substances and begins to experiment with their use, usually in adolescence or young adulthood. Because substance use involves the behavior of ingesting a drug, biology does not ordain destiny. Even in individuals at high biological risk, environmental and other psychosocial factors can influence the development and expression of a substance use disorder. If use does not take place (e.g., some offspring of alcoholics choose to abstain from using alcohol), then biological risk is not expressed in a substance abuse disorder.

Temperament and personality subsume a variety of characteristics ranging from deficits in self-regulation to levels of emotional responsivity. While still popular in lay circles, the notion of an alcoholic or addictive personality has not been supported by research. However, certain temperamental characteristics involving behavioral undercontrol and disregulation have been identified in childhood or early adolescence as predicting substance abuse in adulthood. These include impulsivity, difficulty concentrating, and negative affectivity. Similar characteristics have been identified in adult substance abusers, who often are characterized by high levels of neuroticism (negative affectivity) and low levels of conscientiousness expressed in low behavioral control and regulation (Gollnisch, 1997; McGue, Slutske, & Iacano, 1999). Thus, although specific indicators or measures of temperament and personality differ across different age groups, there seems to be substantial continuity in their underlying contribution to vulnerability for substance abuse.

Social and cultural influences play important roles in both adolescence and adulthood. Social networks (e.g., family and peers) that approve, tolerate, or model substance use encourage use, thereby increasing vulnerability for abuse. The specific sources of influence may vary somewhat at different stages of development. Initially parents/family may serve as models, whereas peers become important during adolescence and partners/spouses become more important during adulthood. The role of the socioeconomic environment is not clear. However, risks related to poverty, deteriorated neighborhoods, high crime, and easy access to drugs are likely to play a role in substance use in both adolescence and adulthood. Similarly, the norms and values of the individual's social context (including advertising and policies related to access and use of licit substances) remain constant influences on substance use and abuse across the lifespan.

Socialization effects also point to similarities across the lifespan. That is, in both adolescence and adulthood, the demands of successful role performance can inhibit substance use. The content of the roles may be different. During adolescence, school and athletic performance might be important inhibitors of substance use, whereas during adulthood, work and parental roles may become important. For example, educational attainment during adolescence is lower in those teens who drink more frequently than in those who drink less frequently (Cook & Moore, 1993). Similarly, married men and women report drinking less (particularly binge drinking) than do their divorced and single counterparts (National Institute on Alcohol Abuse and Alcoholism, 1997). These findings illustrate the fact that disruption of certain roles (e.g., becoming divorced) can increase vulnerability for heavier drinking and other substance use, and also that substance use can impair the successful acquisition of social roles.

Data from both adolescence and adulthood suggest that individuals who have more positive beliefs about the effects of substance use (i.e., positive expectancies) are more likely to use and abuse substances. This phenomenon is well documented for alcohol use (Goldman, Del Boca, & Darkes, 1999). The specific content and organization of expectancies vary with age and experience such that adolescents report more diffuse and generally positive beliefs. As drinking experience increases, these beliefs become more homogeneous and "crystallized" (Christiansen, Goldman, & Inn, 1982), but beliefs about the effects of alcohol and drugs are related to substance use in similar ways for adolescents and adults.

Thus, the literature reveals important commonalities in these vulnerability factors for alcohol and drug abuse/dependence for adolescents and adults. Although manifestations of the disorder may vary in adolescence versus adulthood, several of the underlying issues and sources of vulnerability are similar across the lifespan.

POINTS OF DEPARTURE: APPRECIATING THE UNIQUE THEMES AND ISSUES AT DIFFERENT DEVELOPMENTAL PERIODS

As noted earlier, there is substantial common ground in genetic and biological factors, personality and temperament factors, social-environmental influences, and social-cognitive influences on substance use and abuse across the lifespan. However, there also are points of departure, where it is necessary to consider the features of adolescents as distinct from adults. First, although current practice is to use the same diagnostic criteria across the lifespan, some of these criteria appear to be inappropriate for capturing adolescent substance abuse and dependence. For example, as noted in Collins and Shirley (Chapter 6, this volume), a diagnosis according to the fourth edition of the *Diagnostic and Statistical Manual of Mental Disorders* (DSM-IV; American Psychiatric Association, 1994) includes tolerance, withdrawal, and impairment in life functioning. However, given their relatively brief substance use histories, adolescents do not always have symptoms of tolerance and withdrawal, and they do not have occupational and marital roles to show impairment (Vik, Brown, & Myers, 1997). Thus, future research might focus on creating diagnostic criteria that better reflect the unique nature of adolescent substance abuse and dependence.

Other important distinctions between substance use in adolescence and adulthood are social context and relative social acceptance. This point is particularly salient for alcohol consumption and cigarette smoking, which are illegal behaviors for adolescents but legal and socially acceptable for adults. Theoretical models of "problem behaviors" (including alcohol and drug use) note the age-graded nature of these behaviors: use at younger ages is considered more socially deviant and associated with other forms of deviant behavior than is use at older ages (Jessor & Jessor, 1977; Donovan & Jessor, 1985). The implication of these models is that antisocial behavior and other forms of deviance are more strongly predictive of alcohol use, cigarette smoking, and other drug use for adolescents than for adults.

One important area for theory and empirical research explores the heterogeneity among substance abusers. A substantial body of research on subtypes of alcoholics already exists. However, this literature has been largely confined to studies of adult populations. As reviewed by Collins and Shirley (Chapter 6, this volume), researchers have suggested that there are qualitatively different forms of alcoholism that can be distinguished by their age of onset. Babor's Type B and Cloninger's Type II alcoholism are characterized by early onset, substantial heritability, and significant levels of antisocial behavior. Babor's Type A alcoholism and Cloninger's Type I alcoholism are characterized by later (adult) ages of onset, fewer use-related social consequences, less antisocial behavior, but more affective symptomatology (Babor, 1994; Babor et al., 1992; Cloninger, 1987; Cloninger, Bohman, & Sigvardsson, 1981). In contrast, less research has been devoted to subtyping adolescent substance abuse and dependence, with most researchers assuming that adolescent problems reflect Type II or Type B disorders. Research to explore the heterogeneity of adolescent substance abuse/dependence is harder to conduct because of the lower base rates of clinical disorders. However, in some notable exceptions (Mezzich et al., 1993; Tarter, Kirisci, Hegedus, Mezzich, & Vanyukov, 1994; Tarter, Kirisci, & Mezzich, 1997), subtypes of adolescent alcoholism have been identified, and these subtypes seem to parallel the adult distinctions between antisocial alcoholism and negative affect–related alcoholism. These data suggest that more research on the potential heterogeneity of adolescent substance use disorders is warranted.

Reports of a negative affect subtype of adolescent substance abuse/dependence also raises a somewhat controversial question regarding the relative importance of negative affect as a vulnerability factor in substance abuse/dependence across the lifespan. In the adult literature, this controversy may be somewhat resolved by the notion of primary versus secondary alcoholism, in which secondary alcoholism is seen as motivated by self-medication of depression or anxiety (Schuckit, 1985). Similarly, Zucker (1994) has described negative affect alcoholism as one of four different subtypes of alcoholism, and others have suggested that depression in particular might be particularly important for alcoholism in women (Fillmore et al., 1997). Thus, among adults, the role of negative affect in vulnerability to substance abuse may be important for a subtype of the disorder and might vary with such demographic characteristics as gender.

In adolescence, the importance of negative affect has been questioned repeatedly. Some researchers have argued that adolescent substance abuse/dependence may be motivated by a need to cope with negative emotions, and adolescent substance abuse has been linked with both depression and anxiety (Clark et al., 1997; Deykin, Levy, & Wells, 1987). However, the role of negative affect in adolescent substance abuse/dependence remains controversial (Swaim, Oetting, & Beauvais, 1989), and some researchers suggest that negative affect results from rather than causes substance use (Hansell & White, 1991).

One reason for discrepant findings may be the failure to distinguish between different forms of negative affect (Hussong & Chassin, 1994). It may be that anger, hostility, and irritability are more predictive of later adolescent substance use problems than are anxiety and depression (Block, Block, & Keys, 1988; Forgays, Forgays, Wrzensniewski, & Bonaiuto, 1992; Wills & Filer, 1996). Moreover, for adolescent forms of substance abuse/dependence it may be that negative affect alone is not a vulnerability factor. Adolescents who cope with negative affect by social withdrawal and isolation may be less likely to participate in a peer culture that promotes substance use and thus may be at lower risk for alcohol problems. Even if negative affectivity alone is not a vulnerability factor for adolescents, it may operate in combination with other risk factors. For example, adolescents who both experience negative affect and show poor self-regulation are more likely to engage in antisocial behaviors in general and substance use in particular (Miller, Lochman, Coie, Terry, & Hyman, 1998). It will require prospective research with appropriate measures of negative affect and sufficient base rates of substance use/abuse to test these hypotheses with adolescents and other populations.

LEARNING FROM EACH OTHER: HOW FUTURE RESEARCH CAN BE IMPROVED THROUGH CROSS-FERTILIZATION

Our description of commonalities and points of departure suggests fruitful areas for a lifespan approach to understanding vulnerability to substance abuse. Zucker (1994) has presented such a perspective for understanding alcoholism, which could easily be applied to understanding the use and abuse of a variety of substances. His framework incorporates a developmental biopsychosocial perspective for evaluating multiple etiologies and courses of alcohol disorders. Within this perspective, sources of influence include biological, psychological, peer, familial, and sociocultural factors, and life stages range from prenatal through late adulthood. Over the lifespan, sources of influence interact with risk and protective factors to characterize levels of vulnerability.

There are many ways in which investigators of adolescents and investigators of adults can learn from each other. Researchers on adolescents could benefit from considering the adult literature on subtyping and by looking for heterogeneity in vulnerability to substance abuse disorders. Difficulties with subtyping linked to clinical observations or diagnostic systems might occur because some substance use disorders do not develop until early adulthood. Even so, differences in biological characteristics (e.g., being the offspring of an alcoholic), demographic factors (e.g., gender), patterns of substance use, and the existence of comorbid disorders provide points for differentiating the course and outcome of substance use disorders among adolescents.

The methodologies used in research also provide points for crossfertilization. Much of the existing research on adolescents and adults is cross-sectional, with emphasis on developmental homogeneity. Cross-sectional studies that include age-heterogeneous samples would allow for examination of age differences in vulnerability for substance abuse. Such studies should be based on sound conceptual frameworks that incorporate developmental issues and should use measures that are appropriate for (or comparable across) different age groups. Longitudinal studies provide powerful tests of developmental issues in vulnerability to substance abuse. They can link child and adolescent vulnerability factors to both adolescent onset and adult onset forms of substance use disorders. They also can help to establish the continuity of constructs across developmental stages; for example, such studies can elucidate the ways in which early temperament links to later adult personality. The combination of both designs to study age cohorts (cross-sectional) that represent the lifespan (longitudinal) may be useful.

The research described in the two chapters on substance abuse illustrates the fact that substance use disorders are developmental disorders. Comprehensive models that explicitly incorporate a developmental perspective already exist (e.g., Tarter & Vanyukov, 1994; Zucker, 1994). Although complex, these models provide useful starting points for conceptualizing vulnerability, designing meaningful research, and developing effective intervention strategies.

REFERENCES

American Psychiatric Association. (1994). *Diagnostic and statistical manual of mental disorders* (4th ed.). Washington, DC: Author.
Barbor, T. F. (1994). Introduction: Method and theory in the classification of alcoholics. In T. F. Babor, V. Hesselbrock, R. E. Meyer, & W. Shoemaker (Eds.), *Types of alcoholics: Evidence from clinical, experimental, and genetic research* (pp. 1–6). New York: New York Academy of Sciences.
Barbor, T. F., Dolinsky, Z. S., Meyer, R. E., Hesselbrock, M., Hofmann, M., & Tennen, H. (1992). Types of alcoholics: Concurrent and predictive validity of some common classification schemes. *British Journal of Addictions, 87,* 1415–1431.
Block, J., Block, H., & Keys, S. (1988). Longitudinally foretelling drug usage in adolescence: Early childhood personality and environmental precursors. *Child Development, 59,* 336–355.

Christiansen, B. A., Goldman, M. S., & Inn, A. (1982). Development of alcohol-related expectancies in adolescents: Separating pharmacological from social-learning influences. *Journal of Consulting and Clinical Psychology, 50,* 336–344.

Clark, D., Pollock, N., Buckstein, O., Mezzich, A., Bromburger, J., & Donovan, J. (1997). Gender and comorbid psychopathology in adolescents with alcohol dependence. *Journal of the American Academy of Child and Adolescent Psychiatry, 36,* 1195–1203.

Cloninger, R. (1987). Neurogenetic adaptive mechanisms in alcoholism. *Science, 236,* 410–416.

Cloninger, R., Bohman, M., & Sigvardsson, S. (1981). Inheritance of alcohol abuse. *Archives of General Psychiatry, 38,* 861–868.

Cook, P. J., & Moore, M. J. (1993). Drinking and schooling. *Journal of Health Economics, 12,* 411–429.

Deykin, E., Levy, J., & Wells, V. (1987). Adolescent depression, alcohol, and drug abuse. *American Journal of Public Health, 77,* 178–182.

Donovan, J. E., & Jessor, R. (1985). Structure of problem behavior in adolescence and young adulthood. *Journal of Consulting and Clinical Psychology, 53,* 890–904.

Fillmore, K. M., Golding, J. M., Leino, E. V., Motoyoshi, M., Shoemaker, C., Terry, H., Ager, C. R., & Ferrer, H. P. (1997). Pattern and trends in women's and men's drinking. In R. W. Wilsnack & S. C. Wilsnack (Eds.), *Gender and alcohol* (pp. 21–48). New Brunswick, NJ: Rutgers Center of Alcohol Studies.

Forgays, D., Forgays, D. G., Wrzesniewski, K., & Bonaiuto, P. (1992). Alcohol use and personality: Relationships in U.S. and Polish adolescents. *Journal of Substance Abuse, 4,* 393–402.

Goldman, M. S., Del Boca, F. K., & Darkes, J. (1999). Alcohol expectancy theory: The application of cognitive neurosciences. In K. E. Leonard & H. T. Blane (Eds.), *Psychological theories of drinking and alcoholism* (2nd ed., pp. 203–246). New York: Guilford Press.

Gollnisch, G. (1997). Multiple predictors of illicit drug use in methadone maintenance clients. *Addictive Behaviors, 22,* 353–366.

Hansell, S., & White, H. R. (1991). Adolescent drug use, psychological distress and physical symptoms. *Journal of Health and Social Behavior, 32,* 288–301.

Hussong, A., & Chassin, L. (1994). The stress–negative affect model of adolescent alcohol use: Disaggregating negative affect. *Journal of Studies on Alcohol, 55,* 707–719.

Jessor, R., & Jessor, S. L. (1977). *Problem behavior and psychosocial development: A longitudinal study of youth.* New York: Academic Press.

McGue, M. K., Slutske, W., & Iacono, W. G. (1999). Personality and substance use disorders: II. Alcoholism versus drug use disorders. *Journal of Consulting and Clinical Psychology, 67,* 394–404.

Mezzich, A., Tarter, R., Kirisci, L., Clark, D., Buckstein, O., & Martin, C. (1993). Subtypes of early age onset alcoholism. *Alcoholism: Clinical and Experimental Research, 17,* 767–770.

Miller, S., Lochman, J., Coie, J., Terry, R., & Hyman, C. (1998). Comorbidity of conduct and depressive problems at 6th grade: Substance use outcomes across adolescence. *Journal of Abnormal Child Psychology, 26,* 221–232.

National Institute on Alcohol Abuse and Alcoholism. (1997). *Ninth special report to the U.S. Congress on alcohol and health*. (97–4017). Washington, DC: U.S. Department of Health and Human Services.

Schuckit, M. A. (1985). The clinical implications of primary diagnostic groups among alcoholics. *Archives of General Psychiatry, 42*, 1043–1049.

Swaim, R., Oetting, E., & Beauvais, F. (1989). Links from emotional distress to adolescent drug use: A path model. *Journal of Consulting and Clinical Psychology, 57*, 227–231.

Tarter, R. E., Kirisci, L., Hegedus, A., Mezzich, A., & Vanyukov, M. (1994). Heterogeneity of adolescent alcoholism. *Annals of New York Academy of Sciences, 708*, 182–180.

Tarter, R. E., Kirisci, L., & Mezzich, A. (1997). Multivariate typology of adolescents with alcohol use disorder. *American Journal of the Addictions, 6*, 150–158.

Tarter, R. E., & Vanyukov, M. (1994). Alcoholism: A developmental disorder. *Journal of Consulting and Clinical Psychology, 62*, 1096–1107.

Vik, P. W., Brown, S. A., & Meyers, M. G. (1997). Adolescent substance use problems. In E. J. Mash & L. G. Terdal (Eds), *Assessment of childhood disorders* (3rd ed., pp. 717–748). New York: Guilford Press.

Wills, T., & Filer, M. (1996). Stress–coping model of adolescent substance use. In T. Ollendick & R. Prinz (Eds). *Advances in clinical child psychology* (Vol. 18, pp. 91–132). New York: Plenum.

Zucker, R. A. (1994). Pathways to alcohol problems and alcoholism: A developmental account of the evidence for multiple alcoholisms and for contextual contributions to risk. In R. Zucker, G. Boyd, & J. Howard (Eds.), *The development of alcohol problems: Exploring biopsychosocial matrix of risk* (NIAAA Research Monographs 26, NIH Pub. No. 94-3495, pp. 255–290). Washington, DC: U.S. Government Printing Office.

DEPRESSION

8

Vulnerability to Depression in Childhood and Adolescence

JUDY GARBER
CYNTHIA FLYNN

Despite the fact that the construct of childhood depression has been considered a valid entity only for less than a quarter of a century (Kovacs, 1989), there has been considerable progress toward describing the phenomenon and understanding the processes underlying it (Birmaher, Ryan, Williamson, Brent, Kaufman, Dahl, et al., 1996). This chapter is complementary to the following chapter (Hammen, Chapter 9) and focuses on issues of vulnerability particularly relevant to depression in youth. Many of the definitions, characteristics, and theories are similar for child and adult depression. This chapter highlights the features and empirical findings specific to depression in children and adolescents.

DEFINITIONS AND CHARACTERISTICS OF DEPRESSION IN CHILDREN AND ADOLESCENTS

Phenomenology

In Chapter 9 on adult depression, Hammen describes the affective, behavioral, cognitive, and somatic symptoms that define the diagnosable syndrome of depression. The criteria outlined in the fourth edition of the *Diagnostic and Statistical Manual of Mental Disorders* (DSM-IV; American Psychiatric Association, 1994) that currently define depressive disorders are essentially the same regardless of developmental level. Two minor variations in DSM-IV are that for children and adolescents, irritability is consid-

175

ered a manifestation of dysphoric mood, and the duration of dysthymia is 1 rather than 2 years. Thus, according to DSM-IV there are few real differences in the symptoms that comprise the syndromes of major depression or dysthymia.

Developmental psychopathologists (Cicchetti & Schneider-Rosen, 1984; Cicchetti & Toth, 1998; Weiss & Garber, 2000), however, have suggested that manifestations of depression might depend on an individual's level of cognitive, social, and physiological development, and therefore the symptoms of depression might not be isomorphic across the lifespan. The broad criteria that define depression in adults may "need to be translated into age-appropriate guidelines for children, sensitive to developmental changes in the children's experience and expression of depression" (Cicchetti & Schneider-Rosen, 1984, p. 7). Moreover, although there might be a core set of depressive symptoms common across all ages, there also might be other symptoms that are uniquely associated with the syndrome at different developmental levels (Carlson & Kashani, 1988).

Weiss and Garber (2000) suggested two ways in which there could be developmental differences in depressive symptoms. First, children and adults might differ in how they express particular symptoms, although the basic symptoms would be similar regardless of age. For example, dysphoric mood might be manifest by excessive crying in very young children, nonverbal sadness in schoolage children, irritability in adolescents, and depressed mood in adults, but the core mood symptom is essentially the same across these age-specific expressions.

Second, it is possible that the symptoms that comprise the syndrome actually differ developmentally. That is, different combinations of symptoms would define the syndrome in children versus adults. This could be because a certain level of cognitive or physiological maturation might be necessary for some depressive symptoms to occur and young children might not yet be developmentally capable of experiencing such symptoms. For example, young children think concretely and respond to their immediate circumstances, whereas adolescents and adults are more capable of thinking abstractly about themselves and time (Piaget & Inhelder, 1969). With development comes the increasing capacity to maintain a negative self-view and negative expectations about the future, which then can sustain negative emotions beyond the immediate situation (Bemporad & Wilson, 1978; Harris, 1989; Harter, 1999). Thus, although young children might be able to experience transient sadness, particularly in response to an acute stressor, they might be less likely to experience other symptoms of depression that require a higher level of cognitive development such as guilt, worthlessness, and hopelessness (Weiner, 1985).

The primary implication of this with respect to the phenomenology of depression across development is that some symptoms might be less likely than others to comprise the syndrome at different ages. This would appear as differences between depressed children and adults in the rates of particular depressive symptoms and in the symptom structure of the syndrome. In a meta-analysis of 11 empirical studies that compared the rates of depressive symptoms in different age groups, Weiss and Garber (2000) found that for 18 of the 29 (62%) core and associated depressive symptoms there were developmental effects, although these effects were not consistent across studies. That is, there was significant variability in the magnitude of the developmental effects across studies that was greater than would have been expected due to random effects (Hedges & Olkin, 1985). Thus, there were developmental differences in the rates at which at least some depressive symptoms were endorsed.

Weiss and Garber (2000) also reviewed five studies that had compared the structure of depression at different age levels. Two studies had found a similar factor structure across ages, two had found developmental differences, and one found mixed results. Thus, contrary to current views in the literature (Kashani, Rosenberg, & Reid, 1989; Ryan et al., 1987), the evidence does *not* support the conclusion that there are no developmental differences in the rates of depressive symptoms. Nor is it clear from the limited data currently available whether or not there are differences in the structure of depressive syndrome across development. Goodyer (1996) asserted that "the suggestion that the clinical presentation of major depression varies with age is far from resolved and more developmentally sensitive studies are required" (p. 407).

Such developmental differences in the phenomenology of depression are relevant to the issue of vulnerability because they might be the result of differences in the causal processes that underlie the disorder at different ages. For example, Wickramaratne and Weissman (1998) recently found that whereas childhood-onset depressive disorder was associated with early onset of mood disorders in parents, adolescent-onset depressions were not. They suggested that childhood- and adolescent-onset mood disorders might be etiologically distinct. Therefore, it is possible that different causal processes could result in a different configuration of symptoms. That is, even if children were developmentally capable of experiencing the various symptoms of depression, certain symptoms that are tied more closely to one causal mechanism or another could be more or less a part of depression in children than adults.

Weiss and Garber (2000) suggested several ways in which such differences in causal processes might arise. First, both a specific symptom and the full syndrome of depression may be caused by a common third variable; that is, they may share a mutual causal agent. For instance, the same biochemical imbalance might cause anhedonia as well as the other symptoms of the syndrome (e.g., dysphoric mood, appetite change). Second, an individual symptom might be related to the broader syndrome of depression because the symptom itself may be part of the causal mechanisms, producing the depression. For example, one reason hopelessness is strongly correlated with depression in both adults (e.g., Beck, Steer, Beck, & Newman,

1993) and children (e.g., Asarnow & Guthrie, 1989) might be because hopelessness is part of the causal process for some forms of depression (Abramson, Metalsky, & Alloy, 1989). Third, a specific symptom could be related to the disorder because it is a consequence of other symptoms of the depressive syndrome. For instance, concentration problems, currently considered a symptom of depression (American Psychiatric Association, 1994), might be a result of other symptoms of depression (e.g., distracting cognitions or fatigue).

Thus, developmental differences in the causal processes or consequences of depression could produce differences in the relations among depressive symptoms at different ages. For instance, if the etiology of depression is less biological in children than in adults (e.g., Post, 1992), then the relation between symptoms resulting from these biological processes (e.g., sleep disturbance) and the rest of the syndrome of depression would be greater for adults. This would occur because the causal processes underlying depression would be more responsible (both in absolute terms and relative to the nondepressive causes of the symptom) for intersubject variability in the symptoms (e.g., sleep disturbances). That is, compared to children, in adults a greater proportion of the variance in sleep disturbance would be accounted for by the causal processes underlying depression.

Developmental factors unrelated to depression also could cause age differences in the relations among depressive symptoms. For example, it is possible that even if the causal processes underlying depression were the same in children and adults, some symptoms (e.g., fatigue) could be more a part of depression at one developmental period than another. This could occur because the normative causal processes that produce that symptom change developmentally. For instance, hormonal factors associated with puberty but not with depression could become increasingly responsible for the development of fatigue and sleepiness during adolescence and adulthood (Carskadon, Keenan, & Dement, 1987). Therefore, the causal processes underlying depression would be less of a factor proportionally for intersubject variability in fatigue, and therefore the relation between depression and fatigue would be smaller for children than for adults (Weiss & Garber, 2000). Thus, there are important theoretical and empirical reasons why it is possible that symptoms of depression could differ across development.

In addition to this developmental issue regarding the criteria that define the syndrome of depression, several other important definitional points noted by Hammen are relevant to studying vulnerability to depression in children, particularly the problem of comorbidity and the continuity of depression across levels of severity. Comorbidity of other disorders with depression is very common in children and adolescents (Angold & Costello, 1993). Rates of oppositional/conduct disorders have been found to be between three and nine times higher in depressed than in nondepressed children. Anxiety disorders tend to occur in about 30–70% of depressed children at rates between 2 and 25 times higher than in nondepressed children. Recognizing and explicitly identifying such comorbidity is particularly important in studies of vulnerability because it is possible that some factors that are identified as being risks for depression really could be causes of the comorbid condition instead.

The issue of the continuity of depression across symptoms, syndrome, and disorder also is important to discussions about vulnerability (Compas, Ey, & Grant, 1993). One aspect of this continuity issue concerns how depression in children is measured. Much of the research on depression in children and adolescents has used questionnaires to assess depressive symptoms. The most commonly used instruments are the self-report Children's Depression Inventory (Kovacs, 1981) and the parent-report Child Behavior Checklist (CBCL; Achenbach, 1991). These assessment methods have several limitations. First, there is a problem of comorbidity; that is, such measures assess levels of distress but not other symptoms of psychopathology that the children also might have. Second, typically studies that use such questionnaire methodologies to identify subjects use community (school) samples that generally have lower levels of severity. It is not clear whether the same findings about etiological correlates apply to more severe levels of depression or diagnoses of depressive disorders. Third, parent and teacher report measures such as the CBCL typically include other internalizing symptoms, particularly anxiety, in their assessment of depression. Thus, it is unclear whether the findings are specific to depression in particular or to internalizing symptoms in general.

A second question with regard to continuity is whether the same mechanisms that lead to depressive mood also produce depressive syndrome and disorders. Moreover, how is it that depressive mood develops into more severe and extensive depressive syndrome for some people but not for others? Is it simply that such individuals have more of the causal agent or are there qualitatively different processes occurring that push such persons into the full depressive syndrome and disorder? Compas et al. (1993) suggested that the three levels of depression are hierarchical and depressive disorders are a subset of depressive syndrome, which is a subset of depressed mood. Compas et al. (1993) further proposed that the transition from one level to the next is the result of "dysregulation or dysfunction in biological, stress, and/or coping processes" (p. 336), and that there are likely important developmental changes in all three processes that make adolescence a time of increased vulnerability.

Course and Outcome

In general, the duration of episodes of clinically diagnosed depression in children (Kovacs, Feinberg, Crouse-Novak, Paulauskas, & Finkelstein, 1984; Kovacs, Feinberg, Crouse-Novak, Paulauskas, Pollock, et al., 1984) has been found to be similar to those reported in adults (Coryell et al., 1994). Kovacs, Feinberg, Crouse-Novak, Paulauskas, and Finkelstein (1984) and Kovacs, Feinberg, Crouse-Novak, Paulauskas, Pollock, et al. (1984) reported that in 8- to 13-year-old children, major depressive disorder tended to be acute, had a mean length of episode of about 32 weeks,and the maximal recovery rate of 92% of the sample was reached at about 18 months from onset. Duration of depressive episodes in nonreferred community samples of ado- lescents (Lewinsohn, Clarke, Seeley, & Rohde, 1994), however, tends to be shorter than what has been reported for clinic samples of children and ado- lescents.

With regard to longer-term prognosis, short-term follow-up studies of children have shown that early-onset depressions tend to recur. Kovacs, Feinberg, Crouse-Novak, Paulauskas, Pollock, et al. (1984) reported that the cumulative probability of a recurrent episode of major depression was .72 over the course of 5 years from the onset of the disorder. "Catchup" longitudinal studies (Harrington, Fudge, Rutter, Pickles, & Hill, 1990) have found that individuals who were depressed as children or adolescents tend to have recurrent episodes of depression as adults. Moreover, there tends to be specificity in the continuity of mood disorders. Depressed children were more likely to have subsequent episodes of depression than were those who had other psychiatric disorders (Harrington et al., 1990).

An important question with respect to the issue of vulnerability is what accounts for the observed continuity and recurrence of depression from child- hood to adulthood. It could be that the same underlying processes cause depression across the lifespan such as a biological propensity, chronic envi- ronmental stressors, or the interaction between these. It also is possible that depressions that occur in the same individuals at different age periods are the result of correlated, although different, risk factors such as parental depression and marital discord.

Another possibility is that earlier episodes of depression create a bio- logical and/or psychological scar that sensitizes the individual to later expo- sures to even low levels of the etiological agent(s). Teasdale's (1983, 1988) differential activation hypothesis proposes that vulnerability to subsequent, more severe depressive episodes is influenced by patterns of information processing that occur during earlier, milder depressions. That is, depressive mood states presumably activate negatively biased interpretations of expe- riences that then serve to maintain and exacerbate the dysphoria into fur- ther clinical depression. Post (1992) suggested a kindling hypothesis in which prior episodes of depression "leave behind neurobiological residues that make a patient more vulnerable to subsequent episodes" (p. 1006). A re- lated explanation is that earlier depressions change individuals in some ways, which, then lead to their generating the kinds of stressful environments that are likely to precipitate future episodes (Hammen, 1991a).

Finally, the important distinction between relapse of symptoms within the same episode versus recurrence of symptoms of a totally new episode is relevant to discussions about vulnerability (Prien & Kupfer, 1986). It is not clear that the same processes underlie these different kinds of return of symptoms in depressed patients (Hollon, Evans, & DeRubeis, 1990). Thus, studies of vulnerability need to address the question of what factors maintain depressive symptoms within an episode, account for relapse of the same episode once it has remitted, and underlie the recurrence of depression over time.

Prevalence of Child and Adolescent Depression

Epidemiological studies examining the rates of major depressive disorder (MDD) among community samples have yielded different prevalence estimates primarily due to different methods of case ascertainment. MDD is rare in young children and less common during childhood, but the rates become comparable to adults by middle adolescence (Costello et al., 1996; Fleming & Offord, 1990). Blazer, Kessler, McGonagle, and Swartz (1994) found the 1-month prevalence rates to be highest among individuals between 15 to 24 years old compared to all other age groups studied. Lifetime prevalence rates of MDD in adolescents range from 8.3% to 18.5%: about 24% for females and 11.6% for males (Lewinsohn, Hops, Roberts, Seeley, & Andrews, 1993). It is likely that many adults' mood disorders began during middle to late adolescence, which might be a particularly vulnerable period for first episodes of MDD (Hankin et al., 1998).

Epidemiological studies across cultures repeatedly have found approximately twice the rate of depression in women compared to men (Weissman & Olfson, 1995). This 2-to-1 sex ratio, however, does not become apparent until adolescence. In prepubertal children the rate of MDD is about equal in girls and boys, and in some cases higher among boys (Fleming & Offord, 1990). Ryan et al. (1987) reported that 62% of their depressed prepubertal patients were boys, whereas 54% of their depressed adolescents were girls.

Developmental epidemiologists (Costello, 1989; Rutter, 1988) have noted that epidemiological findings can "capitalize on developmental variations and psychopathologic variations to ask questions about mechanism and processes" (Rutter, 1988, p. 486). For example, why is MDD less common during childhood? What about childhood prevents depression from occurring or what happens during adolescence that increases an individual's risk for depression? What accounts for the change in the sex ratio of depression from childhood to adolescence? Thus, epidemiological data concerning age trends in prevalence rates can serve as a guide to inquiries about mechanisms underlying the disorder.

Secular trends in the rates of depression also might provide clues about underlying processes. Depressive disorders have been found to be relatively higher among those born more recently (Burke, Burke, Rae, & Regier, 1991; Klerman & Weissman, 1989). Burke et al. (1991) compared cohorts of individuals born between 1953 and 1966 with those born between 1937 and 1952 and between 1917 and 1936 and found an increase in depression in each young group compared to the older ones. Klerman and Weissman (1989) argued that such secular trends were not simply due to overreporting by the young or underreporting by older individuals since objective indexes of distress such as suicides and hospitalizations also had been found to have increased. They also suggested that the secular trend was not a memory artifact because studies had not found evidence that recall of more distant depressive experiences were impaired among those known to have been depressed.

Because it is unlikely that the genetic makeup of the population changed substantially during this relatively short period, it is more probable that the secular increase resulted from environmental factors or the interaction of environmental and genetic factors (Gershon, Hamovit, Guroff, & Nurnberger, 1987). Changing cultural trends such as greater social mobility and the breakdown of the family might both create more stress and reduce available resources for coping with them, thereby resulting in more depressions. Thus, any credible and complete theory of depression needs to account for these two important developmental epidemiological findings: (a) age differences in the rates of depression and (2) the birth cohort effect.

METHODS USED TO STUDY
VULNERABILITY TO DEPRESSION

Several methodologies have been used to examine vulnerability to depression in children and adolescents. These methods overlap somewhat with those that have been used with adults (Ingram, Miranda, & Segal, 1998) and include cross-sectional, prospective, offspring, and prevention studies. Although limited with respect to conclusions about causality, cross-sectional studies are used to identify potential risk and vulnerability factors that characterize depressed children in comparison to nondepressed children. A particularly interesting kind of cross-sectional study is one that contrasts never depressed, currently depressed, and formerly depressed individuals. If a stable vulnerability marker has been identified, presumably it should characterize both currently depressed individuals and formerly depressed persons in remission but not the never depressed controls (although see Just, Abramson, & Alloy, in press).

Prospective studies are increasingly being used to demonstrate the temporal relations among potential predictors and both depressive symptoms and disorders in children and adolescents. Whereas most of these longitudinal studies have used continuous measures of depression to show increases in symptoms over time, several recent studies have predicted the onset of depressive disorders as well. Although prospective designs can show that a variable precedes the increase or onset of depressive symptoms and disorders, they are not conclusive with regard to causality because it is still possible that some unmeasured third variable accounts for the link between the vulnerability factor and depressive outcome.

Another strategy for examining vulnerability is to study offspring of depressed parents. There is clear evidence that children of depressed parents are at increased risk for developing mood disorders themselves (Cummings & Davies, 1994a; Downey & Coyne, 1990). If a particular vulnerability factor or factors contribute to the development of such mood disorders, then these high-risk individuals would be more likely to exhibit the vulnerability than would children whose parents have not experienced mood disorders.

Finally, prevention studies can be used to study vulnerability. The basic idea of prevention studies is that if individuals who receive an intervention aimed at changing an identified vulnerability factor show lower rates of depression compared to individuals in the untreated group, then this would be consistent with the view that this vulnerability factor might be a risk factor for depression. Of course, prevention designs can only demonstrate reduction in symptoms and cannot confirm that the identified variable contributed to the original onset of the symptoms.

THEORY AND RESEARCH ON VULNERABILITY TO DEPRESSION

Theories of depression can be divided into the following categories of etiological processes: genetics, neurobiology, stressful life events, negative cognitions, and interpersonal relationships. We discuss each of these perspectives and review empirical findings based on cross-sectional, prospective, high-risk, and prevention studies when such data are available.

Genetic Vulnerability

Family, twin, and adoption studies have yielded varying results regarding genetic contributions to individual differences in depression (Blehar, Weissman, Gershon, & Hirschfeld, 1988). Family studies of depressive disorders have shown that children of depressed parents are three times more likely to experience an episode of depression than are children of normal controls (Beardslee, Versage, & Gladstone, 1998), and they have about a 40% chance of having a depressive episode before the age of 18 (Weissman et al., 1987). In addition, the risk of having a depressive episode is higher in relatives of depressed children than in relatives of psychiatric and normal controls (Harrington, Fudge, Rutter, Bredenkamp, & Pridham, 1993; Puig-Antich et al., 1989).

However, family studies confound genetic effects with shared environmental effects (Rutter, Bolton, et al., 1990). Familiality of depression also could be due to psychosocial factors such as maladaptive parenting styles, marital dysfunction, and stress, which also are associated with parental psychopathology (Goodman & Gotlib, 1999; Hammen, 1991b). Children exposed to these conditions early in development might be especially vulnerable to developing mood disorders. That is, childhood-onset depressions in particular may be associated with more severe environmental stressors or traumas (Nolen-Hoeksema, Girgus, & Seligman, 1992; Post, 1992).

Twin studies with children have yielded heritability estimates comparable to those found in adults (see Hammen, Chapter 9, this volume). In a study of 41 twin pairs ages 6 to 16, Wierzbicki (1987) reported that monozygotic twins more closely resembled each other in depressive symptomatoogy than did dizygotic twins. Heritability estimates were 0.32 for child self-report of depression and 0.93 for parent report of children's symptoms.

The Virginia Twin Study of Adolescent Behavioral Development (Eaves et al., 1997) consists of 1,412 twin pairs ages 8 to 16 years old. Heritability estimates were small (0.15 for girls and 0.16 for boys) and shared environmental effects were small to moderate (0.26 for girls and 0.14 for boys) when using child self-report. However, when using parent report, heritability estimates were much larger (between 0.60 for mothers and 0.65 for fathers) and shared environment effects were negligible. It is possible that higher parent-report heritabilities may be partially due to the greater physical similarities between MZ twins. Parents might see MZ twins as more phenotypically similar than DZ twins across constructs, thus elevating heritability estimates when using parent report.

Thaper and McGuffin (1994) also reported large genetic contributions to individual differences in parent-reported depression ($h^2 = 0.79$) in a sample of 411 twin pairs, ages 8 to 16. Shared environment effects were nonsignificant. In adolescents, the heritability estimate for self-reported depression was also high ($h^2 = 0.70$). However, when they examined only the 8 to 11-year-old pairs, shared environmental effects on parent-reported depression accounted for 77% of the variance and heritability effects were negligible. Child self-report measures were not available for this age group. Thus, genetic and environmental effects on depression may differ as a function of age.

Finally, Eley (cited in Eley, Deater-Deckard, Fombonne, Fulker, & Plomin, 1998), in a sample of 395 twin pairs, 8 to 16 years old, reported similar heritability estimates for both child-reported depression ($h^2 = 0.48$) and parent report of child depression ($h^2 = 0.49$). Shared environment effects were greater in adolescents (0.28) than children (0.08), and heritability estimates were moderate in both groups; $h^2 = 0.34$ for children and $h^2 = 0.28$ for adolescents. These results also suggest age differences but in the opposite direction. In this case, shared environmental effects were stronger in adolescents.

Thus, evidence from twin studies that genes account for approximately 30 to 50% of the variance in child-reported depression. The evidence for environmental effects is mixed. In addition, genetic and environmental influences on individual differences in depression differ with informant (Eaves et al., 1997; Wierzbicki, 1987) and age (Eley, cited in Eley et al., 1998; Thaper & McGuffin, 1994). Early-onset (i.e., < 20 years old) depressions have been found to be associated with greater risk for depression in family members (Weissman, Warner, Wickramaratne, & Prusoff, 1988; Weissman et al., 1984, 1986). Alternatively, childhood depression has been associated with greater environmental contributions (Thaper & McGuffin, 1994). It is unclear whether earlier-onset depression is due to greater genetic influence or factors within the shared environment of families with a depressed proband (Rutter, MacDonald, et al., 1990).

Nonshared environmental factors also influence depressive symptoms. The Virginia Twin Study (Eaves et al., 1997) found that nonshared environmental factors played a moderate role in both child (0.59 for girls, 0.70 for boys) and parent report (0.35 for mothers, 0.40 for fathers) of children's depression. Reiss et al. (1995) found that 37% of the variance in adolescent depressive symptoms was accounted for by nonshared environmental factors in the form of parental negativity directed at the affected twin.

Adoption designs have traditionally been able to directly disentangle shared and nonshared environmental effects. van den Oord, Boomsma, and Verhulst (1994) reported negligible heritability, moderate effects of shared environmental factors, and moderate to large effects of nonshared environmental factors on parent-reported internalizing behaviors in a large sample of young adolescent adoptees. Eley et al. (1998) employed an offspring design combined with a sibling design to assess the variance accounted for by genetic and environmental factors in child-reported and parent-reported depression. Neither the sibling nor the parent–offspring correlations showed a significant genetic effect. There was evidence of some shared environmental effects, although these were greater for parents' reports, indicating inflation possibly due to method bias in the relation between mothers' report of their own and their children's symptoms. The results also suggest a substantial role for nonshared environmental effects.

Thus, findings from twin and adoption studies of childhood depression differ. Whereas twin studies suggest a moderate role for genetic influences on individual differences in depression, adoption studies typically have reported negligible genetic effects. In general, twin studies report nonsignificant effects of shared environment, whereas adoption studies suggest a small but significant effect of shared environment. Both designs provide evidence of moderate to large nonshared environmental influences.

Finally, heritability of depression may vary as a function of symptom heterogeneity. Adult studies generally have found that environmental factors make a greater contribution to mild depressions, and genes play a larger role in more severe depressions (Rutter, MacDonald, et al., 1990). In children, studies that have evaluated differences in genetic and environmental effects have reported mixed results. In two such studies (Eley, 1997; Rende, Plomin, Reiss, & Hetherington; 1993) child report on the Children's Depression Inventory (CDI; Kovacs, 1981) was used to establish groups of varying severity. In a sample of 9- to 18-year-olds, Rende et al. (1993) found smaller genetic effects and significant shared-environment effects in children with greater severity of symptoms. In contrast, Eley (1997) found in a sample of 8- to 16-year-olds similar heritability estimates for severe groups but less influence of shared environmental factors. There were slight differences in age that may explain the conflicting results for environmental effects, suggesting that environmental factors may be more important as children get older. In addition, the cutoff points used to identify the groups fell within the mild to moderate range of depressive symptomatology, (i.e., between 13 and 17 on the CDI). The most contradictory findings in the adult literature have been associated with depressions of moderate severity (Rutter, MacDonald, et al., 1990).

In sum, behavioral genetic designs provide evidence of both genetic and environmental effects (Plomin, 1990). Estimates of heritability tend to be moderate and shared-environment effects tend to be small. However, both tend to vary as a function of informant, age, and severity of depressive symptoms. Although vulnerability to depression clearly has a genetic component, it is not yet clear what is inherited that places an individual at greater risk. Genetic factors may contribute to neurobiological and/or cognitive vulnerabilities, which then interact with the environment to produce depressive symptoms. Nonshared environmental effects, that is, experiences that are unique to individuals within a family, emerge as the largest environmental influence on individual differences in childhood depression (Plomin, 1990). The latter has been found to be true for most forms of psychopathology, as well as for certain personality traits and cognitive abilities (Plomin, 1990). Additional research is needed to illuminate the mechanisms through which genes influence individual differences in depression as well as their potentially complex interactions with environmental factors.

Neurobiological Vulnerability

Psychobiological studies of depression in children and adolescents generally have attempted to replicate results of studies with adults. This research has primarily focused on dysregulation in neuroendocrine and neurochemical systems and in disturbances in sleep architecture (Dahl & Ryan, 1996; Emslie, Weinberg, Kennard, & Kowatch, 1994). In addition, a few studies have investigated functional and anatomical brain differences in depressed children (Botteron, 1999; Dawson, Klinger, Panagiotides, Spieker, & Frey, 1992; Field, Fox, Pickens, & Nawrocki, 1995).

Psychoneuroendocrinology

Within the neuroendocrine system, abnormalities in the hypothalamic–pituitary–adrenal (HPA) axis have been assessed through measures of basal cortisol secretion and the dexamethasone suppression test (DST) (Ryan & Dahl, 1993). Whereas most studies have not found differences in basal cortisol secretion between depressed and normal children (Dahl, Ryan, Puig-Antich, et al., 1991; Kutcher et al., 1991; Puig-Antich et al., 1989), a few have shown elevated cortisol secretion near sleep onset in suicidal and depressed inpatients (Dahl, Ryan, Puig-Antich, et al., 1991). Goodyer et al. (1996) also found differences in evening cortisol secretion between patients with major depressive disorder and normal controls. Moreover, elevated cortisol levels near sleep onset in depressed adolescents have been shown to predict recurrence (Rao et al., 1996). However, baseline cortisol levels generally have not discriminated between depressed children and controls (Ryan, 1998).

In contrast to baseline observations, challenging a regulatory system allows observation of its functioning when stressed. For example, depressive abnormalities in the HPA axis response to physiological stress have been investigated with the DST. Numerous studies with in- and outpatient groups of children and adolescents have found greater sensitivity in children than in adolescents (58% vs. 44%) and in inpatients compared to outpatients (61% vs. 29%) but greater specificity in adolescents; that is, comparisons with psychiatric controls were stronger in adolescent samples (85%) than in child samples (60%) (see Dahl & Ryan, 1996, and Ryan & Dahl, 1993, for reviews).

In addition, DST results have been found to vary as a function of depressive heterogeneity (Dahl & Ryan, 1996). DST nonsuppression has been associated with concurrent suicidal behavior as well as successful suicide (e.g., Pfeffer, Stokes, & Shindledecker, 1991), endogenous subtypes of depression (Robbins, Alessi, Yanchyshyn, & Colfer, 1983), and a prior history of major depressive disorder (Klee & Garfinkel, 1984).

In sum, basal cortisol levels have not been reliably associated with depression in children and adolescents, although evening hypersecretion has been found to be associated with greater severity of symptoms (Dahl, Ryan, Puig-Antich, et al., 1991) and to predict recurrence (Rao et al., 1996). DST nonsuppression distinguishes groups of depressed children from both psychiatric and normal controls, but results are variable and some studies have not found significant sensitivity (Dahl, Kaufman, et al., 1992). Developmental changes in the HPA axis may be responsible for the lack of consistent findings in children as opposed to the stronger findings reported in adults (Halbreich, Asnis, Zumoff, Nathan, & Shindledecker, 1984).

Most studies of HPA axis abnormalities have been cross-sectional comparisons of children with major depressive disorder versus other psychiatric diagnoses and normal controls. In one study (Puig-Antich et al., 1989) that followed a few depressed children who had elevated cortisol levels, only one of four continued to show elevated levels after recovery. Thus, there currently is little evidence that HPA axis dysregulation is a stable vulnerability marker. Prospective studies of HPA axis functioning in children who may be at risk for depression are needed to clarify the role that dysregulation in this system may play in onset of depression in children.

Research on growth hormone regulation in children has been particularly interesting. Growth hormone (GH) is normatively secreted by the pituitary gland and functions as a growth-promoting agent throughout the body. In children, it is mostly secreted during sleep (Ryan & Dahl, 1993). Some studies have found an increase in unstimulated GH secretion at night in depressed children (Puig-Antich, Goetz, et al., 1984) and adolescents (Kutcher et al., 1988), whereas others have found blunted GH secretion throughout the day (Meyer et al., 1991). In response to pharmacological challenges, which attempt to artificially stimulate the growth hormone system, depressed children typically show blunted GH secretion. Studies comparing children with major depressive disorder to normal controls have found a blunted GH response to stimulation with insulin-induced hypoglycemia, arginine, clonidine, and growth hormone releasing hormone (GHRH) (Meyer et al., 1991; Ryan et al., 1994). Jensen and Garfinkel (1990) reported a blunted GH response to L-dopa and clonidine in prepubertal boys compared to normal controls but not in adolescent boys. Depressed and suicidal adolescents have been shown to have a blunted GH response to desmethylimipramine when compared to normals (Ryan et al., 1988) and to hyposecrete GH during sleep (Dahl, Ryan, et al., 1992). Children with endogenous depressions have demonstrated a blunted response to hypoglycemic stimulation in comparison to nondepressed neurotic children (Puig-Antich, Novacenko, Davies, Chambers, et al., 1984), and they continue to hyposecrete GH in response to the insulin tolerance test after remission (Puig-Antich, Novacenko, Davies, Tabrizi, et al., 1984).

In addition, Birmaher et al. (1999) reported that children who have never experienced an episode of depression themselves but have depressed parents (high risk), in comparison to children with no familial psychiatric history (low risk), showed a blunted GH response to administration of GHRH, although there were no baseline GH differences between the groups. Moreover, there were no differences between these high-risk and currently depressed children in GH response. These results suggest that growth hormone system dysregulation may be a vulnerability marker for depression. These high-risk children need to be followed, however, to determine whether they eventually develop depressive disorders.

Neurotransmitters

A second important area of biological dysregulation among depressed patients is in their neurochemistry, with serotonin, norepinephrine, and acetylcholine particularly implicated in the pathophysiology of mood disorders (Gold, Goodwin, & Chrousos; 1988). Depressed adults have been found to have dysregulation of the central serotonergic function (e.g., Maes & Meltzer, 1995). Consistent with this, in comparison to normal controls, depressed children demonstrate hyposecretion of melatonin (Cavallo, Holt, Hejazi, Richards, & Meyer, 1987) and a blunted cortisol response and an increased prolactin response after administration of L-5-hydroxytryptophan, primarily in girls (Ryan et al., 1992). Moreover, similar results have been found in never depressed children with high familial loadings for depression (Birmaher et al., 1997), suggesting a serotonergic system marker for depression.

Investigation into the effectiveness of selective serotonin reuptake inhibitors (SSRIs) in reducing depressive symptoms in children also has implicated serotonergic system dysregulation in childhood depression (Emslie et al., 1997). Overall, there is evidence of neurotransmitter involvement in child and adolescent depression. Moreover, serotonergic system dysregulation may be a risk factor for depression because it has been found in both high risk and currently depressed children.

Functional and Anatomical Brain Differences

Abnormal functioning of the prefrontal cortex–limbic–striatal regions in the brain as well as reduced prefrontal volume has been associated with adult depression (Hammen, Chapter 9, this volume). A few studies have examined functional and structural brain changes in children and adolescents. In a large sample of female adolescent twins who had a history of major depressive disorder but were not necessarily currently depressed, Botteron (1999) reported that twins with a history of moderate to severe depression showed a significant reduction in subgenual prefrontal cortical volume compared to normal controls. This region of the prefrontal cortex is known to be important in the response to reinforced stimuli. Individuals who have subgenual prefrontal cortical lesions tend to become affectively labile, to respond inappropriately to events in the environment, and to have difficulty learning from reinforcement (Botteron, 1999).

Resting frontal brain asymmetry also has been linked with depression in adults and appears to persist into remission (Tomarken & Keener, 1998). In children, a few studies have found left frontal hypoactivation in the infants of depressed mothers compared to infants of nondepressed mothers (Dawson et al., 1992; Field et al., 1995). Tomarken, Simien, and Garber (1994) compared the resting electroencephalograph (EEG) patterns of young adolescents whose mothers either did or did not have histories of mood disorders. The high-risk group demonstrated left frontal hypoactivation relative to the low-risk group, suggesting a possible vulnerability marker for depression that was independent of current mood state or prior depressive episodes. Tomarken and Keener (1998) proposed that the prefrontal cortex is linked to approach/withdrawal systems and that the relative left frontal hypoactivation associated with depression might result in a bias away from approach and in favor of withdrawal. A tendency to favor withdrawal may represent a behavioral precursor to the anhedonia typical of depressed individuals.

Sleep Architecture Abnormalities

Although the subjective report of sleep disturbance has been observed among depressed children and adolescents, sleep EEG results are less consistent in children than in adults (Ryan & Dahl, 1993). Depressed adults show many sleep abnormalities such as decreased sleep efficiency, reduced delta sleep, increased rapid eye movement (REM) density, and shortened REM latency (Kupfer & Reynolds, 1992). Depressed children and adolescents show some of these same kinds of sleep anomalies, including prolonged sleep latencies (Emslie, Rush, Weinberg, Rintelmann, & Roffwarg, 1990; Goetz, et al., 1987), especially suicidal adolescents (Dahl, et al., 1990), reduced REM latencies (Emslie et al., 1990), especially in more severely depressed children (Dahl, Ryan, Birmaher, et al., 1991), and decreased sleep efficiency (Goetz et al., 1987). However, findings are inconsistent across studies, and several studies have failed to find differences between depressed and nondepressed children and adolescents in EEG sleep patterns (Dahl & Ryan, 1996).

The absence of consistent patterns of sleep abnormalities in depressed youth has been attributed to the role of maturational changes. Dahl and Ryan (1996) suggested that the sleep of young children is difficult to disrupt because they are such deep sleepers. During adolescence, however, this protective aspect of sleep begins to decrease. It may not be until adulthood, however, that the sleep disturbances associated with depression become evident.

In summary, there is evidence of neuroendocrine and neurochemical dysregulation in depressed adolescents. Basal cortisol levels do not appear to consistently discriminate between depressed and normal children, whereas the HPA axis response to stress, seen in the DST does appear to differ between depressed and nondepressed children, although these results are also variable. The strongest neuroendocrinological evidence is for dysregulation of the growth hormone system. Moreover, hyposecretion of GH in response to pharmacological challenge has been demonstrated in high-risk children (Birmaher, et al., 1999), suggesting a possible vulnerability marker.

Neurochemical dysregulation has been implicated in childhood depression and serotonergic system dysregulation has been demonstrated in high-risk children (Birmaher et al., 1997), again suggesting a vulnerability for depression. There is also evidence of functional and anatomical brain differences in depressed children and adolescents compared to normal controls and in offspring of depressed mothers. Sleep disturbances, although experientially common in depressed children, have not been consistently found in sleep studies of depressed children and adolescents, possibly due to maturational factors (Dahl & Ryan, 1996). Thus, the neurobiological literature in children and adolescents is more variable although not inconsistent with adult findings.

Stressful Life Events

Stress plays a prominent role in most theories of depression, and there is a clear empirical link between stressful life events and depression in both adults (Brown & Harris, 1989) and children (Compas, 1987; Compas, Grant, & Ey, 1994). A complete review of this literature is beyond the scope of this chapter. Rather, we highlight here results of cross-sectional, prospective, high-risk, and prevention studies supporting the stress–depression relation in youth.

Cross-Sectional Studies

Cross-sectional studies have consistently shown that depressive symptoms and disorders are significantly associated with minor and major undesirable life events in children (Compas, 1987) and are more prevalent among depressed compared to nondepressed children (e.g., Goodyer, Wright, & Altham, 1988). Although the evidence is mixed with respect to the relation between discrete single negative events (e.g., disasters) and depression in children, the findings are stronger regarding the link between cumulative or chronic stressors and depression in children and adolescents (Compas et al., 1994).

Most of this research has used life-events checklists to ascertain information about the occurrence of events. Such checklists, however, have the disadvantage of sometimes confounding symptoms and events and do not distinguish well between subjective reactions and objective consequences of events. In contrast, life-events interviews allow researchers to rate the severity of an event given the context in which it occurred separately from the person's subjective reaction, and to more precisely determine the actual timing of events in relations to symptoms. Studies that have used life-events interviews with adolescents (Garber & Robinson, 1997a; Goodyer et al., 1988; Hammen et al., 1987; Monck & Dobbs, 1985; Williamson et al., 1998) have found that stressful life events are associated with depressive symptoms and disorders. Moreover, Williamson, Birmacher, Anderson, Alshabbout, and Ryan (1995) reported that depressed adolescents had significantly more dependent stressful life events during the previous year than did normal controls. Thus, cross-sectional studies using either checklist or interview methodologies have reliably found a strong link between stress and depression in children and adolescents.

Cross-sectional studies, however, are not informative about the direction of the relation between stress and depression. Given the association between dependent stressors and depression, it is quite possible that depression contributes to the occurrence of stressors. Depressed individuals have been found to generate many of the stressors they encounter, and these stressors then exacerbate and maintain the depressive symptoms (Coyne et al., 1987; Hammen, 1991a). Prospective studies in which stressors are assessed prior to the onset of symptoms are more informative about the temporal relations between stress and depression.

Prospective Studies

Most prospective studies in children and adolescents examining the relation between negative life events and depression have used continuous measures of self- or parent-reported depressive symptoms and life-events checklists. In general, these studies have found that stress predicts increases in depressive symptoms, controlling for prior symptoms (Allgood-Merten, Lewinsohn, & Hops, 1990; Ge, Lorenz, Conger, Elder, & Simons, 1994; Leadbeater, Kuperminc, Blatt, & Hertzog, 1999; Nolen-Hoeksema et al., 1992; Petersen, Sarigiani, & Kennedy, 1991) over a few months (Wagner, Compas, & Howell, 1988) to several years (Velez, Johnson, & Cohen, 1989). The relations tend to be stronger predicting to children's self-reports compared to parents' reports of children's depressive symptoms (Compas, Howell, Phares, Williams, & Giunta, 1989; Stanger, McConaughy, & Achenbach, 1992).

Fewer studies have examined the contribution of negative life events to the first onset of depressive disorders in children and adolescents. Using a modification of Brown and Harris's (1978) contextual threat method to assess stress, Hammen, Adrian, and Hiroto (1988) found that stress significantly predicted depressive disorders among offspring of mothers with histories of mood disorders. Also using a modification of Brown's contextual threat interview, Garber, Martin, and Keiley (1999) conducted a survival analysis and found that as the average number of stressors per week increased, so did the risk of the onset of a first depressive episode in young adolescents. Finally, Lewinsohn and colleagues (Lewinsohn, Allen, Seeley, & Gotlib, 1999; Lewinsohn, Roberts, et al., 1994) also have reported that major stressful life events significantly predicted the first episode of depression during middle adolescence.

Although there is not one specific type of stressful event that invariably leads to depression in children and adolescents, it often involves loss, separation, or interpersonal conflict (Monroe, Rohde, Seeley, & Lewinsohn, 1999; Reinherz et al., 1989; Rueter, Scaramella, Wallace, & Conger, 1999). For example, a recent breakup with a boyfriend or girlfriend has been found to significantly increase the likelihood of a depressive episode in adolescents

(Monroe et al., 1999). Thus, stressors within the interpersonal domain are particularly likely to lead to depression in children and adolescents.

This is especially probable for individuals who tend to be more socially dependent or sociotropic. That is, according to the specific vulnerability hypothesis (Beck, 1983, Blatt, Quinlan, Chevron, McDonald, & Zuroff, 1982), individuals whose self-esteem is derived from interpersonal relationships (sociotropy) are at increased risk for depression when they experience stressors within the social domain; in contrast, those who derive their self-worth from achievement-related goals are at greater risk for depression when they encounter failure.

Studies investigating this specific vulnerability hypothesis in children have been supportive (Hammen & Goodman-Brown, 1990; Little & Garber, in press; Luthar & Blatt, 1995). Luthar and Blatt (1995) reported that adolescents high on interpersonal dependence were more likely to become depressed when they had interpersonal difficulties. In a short-term prospective study, Little and Garber (in press) found that among boys who experienced negative social stressors, those who were high in interpersonal connectedness reported increases in depressive symptoms. For girls, level of social stressors and connectedness each directly and significantly predicted depressive symptoms.

Thus, prospective studies have found considerable support for the contribution of stressful life events to increases in depressive symptoms and the onset of depressive disorders in children and adolescents. When the stressors that occur fall into an individual's particular area of vulnerability, the likelihood of depression is even greater. As we become better at identifying individuals' specific areas of concern, we will improve our ability to predict who is most likely to become depressed and under what circumstances (Monroe & Roberts, 1990).

Offspring Studies

Do offspring of depressed parents experience higher levels of stress and does this increase their vulnerability to depression themselves? Studies have shown that children living with depressed parents are exposed to high levels of stress (Hammen et al., 1987; Hirsch, Moos, & Reischl, 1985). Hammen et al. (1987) reported that compared to families with medically ill or well mothers, families with unipolar depressed mothers had higher levels of negative life events, including marital discord, family conflict, financial problems, and occupational difficulties.

Marriages of depressed individuals have been reported to be especially conflictual, tense, and hostile (e.g., Gotlib & Beach, 1995). The high levels of divorce, marital disruption, and negative spousal interactions observed in depressed patients and their spouses (Gotlib & Hammen, 1992) clearly can be a stressor for children that adversely affects their development

(Cummings & Davies, 1994b; Grych & Fincham, 1990). Indeed, among offspring of depressed parents, those whose parents were divorced have been found to be more likely to have behavioral problems (Fendrich, Warner, & Weissman, 1990; Goodman, Brogan, Lynch, & Fielding, 1993). Such marital discord with its associated hostility and anger may be one mechanism through which maternal depression leads to child psychopathology (Gotlib & Lee, 1990; Rutter & Quinton, 1984).

Thus, offspring of depressed parents are exposed to a variety of acute and chronic stressors that often are a direct result of their parent's psychopathology. Moreover, these children themselves contribute to the occurrence of stressors. Adrian and Hammen (1993) found that compared to children of normal mothers, offspring of depressed mothers had higher levels of dependent life events, particularly interpersonal conflict.

Not only are offspring of depressed mothers exposed to more independent and dependent stressors, but they also may be less competent at dealing with them. Garber, Braafladt, and Zeman (1991) reported that both depressed mothers and their children generated fewer and lower-quality coping strategies than did nondepressed mothers and their children. This lack of adequate coping skills is likely to lead to longer exposure to the negative events and possibly the generation of more stressors.

Prevention

Prevention studies that target stressors typically do not aim to eliminate the occurrence of negative life events per se but, rather, focus on variables that are likely to moderate the impact of these stressors on children's adjustment. Wolchik and Sandler (1997) have suggested that the primary factors that affect children's adaptation to major stressful situations are social environmental resources and children's coping skills. If preventive approaches that target these constructs decrease the likelihood of child distress, this would be consistent with the view that the lack of social support and child coping abilities may play a role in the development of depressive symptoms as well.

Prevention studies have been conducted that specifically target children exposed to various kinds of stressors including parental divorce (Wolchik et al., 1993) and death of a family member (Sandler, West, Baca, & Pillow, 1992). Wolchik et al. (1993) used a parent-based program that focused on improving the mother–child relationship, discipline, negative divorce events, contact with fathers, and support from nonparental adults. They found higher functioning in children in the treatment than in the control group. The Family Bereavement Program of Sandler et al. (1992) targeted improving the warmth and supportiveness of the family environment and maintaining family discussions of grief-related issues. Again, they found decreased levels of depression and other symptoms in children receiving intervention compared to controls.

In another prevention study, Zubernis, Cassidy, Gillham, Reivich, and Jaycox (1999) implemented a program specifically aimed at reducing depression in children from divorced and intact families. This program taught both cognitive and social problem-solving skills. They found that levels of depressive symptoms decreased over time in children from both intact and divorced families, although the effects were not sustained over 24 months in the divorced group.

Thus, prevention programs that target children undergoing specific life events such as divorce or death can reduce the likelihood of maladjustment in children by manipulating moderators of the effects of these stressors. Such prevention programs also should teach both parents and children about their possible role in the generation of stressors in order to decrease the likelihood of their occurring in the first place.

In summary, there clearly is a link between stressors and depression. But by what mechanisms does stress increase an individual's vulnerability to depression? Although stressors often precede mood disorders, not all individuals exposed to stressors become depressed. That is, there is not a perfect correspondence between exposure to negative life events and the onset of depressive symptoms or disorders. Rather, it is how individuals interpret and respond to events that differentiates who does and does not become depressed. Much of the individual variability is due to differences in appraisals of the meaning of the events with regard to the self and future. Such appraisal processes are central to cognitive theories of depression.

Cognitive Vulnerability

According to cognitive theories of depression (Abramson et al., 1989; Beck, 1967), depressed individuals have negative beliefs about themselves and their future and tend to make global, stable, and internal attributions for negative events. When confronted with stressful life events, individuals who have such cognitive tendencies will appraise the stressors and their consequences more negatively, and therefore they are more likely to become depressed than are individuals who do not have such cognitive styles. These are essentially cognitive diathesis–stress models because cognitions are presumed to contribute to the onset of depression primarily in the context of stressful life events.

Cross-Sectional Studies

The empirical literature generally has shown that depressed and nondepressed children and adolescents report the hypothesized depressogenic attributional style, negative expectations and hopelessness, cognitive distortions, and cognitive errors (Garber & Hilsman, 1992; Gladstone & Kaslow, 1995). Although such covariation between negative cognitions and current depression is certainly consistent with there being a cognitive vulnerability, the alternative that cognitions are a concomitant or consequence of a depressive state cannot be ruled out from cross-sectional studies (Barnett & Gotlib, 1988; Haaga, Dyck, & Ernst, 1991). Negative cognitions could be the result of the underlying depressive process and hold no particular causal status. Depressions that are clearly caused by a biological process, such as Cushing's disease, have been found to be characterized by some of the same kinds of negative cognitions found in other depressions (Hollon, 1992). Thus, negative cognitions could simply be a symptom of the depressive disorder.

In addition, the experience of depression itself could lead to depressogenic cognitions. This hypothesis has found mixed support (Lewinsohn, Steinmetz, Larson, & Franklin, 1981). Lewinsohn and colleagues (Lewinsohn et al., 1981; Rohde, Lewinsohn, & Seeley, 1994) have not found that depression permanently affected cognitive style in either adults or adolescents. In contrast, Nolen-Hoeksema et al. (1992) reported that children who experienced relatively higher levels of depressive symptoms had more pessimistic explanatory styles over time than did their less depressed peers. Moreover, explanatory style became more pessimistic over time in the group of children with higher levels of depressive symptoms, even after their level of depression declined. Nolen-Hoeksema et al. (1992) concluded that "a period of depression during childhood can lead to the development of a fixed and more pessimistic explanatory style, which remains with a child after his or her depression has begun to subside" (p. 418). Given the differences in the ages of the subjects studied in the Nolen-Hoeksema et al. versus Lewinsohn studies, it is possible that the "scarring" effect of depression on cognitive style occurs earlier in development.

Some have argued that if cognitive style is a vulnerability to depression, it should be a stable characteristic present both during and after depressive episodes (Barnett & Gotlib, 1988), although others have questioned this assertion (Just et al., in press). If negative cognitions are a stable characteristic of depression-vulnerable individuals, then persons whose depressions have remitted should continue to report a more negative cognitive style than never-depressed individuals, although possibly not at the same level as those who are currently depressed. Whereas some studies have found that compared with nondepressed controls, formerly depressed adults continue to report more negative cognitions even after their depression has remitted (e.g., Eaves & Rush, 1984; Teasdale & Dent, 1987), most studies have found that the cognitions of remitted persons are not significantly different from those of nondepressed controls (Fennell & Campbell, 1984; Hamilton & Abramson, 1983; Lewinsohn et al., 1981; Persons & Miranda, 1992; Rohde, Lewinsohn, & Seeley, 1990). Similarly, studies in children and adolescents have not found cognitive differences between remitted and nondepressed individuals (Asarnow & Bates, 1988; McCauley, Mitchell, Burke, & Moss,

1988). In contrast, Gotlib, Lewinsohn, Seeley, Rohde, and Redner (1993) reported that the cognitions of remitted adolescents did not return to normal levels, although neither did their levels of depressive symptoms.

Taken together, these mixed findings have been used to argue against there being a stable cognitive style that serves as a vulnerability to depression (Barnett & Gotlib, 1988; Segal & Dobson, 1992). Just et al. (in press), however, have noted several limitations of these kinds of "remission" studies, including that (1) treatment could have altered formerly depressed patients' cognitions, (2) the formerly depressed group might have been heterogeneous with regard to cognitive style, and (3) cognitive style might need to be activated to be assessed properly. Thus, the stability of the cognitive vulnerability needs to be studied further.

Prospective Studies

Short-term longitudinal studies examining the contribution of cognitions to the prediction of depression have been both supportive (e.g., Cutrona, 1983; Metalsky, Joiner, Hardin, & Abramson, 1993) and nonsupportive (e.g., Cochran & Hammen, 1985; Lewinsohn et al., 1981). Abramson et al. (1989) argued that these longitudinal results have been mixed because some studies tested a "cognitive trait theory" in which only the relation between the cognitive variables and depression was assessed rather than testing a "cognition–stress interaction theory" in which both the cognitive predisposition and negative life events are considered in interaction with one another. Whereas a cognitive-trait theory would predict that all individuals who have the depressogenic cognitive predisposition should become depressed, the cognitive diathesis–stress model improves predictability by suggesting that cognitively vulnerable individuals will become depressed *when* they are faced with important stressful events.

Several prospective studies have tested the cognitive diathesis–stress model of depression in children (Hilsman & Garber, 1995; Nolen-Hoeksema et al., 1992; Panak & Garber, 1992; Robinson, Garber, & Hilsman, 1995). Garber and colleagues (Hilsman & Garber, 1995; Panak & Garber, 1992; Robinson et al., 1995), in three different short-term longitudinal studies using different stressors (grades, peer rejection, and school transition) and different time periods, found that cognitions (attributions, self-worth) measured before the stressors occurred moderated the effect of the stressors on depressive symptoms in children. That is, among those children who experienced high levels of stress, those with more negative cognitions about the self or causes of events were more likely to show increases in depressive symptoms compared to those without such negative cognitions. Thus, studies that have explicitly tested the cognitive–stress interaction have found support for the cognitive model and for the existence of a cognitive vulnerability.

Offspring Studies

If negative cognitions contribute to the development of mood disorders, then high-risk offspring of depressed parents should be more likely to exhibit a cognitive vulnerability than children whose parents have not experienced mood disorders. Only a few studies have explicitly tested this hypothesis. Jaenicke et al. (1987) found that offspring of unipolar mothers reported significantly lower self-esteem and a more depressogenic attributional style than did children of medically ill and control mothers. Goodman, Adamson, Riniti, and Cole (1994) similarly found that children of depressed mothers reported significantly lower perceived self-worth than did children of well mothers. In a college student sample, Taylor and Ingram (1999) found that when primed, offspring of depressed mothers showed more negative information processing and a less positive self-concept than did offspring of nondepressed mothers.

Finally, Garber and Robinson (1997b) found that high-risk children, particularly offspring of mothers with a more chronic history of depression, reported a significantly more negative cognitive style than did children of mothers with no history of psychiatric disorders. Even when children's current level of depressive symptoms was controlled, high- and low-risk children continued to differ with regard to their attributional style and perceived self-worth. Thus, children who are at risk for depression but who have not yet experienced depression themselves have been found to report a more depressogenic cognitive style that might be a vulnerability to later depression.

Prevention

If cognitive prevention programs that change negative thinking show lower rates of depression in the treated versus the untreated group, this would be consistent with cognitive vulnerability models of depression. Seligman and colleagues (Gillham, Reivich, Jaycox, & Seligman, 1995; Hollon, DeRubeis, & Seligman, 1992; Jaycox, Reivich, Gillham, & Seligman, 1994) have found that a cognitive prevention program that focuses particularly on changing attributional style successfully reduced the rates of depressive symptoms in children and college students.

Clarke et al. (1995) implemented a targeted cognitive prevention program in a sample of adolescents with elevated levels of depressive symptoms. The intervention involved 15 group sessions in which participants were taught cognitive techniques to identify and challenge their negative thoughts. Results of this randomized prevention trial indicated that the incidence rates of depressive disorders in the treatment group were significantly lower than those in the control group.

Thus, cognitive prevention programs that explicitly teach adolescents how to examine and dispute their negative beliefs and attributions appear to successfully reduce the occurrence of depressive symptoms and disorders. Future prevention studies need to examine whether these programs have long-term effects on reducing depressive symptoms and disorders and whether they can be implemented with younger children.

In summary, evidence from correlational, predictive, offspring, and prevention studies indicates that a negative cognitive style may be a vulnerability to depressive symptoms and disorders in children and adolescents. This cognitive style involves negative beliefs about the self and explanations about the causes of negative events. More adequate studies examining the stability of this cognitive vulnerability need to be conducted (Just et al., in press). In addition, the extent to which these cognitions need to be primed in children and adolescents should be explored further (Ingram et al., 1998).

Interpersonal Vulnerability

Interpersonal perspectives on depression emphasize the importance of the social environment and the development of secure attachments (Cummings & Cicchetti, 1990; Gotlib & Hammen, 1992; Joiner & Coyne, 1999). Vulnerability to depression presumably arises in early family environments in which the child's need for security, comfort, and acceptance are not met. Bowlby (1980) argued that children with caretakers who are consistently accessible and supportive will develop cognitive representations, or "working models," of the self and others as positive and trustworthy. In contrast, caretakers who are characterized by unresponsiveness or inconsistency will produce insecure attachments leading to working models that include abandonment, self-criticism, and excessive dependency. Such working models presumably increase individuals' vulnerability to depression, particularly when exposed to new interpersonal stressors.

Over the last decade, there have been several reviews of the literature concerning the relation between the family environment and depression (Beardslee et al., 1998; Chiariello & Orvaschel, 1995; Cummings & Davies, 1994a; Downey & Coyne, 1990; Gelfand & Teti, 1990; Kaslow, Deering, & Racusin, 1994; Keitner & Miller, 1990; McCauley & Myers, 1992). We highlight here consistencies in empirical findings regarding the role of the family environment in increasing an individual's vulnerability to depression.

Cross-Sectional Studies

Families of depressed children and adolescents are characterized by problems with attachment, communication, conflict, and social support. Although few studies have tested Bowlby's attachment model directly in relation to depression, some have reported findings consistent with it. Depressed adolescents have less secure attachments to parents than do nondepressed individuals (Armsden, McCauley, Greenberg, Burke, & Mitchell, 1990; Kenny, Moilanen, Lomax, & Brabeck, 1993; Kobak, Sudler, & Gamble, 1991). Moreover, adolescents undergoing stressful life events are more likely to become depressed if they had insecure attachments to their parents than adolescents with more secure attachments (Hammen et al., 1995; Kobak et al., 1991).

Beyond attachment, other kinds of dysfunctional patterns have been found to characterize families of currently depressed children (Kaslow et al., 1994) and adolescents (Reinherz et al., 1989; Sheeber, Hops, Andrews, Alpert, & Davis, 1998). In observations of mother–child interactions, mothers of depressed children have been described as being less rewarding (Cole & Rehm, 1986) and more dominant and controlling (Amanat & Butler, 1984) than mothers of nondepressed children. In addition, currently depressed adults recall having had more family problems as children (Gerlsma, Emmelkamp, & Arrindell, 1990).

Currently depressed children and adolescents perceive their families to be less cohesive and more conflictual than nondepressed youth (e.g., Stark, Humphrey, Crook, & Lewis, 1990; Walker, Garber, & Greene, 1993). Asarnow, Carlson, and Guthrie (1987), however, did not find differences between depressed and nondepressed inpatients' reports about their family environment, although the suicidal patients did describe their families as more dysfunctional compared to nonsuicidal patients.

Depressed children and adolescents also describe their parents to be more rejecting than do nondepressed youth. In retrospective reports about their childhood, currently depressed adults recall being rejected by parents. In adolescents, self-reported depressive symptoms have been significantly associated with perceived rejection, particularly by fathers (Baron & MacGillivray, 1989), and among those youth high in reassurance seeking (Joiner, 1999).

Depressed children also have significant peer difficulties and social skills deficits (e.g., Altmann & Gotlib, 1988; Blechman, McEnroe, Carella, & Audette, 1986). Self- reported depression significantly correlates with teachers' reports of peer rejection in children (Rudolph, Hammen & Burge, 1994) and low peer ratings in adolescents (Luthar & Blatt, 1995). In laboratory studies, both children (Peterson, Mullins, & Ridley-Johnson, 1985) and adolescents (Connolly, Geller, Marton, & Kutcher, 1992) rated peers displaying depressive symptoms more negatively than peers without symptoms.

Finally, few studies have examined whether interpersonal difficulties persist after depressive symptoms have remitted. In one of the earliest investigations of interpersonal functioning in a clinical sample, Puig-Antich et al. (1985a) reported that currently depressed children were less communicative and more distant with family members. Although the mother–child relationship showed some improvement with symptom remission, the children continued to show interpersonal difficulties even in the absence of depression, particularly with siblings (Puig-Antich et al., 1985b).

Armsden et al. (1990) compared currently depressed, formerly depressed, psychiatric controls, and nonpsychiatric controls with regard to their reported attachment to parents and peers. The currently depressed group reported significantly less secure parent and peer attachment compared to nondepressed controls, whereas adolescents with resolved depression reported scores that fell in between these groups and were not significantly different from either. Thus, there might be some improvement in perceptions about interpersonal attachment after depressive symptoms remit, although not back to the same level of nondepressed youth.

In summary, depression in children is associated with high levels of interpersonal conflict and rejection from various members in their social domain including family, friends, and peers. It is likely that the link between interpersonal vulnerability and depression is bidirectional. Prospective studies can help untangle this issue by exploring the temporal relations between interpersonal difficulties and depression.

Prospective Studies

Prospective studies have examined the contribution of family dysfunction, parent–child conflict, peer difficulties, and interpersonal rejection to increases in and maintenance of depressive symptoms in children and adolescents. These studies have shown both that social problems temporally precede depression, and that depression contributes to interpersonal difficulties. Longitudinal studies have found that family dysfunction in the form of perceived lack of family cohesion or parental attachment (Garrison et al., 1997; Leadbeater et al., 1999), parent–adolescent conflict, (Buchanan & Brinke, 1998; Lewinsohn, Roberts, et al., 1994; Rueter et al., 1999), hostile child-rearing attitudes (Katainen, Raikkonen, Keskivaara, & Keltikangas-Jarvinen, 1999), and maternal criticism (Garber et al., 1999) significantly predict increases in depressive symptoms or the onset of depressive disorders in children and adolescents. For example, Rueter et al. (1999) reported that increasing disagreements between parents and adolescents over time predicted increases in internalizing symptoms, and, conversely, decreasing disagreements predicted symptom decline. Thus, there was a clear association between interpersonal conflict and changes in symptoms.

Several studies also have shown that social adversities contribute to the maintenance or relapse of depressive disorders in youth. Such interpersonal difficulties as persistent poor friendships, low involvement of fathers, stressful family environments, and lack of responsiveness to maternal discipline significantly predict persistent depression (Goodyer, Germany, Gowrusankur, & Altham, 1991; Goodyer, Herbert, Tamplin, Secher, & Pearson, 1997; McCauley et al., 1993; Sanford et al., 1995). In addition, negative attitudes by family members toward depressed children have been found to predict relapse (Asarnow, Goldstein, Tompson, & Guthrie, 1993).

A few prospective studies have demonstrated that rejection by parents and peers predicts subsequent depressive symptoms in children and adolescents. Lefkowitz and Tesiny (1984) reported that rejection by fathers predicted later depression in girls but not boys. However, they did not control for prior depressive symptoms so it is not possible to determine whether rejection contributed beyond initial depression. Wichstrom, Anderson, Holte, and Wynne (1996) reported that children subjected to disqualifying communications from family members showed increases in psychological distress.

With regard to peer rejection, French, Conrad, and Turner (1995) noted that rejection by peers predicted higher levels of self-reported depressive symptoms among antisocial but not among nonantisocial youth. Panak and Garber (1992) found that increases in peer-rated aggression predicted increases in self-reported depression through the mediator of increases in peer-reported rejection. Moreover, the relation between peer-rated rejection and self-reported depression was mediated by perceived rejection. Kistner, Balthazor, Risi, and Burton (1999) similarly found that perceived rejection predicted increases in depressive symptoms during middle childhood.

Two studies have examined both rejection and depression as prospective predictors of one another in adolescents. Vernberg (1990) found that controlling for prior levels of self-reported depressive symptoms, increases in perceived peer rejection significantly predicted depression 6 months later. Moreover, self-reported depression predicted perceived peer rejection, controlling for prior perceived rejection. Similarly, in a 3-year longitudinal study, Nolan and Garber (2000) found that rejection and depression, measured with multiple informants, each significantly predicted the other, controlling for prior levels. Thus, consistent with Coyne's (1976) interpersonal model of depression, rejection by both family and peers appears to be a risk factor for depression in children and adolescents, and expressions of depressive symptoms contribute to the likelihood of being rebuffed by others in one's social network.

Offspring Studies

Relationships between depressed parents and their children consistently have been found to be disrupted (Goodman & Gotlib, 1999; Hammen, 1991b). Offspring of depressed caregivers have been found to have more insecure attachments compared to offspring of well mothers (DeMulder & Radke-Yarrow, 1991; Teti, Gelfand, Messinger, & Isabella, 1995). Moreover, insecurely attached offspring of depressed mothers tend to have difficulties in their relationships with peers (Rubin et al., 1991).

Observations of depressed mothers interacting with their children reveal that these mothers are more negative (Garber et al., 1991; Lovejoy, 1991), more controlling (Kochanska, Kuczynski, Radke-Yarrow, & Welsh, 1987), and less responsive and affectively involved (Cohn & Tronick, 1989; Goodman & Brumley, 1990), and they use less productive communications (Gordon et al., 1989). In addition, negative reciprocal interaction patterns have been observed between depressed mothers and their children (Hammen, Burge, & Stansbury, 1990; Hops et al., 1987; Radke-Yarrow & Nottelman, 1989).

Such nonsupportive and negative family environments increase children's vulnerabilities for depression in several ways. First, through modeling and direct feedback from their depressed parents, children learn inadequate patterns of social interactions, problem solving, and affect regulation. Second, such negative exchanges with parents teach children about their own worth and about the extent to which others can be trusted and counted on for support (Garber & Flynn, 1998). These dysfunctional working models of themselves and others increase their risk of depression, particularly when they encounter new interpersonal challenges.

Prevention

Although no prevention program has been implemented that specifically targets all the various aspects of interpersonal vulnerability to depression described here, components of several treatment and prevention programs could be used to design such an intervention. For example, social skills training programs that teach children appropriate ways of interacting with peers have been effective in reducing social problems in children (Bierman, Greenberg, & Conduct Problems Prevention Research Group, 1996). Treatment programs with depressed children that have included a social skills training component have been found to reduce depressive symptoms (Butler, Miezitis, Friedman, & Cole, 1980). Such interventions support the notion that social skills deficits may be part of the interpersonal vulnerability to depression in children.

Beardslee (1998) developed one important family-based depression preventive intervention. It is a psychoeducational program that targets offspring of parents with mood disorders. The aims of the program are to (1) educate all family members about affective disorders and about risks and resilience in children, (2) link the psychoeducational material to the family's own life experience, (3) decrease feelings of guilt and blame in children, (4) help the children develop relationships both within and outside the family, and (5) facilitate their independent functioning in school and outside the home. Outcome studies have shown that the intervention positively changes family functioning, and that in those families in which family functioning has improved, the adolescents show better adjustment (Beardslee, Wright, Rothberg, Salt, & Versage, 1996; Beardslee et al., 1997). The success of this prevention program provides support for the possible role that the family plays in adolescent depression among offspring of parents with mood disorders.

In summary, two important findings emerge regarding the link between interpersonal vulnerability and depression in children and adolescents. First, families with a depressed member tend to be characterized by less support and more conflict, and such family dysfunction increases children's risk of developing depression. Second, depressed children and adolescents are themselves more interpersonally difficult, which results in greater problems in their social network. Thus, the relation between child depression and interpersonal dysfunction is bidirectional. That is, family and peer environments clearly are important and sometimes stressful contexts in which children develop schema about themselves and others, which then can serve as a vulnerability to depression. In addition, children's own reactions to these environments can exacerbate and perpetuate negative social exchanges, which furthers the interpersonal vicious cycle, thereby resulting in more rejection and depression (Coyne, 1976). Thus, a transactional model of mutual influence probably best characterizes the association between depressed individuals and their social environment (Sameroff & Chandler, 1975).

Other Risk Factors

Several other factors have been identified that increase risk for depression. Risk indicates the increased probability of an outcome, but it does not imply causation. Thus, risk factors differ from vulnerability variables because they do not explain mechanisms by which they produce the disorder. Two risk factors that often have been linked with depressive disorders include female gender and prior depressive symptoms.

Gender

Being female clearly increases risk for depression (Weissman & Olfson, 1995); this sex difference emerges during adolescence (Hankin et al., 1998; Lewinsohn, Roberts, et al., 1994). Several theorists (Cyranowski, Frank, Young, & Shear, 2000; Leadbeater, Blatt, & Quinlan, 1995; Nolen-Hoeksema & Girgus, 1994; Rutter, 1986) have speculated about why women are at greater risk than men and about what accounts for the change in the sex ratio of depression from childhood to adolescence.

Nolen-Hoeksema and Girgus (1994) proposed three developmental models to explain sex differences in depression that emerge during adolescence: (1) the causes of depression are the same in girls and boys, but girls have more of these causal agents; (2) different processes cause depression in girls and boys, and the causal agents in girls might be more prevalent during adolescence; or (3) the causes of depression are the same in girls and boys, but girls have more of these factors prior to adolescence, and depression does not onset until these earlier causal agents interact with other variables (e.g., stress) that occur during adolescence.

Rutter (1986) outlined several potential mechanisms that may contribute to the emergence of sex differences in depression during adolescence, including (1) hormonal changes accompanying puberty, (2) genetic regulatory processes, (3) alterations in the frequency of environmental stressors, (4) developmental changes in the availability of social support, (5) developing cognitive processes such as attributional style, and (6) the manner in which emotions are experienced, expressed, and regulated.

Results of studies examining the relation between puberty and depression have been mixed (Angold, Costello, & Worthman, 1998; Angold & Rutter, 1992; Brooks-Gunn & Warren, 1989). Angold et al. (1998) conducted a careful assessment of both morphological development and diagnoses of depression and found that pubertal status was a better predictor than age of the emergence of sex differences in depression. Girls were more likely than boys to be depressed only after the transition to Tanner Stage III and above (mid-puberty), whereas boys had higher rates before Tanner Stage III. Angold et al. (1998) noted that pubertal status is just a marker of risk and does not explain the mechanism underlying the link between puberty and depression in girls. The hormonal, cognitive, and socioemotional changes that occur in girls and boys with puberty need to be explored further to better understand the emergence of sex differences in depression.

Prior Depressive Symptoms

One of the strongest predictors of subsequent depression is prior depression. Compas et al. (1993) suggested that depressed mood may be a marker of risk for subsequent depressive syndromes. Studies have found that subsyndromal levels of depressive symptoms significantly increase the risk of having a full major depressive episode in adults (Horwath, Johnson, Klerman, & Weissman, 1992; Judd, Akiskal, & Paulus, 1997) and adolescents (Lewinsohn et al., 1999; Pine, Cohen, Cohen, & Brook, 1999; Rueter et al., 1999). Rueter et al. (1999) found that adolescents reporting high levels of internalizing symptoms were at increased risk for the subsequent first onset of a mood disorder. Similarly, Pine et al. (1999) reported that having depressive symptoms during adolescence predicted a two- to threefold greater risk of an episode of major depression in adulthood.

By what mechanisms do prior depressive symptoms lead to more symptoms later? It could be that prodomal symptoms weaken an individual's resources to deal with the everyday events and stressors that occur. Such individuals would have a lower threshold for stress; that is, fewer or less severe negative life events would set off a depressive episode.

Another possibility is that the subsyndromal symptoms themselves produce more stressors, which lead to the onset of a depressive episode. For
example, irritable adolescents are more likely to get into interpersonal conflicts with parents and peers. Concentration difficulties or low self-esteem
might interfere with school performance, leading to more academic
stressors. This view is consistent with the stress-generation hypothesis suggested by Hammen (1991a). An important issue for future research is to
explain what starts and maintains subsyndromal levels of depressive symptoms and by what processes they intensify and expand into the full depressive syndrome.

CONCLUSIONS AND FUTURE DIRECTIONS

This chapter highlights what is known and what still needs to be studied
with regard to vulnerabilities for depression. Most knowledge has come
from cross-sectional studies that compared depressed and nondepressed individuals. Prospective studies have shown that stress, cognitions, and social
difficulties temporally precede depressive symptoms and disorders. High-
risk designs have demonstrated that the offspring of depressed parents have
neurobiological, cognitive, and interpersonal vulnerabilities that put them
at risk for developing depression. Early prevention efforts have provided
some support for the use of interventions that teach cognitive and coping
skills for reducing the likelihood of depression in children and adolescents.

Thus, some evidence supports each of the different vulnerability models of depression that have been articulated. How can all these theories be
right? One way to deal with such etiological heterogeneity has been to suggest specific subtypes that map on to different causal processes (Abramson
et al., 1989; Winokur, 1997). Winokur (1997) suggested that unipolar depression can be divided into endogenous, reactive, and emotionally unstable
on the basis of differences in clinical, follow-up, personality, familial, and
treatment variables.

Another approach has been to formulate integrated models of depression that include the additive or interactive effects of multiple vulnerability
factors (e.g., Abramson et al., 1989; Akiskal & McKinney, 1975; Gotlib &
Hammen, 1992). In an earlier integrated model, Akiskal and McKinney
(1975) suggested that most distal causal processes such as stressors and low
rates of positive reinforcement went through a common final neuroanatomical pathway. Diathesis–stress models highlight the interaction of person characteristics such as genetic or cognitive vulnerability with the experience of environmental stressors (Abramson et al., 1989; Beck, 1976; Kendler
et al., 1995; Monroe & Simons, 1991). Interpersonal cognitive approaches
(e.g., Gotlib & Hammen, 1992; Safran & Segal, 1990) suggest that individuals' cognitions about important social relationships can be a vulnerability to depression when negative interpersonal events occur. Moreover,

negative cognitive schema about the self and others are the result of earlier attachment and interpersonal difficulties. Ingram et al. (1998), on the other hand, emphasized that cognitive processes were the common final pathway through which all social as well as nonsocial information was processed and linked to depression.

It is likely that a broad biopsychosocial model of depression is needed that will incorporate most of the vulnerability processes discussed here (Gotlib & Hammen, 1992; Petersen et al., 1993). Such a model would suggest that children are born with certain biological propensities and tendencies, such as stress-reactivity or an irritable temperament, that make them more vulnerable to the effects of negative life events or less able to obtain help from others to deal with stressors. As children grow they learn, in part, through interactions with important others, that they either are or are not capable of coping with the stressors of life and that others either can or cannot be counted on for support. Exposure to stressful life events can activate negative affective structures that connect with developing negative schema about the self and others (Ingram et al., 1998). A cycle begins in which they develop some symptoms of depression (e.g., low self-esteem; anhedonia) that then lead to their being exposed to further stressors such as interpersonal rejection and academic failures. Also, exposure to chronic or severe stressors can produce biological changes that further maintain or exacerbate the depressive symptoms. Over time, depressions might become more autonomous (Post, 1992), but at least during childhood and adolescence depression likely is more closely linked with exposure to stress.

What needs to be done from here? First, future studies should examine multivariate vulnerability models. Such investigations should not simply examine the independent contribution of individual risk factors but should test more complex moderator and mediation models that explore how these vulnerability factors synergistically combine to explain the onset of depression. Second, by testing such multivariate models, we will be better able to address questions of specificity. Just because a particular risk factor (e.g., stress) predicts more than one disorder (e.g., anxiety and depression), it does not mean that the risk factor cannot be part of a more complex causal model (Garber & Hollon, 1991). It will only be possible to address the issue of specificity by comparing vulnerability models rather than individual risk factors.

Third, the various research strategies described here should be combined. For example, studies should compare currently depressed, remitted, high-risk, and never depressed children with regard to these multivariate models. In addition, these groups should be followed over time in order to address the question of temporal precedence in the relations among the vulnerability predictors and depressive outcomes. Finally, experimental designs that randomly assign children from each of these groups (i.e., currently depressed, remitted, high-risk, and never depressed) to singular as well as to multimodal interventions are needed to examine questions of change. In addition, more laboratory analogue studies that experimentally manipulate specific processes are needed to understand the causal mechanisms.

Several important developmental questions remain regarding vulnerability to depression. Theories of depression need to account for differences in the phenomenology of depression in children and adults and in changes in the rates of depression from childhood to adolescence, particularly in girls. Are the processes that underlie childhood-onset depressions different from those that explain depressions that have their first onset during adolescence or adulthood? Are vulnerabilities different for first versus recurrent episodes of depression? How do we account for the recurrent nature of depression across the lifespan? Do depressive vulnerabilities change with development, and if so, how? When and how do depressive vulnerabilities develop and unfold?

One final fundamental question that remains is whether depressive vulnerabilities are permanent characteristics of individuals and by what internal and external mechanisms are they turned on and off. That is, what biological, psychosocial, or environmental processes set off vulnerabilities to produce depressive symptoms and episodes of disorder, and, conversely, how do we explain the remission of symptoms? Do vulnerable individuals no longer have the risk factor(s) or do they develop mechanisms for compensating for them?

ACKNOWLEDGMENTS

Judy Garber was supported in part by grants from the National Institute of Mental Health (No. R01-MH57822-01A1) and from the William T. Grant Foundation (No. 96173096) during completion of this work. Cynthia Flynn was supported in part from an NIMH training grant (No. T32-MH18921).

REFERENCES

Abramson, L. Y., Metalsky, G. I., & Alloy, L. B. (1989). Hopelessness depression: A theory-based subtype of depression. *Psychological Review, 96,* 358–372.

Achenbach, T. M. (1991). *Manual for the Child Behavior Checklist 4–18 and Revised 1991 Child Behavior Profile.* Burlington: University of Vermont, Department of Psychiatry.

Adrian, C., & Hammen, C. (1993). Stress exposure and stress generation in children of depressed mothers. *Journal of Consulting and Clinical Psychology, 61,* 354–359.

Akiskal, H. S., & McKinney, W. T. (1975). Overview of recent research in depression: Integration of ten conceptual models into a comprehensive clinical framework. *Archives of General Psychiatry, 32,* 285–305.

Allgood-Merten, B., Lewinsohn, P. M., & Hops, H. (1990). Sex differences and adolescent depression. *Journal of Abnormal Psychology, 99,* 55–63.

Altmann, E. O., & Gotlib, I. H. (1988). The social behavior of depressed children: An observational study. *Journal of Abnormal Child Psychology, 16,* 29–44.

Amanat, E., & Butler, C. (1984). Oppressive behaviors in the families of depressed children. *Family Therapy, 11,* 65–75.

American Psychiatric Association. (1994). *Diagnostic and statistical manual of mental disorders* (4th ed.). Washington, DC: Author.

Angold, A., & Costello, E. J. (1993). Depressive comorbidity in children and adolescents: Empirical, theoretical, and methodological issues. *American Journal of Psychiatry, 150,* 1779–1791.

Angold, A., Costello, E. J., & Worthman, C. M. (1998). Puberty and depression: The roles of age, pubertal status, and pubertal timing. *Psychological Medicine, 28,* 51–61.

Angold, A., & Rutter, M. (1992). Effects of age and pubertal status on depression in a large clinical sample. *Development and Psychopathology, 4,* 5–28.

Armsden, G. C., McCauley, E., Greenberg, M. T., Burke, P. M., & Mitchell, J. R. (1990). Parent and peer attachment in early adolescent depression. *Journal of Abnormal Child Psychology, 18,* 683–698.

Asarnow, J. R., & Bates, S. (1988). Depression in child psychiatric inpatients: Cognitive and attributional patterns. *Journal of Abnormal Child Psychology, 16,* 601–615.

Asarnow, J. R., Carlson, G. A., & Guthrie, D. (1987). Coping strategies, self- perceptions, hopelessness, and perceived family environments in depressed and suicidal children. *Journal of Consulting and Clinical Psychology, 55,* 361–366.

Asarnow, J. R., Goldstein, M. J., Tompson, M., & Guthrie, D. (1993). One-year outcomes of depressive disorders in child psychiatric in-patients: Evaluation of the prognostic power of a brief measure of expressed emotion. *Journal of Child Psychology and Psychiatry, 34,* 129–137.

Asarnow, J. R., & Guthrie, D. (1989). Suicidal behavior, depression, and hopelessness in child psychiatric inpatients: A replication and extension. *Journal of Clinical Child Psychology, 18,* 129–136.

Barnett, P. A., & Gotlib, I. H. (1988). Psychosocial functioning and depression: Distinguishing among antecedents, concomitants, and consequences. *Psychological Bulletin, 104,* 97–126.

Baron, P., & MacGillivray, R. G. (1989). Depressive symptoms in adolescents as a function of perceived parental behavior. *Adolescent Research, 4,* 50–62.

Beardslee, W. R. (1998). Prevention and the clinical encounter. *American Journal of Orthopsychiatry, 68,* 521–533.

Beardslee, W. R., Versage, E. M., & Gladstone, T. R. G. (1998). Children of affectively ill parents: A review of the past 10 years. *Journal of the American Academy of Child and Adolescent Psychiatry, 37,* 1134–1141.

Beardslee, W. R., Wright, E., Rothberg, P. C., Salt, P., & Versage, E. (1996). Response of families to two preventive interveion strategies: Long-term differences in behavior and attitude change. *Journal of the American Academy of Child and Adolescent Psychiatry, 35,* 774–782.

Beardslee, W. R., Wright, E., Salt, P., Drezner, K., Gladstone, T. R. G., Versage, E. M., & Rothberg, P. C. (1997). Examination of children's responses to tow preventive intervention strategies over time. *Journal of the American Academy of Child and Adolescent Psychiatry, 36,* 196–204.

Beck, A. T. (1967). *Depression: Clinical, experiential, and theoretical aspects.* New York: Harper & Row.

Beck, A. T. (1976). *Cognitive therapy and the emotional disorders.* New York: International Universities Press.

Beck, A. T. (1983). Cognitive therapy of depression: New perspectives. In P.J. Clayton & J.E. Barrett (Eds.), *Treatment of depression: Old controversies and new approaches* (pp. 265–290). New York: Raven Press.

Beck, A. T., Steer, R. A., Beck, J. S., Newman, C. F. (1993). Hopelessness, depression, suicidal ideation, and clinical diagnosis of depression. *Suicide and Life Threatening Behavior, 23,* 139–145.

Bemporad, J. R., & Wilson, A. (1978). A developmental approach to depression in childhood and adolescence. *Journal of the American Academy of Psychoanalysis, 6,* 325–352.

Bierman, K. L., Greenberg, M. T., & Conduct Problems Prevention Research Group. (1996). Social skills training in the Fast Track program. In R. D. Peters & R. J. McMahon (Eds.), *Preventing childhood disorders, substance abuse, and delinquency* (pp. 65–89). Thousand Oaks, CA: Sage.

Birmaher, B., Dahl, R. E., Williamson, D. E., Perel, J. M., Brent, D. A., Axelson, D. A., Kaufman, J., Dorn, L. D., Stull, S., Rao, U., & Ryan, N. (1999). *Biological correlates in children at high risk to develop depression.* Paper presented at the Child and Adolescent Depression Consortium, Western Psychiatric Institute and Clinic, Pittsburgh, PA.

Birmaher, B., Kaufman, J., Brent, D. A., Dahl, R. E., Perel, J. M., Al-Shabbout, M., Nelson, B., Stull, S., Rao, U., Waterman, G. S., Williamson, D. E., & Ryan, N. D. (1997). Neuroendocrine response to 5-hydroxy-l-tryptophan in prepubertal children at high risk of major depressive disorder. *Archives of General Psychiatry, 54,* 1113–1119.

Birmaher, B., Ryan, N. D., Williamson, D. E., Brent, D. A., Kaufman, J., Dahl, R. E., Perel, J., & Nelson, B. (1996). Childhood and adolescent depression: A review of the past ten years. Part I. *Journal of the American Academy of Child and Adolescent Psychiatry, 35,* 1427–1439.

Blatt, S. J., Quinlan, D. M., Chevron, E. S., McDonald, C., & Zuroff, D. (1982). Dependency and self-criticism: Psychological dimensions of depression. *Journal of Consulting and Clinical Psychology, 50,* 113–124.

Blazer, D. G., Kessler, R. C., McGonagle, K. A., & Swartz, M. S. (1994). The prevalence and distribution of major depression in a national community sample: The national comorbidity survey. *American Journal of Psychiatry, 151,* 979–986.

Blechman, E. A., McEnroe, M. J., Carella, E. T., & Audette, D. P. (1986). *Journal of Abnormal Psychology, 95,* 223–227.

Blehar, M. C., Weissman, M. M., Gershon, E. S., & Hirschfeld, R. M. A. (1988). Family and genetic studies of affective disorders. *Archives of General Psychiatry, 45,* 289–292.

Botteron, K. (1999). *The role of the medial prefrontal cortex in early onset depression: Current results from an epidemiologic twin study.* Paper presented at the Child and Adolescent Depression Consortium, Western Psychiatric Institute and Clinic, Pittsburgh, PA.

Bowlby, J. (1980). *Attachment and loss: Vol 3. Loss, sadness, and depression.* New York: Basic Books.

Brooks-Gunn, J., & Warren, M. P. (1989). Biological and social contributions to negative affect in young adolescent girls. *Child Development, 60*, 40–55.

Brown, G. W., & Harris, T. O. (1978). *Social origins of depression: A study of psychiatric disorder in women.* London: Tavistock.

Brown, G. W., & Harris, T. O. (Eds.). (1989). *Life events and illness.* New York: Guilford Press.

Buchanan, A., & Brinke, J. T. (1998). Measuring outcomes for children: Early parenting experiences, conflict, maladjustment, and depression in adulthood. *Children and Youth Services Review, 20*, 251–278.

Burke, K. C., Burke, J. D., Rae, D., & Regier, D. A. (1991). Comparing age at onset of major depression and other psychiatric disorders by birth cohorts in five US community populations. *Archives of General Psychiatry, 48*, 789–795.

Butler, L., Miezitis, S., Friedman, R., & Cole, E. (1980). The effect of two school-based intervention programs on depressive symptoms in preadolescents. *American Educational Research Journal, 17*, 111–119.

Carlson, G. A., & Kashani, J. H. (1988). Phenomenology of major depression from childhood through adulthood: Analysis of three studies. *American Journal of Psychiatry, 137*, 445–449.

Carskadon, M. A., Keenan, S., & Dement, W. C. (1987). Nighttime sleep and daytime sleep tendency in preadolescents. In C. Guilleminault (Ed.), *Sleep and its disorders* (pp. 43–52). New York: Raven Press.

Cavallo, A., Holt, K. G., Hejazi, M. S., Richards, G. E., & Meyer, W. J. (1987). Melatonin circadian rhythm in childhood depression. *Journal of the American Academy of Child and Adolescent Psychiatry, 26*, 395–399.

Chiariello, M. A., & Orvaschel, H. (1995). Patterns of parent–child communication: Relationship to depression. *Clinical Psychology Review, 15*, 395–407.

Cicchetti, D., & Schneider-Rosen, K. (Eds.). (1984). Childhood depression. *New Directions in Child Development.* San Francisco: Jossey-Bass.

Cicchetti, D., & Toth, S. L. (1998). The development of depression in children and adolescents. *American Psychologist, 53*, 221–241.

Clarke, G. N., Hawkins, W., Murphy, M., Sheeber, L. B., Lewinsohn, P. M., & Seeley, J. R. (1995). Targeted prevention of unipolar depressive disorder in an at-risk sample of high school adolescents: A randomized trial of a group cognitive intervention. *Journal of the Academy of Child and Adolescent Psychiatry, 34*, 312–321.

Cochran, S. D., & Hammen, C. L. (1985). Perceptions of stressful life events and depression: A test of attributional models. *Journal of Personality and Social Psychology, 48*, 1562–1571.

Cohn, J. F., & Tronick, E. (1989). Specificity of infants' response to mothers' affective behavior. *Journal of the American Academy of Child and Adolescent Psychiatry, 28*, 242–249.

Cole, D. A., & Rehm, L. P. (1986). Family interaction patterns and childhood depression. *Journal of Abnormal Child Psychology, 14*, 297–314.

Compas, B. E. (1987). Stress and life events during childhood and adolescence. *Clinical Psychology Review, 7*, 275–302.

Compas, B. E., Ey, S., & Grant, K. (1993). Taxonomy, assessment, and diagnosis of depression during adolescence. *Psychological Bulletin, 114*, 323–344.

Compas, B. E., Grant, K., & Ey, S. (1994). Psychosocial stress and child/adolescent depression: Can we be more specific? In W. M. Reynolds & H. F. Johnston

(Eds.), *Handbook of depression in children and adolescents* (pp. 509–523). New York: Plenum.

Compas, B. E., Howell, D. C., Phares, V., Williams, R. A., & Giunta, C. T. (1989). Risk factors for emotional/behavioral problems in young adolescents: A prospective analysis of parent and adolescent stress and symptoms. *Journal of Consulting and Clinical Psychology, 57,* 732–740.

Connolly, J., Geller, S., Marton, P., & Kutcher, S. (1992). Peer responses to social interaction with depressed adolescents. *Journal of Personality and Social Psychology, 55,* 410–419.

Coryell, W., Akiskal, H. S., Leon, A. C., Winokur, G., Maser, J. D., Mueller, T., & Keller, M. B. (1994). The time course of nonchronic major depressive disorder: Uniformity across episodes and samples. *Archives of General Psychiatry, 51,* 405–410.

Costello, E. J. (1989). Developments in child psychiatric epidemiology. *Journal of the American Academy of Child and Adolescent Psychiatry, 28,* 836–841.

Costello, E. J., Angold, A., Burns, B. J., Stangl, D. K., Tweed, D. L., Erkanli, A., & Worthman, C. M. (1996). The Great Smoky Mountains study of youth: Goals, design, methods, and prevalence of DSM-III-R disorders. *Archives of General Psychiatry, 53,* 1129–1136.

Coyne, J. C. (1976). Toward an interactional description of depression. *Psychiatry, 39,* 28–40.

Coyne, J. C., Kessler, R. C., Tal, M., Turnbull, J., Wortman, C. B., & Greden, J. F. (1987). Living with a depressed person. *Journal of Consulting and Clinical Psychology, 55,* 347–352.

Cummings, E. M., & Cicchetti, D. (1990). Toward a transactional model of relations between attachment and depression. In M. T. Greenberg, D. Cicchetti, & E. M. Cummings (Eds.), *Attachment in the preschool years: Theory, research and intervention* (pp. 339–372). Chicago: University of Chicago Press.

Cummings, E. M., & Davies, P. T. (1994a). Maternal depression and child development. *Journal of Child Psychology and Psychiatry, 35,* 73–112.

Cummings, E. M., & Davies, P. T. (1994b). *Children and marital conflict: The impact of family dispute and resolution.* New York: Guilford Press.

Cutrona, C. E. (1983). Causal attributions and perinatal depression. *Journal of Abnormal Psychology, 92,* 161–172.

Cyranowski, J. M., Frank, E., Young, E., & Shear, M. K. (2000). Adolescent onset of the gender difference in lifetime rates of major depression. *Archives of General Psychiatry, 57,* 21–27.

Dahl, R. E., Kaufman, J., Ryan, N. D., Perel, J., Al-Shabbout, M., Birmaher, B., Nelson, B., & Puig-Antich, J. (1992). The dexamethasone suppression test in children and adolescents: A review and controlled study. *Biological Psychiatry, 32,* 109–126.

Dahl, R. E., Puig-Antich, J., Ryan, N. D., Nelson, B., Dachille, S., Cunningham, S. L., Trubnick, L., & Klepper, T. P. (1990). EEG sleep in adolescents with major depression: The role of suicidality and inpatient status. *Journal of Affective Disorders, 19,* 63–75.

Dahl, R. E., & Ryan, N. D. (1996). The psychobiology of adolescent depression. In. D. Cicchetti & S. L. Toth (Eds.), *Adolescence: Opportunities and challenges* (pp. 197–232). Rochester, NY: University of Rochester Press.

Dahl, R. E., Ryan, N. D., Birmaher, B., Al-Shabbout, M., Williamson, D. E., Neidig,

M., Nelson, B. & Puig-Antich, J. (1991). Electroencephalographic sleep measures in prepubertal depression. *Psychiatry Research, 38,* 201–214.

Dahl, R. E., Ryan, N. D., Puig-Antich, J., Nguyen, N. A., Al-Shabbout, M., Meyer, V. A., & Perel J. (1991). 24-hour cortisol measures in adolescents with major depression: A controlled study. *Biological Psychiatry, 30,* 25–36.

Dahl, R. E., Ryan, N. D., Williamson, D. E., Ambrosini, P. J., Rabinovich, H., Novacenko, H., Nelson, B., & Puig-Antich, J. (1992). Regulation of sleep and growth hormone in adolescent depression. *Journal of the American Academy of Child & Adolescent Psychiatry, 31,* 615–621.

Dawson, G., Klinger, L. G., Panagiotides, H., Spieker, S., & Frey, K. (1992). Infants of mothers with depressive symptoms: Electroencephalographic and behavioral findings related to attachment status. *Development and Psychopathology, 4,* 67–80.

DeMulder, E. K., & Radke-Yarrow, M. (1991). Attachment with affectively ill and well mothers: Concurrent behavioral correlates. *Development and Psychopathology, 3,* 227–242.

Downey, G., & Coyne, J. C. (1990). Children of depressed parents: An integrative review. *Psychological Bulletin, 108,* 50–76.

Eaves, G., & Rush, A. J. (1984). Cognitive patterns in symptomatic and remitted unipolar depression. *Journal of Abnormal Psychology, 93,* 31–40.

Eaves, L. J., Silberg, J. L., Meyer, J. M., Maes, H. H., Simonoff, E., Pickles, A., Rutter, M., Neale, M. C., Reynolds, C. A., Erikson, M. T., Heath, A. C., Loeber, R., Truett, K. R., & Hewitt, J. K. (1997). Genetics and developmental psychopathology: 2. The main effects of genes and environment on behavioral problems in the Virginia Twin Study of Adolescent Behavioral Development. *Journal of Child Psychology and Psychiatry, 38,* 965–980.

Eley, T. C. (1997). Depressive symptoms in children and adolescents: Etiological links between normality and abnormality: A research note. *Journal of Child Psychology and Psychiatry, 38,* 861–865.

Eley, T. C., Deater-Deckard, K., Fombonne, E., Fulker, D. W., & Plomin, R. (1998). An adoption study of depressive symptoms in middle childhood. *Journal of Child Psychology and Psychiatry, 39,* 337–345.

Emslie, G. J., Rush, A. J., Weinberg, W. A., Kowatch, R. A., Hughes, C. W., Carnody, T., & Rintelmann, J. (1997). A double-blind, randomized, placebo-controlled trial of Fluoxetine in children and adolescents with depression. *Archives of General Psychiatry, 54,* 1031–1037.

Emslie, G. J., Rush, A. J., Weinberg, W. A., Rintelmann, J. W., & Roffwarg, H. P. (1990). Children with major depression show reduced rapid eye movement latencies. *Archives of General Psychiatry, 47,* 119–124.

Emslie, G. J., Weinberg, W. A., Kennard, B. D., & Kowatch, R. A. (1994). Neurobiological aspects of depression in children and adolescents. In W. M. Reynolds & H. E. Johnston (Eds.), *Handbook of depression in children and adolescents* (pp. 143–165). New York: Plenum.

Fendrich, M., Warner, V., & Weissman, M. M. (1990). Family risk factors, parental depression, and psychopathology in offspring. *Developmental Psychology, 26,* 40–50.

Fennell, M. J. V., & Campbell, E. A. (1984). The Cognitions Questionnaire: Specific thinking errors in depression. *British Journal of Clinical Psychology, 23,* 81–92.

Gotlib, I. H., Lewinsohn, P. M., Seeley, J. R., Rohde, P., & Redner, J. E. (1993). Negative cognitions and attributional style in depressed adolescents: An examination of stability and specificity. *Journal of Abnormal Psychology, 102,* 607–615.

Grych, J. H., & Fincham, F. D. (1990). Marital conflict and children's adjustment: A cognitive–contextual framework. *Psychological Bulletin, 108,* 267–290.

Haaga, D., Dyck, M., & Ernst, D. (1991). Empirical status of cognitive theory of depression. *Psychological Bulletin, 110,* 215–236.

Halbreich, U., Asnis, G. M., Zumoff, B., Nathan, R. S., & Shindledecker, R. (1984). Effect of age and sex on cortisol secretion in depressives and normals. *Psychiatry Research, 13,* 221–229.

Hamilton, E. W., & Abramson, L. Y. (1983). Cognitive patterns and major depressive disorder: A longitudinal study in a hospital setting. *Journal of Abnormal Psychology, 92,* 173–184.

Hammen, C. L. (1991a). The generation of stress in the course of unipolar depression. *Journal of Abnormal Psychology, 100,* 555–561.

Hammen, C. L. (1991b). *Depression runs in families: The social context of risk and resilience in children of depressed mothers.* New York: Springer-Verlag.

Hammen, C. L., Adrian, C., & Hiroto, D. (1988). A longitudinal test of the attributional vulnerability model in children at risk for depression. *British Journal of Clinical Psychology, 27,* 37–46.

Hammen, C. L., Burge, D., Daley, S. E., Davila, J., Paley, B., & Rudolph, K. D. (1995). Interpersonal attachment cognitions and prediction of symptomatic responses to interpersonal stress. *Journal of Abnormal Psychology, 104,* 436–443.

Hammen, C. L., Burge, D., & Stansbury, K. (1990). Relationship of mother and child variables to child outcomes in a high-risk sample: A causal modeling analysis. *Developmental Psychology, 26,* 24–30.

Hammen, C. L., & Goodman-Brown, T. (1990). Self-schemas and vulnerability to specific life stress in children at risk for depression. *Cognitive Therapy and Research, 14,* 215–227.

Hammen, C. L., Gordon, D., Burge, D., Adrian, C., Jaenicke, C., & Hiroto, D. (1987). Maternal affective disorders, illness, and stress: Risk for children's psychopathology. *American Journal of Psychiatry, 144,* 736–741.

Hankin, B. L., Abramson, L. Y., Moffitt, T. E., Silva, P. A., McGee, R., & Angell, K. E. (1998). Development of depression from preadolescence to young adulthood: Emerging gender differences in a 10-year longitudinal study. *Journal of Abnormal Psychology, 107,* 128–140.

Harrington, R. C., Fudge, H., Rutter, M. L., Bredenkamp, C. G., Groothues, C., & Pridham, J. (1993). Child and adult depression: A test of continuities with data from a family study. *British Journal of Psychiatry, 162,* 627–633.

Harrington, R., Fudge, H., Rutter, M., Pickles, A., & Hill, J. (1990). Adult outcomes of childhood and adolescent depression. *Archives of General Psychiatry, 47,* 465–473.

Harris, P. L. (1989). *Children and emotion: The development of psychological understanding.* Oxford: Basil Blackwell.

Harter, S. (1999). *The construction of the self: A developmental perspective.* New York: Guilford Press.

Hedges, L. V., & Olkin, I. (1985). *Statistical methods for meta-analysis.* Orlando: Academic Press.

Hilsman, R., & Garber, J. (1995). A test of the cognitive diathesis–stress model in children: Academic stressors, attributional style, perceived competence and control. *Journal of Personality and Social Psychology, 69,* 370–380.

Hirsch, B. J., Moos, R. H., & Reischl, T. M. (1985). Psychosocial adjustment of adolescent children of a depressed, arthritic, or normal parent. *Journal of Abnormal Psychology, 94,* 154–164.

Hollon, S. D. (1992). Cognitive models of depression from a psychobiological perspective. *Psychological Inquiry, 3,* 250–253.

Hollon, S. D., DeRubeis, R. J., & Seligman, M. E. P. (1992). Cognitive therapy and the prevention of depression. *Applied and Preventive Psychology, 1,* 89–95.

Hollon, S. D., Evans, M. D., & DeRubeis, R. J. (1990).Cognitive mediation of relapse prevention following treatment for depression: Implications of differential risk. In R.E. Ingram (Ed.), *Contemporary psychological approaches to depression* (pp. 117–136). New York: Plenum.

Hops, H., Biglan, A., Sherman, L., Arthur, J., Friedman, L., & Osteen, V. (1987). Mome observations of family interactions of depressed women. *Journal of Consulting and Clinical Psychology, 55,* 341–346.

Howarth, E., Johnson, J., Klerman, G. L., & Weissman, M. M. (1992). Depressive symptoms as relative and attributable risk factors for first-onset major depression. *Archives of General Psychiatry, 49,* 817–823.

Ingram, R. E., Miranda, J., & Segal., Z. V. (1998). *Cognitive vulnerability to depression.* New York: Guilford Press.

Jaenicke, C., Hammen, C. L., Zupan, B., Hiroto, D., Gordon, D., Adrian, C., & Burge, D. (1987). Cognitive vulnerability in children at risk for depression. *Journal of Abnormal Child Psychology, 15,* 559–572.

Jaycox, L. H., Reivich, K., Gillham, J., & Seligman, M. E. P. (1994). Prevention of depressive symptoms in school children. *Behavior Research and Therapy, 32,* 801–816.

Jensen, J. B., & Garfinkel, B. D. (1990). Growth hormone dysregulation in children with major depressive disorder. *Journal of the American Academy of Child and Adolescent Psychiatry, 29,* 295–301.

Joiner, T. E. (1999). A test of interpersonal theory of depression in youth psychiatric inpatients. *Journal of Abnormal Child Psychology, 27,* 77–85.

Joiner, T. E., & Coyne, J. C. (Eds.). (1999). *The interactional nature of depression: Advances in interpersonal approaches.* Washington, DC: American Psychological Association.

Judd, L. L., Akiskal, H. S., & Paulus, M. P. (1997). The role and clinical significance of subsyndromal depressive symptoms (SSD) in unipolar major depressive disorder. *Journal of Affective Disorders, 45,* 5–18.

Just, N., Abramson, L. Y., & Alloy, L. B. (in press). Remitted depression studies as tests of the cognitive vulnerability hypothesis of depression onset: A critique and conceptual analysis. *Clinical Psychology Review.*

Kashani, J. H., Rosenberg, T. K., & Reid, J. C. (1989). Developmental perspectives in child and adolescent depressive symptoms in a community sample. *American Journal of Psychiatry, 146,* 871–875.

Kaslow, N. J., Deering, C. G., & Racusin, G. R. (1994). Depressed children and their families. *Clinical Psychology Review, 14,* 39–59.

Katainen, S., Raikkonen, K., Keskivaara, P., & Keltikangas-Jarvinen, L. (1999). Maternal child-rearing attitudes and role satisfaction and children's temperament as antecedents of adolescent depressive tendencies: Follow-up study of 6- to 15-year olds. *Journal of Youth and Adolescence, 28,* 139–163.

Keitner, G. I., & Miller, I. W. (1990). Family functioning and major depression: An overview. *American Journal of Psychiatry, 147,* 1128–1137.

Kendler, K. S., Kessler, R. C., Walters, E. E., MacLean, C., Neale, M. C., Heath, A. C., & Eaves, L. J. (1995). Stressful life events, genetic liability, and onset of an episode of major depression in women. *American Journal of Psychiatry, 152,* 833–842.

Kenny, M. E., Moilanen, D. L., Lomax, R., & Brabeck, M. M. (1993). Contributions of parental attachments to views of self and depressive symptoms among early adolescents. *Journal of Early Adolescence, 13,* 408–430.

Kistner, J., Balthazor, M., Risi, S., & Burton, C. (1999). Predicting dysphoria in adolescence from actual and perceived peer acceptance in childhood. *Journal of Clinical Child Psychology, 28,* 94–104.

Klee, S. H., & Garfinkel, B. D. (1984). Identification of depression in children and adolescents: The role of the dexamethasone suppression test. *Journal of the American Academy of Child Psychiatry, 23,* 410–415.

Klerman, G. L., & Weissman, M. M. (1989). Increasing rates of depression. *Journal of the American Medical Association, 261,* 2229–2235.

Kobak, R. R., Sudler, N., & Gamble, W. (1991). Attachment and depressive symptoms during adolescence: A developmental pathways analysis. *Development and Psychopathology, 3,* 461–474.

Kochanska, G., Kuczynski, L., Radke-Yarrow, M., & Welsh, J. D. (1987). Resolutions of control episodes between well and affectively ill mothers and their young children. *Journal of Abnormal Child Psychology, 15,* 441–456.

Kovacs, M. (1981). Rating scales to assess depression in school-aged children. *Acta Paedopsychiatrica, 46,* 305–315.

Kovacs, M. (1989). Affective disorders in children and adolescents. *American Psychologist, 44,* 209–215.

Kovacs, M., Feinberg, T. L., Crouse-Novak, M. A., Paulauskas, S. L., & Finkelstein, R. (1984). Depressive disorders in childhood. I. A longitudinal prospective study of characteristics and recovery. *Archives of General Psychiatry, 41,* 229–237.

Kovacs, M., Feinberg, T. L., Crouse-Novak, M., Paulauskas, S. L., Pollock, M., & Finkelstein, R. (1984). Depressive disorders in childhood. II. A longitudinal study of the risk for a subsequent major depression. *Archives of General Psychiatry, 41,* 653–649.

Kupfer, D. J., & Reynolds, C. F. (1992). Sleep and affective disorders. In E. S. Paykel (Ed.), *Handbook of affective disorders* (2nd ed., pp. 311–323). New York: Guilford Press.

Kutcher, S. P., Malkin, D., Silverberg, J., Marton, P., Williamson, P., Malkin, A., Szalai, J., & Katic, M. (1991). Nocturnal cortisol, thyroid stimulating hormone and growth hormone secreting properties in depressed adolescents. *Journal of the American Academy of Child and Adolescent Psychiatry, 30,* 407–414.

Kutcher, S., Williamson, P., Silverberg, J., Marton, P., Malkin, D., & Malkin, A. (1988). Nocturnal growth hormone secretion in depressed older adolescents. *Journal of the American Academy of Child & Adolescent Psychiatry, 27,* 751–754.

Leadbeater, B. J., Blatt, S. J., & Quinlan, D. M. (1995). Gender-linked vulnerabilities to depressive symptoms, stress, and problem behaviors in adolescents. *Journal of Research on Adolescence, 5,* 1–29.

Leadbeater, B. J., Kuperminc, G. P., Blatt, S. J., & Hertzog, C. (1999). A multivariate model of gender differences in adolescents' internalizing and externalizing problems. *Developmental Psychology, 35,* 1268–1282.

Lefkowitz, M. M., & Tesiny, E. P. (1984). Rejection and depression: Prospective and contemporaneous analyses. *Developmental Psychology, 20,* 776–785.

Lewinsohn, P. M., Allen, N. B., Seeley, J. R., & Gotlib, I. H. (1999). First onset versus recurrence of depression: Differential processes of psychosocial risk. *Journal of Abnormal Psychology, 108,* 483–489.

Lewinsohn, P. M., Clarke, G. N., Seeley, J. R., & Rohde, P. (1994). Major depression in community adolescents: Age at onset, episode duration, and time to recurrence. *Journal of the American Academy of Child and Adolescent Psychiatry, 33,* 809–818.

Lewinsohn, P. M., Hops, H., Roberts, R. E., Seeley, J. R., & Andrews, J. A. (1993). Adolescent psychopathology: I. Prevalence and incidence of depression and other DSM-III-R disorders in high school students. *Journal of Abnormal Psychology, 102,* 133–144.

Lewinsohn, P. M., Roberts, R. E., Seeley, J. R., Rohde, P., Gotlib, I. H., & Hops, H. (1994). Adolescent psychopathology: II. Psychosocial risk factors for depression. *Journal of Abnormal Psychology, 103,* 302–315.

Lewinsohn, P. M., Steinmetz, J. L., Larson, D. W., & Franklin, J. (1981). Depression related cognitions: Antecedent or consequence? *Journal of Abnormal Psychology, 91,* 213–219.

Little, S. A., & Garber, J. (in press). Interpersonal and achievement orientations and specific hassles predicting depressive and aggressive symptoms in children. *Cognitive Therapy and Research.*

Lovejoy, M.C. (1991). Maternal depression: Effects on social cognition and behavior in parent–child interactions. *Journal of Abnormal Child Psychology, 19,* 693–706.

Luthar, S., & Blatt, S. J. (1995). Differential vulnerability of dependency and self-criticism among disadvantaged teenagers. *Journal of Research on Adolescence, 5,* 431–449.

Maes, M., & Meltzer, H. (1995). The serotonin hypothesis of major depression. In F. E. Bloom & D. J. Kupfer (Eds.), *Psychopharmacology: The fourth generation of progress* (pp. 933–944). New York: Raven Press.

McCauley, E., Mitchell, J. R., Burke, P., & Moss, S. (1988). Cognitive attributes of depression in children and adolescents. *Journal of Consulting and Clinical Psychology, 56,* 903–908.

McCauley, E., & Myers, K. (1992). Family interactions in mood-disordered youth. *Child and Adolescent Psychiatric Clinics of North America, 1,* 111–127.

McCauley, E., Myers, K., Mitchell, J., Calderon, R., Schloredt, K., & Treder, R. (1993). Depression in young people: Initial presentation and clinical course. *Journal of the American Academy of Child and Adolescent Psychiatry, 32,* 714–722.

Metalsky, G. I., Joiner, T. E., Hardin, T. S., & Abramson, L. Y. (1993). Depressive reactions to failure in a naturalistic setting: A test of the hopelessness and self-esteem theories of depression. *Journal of Abnormal Psychology, 102,* 101–109.

Meyer, W. J., Richards, G. E., Cavallo, A., Holt, K. G., Hejazi, M. S., Wigg, C., & Rose, R. M. (1991). Depression and growth hormone. *Journal of the American Academy of Child and Adolescent Psychiatry, 30,* 335.

Monck, E., & Dobbs, R. (1985). Measuring life events in an adolescent population: Methodological issues and related findings. *Psychological Medicine, 15,* 841–850.

Monroe, S. M., & Roberts, J. R. (1990). Definitional and conceptual issues in the measurement of life stress: Problems, principles, procedures, progress. *Stress Medicine, 6,* 209–216.

Monroe, S. M., Rohde, P., Seeley, J. R., & Lewinsohn, P. M. (1999). Life events and depression in adolescence: Relationship loss as a prospective risk factor for first-onset of major depressive disorder. *Journal of Abnormal Psychology, 108,* 606–614.

Monroe, S. M., & Simons, A. D. (1991). Diathesis–stress theories in the context of life stress research: Implications for the depressive disorders. *Psychological Bulletin, 110,* 406–425.

Nolan, S., & Garber, J. (2000). *The relation of rejection to depression in adolescents.* Manuscript submitted for publication.

Nolen-Hoeksema, S., & Girgus, J. (1994). The emergence of gender differences in depression during adolescence. *Psychological Bulletin, 115,* 424–441.

Nolen-Hoeksema, S., Girgus, J., & Seligman, M. E. P. (1992). Predictors and consequences of childhood depressive symptoms: A 5-year longitudinal study. *Journal of Abnormal Psychology, 101,* 405–422.

Panak, W., & Garber, J. (1992). Role of aggression, rejection, and attributions in the prediction of depression in children. *Development and Psychopathology, 4,* 145–165.

Persons, J. B., & Miranda, J. (1992). Cognitive theories of vulnerability to depression: Reconciling negative evidence. *Cognitive Therapy and Research, 16,* 485–502.

Petersen, A. C., Compas, B. E., Brooks-Gunn, J., Stemmler, M., Ey, S., & Grant, K. E. (1993). Depression in adolescence. *American Psychologist, 48,* 155–168.

Petersen, A. C., Sarigiani, P. A., & Kennedy, R. E. (1991). Adolescent depression: Why more girls? *Journal of Youth and Adolescence, 20,* 247–271.

Peterson, L., Mullins, L. L., & Ridley-Johnson, R. (1985). Childhood depression: Peer reactions to depression and life stress. *Journal of Abnormal Child Psychology, 13,* 597–609.

Pfeffer, C. R., Stokes, P., & Shindledecker, R. (1991). Suicidal behavior and hypothalamic–pituitary–adrenocortical axis indices in child psychiatric inpatients. *Biological Psychiatry, 29,* 909–917.

Piaget, J., & Inhelder, B. (1969). *The psychology of the child.* New York: Basic Books.

Pine, D. S., Cohen, E., Cohen, P., & Brook, J. (1999). Adolescent depressive symptoms as predictors of adult depression: Moodiness or mood disorder? *American Journal of Psychiatry, 156,* 133–135.

Plomin, R. (1990). Nature and nurture: An introduction to human behavioral genetics. Pacific Grove, CA: Brooks/Cole.

Post, R. M. (1992). Transduction of psychosocial stress into the neurobiology of recurrent affective disorder. *American Journal of Psychiatry, 149,* 999–1010.

Prien, R. F., & Kupfer, D. J. (1986). Continuation drug therapy for major depressive episodes: How long should it be maintained? *American Journal of Psychiatry, 143*, 18–23.

Puig-Antich, J., Dahl, R. E., Ryan, N. D., Novacenko, H., Goetz, D., Goetz, R., Twomey, J., & Klepper, T. (1989). Cortisol secretion in prepubertal children with major depressive disorder: Episode and recovery. *Archives of General Psychiatry, 46*, 801–809.

Puig-Antich, J., Goetz, R., Davies, M., Tabrizi, M. A., Novacenko, H., Hanlon, C., Sachar, E. J., & Weitzman, E. D. (1984). Growth hormone secretion in prepubertal children with major depression: IV. Sleep-related plasma concentrations in a drug-free, fully recovered clinical state. *Archives of General Psychiatry, 41*, 479–483.

Puig-Antich, J., Lukens, E., Davies, M., Goetz, D., Brennan-Quattrock, J., & Todak, G. (1985a). Psychosocial functioning in prepubertal major depressive disorder. I. Interpersonal relatinships during the depressive episode. *Archives of General Psychiatry, 42*, 500–507.

Puig-Antich, J., Lukens, E., Davies, M., Goetz, D., Brennan-Quattrock, J., & Todak, G. (1985b). Psychosocial functioning in prepubertal major depressive disorder. II. Interpersonal relatinships after sustained recovery from affective episode. *Archives of General Psychiatry, 42*, 511–517.

Puig-Antich, J., Novacenko, H., Davies, M., Chambers, W. J., Tabrizi, M. A., Krawiec, V., Ambrosini, P. J., & Sachar, E. J. (1984). Growth hormone secretion in prepubertal children with major depression: I. Final report on response to insulin-induced hypoglycemia during a depressive episode. *Archives of General Psychiatry, 41*, 455–460.

Puig-Antich, J., Novacenko, H., Davies, M., Tabrizi, M. A., Ambrosini, P. J., Goetz, R., Bianca, J., Goetz, D., & Sachar, E. J. (1984). Growth hormone secretion in prepubertal children with major depression: III. Response to insulin-induced hypoglycemia after recovery from a depressive episode and in a drug-free state. *Archives of General Psychiatry, 41*, 471–475.

Radke-Yarrow, M., & Nottelmann, E. (1989, April). *Affective development in children of well and depressed mothers.* Paper presented at the meeting of the Society for Research in Child Development, Kansas City, MO.

Rao, U., Dahl, R. E., Ryan, N.D., Birmaher, B., Williamson, D.E., Giles, D.E., Rao, R., Kaufman, J., & Nelson, B. (1996). The relationship between longitudinal clinical course and sleep and cortisol changes in adolescent depression. *Biological Psychiatry, 40*, 474–484.

Reinherz, H. Z., Stewart-Berghauer, G., Pakiz, B., Frost, A. K., Moeykens, B. A., & Holmes, W. M. (1989). The relationship of early risk and current mediators to depressive symptomatology in adolescence. *Journal of the American Academy of Child and Adolescent Psychiatry, 28*, 942–947.

Reiss, D., Hetherington, M., Plomin, R., Howe, G.W., Simmens, S. J., Henderson, S. H., O'Connor, T. J., Bussell, D. A., Anderson, E. R., & Law, T. (1995). Genetic questions for environmental studies: Differential parenting and psychopathology in adolescence. *Archives of General Psychiatry, 52*, 925–936.

Rende, R. D., Plomin, R., Reiss, D., & Hetherington, E. M. (1993). Genetic and environmental influences on depressive symptomatology in adolescence: Individual differences and extreme scores. *Journal of Child Psychology and Psychiatry, 34*, 1387–1398.

Robbins, D. R., Alessi, N. E., Yanchyshyn, G. W., & Colfer, M. V. (1983). The dexamathasone suppression test in psychiatrically hospitalized adolescents. *Journal of the American Academy of Child Psychiatry, 22,* 467–469.

Robinson, N. S., Garber, J., & Hilsman, R. (1995). Cognitions and stress: Direct and moderating effects on depressive versus externalizing symptoms during the junior high school transition. *Journal of Abnormal Psychology, 104,* 453–463.

Rohde, P., Lewinsohn, P. M., & Seeley, J. R. (1990). Are people changed by the experience of having an episode of depression? A further test of the scar hypothesis. *Journal of Abnormal Psychology, 99,* 264–271.

Rohde, P., Lewinsohn, P. M., & Seeley, J. R. (1994). Are adolescents changed by an episode of major depression? *Journal of the American Academy of Child and Adolescent Psychiatry, 33,* 1289–1298.

Rubin, K., Booth, L., Zahn-Waxler, C., Cummings, E. M., & Wilkinson, M. (1991). Dyadic play behaviors of children of well and depressed mothers. *Development and Psychopathology, 3,* 243–251.

Rudolph, K. D., Hammen, C. L., & Burge, D. (1994). Interpersonal functioning and depressive symptoms in childhood: Addressing the issue of specificity and comorbidity. *Journal of Abnormal Child Psychology, 22,* 355–371.

Rueter, M. A., Scaramella, L., Wallace, L. E., & Conger, R. D. (1999). First onset of depressive or anxiety disorders predicted by the longitudinal course of internalizing symptoms and parent–adolescent disagreements. *Archives of General Psychiatry, 56,* 726–732.

Rutter, M. (1986). The developmental psychopathology of depression: Issues and perspectives. In M. Rutter, C. E. Izard, & P. B. Read (Eds.), *Depression in young people: Developmental and clinical perspectives* (pp. 3–30). New York:Guilford Press.

Rutter, M. (1988). Epidemiological approaches to developmental psychopathology. *Archives of General Psychiatry, 45,* 486–495.

Rutter, M., Bolton, P., Harrington, R., Le Couteur, A., Macdonald, H., & Simonoff, E. (1990). Genetic factors in child psychiatric disorders—I. A review of research strategies. *Journal of Child Psychology and Psychiatry, 31,* 3–37.

Rutter, M., Macdonald, H., Le Couteur, A., Harrington, R., Bolton, P. & Bailey, A. (1990). Genetic factors in child psychiatric disorders—II. Empirical findings. *Journal of Child Psychology and Psychiatry, 31,* 39–83.

Rutter, M., & Quinton, P. (1984). Parental psychiatric disorder: Effects on children. *Psychological Medicine, 14,* 853–880.

Ryan, N. D. (1998). Psychoneuroendocrinology of children and adolescents. *Psychiatric Clinics of North America, 21,* 435–441.

Ryan, N. D., Birmaher, B., Perel, J. M., Dahl, R. E., Meyer, V., Al-Shabbout, M., Iyengar, S., & Puig-Antich, J. (1992). Neuroendocrine response to L-5-Hydroxytryptophan challenge in prepubertal major depression: Depressed vs. normal children. *Archives of General Psychiatry, 49,* 843–851.

Ryan, N. D., & Dahl, R. (1993). The biology of depression in children and adolescents. In J. J. Mann & D. J. Kupfer (Eds.), *Biology of depressive disorders, Part B: Subtypes of depression and comorbid disorders* (pp. 37–58). New York: Plenum.

Ryan, N. D., Dahl, R. E., Birmaher, B., Williamson, D. E., Iyengar, S., Nelson, B., Puig-Antich, J., & Perel, J. M. (1994). Stimulatory tests of growth hormone secretion inprepubertal major depression: Depressed versus normal children.

Journal of the American Academy of Child and Adolescent Psychiatry, 33, 824–833.

Ryan, N. D., Puig-Antich, J., Ambrosini, P., Rabinovich, H., Robinson, D., Nelson, B., Iyengar, S., & Twomey, J. (1987). The clinical picture of major depression in children and adolescents. *Archives of General Psychiatry, 44,* 854–861.

Ryan, N. D., Puig-Antich, J., Rabinovich, H., Ambrosini, P., Robinson, D., Nelson, B., & Novacenko, H. (1988). Growth hormone response to desmethylimipramine in depressed and suicidal adolescents. *Journal of Affective Disorders, 15,* 323–337.

Safran, J. D., & Segal, Z. V. (1990). *Interpersonal process in cognitive therapy.* New York: Basic Books.

Sameroff, A. J., & Chandler, M. J. (1975). Reproductive risk and the continuum of caretaking casualty. In F.D. Horowitz (Ed.), *Review of child development research* (Vol. 4, pp. 187–244). Chicago: University of Chicago Press.

Sandler, I. N., Wes, S. G., Baca, L., & Pillow, D. R. (1992). Linking empirically based theory and evaluation: The Family Bereavement Program. *American Journal of Community Psychology, 20,* 491–521.

Sanford, M., Szatmari, P., Spinner, M., Munroe-Blum, H., Jamieson, E., Walsh, C., & Jones, D. (1995). Predicting the one-year course of adolescent major depression. *Journal of the American Academy of Child and Adolescent Psychiatry, 34,* 1618–1628.

Segal, Z. V., & Dobson, K. S. (1992). Cognitive models of depression: Report from a Consensus Development Conference. *Psychological Inquiry, 3,* 214–224.

Sheeber, L., Hops, H., Andrews, J., Alpert, T., & Davis, B. (1998). Interactional processes in families with depressed and nondepressed adolescents: Reinforcement of depressive behavior. *Behavior Research and Therapy, 36,* 417–427.

Stanger, C., McConaughy, S. H., & Achenbach, T. M. (1992). Three-year course of behavioral/emotional problems in a national sample of 4- to 16-year-olds. II. Predictors of syndromes. *Journal of the American Academy of Child and Adolescent Psychiatry, 31,* 941–950.

Stark, K. D., Humphrey, L. L., Crook, K., & Lewis, K. (1990). Perceived family environments of depressed and anxious children. Child's and maternal figure's perspective. *Journal of Abnormal Child Psychology, 18,* 527–547.

Taylor, L., & Ingram, R. E. (1999). Cognitive reactivity and depressotypic information processing in children of depressed mothers. *Journal of Abnormal Psychology, 108,* 202–210.

Teasdale, J. D. (1983). Negative thinking in depression: Cause, effect or reciprocal relationship? *Advances in Behavior Research and Therapy, 5,* 3–25.

Teasdale, J. D. (1988). Cognitive vulnerability to persistent depression. *Cognition and Emotion, 2,* 247–274.

Teasdale, J. D., & Dent, J. (1987). Cognitive vulnerability to depression: An investigation of two hypotheses. *British Journal of Clinical Psychology, 26,* 113–126.

Teti, D., Gelfand, D., Messinger, D., & Isabella, R. (1995). Maternal depression and the quality of early attachment: An examination of infants, preschoolers, and their mothers. *Developmental Psychology, 31,* 364–376.

Thaper, A., & McGuffin, P. (1994). A twin study of depressive symptoms in childhood. *British of Psychiatry, 165,* 259–265.

Tomarken, A. J., & Keener, A. D. (1998). Frontal brain asymetry and depression: A self-regulatory perspective. *Cognition and Emotion, 12,* 387–420.

Tomarken, A. J., Simien, C., & Garber, J. (1994). Resting frontal brain asymmetry discriminates adolescent children of depressed mothers from low risk controls. *Psychophysiology, 3,* S97–S98.

van den Oord, E. J. C. G., Boomsma, D. I., & Verhulst, F. C. (1994). A study of problem behaviors in 10- to 15-year-old biologically related and unrelated international adoptees. *Behavior Genetics, 24,* 193–205.

Velez, C. N., Johnson, J., & Cohen, P. (1989). A longitudinal analysis of selected risk factors for childhood psychopathology. *Journal of the American Academy of Child and Adolescent Psychiatry, 28,* 861–864.

Vernberg, E. M. (1990). Psychological adjustment and experiences with peers during early adolescence: Reciprocal, incidental, or unidirectional relationships? *Journal of Abnormal Child Psychology, 18,* 187–198.

Wagner, B., Compas, B., & Howell, D. C. (1998). Daily and major life events: A test of an integrative model of psychosocial stress. *American Journal of Community Psychology, 16,* 189–205.

Walker, L. S., Garber, J., & Greene, J. (1993). Psychosocial correlates of recurrent childhood pain: A comparison of pediatric patients with recurrent abdominal pain, organic illness, and psychiatric disorders. *Journal of Abnormal Psychology, 102,* 248–258.

Weiner, B. (1985). An attributional theory of achievement motivation and emotion. *Psychological Review, 92,* 548–573.

Weiss, B., & Garber, J. (2000). *Developmental differences in the phenomenology of depression.* Manuscript submitted for publication.

Weissman, M. M., Gammon, G. D., John, K., Merikangas, K. R., Warner, V., Prusoff, B. A., & Sholomskas, D. (1987). Children of depressed parents: Increased psychopathology and early onset of major depression. *Archives of General Psychiatry, 44,* 847–853.

Weissman, M. M., Merikangas, K. R., Wickramaratne, P., Kidd, K. K., Prusoff, B. A., Leckman, J. F. & Pauls, D. L. (1986). Understanding the clinical heterogeneity of major depression using family data. *Archives of General Psychiatry, 43,* 430–434.

Weissman, M. M., & Olfson, M. (1995). Depression in women: Implications for health care research. *Science, 269,* 799–801.

Weissman, M. M., Warner, V., Wickramaratne, P., & Prusoff, B. A. (1988). Early-onset major depression in parents and their children. *Journal of Affective Disorders, 15,* 269–277.

Weissman, M. M., Wickramaratne, P., Merikangas, K. R., Leckman, J. F., Prusoff, B. A., Caruso, K. A., Kidd, K. K., & Gammon, G.D. (1984). Onset of major depression in early adulthood: Increased familial loading and specificity. *Archives of General Psychiatry, 41,* 1136–1143.

Wichstron, L., Anderson, A. M. C., Holte, A., & Wynne, L. C. (1996). Disqualifying family communication and childhood social competence as predictors of offspring's mental health and hospitalization: A 10- to 14-year longitudinal study of children at risk of psychopathology. *Journal of Nervous and Mental Disease, 184,* 581–588.

Wickramaratne, P. J., & Weissman, M. M. (1998). Onset of psychopathology in offspring by developmental phase and parental depression. *Journal of the American Academy of Child and Adolescent Psychiatry, 37*, 933–942.

Wierzbicki, M. (1987). Similarity of monozygotic and dizygotic child twins in level and lability of subclinically depressed mood. *American Journal of Orthopsychiatry, 57*, 33–40.

Williamson, D. E., Birmaher, B., Anderson, B. P., Al-Shabbout, M., & Ryan, N. D. (1995). Stressful life events in depressed adolescents: The role of dependent events during the depressive episode. *Journal of the American Academy of Child and Adolescent Psychiatry, 34*, 591–598.

Williamson, D. E., Birmaher, B., Frank, E., Anderson, B. P., Matty, M. K., & Kupfer, D. J. (1998). Nature of life events and difficulties in depressed adolescents. *Journal of the American Academy of Child and Adolescent Psychiatry, 37*, 1049–1057.

Winokur, G. (1997). All roads lead to depression: Clinically homogeneous, etiologically heterogeneous. *Journal of Affective Disorders, 45*, 97–108.

Wolchik, S. A., & Sandler, I. N. (Eds.). (1997). *Handbook of children's coping: Linking theory and intervention.* New York: Plenum.

Wolchik, S. A., West, S. G., Westover, S., Sandler, I., Martin, A., Lustig, J., Tein, J., & Fisher, J. (1993). The children of divorce parenting intervention: Outcome evaluation of an empirically-based program. *American Journal of Community Psychology, 21*, 293–331.

Zubernis, L. S., Cassidy, K. W., Gillham, J. E., Reivich, K. J., & Jaycox, L. H. (1999). Prevention of depressive symptoms in preadolescent children of divorce. *Journal of Divorce and Remarriage, 30*, 11–36.

9

Vulnerability to Depression in Adulthood

CONSTANCE HAMMEN

This chapter highlights research on adult depression, presenting definitions and features of depression in adults, assessment methods, historical trends in vulnerability research, and current models and findings. It should be noted at the outset, however, that vulnerability is assumed to arise in childhood in most cases of depression. Thus, the major distinction between this chapter and the chapter on vulnerability to depression in childhood and adolescence (Garber & Flynn, Chapter 8, this volume) is the age of the research populations studied. It may be assumed that the vulnerability factors are the same, although the child and adult literatures differ in emphasis and methods. This chapter is limited to research conducted on adults—many of whom actually may have experienced their first depressive experiences as children or adolescents.

DEFINITIONS AND CHARACTERISTICS OF DEPRESSION

Most research on vulnerability to adult depression has focused on conditions that are marked by four features considered essential to a working definition: a constellation of symptoms defining a depressive syndrome rather than single symptom such as mood; a sustained period of symptoms over days, weeks, or months; some degree of impaired functioning; and a nonbipolar course. The specific *methods* of defining depression, such as self-reports on questionnaires or systematic interviews, as well as different samples surveyed such as patients or community members, may yield important differences that have implications for our understanding of vulnerability. These issues are discussed in more detail later.

Diagnosable syndromes of depression include affective, behavioral, somatic, and cognitive symptoms. Affective symptoms may include depressed mood or sadness and feelings of loss of pleasure in typically enjoyable activities; irritability and anger may also be apparent. Behavioral symptoms include decreased activity such as withdrawal from typical pursuits and social interactions and may include changes in movement such as slowed talking and reduced gestures, slumped posture, and sad facial expressions. On the other hand, some depressed people are agitated, with pacing, hand wringing, and difficulty sitting still. Somatic signs may be especially pronounced in more severe depression, including significant weight changes associated with either increased or decreased appetite, sleep changes including increased or decreased hours of sleep, loss of energy, fatigue, and lethargy. Cognitive symptoms include subjective experiences of worthlessness, futility, helplessness, hopelessness, loss of motivation, pessimism, and suicidal thoughts. Changes in intellectual activity may also be noticed, including poor memory and difficulty concentrating and making decisions.

Many investigators have held the *Diagnostic and Statistical Manual of Mental Disorders* (DSM)-based *major depressive disorder* (MDD) as the gold standard for inclusion in research samples. The DSM-IV (American Psychiatric Association, 1994) criteria require a 2-week minimum and five of nine symptoms at least one of which is depressed mood or loss of pleasure, plus clinically significant distress or impairment in important roles. The nine listed symptoms include many somatic features. Less often, research has also included DSM-defined *dysthymic disorder*, a milder degree of depression over a prolonged period (at least 2 years of nearly constant depressive symptoms).

Although there is much to be said for use of standardized criteria for defining research samples, there has been a tendency to reify major depressive disorder as an "illness" with distinct boundaries. Two important features of depressive experiences are coming to light based on recent research findings that call the categorical approach into question. One is that substantial morbidity may accompany "subsyndromal" forms of depression (e.g., Gotlib, Lewinsohn, & Seeley, 1995; Wells et al., 1989). Such states of milder depression are also frequently associated with excessive use of community resources (e.g., Johnson, Weissman, & Klerman, 1992) and have a high probability of developing into more severe depressive conditions (e.g., Horwath, Johnson, Klerman, & Weissman, 1992). A second feature is that over the long term, the course of major depression is markedly dynamic, changing between MDD and subsyndromal levels, suggesting a single underlying process with a highly varying continuum of severity (Judd et al., 1998; see also Sherbourne, Hays, & Wells, 1995).

Based on such research, it appears that a full understanding of the vulnerability to depressive experiences should include samples and definitions not constrained by DSM categories but perhaps supplemented by studies of samples selected by course features and symptom profiles (e.g., Clark, Cook,

& Snow, 1998). Indeed, increasing evidence points to the utility of considering continuous broad-band symptom constellations such as "internalizing" disorders (Krueger, Caspi, Moffitt, & Silva, 1998) or "negative affectivity" that, according to the tripartite model of emotional distress, is unique to depression (e.g., Watson et al., 1995).

Several additional definitional issues affect our interpretation of research findings on depression vulnerability. Comorbidity of depression with other disorders has emerged into depression researchers' awareness, supported in part by the finding that more than half of those with major depressive episode (MDE) had at least one other diagnosable condition (Blazer, Kessler, McGonagle, & Swartz, 1994). Numerous studies have shown that individuals with histories of major depression are also likely to suffer from anxiety disorders, substance use disorders, and eating disorders—and a significant subset experience more than two diagnoses. Moreover, Axis II pathology is extremely common among depressed individuals, with rates across different studies ranging from 23% to 87% (Shea, Widiger, & Klein, 1992), including 74% in the National Institute of Mental Health (NIMH) Treatment of Depression Collaborative Research Project (Shea et al., 1990). Comorbidity raises numerous conceptual and methodological issues, not the least of which is whether studies of vulnerability to depression are really about "depression" or about comorbid conditions. Demographic risk factors, for example, differ for pure and comorbid depression (e.g., Blazer et al., 1994), but relatively few other studies have distinguished between such groups.

A central issue that affects the future of vulnerability research in depression, therefore, is what we mean by "depression" and how we disentangle its unique attributes from those contributed merely by severity of symptoms or by coexisting psychopathology. Moreover, conceptualizing depression as a disease entity—or as an empirically defined construct—will likely lead in different directions. Over time we will be able to evaluate the yield of each approach. Also, currently, whether depression is a single disorder varying in severity with a presumed single cause (e.g., Judd, 1997) or a heterogeneous set of disorders with multiple etiologies remains an issue to be resolved.

Course of Depression

Increasingly, major depression is understood as a highly recurrent and even chronic condition. More than 80% of people experience at least one recurrence—a figure increasing to 100% if minor or subsyndromal episodes are included; and the median number of MDEs is four (reviewed in Judd, 1997). Recurrent episodes of MDE last about 20 weeks (Solomon et al., 1997). Although individuals do tend to recover from episodes of major depression, many have continuing or repeated periods of subclinical depressive symptoms (Judd et al., 1998). The fact of recurrence or chronicity of depression is critically important to research on vulnerability. When selecting a study sample of depressed people, many investigators have not distinguished between those with first onset and the more prevalent group of those with a recurrence episode. Predictors of onset and recurrence may be different, as many have noted. Moreover, the frequent demonstration that past episodes are the strongest predictor of future depression in both clinical and community samples (e.g., Coyne, Pepper, & Flynn, 1999; Daley, Hammen, & Rao, in press) requires vulnerability models to be explicit in addressing this issue, as discussed later.

Age of onset appears to be in the 20s for treated samples, but women in particular appear to have a liability for onset between 15 and 19 in U.S. community samples (Burke, Burke, Regier, & Rae, 1990). Ample evidence points to increasing rates of MDD in younger populations, as noted in Chapter 8 (Garber & Flynn, this volume). Onset in the teens and early 20s, therefore, is an additional issue for vulnerability models to address.

Epidemiology and Demographics of Depression

Cross-national studies show rates of current MDE ranging between 4.6% and 7.4% (Smith & Weissman, 1992). In the United States, the most recent national epidemiological study found 4.9% (Blazer et al., 1994). Current dysthymic disorder affects 2 to 4% of the population based on cross-national studies (Smith & Weissman, 1992). Lifetime rates of MDD are estimated at 17.1% in the National Comorbidity Study (Blazer et al., 1994). Depression rates are significantly higher for females than for males worldwide (Weissman & Olfson, 1995), another striking feature of depression that must be addressed by vulnerability models. Hispanic ethnicity, younger age, lower education, lower income, and separated/divorced status are all significantly associated with higher rates of MDE (Blazer et al., 1994). It is important to note that variations in the screening questions in an interview for DSM-based depression used in two U.S. epidemiological studies may have contributed to considerably different estimates of prevalence (Regier et al., 1998). This issue is a reminder that research findings and conclusions may be substantially affected by assessment methods, a discussion of which is beyond the scope of this chapter.

HISTORICAL APPROACHES TO DEPRESSION VULNERABILITY

Three major models of depression have dominated the scene for centuries, and each has also risen and fallen in prominence in the 20th century, based on historical/political tides and methodological advances. These themes are biological, intrapsychic, and environmental approaches. Biological models have always suggested that depression results from an imbalance of "humors," neurotransmitters, or other brain-related dysfunction. In recent years after a period of relative eclipse, the biological models are again ascendant, buoyed by successes in pharmacological treatment that often lead to the logically erroneous conclusion that depression must therefore have been an "illness" caused by a fundamental biological defect. Nowadays, however, reductionistic models, while present, coexist with relatively sophisticated diathesis–stress approaches and perspectives that are highly aware of the enormous complexity of potential vulnerability processes (e.g., Gold, Goodwin, & Chrousos, 1988).

Modern versions of intrapsychic models originated, of course, with psychodynamic theorizing and Freudian assumptions about disorders arising from internal conflicts based on early childhood experiences. The more modern versions of intraindividual perspectives, such as Beck's cognitive model, or Blatt's model of depressive personality styles, focus largely on the individual's self-schemas and *interpretations* of the world acquired as a product of learning experiences. These models have themselves been increasingly elaborated and refined. The third model, the environmental approach, evolved from ancient common understanding of depression as a response to overwhelming perils such as Job's afflictions. In more modern times, it has taken various forms: sociodemographic statistical risk-factor models, efforts to understand stressors as triggers of depressive reactions, and a more recent interpersonal focus on depression as arising from the transactions of individuals embedded in their social worlds. Probably the only conclusion that can be drawn about these trends is that models are bound to change in prominence, but the longevity of each through multiple reincarnations across cultures and centuries suggests the necessity and validity of all three perspectives.

METHODS OF STUDYING DEPRESSION VULNERABILITY

It would be impossible to give a complete and accurate accounting of all the methods used in studying vulnerability from the perspective of the major models. However, several methodological themes are worth noting, briefly reflecting increasing appreciation for the need to understand vulnerability processes. Ingram, Miranda, and Segal (1998) discussed a number of similar issues in their book, *Cognitive Vulnerability to Depression.*

First, there has been increasing movement away from cross-sectional studies to more longitudinal designs, attempting to replace correlation-based inferences with temporal order of variables as a basis for inferring causality. Such designs have revealed the transitory nature of vulnerability factors that previously had been assumed to be stable and have sharpened our search for phenotypic trait markers of depression instead of state indicators. A more recent version of cross-sectional studies includes comparisons of currently remitted depressed people with nondepressed individuals as a method of evaluating vulnerability independent of current depressed mood. A second development has been the increasing use of "challenge" situations or experimental manipulations as a supplement to naturalistic, descriptive studies of depression. Whereas psychology has always applied experimental approaches to some extent, biological psychiatry has become increasingly experimental within the constraints of ethical concerns. Psychological investigations continue to develop challenge tasks, such as mood induction or priming experiments.

A third trend has been the gradual development of designs to go beyond tests of single variables toward more truly integrative, diathesis–stress tests. Even if initially an implicit diathesis–stress model, many approaches did not literally examine vulnerability factors in a stress context (e.g., cognitive models), and even today many biological models do not include tests of the diathesis–stress approach. It is increasingly apparent that even more fully integrative models are needed to test vulnerability hypotheses, and although this trend is slow in developing it is to be hoped that such integration will increasingly occur.

It might be noted that the issue of sample selection has also undergone shifts during the history of research on depression vulnerability. As noted earlier, the gold standard in biological psychiatry continues to be treatment-seeking samples with DSM diagnoses. However, it is increasingly recognized that such samples may be "atypical" in the severity and likely comorbidity of their disorders, so that epidemiological research on community samples has gained in prominence. Given that most people who meet criteria for depressive disorders do not seek specialized mental health treatment, depression defined in primary-care settings has also gained attention. College undergraduates continue to be a convenience sample for some studies of depressive vulnerability processes, but the burden is on investigators to demonstrate that such samples meet the basic working definitions of depression stated earlier.

Finally, there appears to be increasing interest not only in identifying risk factors for depression but also in studying vulnerability processes, a distinction well articulated by Ingram et al. (1998). Investigators in both the biological and psychosocial worlds are increasingly attempting to understand *how* dysfunctional characteristics eventuate in depressive disorder.

All these themes are driven by advances in knowledge and technology that have been the direct by-products of the massive amount of research on depressive disorders conducted in just the past two and a half decades. Spurred by developments in diagnostic criteria, effective treatments, and new conceptual models, the field has shown remarkable growth, and we turn now to a consideration of findings on vulnerability to depressive disorders.

THEORY AND RESEARCH ON VULNERABILITY

Biological Vulnerability

Historically, the study of depression reveals a long-standing belief that among the various forms of depression, some are biologically caused while others are psychogenic in origin. This distinction has given rise to the variously termed neurotic–psychotic, endogenous–reactive, endogenous–neurotic, and endogenous–nonendogenous subtypes. Further, as Zimmerman, Coryell, Stangl, and Pfohl (1987) noted, labels for "endogenous" depression have included vital, severe, major, incapacitating, psychotic, primary, retarded, melancholic, autonomous, and endogenomorphic, whereas "nonendogenous" depressions have been variously called neurotic, reactive, characterological, atypical, secondary, mild, psychogenic, situational, and nonmelancholic. Further confusion has arisen because "endogenous" is a term that variously applied not just to the presumed biological origins but to the qualitative symptoms of depression, or to the apparent absence of stress precipitation.

In the modern research milieu, no clear support has arisen for a distinction between types of depression based on biological or nonbiological etiology. Instead, the term "melancholic" has been retained in DSM-IV to represent a qualitative distinction in MDEs, including features such as psychomotor change, diurnal variation, weight and appetite loss, and excessive guilt. It is not intended to signify a different etiology based on biological factors but does appear to predict positive response to electroconvulsive therapy and antidepressant medications (Rush & Weissenberger, 1994). It may in fact represent more a severity than qualitative distinction, but to many clinicians "melancholic depression" continues to imply a biological subtype.

On the other hand, there are many in biological psychiatry—and the general community—that appear to view *all* clinically significant depressions as biologically based disease processes. Supported in part by the knowledge that certain medical illnesses and medications cause depressive symptoms, the somatic symptoms of the depression syndrome itself, and the apparent effectiveness of antidepressant medications, many are convinced that the origin of depression is fundamentally biological, a "disease of the brain" (e.g., Judd, 1997). In this chapter, however, I argue that the evidence for biological factors in depression at best supports a vulnerability model—for some forms of depression—in which certain factors constitute diatheses requiring additional, largely psychosocial stress factors in the classic diathesis–stress model. However, given the limited research that is mostly based on cross-sectional, correlational designs, many observed differences between depressed and comparison groups may be consequences of depression or markers of other processes not yet clarified. Having noted these cautions, it is also important to suggest that several areas of biological research are extremely intriguing and promise to promote further understanding of human behavior generally and are not limited just to depressive syndromes.

Genetic Vulnerability to Depression

Depression undeniably runs in families. Gershon (1990) reviewed 10 studies of families of adult unipolar depressed probands and found rates of depression in first-degree relatives ranging between 7 and 30% across the studies, all considerably higher than in the general population. Findings from the Collaborative Depression Study of nearly 900 patients and controls found that 10.4% of patients' relatives had depression that involved hospitalization, incapacitation, or psychosis, compared with 4.9% of controls' relatives (Winokur, Coryell, Keller, Endicott, & Leon, 1995). Studies of the offspring of depressed parents have also revealed that having a depressed parent is one of the strongest predictors of depression in youth (reviewed in Beardslee, Versage, & Gladstone, 1998).

Family studies do not, of course, prove a genetic mechanism of transmission, and in later sections of this chapter I discuss the psychosocial processes. Alternative genetic strategies that are less confounded with environmental factors are also suggestive. Marker and linkage studies have not proven to be successful because unipolar depression is regarded as a heterogeneous disorder lacking a single major gene mode of transmission and including many nongenetic "phenocopies" that obscure current linkage methods (Blehar, Weissman, Gershon, & Hirschfeld, 1988). However, twin studies using modern biometric model-testing analyses have proven to be informative, as exemplified by two recent samples. Kendler and colleagues (e.g., Kendler, Neale, Kessler, Heath, & Eaves, 1992) have published a series of studies based on a population-based twin registry in Virginia. Initially focused on female twins (Kendler et al., 1992), the authors found significantly higher monozygotic (MZ) concordance than dizygotic (DZ) concordance. Recently extending the sample to include male twins, Kendler and Prescott (1999) reported on 3,790 twin pairs. Biometric twin modeling analyses to evaluation heritability and environmental factors for major depression concluded that the genetic liability accounted for 39% of the risk for MDE in both male and female twin pairs, with the remaining 61% of the variance attributable to individual-specific factors (such as stressful events). McGuffin, Katz, Watkins, and Rutherford (1996) obtained more than 200 twin pairs from inpatient treatment for depression in England and also reported significantly higher MZ than DZ concordance. Like Kendler and colleagues, McGuffin et al. (1996) concluded that genetic factors play a moderate role in family patterns of major depression.

Regarding the issue of whether particular subtypes or clinical courses of depression mark a particularly heritable form, the data are inconclusive. McGuffin et al. (1996) found genetic transmission to be especially associated with recurrent depressions with melancholic features. Kendler, Gardner, and Prescott (1999) found heritability in their twin sample to be most associated with intermediate levels of recurrence (e.g., seven to nine episodes, but not higher), longer durations, and high levels of impairment (see also Lyons et al., 1998, who found higher heritability among more severe subtypes of depression in their male community twin sample). Kendler et al. (1999) did not find higher heritability in earlier age of onset—a finding that contrasts with several earlier genetic studies.

Only one genetic study to date has explicitly tested a diathesis–stress model of depression. Kendler et al. (1995) examined the occurrence of stressful life events in the year prior to onset of major depression and found a significant interaction. The highest levels of depression were found in those exposed to severe stressors who were also most genetically at risk for depression (e.g., were identical cotwins of depressed women), whereas women at lowest genetic risk for depression who experienced a severe life event were less likely to become depressed. Interestingly, McGuffin, Katz, and Bebbington (1988) demonstrated an apparent gene–environment correlation in which relatives of depressed probands not only had elevated rates of depression but also elevated rates of stressful life events and adversities compared to the general population. A common familial factor may have contributed both to depression and to a tendency to experience (generate) stressful life events.

Psychoneuroendocrinology of Depression

Even though suggestive, genetic studies to date do not tell what it is that might be transmitted. Brain functioning and neuroendocrine processes may provide possible mechanisms. Considerable evidence implicates dysregulation of the human stress response of the hypothalamic–pituitary–adrenal (HPA) axis in depressive disorders. Numerous studies have found elevated levels of cortisol, a hormone resulting in various forms of physical arousal and activation, in acutely depressed people compared to nondepressed (as well as increased levels of CRF, corticotropin-releasing factor). When no longer depressed, cortisol levels return to normal.

In addition to hypersecretion of cortisol, investigators have observed abnormalities in the regulation of cortisol. Specifically, when the HPA axis is "challenged" by administration of a synthetic cortisol called *dexamethasone*, normal people show a temporary suppression of natural cortisol. However, many depressed individuals show an abnormal reaction consisting of "early escape" from the expected suppression of cortisol. When tested a certain time after the administration of dexamethasone, they have higher cortisol levels than do nondepressed persons. Initially, clinicians welcomed the dexamethasone suppression test (DST) as a potential diagnostic aid and believed that it might indicate a particular biological form of depression likely to respond to medication (e.g., Carroll et al., 1981; Holsboer, 1992). The apparent dysregulation of the underlying HPA axis was thought to play a causal role in depression. However, it has become apparent that abnormal DST reactions not only do not occur in all persons with major depression but also frequently occur in other patient groups, such as schizophrenics, as well (e.g., American Psychiatric Association Task Force, 1987). Moreover, the abnormal DST response is typically observed only in depressive states and appears normal when the person is no longer depressed.

Whether DST nonsuppression predicts response to treatment or future depressive status has been addressed in various studies. A recent review of more than 100 such studies drew several conclusions (Ribeiro, Tandon, Grunhaus, & Greden, 1993). First, pretreatment DST status was unrelated to treatment outcome and status following hospital discharge. Second, when depressed persons continued to show abnormal DST results (nonsuppression) even after treatment, they were more likely to relapse quickly and generally had a poorer prognosis than patients whose cortisol functions returned to normal after treatment. These patterns may suggest that depressed persons with abnormal cortisol mechanisms are "sicker" and therefore less responsive to treatment—or that there may be a subset of patients whose underlying disorder stems from dysregulation of the HPA.

A second line of speculation concerning neuroendocrine processes in depression focuses on the potential effects of early childhood adversity (possibly interacting with genetic predisposition) on the brain. Plotsky, Owens, and Nemeroff (1998) recently reviewed research on stress and HPA-related hormones and their effects on the brain (see also Benes, 1994; Sapolsky, 1996). They speculated that early stress experiences may sensitize specific neural circuits, resulting in depressive reactions in later life in response to stressful life events (see also Gold et al., 1988). Most of the relevant research has been conducted on animals, but a growing body of human research has shown abnormal HPA axis functioning associated with adverse childhood experiences such as insecure attachment and abuse experiences (e.g., Gunnar, 1998; Heim, Ehlert, Hanker, & Hellhammer, 1998). However, information about continuity of effects into childhood or their direct and specific link with depressive reactions has yet to be established.

Neurotransmitters and Depression Vulnerability

There has been considerable historical interest in the potential role of monoamine neurotransmitters (e.g., serotonin, norepinephrine, and dopamine) in mood disorders. These neurotransmitters are especially important in the limbic system of the brain, areas affecting drives and emotions, and pathways to other parts of the brain. The original catecholamine hypothesis of depression (Schildkraut, 1965) emphasizing relative deficits of the substances has proven to be far too simplistic, yielding to greater focus on amine receptor systems (McNeal & Cimbolic, 1986), and models of dysregulation of neurotransmitters (e.g., Siever & Davis, 1985). Recently, attention has turned particularly to serotonin (5-HT) models of depression (reviewed in Maes & Meltzer, 1995), suggesting that vulnerability to depression may arise from alterations in presynaptic 5-HT activity and postsynaptic serotonin receptor functioning. Moreover, because the hippocampus is a site of serotonergic innervation of the regulation of the HPA axis, it has been speculated that lowered central 5-HT activity in depression may attenuate hippocampal feedback control over the HPA axis, inducing excessive corticosteroid secretion (Maes & Meltzer, 1995). Because serotonin synthesis in the brain depends on availability of the precursor amino acid, tryptophan, experimental manipulation of tryptophan through dietary control has provided intriguing evidence of serotonin's association with depressed mood. A number of studies have demonstrated that rapid depletion of tryptophan in remitted depressed patients induces temporary but significant symptoms of depression (e.g., Bremner et al., 1997; Smith, Fairburn, & Cowen, 1997), although it does not affect stably nondepressed persons, providing suggestive causal evidence that serotonin may be implicated in depression onset.

Recent data also implicate catecholamine functioning. State-related changes in catecholamines have been associated with depressive conditions (e.g., the antihypertensive drug reserpine induces depression by depleting monoamines), but a recent study suggests a trait marker may be associated with history of depression. Berman et al. (1999) induced depletion of catecholamines in recovered, medication-free depressives, which led to clinically significant depressive symptoms. The authors suggest that this effect may reflect an abnormality in postsynaptic alpha-adrenergic functioning, which represents a vulnerability for depression (and may interact with other neurotransmitters and the HPA axis). Further studies and replication are needed to determine the validity of the claim that a "phenotypic trait marker for depression" has been found.

Functional and Structural Brain Changes in Depression

A number of medical conditions associated with known brain lesions cause depression. For example, poststroke depression and neurodegenerative diseases such as Parkinson's and Huntington's disease, have prompted the search for specific regions of the brain associated with depressive symptoms. Neuroimaging studies have reported some evidence of structural abnormalities in the brains of depressed people, such as reduced frontal volume (Coffey et al., 1993; see review by Powell & Miklowitz, 1994). Functional neuroimaging studies using PET scans have examined currently depressed patients as well as the effects of experimental mood manipulations and pharmacological challenges. A review by Kennedy, Javanmard, and Vaccarino (1997) concludes that the evidence shows reduced metabolic rate and reduced blood flow during depressive states and consistent evidence of abnormalities in the functions of the prefrontal and cigulate cortex—areas closely linked with limbic and paralimbic structures. Interestingly, a study of tryptophan depletion during PET (positron emission tomography) scanning indicated decreased metabolism in certain brain areas (Bremner et al., 1997). These investigators speculated that prefrontal cortex–limbic–striatal regions comprise a neural circuit that may function abnormally in depressed patients, playing a role in the etiology of depression. Clearly, considerable work is ongoing that will further clarify potential brain areas affected in depression and whether abnormalities have causal significance or mostly describe depressive process.

Electrophysiological research on frontal brain activity by Davidson and colleagues has resulted in a model of emotional reactivity that may have considerable promise as a vulnerability factor in negative emotional states such as depression (e.g., Davidson, 1993). He observed that depressed patients and even previously depressed but remitted patients showed relative left frontal hypoactivation. Davidson proposed that decreased left prefrontal activation represents an underactivation of an approach system, thus reducing the person's propensity to experience pleasure and to develop a positive engagement with the environment and increases the likelihood of developing depressive symptoms. Further developing the model, Davidson (1994) reviewed evidence suggesting the role of left prefrontal activation in inhibiting processing of negative information. He proposed that both prenatal stress and early childhood experiences influence affective structures and mold brain function. Interestingly—and as discussed more fully in Chapter 8 (this volume)—several studies have found that infants and toddlers of depressed mothers display relative left frontal hypoactivation (e.g., Dawson, Klinger, Panagiotides, Spieker, & Frey, 1992; Jones, Field, Fox, Lundy, & Davalos, 1997). Jones et al. (1997) observed the patterns in infants as young as 1 month old and found that it was related to sad facial expression and other behavioral indicators of "depressive" responses. They argue that these patterns may be genetically transmitted as a vulnerability for negative affect or may be acquired prenatally or even in early interactions with a depressed mother. Further research is clearly warranted to determine the origins and consequences of frontal asymmetry and whether its effects are general to emotional disorders or specific for depression.

Additional Topics in Biological Factors

Limited by space, two additional promising research areas are briefly noted. Depressive disorders have been hypothesized to result from the desynchronization of the circadian rhythms such as the sleep–wake cycle, cortisol secretion, and other bodily processes. Bolstered in part by consistent findings of sleep disturbances in depressed patients, including REM and slow-wave patterns—as well as by seasonal patterns of depression in some persons (seasonal affective disorder and normal seasonal variations in activity levels resembling some of the symptoms of depression)—investigators have long speculated a vulnerability to mood disorders based on circadian rhythms (e.g., Goodwin & Jamison, 1990). Despite apparently effective treatment of some forms of depression with exposure to light (e.g., Wirz-Justice, 1998) and sleep deprivation (e.g., Wu & Bunney, 1990), the vulnerability mechanisms are not understood, but circadian rhythm abnormalities continue to be actively investigated.

Those who note the universally higher rates of depression among women than men have frequently postulated the role of female hormones in depression. However, it has been noted that even massive changes in hormonal levels such as those accompanying childbirth are associated with only minor depressive symptoms, called postpartum blues. A recent review of hormone changes such as progesterone, estrogen, prolactin, and others associated with postpartum major depression notes the negative or inconsistent findings (Hendrick, Altshuler, & Suri, 1998). The authors conclude that although there is no evidence of an etiological role for the hormones, some women may experience mood changes because they are extremely sensitive to hormone levels. It is noteworthy that this field of study has focused mainly on levels of hormones while degree of change, as well as the interactions among ovarian and stress-related hormones, are topics meriting further methodological development.

Cognitive Vulnerability

Ingram et al. (1998) wrote an excellent volume devoted to an extensive analysis of conceptual and empirical aspects of the cognitive model of depression. In this chapter, therefore, the relatively brief and limited focus is on key developments and the most recent empirical status of the cognitive approach to vulnerability. Beck's (1967) original cognitive model of depression was the first to illuminate the characteristically negative thinking of depressed people and to assign causal significance in the phenomenology of depressive disorders to self-critical, pessimistic, helpless, and hopeless interpretations of the self and the world. Beck's approach gave rise to a veritable paradigm shift in clinical science in its focus on the significance and measurement of conscious thoughts and cognitive processes in psychopathology and, of course, also spawned a powerful and effective brief treatment of a disorder that had generally eluded clinicians.

Beck's own model evolved over time and also gave rise to a number of different versions, focusing variously on three cognitive aspects defined by Ingram et al. (1998): structural and propositional models (e.g., Beck, 1967; Blatt, 1974; Teasdale & Barnard, 1993), operational models (e.g., Nolen-Hoeksema, 1987), and product models (e.g., Abramson, Seligman, &

Teasdale, 1978; Abramson, Metalsky, & Alloy, 1989). Ingram et al. (1998) note that virtually all these models are primarily about self-related processing of information.

Considerable evidence has been amassed to support the hypothesis that depressed people think and interpret information in negative ways compared to nondepressed individuals, and that these modes of thinking are dysfunctional if not distorted (e.g., reviewed in Hammen, 1997; Segal & Ingram, 1994). However, there have been several roadblocks in the demonstration of depressogenic cognitions as vulnerability factors for depression. One is that few studies actually tested the causal propositions in the form of the diathesis–stress model and relatively little actual supportive evidence was found (reviewed in Barnett & Gotlib, 1988; Haaga, Dyck, & Ernst, 1991; see also Ingram et al., 1998).

Relatedly, another difficulty that emerged was the observation that cognitive dysfunctions that were presumed to put individuals at risk for the development of depression turned out not to be stable and measurable in the nondepressed state. Findings of "state-dependent" cognitions examined by comparing remitted depressed persons with controls (e.g., reviewed in Hammen, 1997; Ingram et al., 1998; Segal & Ingram, 1994) called into question the assumptions of continuously active depressive schemas. However, it should be noted that recent research (e.g., Zuroff, Blatt, Sanislow, Bondi, & Pilkonis, 1999) has revisited the issue, demonstrating that Dysfunctional Attitude Scale subscores displayed considerable stability over time despite overall decreases. These authors suggest a "state–trait vulnerability model" that they believe is a more accurate representation of Beck's and Blatt's models than the pure trait models sometimes attributed to them.

Findings of normalization of negative cognitions in many individuals during remission led to recent theoretical and methodological developments that hypothesize that dysfunctional schemas are "latent" and need to be activated before they can be measured. Activation by "priming" techniques such as depressed mood induction (e.g., Hedlund & Rude, 1995; Miranda & Persons, 1988) has generally demonstrated that formerly depressed individuals differ from nondepressed in the negativity of their responses on information-processing tasks or attitude questionnaires. However, with few exceptions (e.g., Segal, Gemar, & Williams, 1999) such studies have not actually tested the association of such negativity with risk for subsequent depression—nor tested the model's validity in identifying vulnerability for onset of depression.

A recent alternative test of depressive cognition as a true vulnerability factor is based on the hopelessness model of depression, the Abramson et al. (1989) revision of the earlier attribution model of depression (Abramson et al., 1978). Abramson et al. (1989) hypothesized that individuals whose depressive attributional style leads to negative inferences about the cause, consequences, and self-implications of any particular negative life event they confront, thereby increases the likelihood that they will develop hopelessness and, in turn, the symptoms of depression, particularly hopelessness depression (Abramson et al., 1999). Using a behavioral high-risk paradigm, these investigators identified university undergraduates who were not currently depressed but had high or low scores on a version of the Attribution Style Questionnaire, called the Cognitive Style Questionnaire, and Beck's Dysfunctional Attitude Scale (Weissman & Beck, 1978) and followed them longitudinally. Abramson et al. (1999) report that the high-risk students had a 17% rate of first onset of MDD, compared to 1% for the low-risk students, and among those with prior depressive episodes, the high-risk group also was more likely to have recurrences than was the low-risk group. These results held true even when initial subsyndromal symptom levels of depression were controlled. The high- and low-risk students also demonstrated predicted differences in information-processing tasks (Alloy, Abramson, Murray, Whitehouse, & Hogan, 1997). Further analyses are under way to test the diathesis–stress model of depression specifically by including stressful life event occurrence and whether hopelessness cognitions are the proximal causes (mediators) of depressive reactions to stressors. Also, insofar as high-risk students may have had prior (but not current) depressive diagnoses or elevated symptoms, it was not possible to rule out depressive cognitions as a consequence rather than cause of depression.

As the dominant psychological model of vulnerability to depression for nearly 30 years, how might we assess the contributions and future directions of the cognitive model? To the extent that the cognitive perspective is a diathesis–stress model, it makes considerable intuitive sense that it is individuals' appraisals of the meaning and consequences of stressors—rather than simply occurrence of stressors—that determines whether they become depressed or not when misfortunes befall them. It also makes common sense that some individuals are more likely than others to magnify the significance of negative events, to feel diminished or incompetent in ways they may believe cannot be repaired, and to suffer feelings of loss or defeat that induce depression. However, the cognitive models have fallen short in empirically substantiating several key assumptions: that cognitive vulnerabilities exist prior to depression experiences, that negative cognitions play a causal role in onset of first depression as well as recurrences, and that if they are causal rather than merely concomitants or consequences of depression, their contribution is *necessary, substantial, and specific to depression.*

The argument may be made (e.g., Hammen, 1992) that the cognitive models have been overly focused on internal processes to the relative neglect of developmental and contextual factors that contribute to depression. While negative cognitions—such as hopelessness—may indeed be proximal triggers of depressive reactions, their study in relative isolation contributes only a limited amount to our understanding of vulnerability processes. Accordingly, integrative models that include, but are not largely limited to, thinking styles may mark the contributions of this approach in the future. Moreover, another intriguing contribution of cognitive models might be fuller examination of the development and operation of dysfunctional schemas. The study of how adverse childhood experiences are translated into maladaptive "working models" of the self and others (e.g., Cummings & Cicchetti, 1990) and affective networks in memory (e.g., Teasdale, 1988) holds enormous promise for our understanding of the psychopathology of emotional disorders.

Life Stress Approaches to Depression Vulnerability

This section notes several approaches to depression that emphasize reactions to stressful life events.

Stressful Life Events and Depression

Like the cognitive models, research on the role of stress in depression has evolved and taken various forms. Early research relied largely on questionnaire-based retrospective assessments of life events and symptoms, demonstrating overall statistically significant associations. Recent approaches are considerably more sophisticated in methodology, disentangling symptoms and reports of events while also using short-term retrospective or prospective designs. Based on such improved methods, there is strong empirical support for an association between significant stressful life events and depressive syndromes, in both community and clinical samples (e.g., Dohrenwend, Shrout, Link, Martin, & Skodol, 1986; Shrout et al., 1989; reviewed in Brown & Harris, 1989). For instance, in Brown and Harris's (1989) review of seven community studies, approximately 70 to 95% of individuals who developed cases of depression experienced a prior severe life event compared to 25 to 40% among those who did not develop depression.

Although these studies indicate that most depressions are triggered by a significant negative life event, the obverse raises the critical question of vulnerability: Most people who do experience even major negative events do not become depressed. Why do some people become depressed and others do not? One approach that might be characterized as a multiple risk factor perspective was adopted by several large-scale studies that demonstrated a significant association between stressful events and depression in models emphasizing not only negative events but also chronic stressful conditions and social supports (e.g., Billings, Cronkite, & Moos, 1983; Holahan & Moos, 1991; Lewinsohn, Hoberman, & Rosenbaum, 1988; Moos, Cronkite, & Moos, 1998). To a great extent, these approaches suggest that depression is a reaction to adverse life events, mediated by resources for coping with the events; however, mechanisms linking the risk and protective factors specifically to depression have not been clarified.

George Brown, the British sociologist, and his colleagues have pursued the vulnerability question based on their extensive and detailed analyses of the context in which stressors occur in the lives of the women in their studies. Brown and Harris (1978) hypothesized that the meaning of an event is critical to depression and initially determined that several empirically based "vulnerability" factors increased the negative implications of a stressful event or chronic difficulty. Vulnerability factors included lack of a confiding relationship, loss of the mother before age 11, having three or more young children at home, and lack of employment outside the home (Brown & Harris, 1978).

Brown, Bifulco, and Harris (1987) refined the model by specifying that an event had to represent a loss (such as an important person, belief, role, object, health) and it had to "match" a particular role to which a woman was committed. According to the more general model (e.g., Brown & Harris, 1989), the important mediator of the link between stressors and depression is the meaning of the event. Specifically, severe events that give rise to a lack of hope for better things induce depression; low self-esteem prior to the event is likely to give rise to hopelessness. Several studies have shown, for example, that low self-esteem is a risk factor for depression (Brown, Andrews, Harris, Adler, & Bridge, 1986). Low self-esteem is hypothesized to be the outcome of the vulnerability factors, particularly social support factors such as the lack of a confiding relationship or poor quality of the woman's close relationships (Andrews & Brown, 1988). Although Brown's model is different from Beck's in its focus on the nature and context of life events, both models are somewhat similar in their emphasis on cognitive mediation of the effects of stress. Brown and Harris (1989), like Beck, emphasize the interpretation of the event as a depletion of the sense of self-worth and identity. In Brown's research such cognitions are inferred and rated by the investigator through discussions with the subject about her life circumstances, whereas more traditional cognitive researchers have generally elicited direct reports from the subject. However, a major point of disagreement is the extent to which the individual is viewed as having distorted interpretations of events, with Brown and others arguing that depression results from severe negative events and adversity and the contexts in which they occur—not potentially minor misfortunes exaggerated or distorted in the depressed person's interpretations.

Perhaps surprisingly, few studies of adults have included biological vulnerability to predict depressive reactions to stressors. As noted earlier, Kendler et al. (1995) found that the risk for onset of major depression was highest among women who had both a genetic liability for depression (e.g., MZ cotwins of women with a history of depression) and a recent severe stressor. Although the investigators have speculated that the genetic diathesis may alter the threshold at which stressors trigger depression, the actual mechanisms of vulnerability are not known.

Personality and Depressive Reactions to Specific Life-Event Types

Beck (1983) and others including psychodynamically oriented theorists (e.g., Arieti & Bemporad, 1980; Blatt, Quinlan, Chevron, McDonald, & Zoroff, 1982) proposed that individuals may be particularly vulnerable to some stressors more than others. Specifically, individuals differ in the sources of their self-esteem and sense of mastery, with some individuals experiencing personal worth as deriving from the achievement of highly valued goals and control while others are more likely to invest themselves and their self-definitions in personal relationships with others. The former type is variously termed "autonomous," "dominant goal-oriented," or "self-critical," the latter may be termed "sociotropic," "dominant-other oriented," or "dependent" (reviewed in Nietzel & Harris, 1990). Vulnerability, therefore, might consist of attitudes, beliefs, and values such that a major stressor that was interpreted as representing a depletion in the sense of worth or competence would provoke a depressive reaction.

Several studies have tested this model, refining the depression–life stress link to include those events whose content matches the presumed underlying vulnerability as assessed in various self-report or experimental methods (e.g., Hammen, Marks, Mayol, & deMayo, 1985; Hammen, Ellicott, Gitlin, & Jamison, 1989; Robins & Block, 1988; Segal, Shaw, Vella, & Katz, 1992; Zuroff & Mongrain, 1987). These studies have supported the "vulnerability matching" hypothesis, with generally strongest support for the combination of sociotropy or dependency and interpersonal negative events triggering depression. These studies refine the overall stress–depression link and appear to support a cognitive diathesis–stress approach to understanding of the mechanisms of depression (but see Coyne & Whiffen, 1995, for a critique).

Stress Sensitization

Although stress has typically been studied as a precipitant in classic diathesis–stress models, an alternative perspective is that stress exposure is itself part of the diathesis for depression. An emerging "sensitization" perspective in the biological models of depression reviewed earlier suggests that early childhood adversity may alter neural circuits in ways that sensitize the brain to respond maladaptively when triggered by provoking events such as current stress. Post (1992), discussing recurrent mood disorders of both unipolar and bipolar types, has proposed that episodes themselves—or possibly repeated exposure to stress—may sensitize the organism to react to lower levels of stress, similar to kindling or behavioral sensitization. However, as Segal, Williams, Teasdale, and Gemar (1996) argue, the kindling phenomenon may have an alternative explanation as increasing levels of accessibility of negative schemas due to repetition and frequency of past usage. Thus, minor events or negative moods may come to be sufficient to trigger the negative patterns of information processing that intensify depressive moods and symptoms.

The sensitization perspective clearly requires empirical support but is intriguing not only for suggesting that the stress becomes the diathesis but also because it represents a dynamic model rather than the typically static views of most depression models—a conceptual issue addressed further later.

Interpersonal Approaches to Vulnerability

Life-stress researchers insisted that understanding depression requires focus on the context of events and conditions that trigger depressive reactions in those vulnerable to the disorder, but a developing paradigm places particular emphasis on the *interpersonal* context of people's lives. This perspective has emerged from growing awareness of the many ways in which social relationships affect, and are affected by, depression. Also, in my case, the interpersonal interest stemmed from various conceptual and empirical developments, including reaction to the overly intraindividual focus of the original cognitive models, pondering gender differences and the experiences of women that place them at particular risk for depression, and interest in the developmental psychopathology of depression including the impact of early parent–child relationships (Hammen, 1999). Gotlib and Hammen (1992) wrote *Psychological Aspects of Depression: Toward a Cognitive– Interpersonal Integration,* detailing many of these issues (see also Joiner & Coyne, 1999).

The interpersonal approach is more an emphasis and research philosophy with diverse targets and contents than it is a theory or model. It argues for an understanding of depression in individuals embedded in their contexts, focusing on transactions and interactions between individuals, creating a dynamic process that changes over time (Hammen, 1999). Several research themes are discussed briefly.

Effects of Depression on Others

Coyne (1976) was one of the first to articulate a perspective in which the depressed person seeks reassurance and initially elicits sympathetic responses, but excessive need for comfort eventually is perceived as aversive and increasingly elicits rejection, which in turn may increase or perpetuate the symptoms of depression. Numerous studies demonstrated that, indeed, interactions with a depressed person—both real and simulated interactions— elicited rejection and negative attitudes (e.g., reviewed in Gotlib & Hammen, 1992). Many of these studies involved interactions with strangers in contrived situations, and therefore the validity of the hypotheses needed to be tested in real-life situations. Thus, a series of studies by Hokanson and colleagues demonstrated that depressed students over time elicited negative emotions, negative attitudes, and less social interaction in their roommates (e.g., Howes, Hokanson, & Loewenstein, 1985; Hokanson, Rubert, Welker, Hollander, & Hedeen, 1989; Hokanson, Hummer, & Butler, 1991).

These early explorations into the effects of depressed people on others raised awareness about the social context of depression but did not illuminate the meaning of such interactional phenomena in understanding risk for depression. For instance, while Coyne speculated that excessive reassurance seeking was the major cause of rejection, this approach implies that the behavior is but another dysfunctional symptom of depression. Rather than serving an etiological role, reassurance seeking was viewed as a contributor to the downward spiral of depression once a person was already dysphoric.

Dependency and Reassurance Seeking

Recently, Joiner and colleagues speculated that reassurance seeking may in fact be an individual difference variable that serves as a vulnerability to develop depression. Joiner and Metalsky (1995; see also Potthoff, Holahan, & Joiner, 1995) showed that a measure of reassurance seeking predicted future depressive symptoms in students experiencing stressful situations. Reassurance seeking is related to the construct of "dependency"—emotional reliance on others and the belief that affection, acceptance, and support of others is essential to well-being. Dependency has long been recognized as a concomitant and risk factor for depression—as a trait or as the diathesis in a diathesis–stress interaction (e.g., reviews by Barnett & Gotlib, 1988; Nietzel & Harris, 1990). As noted earlier, measures of "sociotropy" or dependency represent beliefs and schemas about the importance of contact and value by others, and when individuals high in such cognitions encounter negative interpersonal relationships, depressive reactions may ensue mediated by interpretations of loss, abandonment, or incompetence.

Dysfunctional Relationships in Depression

A considerable body of literature has demonstrated that maladaptive relationships commonly accompany depressive disorders. For instance, divorce, marital disruption, and negative spousal interactions have frequently been observed (e.g., reviewed in Gotlib & Hammen, 1992). Similarly, dysfunctional interactions between depressed mothers and their children and between depressed children and their mothers have also been extensively documented (e.g., reviewed in Kaslow, Deering, & Racusin, 1994; Downey & Coyne, 1990).

The direction of causality works both ways, with depressed people behaving negatively toward others because they are depressed and becoming depressed in response to others' negative behavior. However, a number of studies have suggested that for many depressive individuals, dysfunctional relationships are not specific to depressive states and often persist even during periods of relative remission (e.g., Billings & Moos, 1985a, 1985b; Hammen, 1991a; Keitner & Miller, 1990, but see Moos et al., 1998). If the dysfunctional patterns persist, they may reflect interpersonal skill deficits, enduring maladaptive cognitions about others, or (and) a continuing social milieu in which aversive participants contribute to the negative interactions.

Maladaptive interaction patterns may create stressful environments that precipitate depressive reactions. Findings indicate that depressed people respond to negative reactions or attitudes by becoming depressed or experiencing relapses. For instance, negative attitudes by spouses and relatives predict a more protracted course of depression or relapses in depressed patients (Hooley, Orley, & Teasdale, 1986; Hooley & Teasdale, 1989; Keitner et al., 1995).

Stress Generation

In a related theme, Hammen (1991b) observed during life-stress interviews with depressed women that many reported highly stressful events that were attributed in part to their own actions, attitudes, and characteristics. A comparison of stressful life events over a 1-year period in groups of unipolar, bipolar, medically ill, and non-ill women indicated significant differences between the groups in terms of stressful life events. The unipolar depressed women—even in remission—reported significantly more events to which they had contributed (nonindependent events), especially interpersonal events and a subcategory, interpersonal conflict. This pattern has subsequently been replicated in children of depressed women (Adrian & Hammen, 1993) and in young women in the community with histories of depression and depression comorbidity (Daley et al., 1997; Davila, Hammen, Burge, Daley, & Paley, 1995). Even when not currently depressed, such individuals engage in interactions that are disruptive, conflicted, and stressful. In turn, such events may precipitate depressive reactions (e.g., Davila et al., 1995). We speculate that for many who develop depression, the vulnerability consists of maladaptive cognitions about attachment and dysfunctional interpersonal skills that contribute to the "creation" of a social milieu that heightens the likelihood of stressful experiences. In turn, the stressors may precipitate or maintain depressive symptoms because of heightened dependency needs and self-deprecating cognitions in the face of interpersonal strife.

Commentary and Future Directions on Interpersonal Approaches

There are many additional facets of interpersonal functioning in depression (see Joiner & Coyne, 1999). It should be emphasized, however, that not all depression arises in an interpersonal context or because of vulnerability based on dependency schemas. Nevertheless, interpersonal perspectives may contribute significantly to an understanding of three of the strongest empirical "truths" about depression: It is highly prevalent in women; depression runs in families; past depression predicts future depression. To the extent that women are socialized to assign particular importance to their interpersonal roles, they may acquire schemas that base self-worth on attachment to others. When coupled with maladaptive skills for resolving interpersonal difficulties or with poor self-esteem, even minor negative social events may take on excessive importance. Depression runs in families not only due to genetic factors but also because dysfunctional parent–child interactions due to maternal depression may create a heritage of negative cognitions and skills. Such experiences may lead to dysfunctional mate selection or to exposure to interpersonal conditions that perpetuate depression and provide a milieu in which children are born and perpetuate the cycle.

The effects of past depression on future depression are a considerable challenge to understand. Past depression may simply reflect the continuing presence of vulnerability factors that lead to future depression. However, effects of past depression could also operate in a much more dynamic fashion. For instance, the continuing residual symptoms of depression may influence how one behaves interpersonally, contributing to a dysfunctional milieu that increases the risk for continuing episodes. Alternatively, depressive experiences may alter an individual both neurochemically and cognitively in ways that lower the threshold for depressive reactions to stressors as discussed in previous sections (e.g., Post, 1992; Segal et al., 1996). Consequently, the individual becomes more vulnerable to the effects of stress.

IMPLICATIONS FOR PREVENTION AND TREATMENT

A variety of effective treatments are now available for both major depressive episodes and dysthymic disorder. New-generation antidepressant drugs, although no more effective than earlier tricyclic antidepressants, have attained widespread use because of ease of administration and relatively fewer side effects (reviewed in Gitlin, 1996). By altering levels of key neurotransmitters both directly and through changes in receptor density and sensitivity, the medications help to reregulate neurochemical changes that underlie depression (although, of course, such neurochemical mechanisms may not themselves be the etiological mechanism causing depression). Presumably further analysis of genetic mechanisms of depression or other neurobiological processes will illuminate more precise, direct targets for intervention or treatment. Theoretically, biological tests could be developed from genetic markers or neurochemical factors that could indicate risk for development of depressive reactions, thereby identifying those who would profit from prevention or early intervention.

Cognitive-behavioral and interpersonal mechanisms of depression lend themselves to treatment and prevention models. The well-established cognitive-behavioral therapy (Beck, Rush, Shaw, & Emery, 1979) and interpersonal psychotherapy (Klerman, Weissman, Rounsaville, & Chevron, 1984) brief treatments, for instance, purport to target the maladaptive cognitive-behavioral patterns or interpersonal role difficulties, respectively, that are thought to play an etiological role in depression—or at least in the maintenance and intensification of depression (e.g., reviewed in Hollon, Shelton, & Davis, 1993; Weissman & Markowitz, 1994). Preventive interventions have begun to appear based on research on cognitive vulnerability to depression (e.g., Clarke et al., 1995; Jaycox, Reivich, Gillham, & Seligman, 1994) and on children's risk due to parental depression (e.g., Beardslee et al., 1993).

Less well studied but of potential importance would be preventive interventions based on interpersonal vulnerabilities, such as dependency or excessive reassurance seeking. Certainly the identification of dysfunctional self-schemas based on extreme sociotropic values could help treatments in tailoring specifically to help individuals avoid or cope effectively with interpersonal stressors that might otherwise trigger depressive reactions. The development of effective treatments for depression occurring in the context of marital difficulties is also an important strategy not only for reducing risk of depression and relapse but potentially also for preventing risk of children born into such families (e.g., Jacobson, Fruzzetti, Dobson, Whisman, & Hops, 1993).

FUTURE DIRECTIONS FOR RESEARCH

Throughout this chapter a number of issues have been highlighted for further research and analysis. Starting with the fundamental issue of what depression *is*, considerable work remains to be done to determine the unique and specific effects and origins of depression given its common co-occurrence with other Axis I and Axis II disorders. Basic questions about the potential effects of different degrees of severity and course, as well as potential subtypes of depression with different causes and consequences, remain. Depression heterogeneity poses a conceptual and methodological challenge and in practical terms may limit the scope of research accomplishments if they can be generalized only to certain forms and levels of depression.

Regarding models of vulnerability, there is an overarching need for integrative models that link biological and psychosocial processes so that theories are not artificially in competition. Similarly, relatively few models have tested their etiological elements in longitudinal designs—with the vast majority of studies describing current features. Specific tests of vulnerability models in a diathesis–stress design are remarkably rare. Models also need to capture the potentially dynamic nature of vulnerability processes, based on the supposition that depression and other personal experiences alter the person and change the relationship among stress and diathesis factors over time. The content of vulnerability models continues to emphasize cognitive and interpersonal factors, and exciting developments in the ways in which these processes are measured and understood have evolved. Nevertheless, critical questions remain about the etiological significance of such factors. Even at the level of understanding cognitive and social processes, remarkably little is known about their acquisition and operation in normal individuals as well as in those suffering from susceptibility to mood disorders.

Finally, it is worth repeating that further attention needs to be given to the three most robust findings to date in the depression field: It is most common in women, past depression is the strongest predictor of future depression, and depression runs in families. There is much to be extracted from these realities, and future theoretical and practical developments will profit from setting their sights on providing explication.

REFERENCES

Abramson, L. Y., Alloy, L. B., Hogan, M. E., Whitehouse, W. G., Donovan, P., Rose, D. T., Panzarella, C., & Raniere, D. (1999). Cognitive vulnerability to depression: Theory and evidence. *Journal of Cognitive Psychotherapy, 13,* 5–20.

Abramson, L. Y., Metalsky, G. I., & Alloy, L. B. (1989). Hopelessness depression: A theory-based subtype of depression. *Psychological Review, 96,* 358–372.

Abramson, L. Y., Seligman, M. E. P., & Teasdale, J. (1978). Learned helplessness in humans: Critique and reformulation. *Journal of Abnormal Psychology, 87,* 49–74.

Adrian, C., & Hammen, C. (1993). Stress exposure and stress generation in children of depressed mothers. *Journal of Consulting and Clinical Psychology, 61,* 354–359.

Alloy, L. B., Abramson, L. Y., Murray, L. A., Whitehouse, W. G., & Hogan, M. E. (1997). Self-referent information-processing in individuals at high and low cognitive risk for depression. *Cognition and Emotion, 11,* 539–568.

American Psychiatric Association. (1994). *Diagnostic and statistical manual of mental disorders* (4th ed.). Washington, DC: Author.

American Psychiatric Association Task Force on Laboratory Tests in Psychiatry. (1987). The dexamethasone suppression test: An overview of its current status in psychiatry. *American Journal of Psychiatry, 144,* 1253–1262.

Andrews, B., & Brown, G. W. (1988). Social support, onset of depression and personality: An exploratory analysis. *Social Psychiatry and Psychiatric Epidemiology, 23,* 99–108.

Arieti, S., & Bemporad, J. (1980). The psychological organization of depression. *American Journal of Psychiatry, 137*, 1360–1365.

Barnett, P. A., & Gotlib, I. H. (1988). Psychosocial functioning and depression: Distinguishing among antecedents, concomitants, and consequences. *Psychological Bulletin, 104*, 97–126.

Beardslee, W. R., Salt, P., Porterfield, K., Rothberg, P. C., van de Velde, P., Swatling, S., Hoke, L., Moilanen, D. L., & Wheelock, I. (1993). Comparison of preventive interventions for families with parental affective disorder. *Journal of the American Academy of Child and Adolescent Psychiatry, 32*, 254–263.

Beardslee, W. R., Versage, E. M., & Gladstone, T. R. G. (1998). Children of affectively ill parents: A review of the past 10 years. *Journal of the American Academy of Child and Adolescent Psychiatry, 37*, 1134–1141.

Beck, A. T. (1967). *Depression: Clinical, experimental, and theoretical aspects.* New York: Harper & Row.

Beck, A. T. (1983). Cognitive therapy of depression: New perspectives. In P. J. Clayton & J. E. Barrett (Eds.), *Treatment of depression: Old controversies and new approaches* (pp. 265–290). New York: Raven Press.

Beck, A. T., Rush, A. J., Shaw, B. F., & Emery, G. (1979). *Cognitive therapy of depression.* New York: Guilford Press.

Benes, F. M. (1994). Developmental changes in stress adaptation in relation to psychopathology. *Development and Psychopathology, 6*, 723–739.

Berman, M. R., Narasimhan, M., Miller, H. L., Anand, A., Cappiello, A., Oren, D. A., Heninger, G. R., & Charney, D. S. (1999). Transient depressive relapse induced by catecholamine depletion. *Archives of General Psychiatry, 56*, 395–403.

Billings, A. G., Cronkite, R., & Moos, R. (1983). Social–environmental factors in unipolar depression: Comparisons of depressed patients and nondepressed controls. *Journal of Abnormal Psychology, 93*, 119–133.

Billings, A. G., & Moos, R. H. (1985a). Life stressors and social resources affect posttreatment outcomes among depressed patients. *Journal of Abnormal Psychology, 94*, 140–153.

Billings, A. G., & Moos, R. H. (1985b). Psychosocial processes of remission in unipolar depression: Comparing depressed patients with matched community controls. *Journal of Consulting and Clinical Psychology, 53*, 314–325.

Blatt, S. (1974). Levels of object representation in anaclitic and introjective depression. *Psychoanalytic Study of the Child, 29*, 107–157.

Blatt, S., Quinlan, D., Chevron, E., McDonald, C., & Zuroff, D. (1982). Dependency and self criticism: Psychological dimensions of depression. *Journal of Consulting and Clinical Psychology, 50*, 113–124.

Blazer, D. G., Kessler, R. C., McGonagle, K. A., & Swartz, M. S. (1994). The prevalence and distribution of major depression in a national community sample: The National Comorbidity Survey. *American Journal of Psychiatry, 151*, 979–986.

Blehar, M. C., Weissman, M. M., Gershon, E. S., & Hirschfeld, R. M. A. (1988). Family and genetic studies of affective disorders. *Archives of General Psychiatry, 45*, 289–292.

Bremner, J. D., Innis, R. B., Salomon, R. M., Staib, L. H., Ng, C. K., Miller, H. L., Bronen, R. A., Krystal, J. H., Duncan, J., Rich, D., Price, L. H., Malison, R., Dey, H., Soufer, R., & Charney, D. S. (1997). Positron emission tomography measurement of cerebral metabolic correlates of tryptophan depletion-induced depressive relapse. *Archives of General Psychiatry, 54,* 364–374.

Brown, G. W., Andrews, B., Harris, T. O., Adler, Z., & Bridge, L. (1986). Social support, self-esteem, and depression. *Psychological Medicine, 16,* 813–831.

Brown, G. W., Bifulco, A., & Harris, T. O. (1987). Life events, vulnerability and onset of depression: Some refinements. *British Journal of Psychiatry, 150,* 30–42.

Brown, G. W., & Harris, T. (1978). *Social origins of depression.* London: Free Press.

Brown, G. W., & Harris, T. O. (1989). Depression. In G. W. Harris & T. O. Harris (Eds.), *Life events and illness* (pp. 49–93). New York: Guilford Press.

Burke, K. C., Burke, J. D., Regier, D. A., & Rae, D. S. (1990). Age at onset of selected mental disorders in five community populations. *Archives of General Psychiatry, 47,* 511–518.

Carroll, B. J., Feinberg, M., Greden, J. F., Tarika, J., Albala, A. A., Haskett, R. F., James, N., Kronfol, Z., Lohr, N., Steiner, M., de Vigne, J. P., & Young, E. (1981). A specific laboratory test for the diagnosis of melancholia. *Archives of General Psychiatry, 38,* 15–22.

Clark, D. A., Cook, A., & Snow, D. (1998). Depressive symptoms difference in hospitalized, medically ill, depressed, psychiatric inpatients and nonmedical controls. *Journal of Abnormal Psychology, 107,* 38–48.

Clarke, G., Hawkins, W., Murphy, M., Sheeber, L., Lewinsohn, P., & Seeley, J. (1995). Targeted prevention of unipolar depressive disorder in an at-risk sample of high school adolescents: A randomized trial of a group cognitive intervention. *Journal of the American Academy of Child and Adolescent Psychiatry, 34,* 312–321.

Coffey, C. E., Wildinson, W. E., Weiner, R. D., Parashos, I. A., Djang, W. T., Webb, M. C., Figiel, G. S., & Spritzer, C. E. (1993). Quantitative cerebral anatomy in depression: A controlled magnetic resonance imaging study. *Archives of General Psychiatry, 50,* 7–16.

Coyne, J. C. (1976). Depression and the response of others. *Journal of Abnormal Psychology, 85,* 186-193.

Coyne, J. C., Pepper, C. M., & Flynn, H. (1999). Significance of prior episodes of depression in two patient populations. *Journal of Consulting and Clinical Psychology, 67,* 76–81.

Coyne, J. C., & Whiffen, V. E. (1995). Issues in personality as diathesis for depression: The case of sociotropy–dependency and autonomy–self criticism. *Psychological Bulletin, 118,* 358–378.

Cummings, E. M., & Cicchetti, D. (1990). Toward a transactional model of relations between attachment and depression. In M. Greenberg & D. Cicchetti (Eds.), *Attachment in the preschool years: Theory, research, and intervention* (pp. 339–372). Chicago: University of Chicago Press.

Daley, S., Hammen, C., Burge, D., Davila, J., Paley, B., Lindberg, N., & Herzberg, D. (1997). Predictors of the generation of episodic stress: A longitudinal study of late adolescent women. *Journal of Abnormal Psychology, 106,* 251–259.

Daley, S., Hammen, C., & Rao, U. (in press). Predictors of first onset and recurrence of major depression in young women during the five years following high school graduation. *Journal of Abnormal Psychology.*

Davidson, R. J. (1993). Cerebral asymmetry and emotion: Conceptual and methodological conundrums. *Cognition and Emotion, 7,* 115–138.

Davidson, R. J. (1994). Asymmetric brain function, affective style, and psychopathology: The role of early experience and plasticity. *Development and Psychopathology, 6,* 741–758.

Davila, J., Hammen, C., Burge, D., Daley, S. E., & Paley, B. (1995). Poor interpersonal problem solving as a mechanism of stress generation in depression among adolescent women. *Journal of Abnormal Psychology, 104,* 592–600.

Dawson, G., Klinger, L. G., Panagiotides, H., Spieker, S., & Frey, K. (1992). Infants of mothers with depressive symptoms: Electroencephalographic and behavioral findings related to attachment status. *Development and Psychopathology, 4,* 67–80.

Dohrenwend, B. P., Shrout, P. E., Link, B., Martin, J., & Skodol, A. (1986). Overview and initial results from a risk-factor study of depression and schizophrenia. In J. E. Barrett (Ed.), *Mental disorder in the community: Progress and challenges.* New York: Guilford Press.

Downey, G., & Coyne, J. C. (1990). Children of depressed parents: An integrative review. *Psychological Bulletin, 108,* 50–76.

Gershon, E. S. (1990). Genetics. In F. K. Goodwin & K. R. Jamison (Eds.), *Manic–depressive illness* (pp. 373–401). New York: Oxford University Press.

Gitlin, M. J. (1996). *The psychotherapist's guide to psychopharmacology* (2nd ed.). New York: Free Press.

Gold, P. W., Goodwin, F. K., & Chrousos, G. P. (1988). Clinical and biochemical manifestations of depression: Relation to the neurobiology of stress. *New England Journal of Medicine, 319,* 348–419.

Goodwin, F. K., & Jamison, K. R. (Eds.). (1990). *Manic–depressive illness.* New York: Oxford University Press.

Gotlib, I. H., & Hammen, C. L. (1992). *Psychological aspects of depression: Toward a cognitive–interpersonal integration.* London: Wiley.

Gotlib, I. H., Lewinsohn, P. M., & Seeley, J. R. (1995). Symptoms versus a diagnosis of depression: Differences in psychosocial functioning. *Journal of Consulting and Clinical Psychology, 65,* 90–100.

Gunnar, M. (1998). Quality of early care and buffering of neuroendocrine stress reactions: Potential effects on the developing human brain. *Preventive Medicine, 27,* 208–211.

Haaga, D. A., Dyck, M. J., & Ernst, D. (1991). Empirical status of cognitive theory of depression. *Psychological Bulletin, 110,* 215–236.

Hammen, C. L. (1991a). *Depression runs in families: The social context of risk and resilience in children of depressed mothers.* New York: Springer-Verlag.

Hammen, C. L. (1991b). The generation of stress in the course of unipolar depression. *Journal of Abnormal Psychology, 100,* 555–561.

Hammen, C. L. (1992). Cognitions and depression: Some thoughts about new directions. *Psychological Inquiry, 3,* 247–250.

Hammen, C. (1997). *Depression.* London: Psychology Press.

Hammen, C. (1999). The emergence of an interpersonal approach to depression. In T. Joiner & J. Coyne (Eds.), *The interactional nature of depression: Advances in interpersonal approaches* (pp. 21–35). Washington, DC: American Psychological Association.

Hammen, C. L., Ellicott, A., Gitlin, M., & Jamison, K. R. (1989). Sociotropy/

autonomy and vulnerability to specific life events in unipolar and bipolar patients. *Journal of Abnormal Psychology, 98,* 154–160.

Hammen, C. L., Marks, T., Mayol, A., & deMayo, R. (1985). Depressive self-schemas, life stress, and vulnerability to depression. *Journal of Abnormal Psychology, 94,* 308–319.

Hedlund, S., & Rude, S. S. (1995). Evidence of latent depressive schemas in formerly depressed individuals. *Journal of Abnormal Psychology, 104,* 517–525.

Heim, C., Ehlert, U., Hanker, J. P., & Hellhammer, D. H. (1998). Abuse-related posttraumatic stress disorder and alterations of the hypothalamic-pituitary-adrenal axis in women with chronic pelvic pain. *Psychosomatic Medicine, 60,* 309–318.

Hendrick, V., Altshuler, L. L., & Suri, R. (1998). Hormonal changes in the postpartum and implications for postpartum depression. *Psychosomatics, 39,* 93–101.

Hokanson, J. E., Hummer, J. T., & Butler, A. C. (1991). Interpersonal perceptions by depressed college students. *Cognitive Therapy and Research, 15,* 443–457.

Hokanson, J. E., Rubert, M. P., Welker, R. A., Hollander, G. R., & Hedeen, C. (1989). Interpersonal concomitants and antecedents of depression among college students. *Journal of Abnormal Psychology, 98,* 209–217.

Holahan, C. J., & Moos, R. H. (1991). Life stressors, personal and social resources, and depression: A 4-year structural model. *Journal of Abnormal Psychology, 100,* 31–38.

Hollon, S. D., Shelton, R. C., & Davis, D. D. (1993). Cognitive therapy for depression: Conceptual issues and clinical efficacy. *Journal of Consulting and Clinical Psychology, 61,* 270–275.

Holsboer, F. (1992). The hypothalamic–pituitary–adrenocortical system. In E. S. Paykel (Ed.), *Handbook of affective disorders* (2nd ed., pp. 267–287). New York: Guilford Press.

Hooley, J. M., Orley, J., & Teasdale, J. D. (1986). Levels of expressed emotion and relapse in depressed patients. *British Journal of Psychiatry, 148,* 642–647.

Hooley, J. M., & Teasdale, J. D. (1989). Predictors of relapse in unipolar depressives: Expressed emotion, marital distress, and perceived criticism. *Journal of Abnormal Psychology, 98,* 229–237.

Horwath, E., Johnson, J., Klerman, G. L., & Weissman, M. M. (1992). Depressive symptoms as relative and attributable risk factors for first-onset major depression. *Archives of General Psychiatry, 49,* 817–823.

Howes, M. J., Hokanson, J. E., & Loewenstein, D. A. (1985). Induction of depressive affect after prolonged exposure to a mildly depressed individual. *Journal of Personality and Social Psychology, 49,* 1110–1113.

Ingram, R. E., Miranda, J., & Segal, Z. V. (1998). *Cognitive vulnerability to depression.* New York: Guilford Press.

Jacobson, N. S., Fruzzetti, A. E., Dobson, K., Whisman, M., & Hops, H. (1993). Couple therapy as a treatment for depression: II. The effects of relationship quality and therapy on depressive relapse. *Journal of Consulting and Clinical Psychology, 61,* 516–519.

Jaycox, L. H., Reivich K. J., Gillham J., & Seligman M. E. P. (1994). Prevention of depressive symptoms in school children. *Behavior Research Therapy, 32,* 801–816.

Johnson, J., Weissman, M. M., & Klerman, G. (1992). Service utilization and social morbidity associated with depressive symptoms in the community. *Journal of the American Medical Association, 267,* 1478–1483.

Joiner, T., & Coyne, J. C. (Eds.). (1999). *The interactional nature of depression: Advances in interpersonal approaches.* Washington, DC: American Psychological Association.

Joiner, T. E., Jr., & Metalsky, G. I. (1995). A prospective test of an integrative interpersonal theory of depression: A naturalistic study of college roommates. *Journal of Personality and Social Psychology, 69,* 778–788.

Jones, N. A., Field, T., Fox, N. A., Lunday, B., & Davalos, M. (1997). EEG activation in 1-month-old infants of depressed mothers. *Development and Psychopathology, 9,* 491–505.

Judd, L. L. (1997). The clinical course of unipolar major depressive disorders. *Archives of General Psychiatry, 54,* 989–991.

Judd, L. J., Akiskal, H. S., Maser, J. D., Zeller, P. J., Endicott, J., Coryell, W., Paulus, M. P., Kunovac, J. L., Leon, A. C., Mueller, T. I., Rice, J. A., & Keller, M. B. (1998). A prospective 12-year study of subsyndromal and syndromal depressive symptoms in unipolar major depressive disorders. *Archives of General Psychiatry, 55,* 694–700.

Kaslow, N. J., Deering, C. G., & Racusin, G. R. (1994). Depressed children and their families. *Clinical Psychology Review, 14,* 39–59.

Keitner, G. I., & Miller, I. W. (1990). Family functioning and major depression: An overview. *American Journal of Psychiatry, 147,* 1128–1137.

Keitner, G. I., Ryan, C. E., Miller, I. W., Kohn, R., Bishop, D. S., & Epstein, N. B. (1995). Role of the family in recovery and major depression. *American Journal of Psychiatry, 152,* 1002–1008.

Kendler, K. S., Gardner, C. O., & Prescott, C. A. (1999). Clinical characteristics of major depression that predict risk of depression in relatives. *Archives of General Psychiatry, 56,* 322–327.

Kendler, K. S., Kessler, R. C., Walters, E. E., MacLean, C., Neale, M. C., Heath, A. C., & Eaves, L. J. (1995). Stressful life events, genetic liability, and onset of an episode of major depression in women. *American Journal of Psychiatry, 152,* 833–842.

Kendler, K. S., Neale, M. C., Kessler, R. C., Heath, A. C., & Eaves, L. J. (1992). A population-based twin study of major depression in women. *Archives of General Psychiatry, 49,* 257–266.

Kendler, K. S., & Prescott, C. A. (1999). A population-based twin study of lifetime major depression in men and women. *Archives of General Psychiatry, 56,* 39–44.

Kennedy, S. H., Javanmard, M., & Vaccarino, F. J. (1997). A review of functional neuroimaging in mood disorders: Positron emission tomography and depression. *Canadian Journal of Psychiatry, 42,* 467–475.

Klerman, G. L., Weissman, M. M., Rounsaville, B. J., & Chevron, E. (1984). *Interpersonal psychotherapy of depression.* New York: Basic Books.

Krueger, R. F., Caspi, A., Moffitt, T. E., & Silva, P. A. (1998). The Structure and Stability of Common Mental Disorders (DSM-III-R): A longitudinal–epidemiological study. *Journal of Abnormal Psychology, 107,* 216–227.

Lewinsohn, P. M., Hoberman, H., & Rosenbaum, M. (1988). A prospective study of risk factors for unipolar depression. *Journal of Abnormal Psychology, 97,* 251–264.

Lyons, M. J., Eisen, S. A., Goldberg, J., True, W., Lin, N., Meyer, J. M., Toomey, R., Faraone, S. V., Merla-Ramos, M., & Tsuang, M. T. (1998). A registry-based twin study of depression in men. *Archives of General Psychiatry, 55,* 468–472.

Maes, M., & Meltzer, H. Y. (1995). The serotonin hypothesis of major depression. In F. E. Bloom & D. J. Kupfer (Eds.), *Psychopharmacology: The fourth generation of progress* (pp. 933–944). New York: Raven Press.

McGuffin, P., Katz, R., & Bebbington, P. (1988a). The Camberwell Collaborative Depression Study: II. Investigation of family members. *British Journal of Psychiatry, 152,* 766–774.

McGuffin, P., Katz, R., Watkins, S., & Rutherford, J. (1996). A hospital-based twin registry study of the heritability of DSM-IV unipolar depression. *Archives of General Psychiatry, 53,* 129–136.

McNeal, E. T., & Cimbolic, P. (1986). Antidepressants and biochemical theories of depression. *Psychological Bulletin, 99,* 361–374.

Miranda, J., & Persons, J. B. (1988). Dysfunctional attitudes are mood-state dependent. *Journal of Abnormal Psychology, 97,* 76–79.

Moos, R. H., Cronkite, R. C., & Moos, B. S. (1998). Family and extrafamily resources and the 10-year course of treated depression. *Journal of Abnormal Psychology, 107,* 450-460.

Nietzel, M. T., & Harris, M. J. (1990). Relationship of dependency and achievement/autonomy to depression. *Clinical Psychology Review, 10,* 279–297.

Nolen-Hoeksema, S. N. (1987). Sex differences in unipolar depression: Evidence and theory. *Psychological Bulletin, 101,* 259–282.

Plotsky, P. M., Owens, M. J., & Nemeroff, C. B. (1998). Psychoneuroendocrinology of depression. *Psychoneuroendocrinology, 21,* 293–307.

Post, R. M. (1992). Transduction of psychosocial stress into the neurobiology of recurrent affective disorder. *American Journal of Psychiatry, 149,* 999–1010.

Potthoff, J. G., Holahan, C. J., & Joiner, T. E., Jr. (1995). Reassurance-seeking, stress generation, and depressive symptoms: An integrative model. *Journal of Personality and Social Psychology, 68,* 664-670.

Powell, K. B., & Miklowitz, D. J. (1994). Frontal lobe dysfunction in the affective disorders. *Clinical Psychology Review, 14,* 525–546.

Regier, D. A., Kaelber, C. T., Rae, D. S., Farmer, M. E., Knauper, B., Kessler, R. C., & Norquist, G. S. (1998). Limitations of diagnostic criteria and assessment instruments for mental disorders. *Archives of General Psychiatry, 55,* 109–115.

Ribeiro, S. C. M., Tandon, R., Grunhaus, L., & Greden, J. F. (1993). The DST as a predictor of outcome in depression: A meta-analysis. *American Journal of Psychiatry, 150,* 1618–1629.

Robins, C. J., & Block, P. (1988). Personal vulnerability, life events, and depressive symptoms: A test of a specific interational model. *Journal of Personality and Social Psychology, 54,* 847–852.

Rush, A. J., & Weissenburger, J. E. (1994). Melancholic symptom features and DSM-IV. *American Journal of Psychiatry, 151,* 489–498.

Sapolsky, R. M. (1996). Why stress is bad for your brain. *Science, 273,* 749–750.

Schildkraut, J. J. (1965). The catecholamine hypothesis of affective disorders: A review of supporting evidence. *American Journal of Psychiatry, 122,* 509-522.

Segal, Z. V., Gemar, M., & Williams, S. (1999). Differential cognitive response to a mood challenge following successful cognitive therapy or pharmacotherapy for unipolar depression. *Journal of Abnormal Psychology, 108,* 3–10.

Segal, Z. V., & Ingram, R. E. (1994). Mood priming and construct activation in tests of cognitive vulnerability to unipolar depression. *Clinical Psychology Review, 14,* 663–695.

Segal, Z. V., Shaw, B. F., Vella, D. D., & Katz, R. (1992). Cognitive and life stress predictors of relapse in remitted unipolar depressed patients: A test of the congruency hypothesis. *Journal of Abnormal Psychology, 101,* 26–36.

Segal, Z. V., Williams, J. M., Teasdale, J. D., & Gemar, M. (1996). A cognitive science perspective on kindling and episode sensitization in recurrent affective disorder. *Psychological Medicine, 26,* 371–380.

Shea, M. T., Pilkonis, P. A., Beckham, E., Collins, J. F., Elkin, I., Sotsky, S. M., & Docherty, J. P. (1990). Personality disorders and treatment outcome in the NIMH Treatment of Depression Collaborative Research Program. *American Journal of Psychiatry, 98,* 468–477.

Shea, M. T., Widiger, T. A., & Klein, M. H. (1992). Comorbidity of personality disorders and depression: Implications for treatment. *Journal of Consulting and Clinical Psychology, 60,* 857–868.

Sherbourne, C. D., Hays, R. D., & Wells, K. B. (1995). Personal and psychosocial risk factors for physical and mental health outcomes and course of depression among depressed patients. *Journal of Consulting and Clinical Psychology, 63,* 345–355.

Shrout, P. E., Link, B. G., Dohrenwend, B. P., Skodol, A. E., Stueve, A., & Mirttznik, J. (1989). Characterizing life events as risk factors for depression: The role of fateful loss events. *Journal of Abnormal Psychology, 98,* 460–467.

Siever, L. J., & Davis, K. L. (1985). Overview: Toward a dysregulation hypothesis of depression. *American Journal of Psychiatry, 142,* 1017–1031.

Smith, A. L., & Weissman, M. M. (1992). Epidemiology. In E. S. Paykel (Ed.), *Handbook of affective disorders* (pp. 111–129). New York: Guilford Press.

Smith, K. A., Fairburn, C. G., & Cowen P. J. (1997). Relapse of depression after rapid depletion of tryptophan. *Lancet, 349,* 915–919.

Solomon, D. A., Keller, M. B., Leon, A. C., Mueller, T. I., Shea, M. T., Warshaw, M., Maser, J. D., Coryell, W., & Endicott, J. (1997). Recovery from major depression. A 10-year prospective follow-up across multiple episodes. *Archives of General Psychiatry, 54,* 1001–1006.

Teasdale, J. D. (1988). Cognitive vulnerability to persistent depression. *Cognition and Emotion, 2,* 247–274.

Teasdale, J. D., & Barnard, P. J. (1993). *Affect, cognition and change: Re-modeling depressive thought.* Hillsdale, NJ: Erlbaum.

Watson, D., Weber, K., Assenheimer, J. S., Clark, L. A., Strauss, M., & McCormick, R. (1995). Testing a tripartite model: I. Evaluating the convergent and dicriminant validity of anxiety and depression symptoms scales. *Journal of Abnormal Psychology, 104,* 3–14.

Weissman, A., & Beck, A. T. (1978). *Development and validation of the Dysfunctional Attitude Scale: A preliminary investigation.* Paper presented at the annual meeting of the American Educational Research Association, Toronto, Canada.

Weissman, M. M., & Markowitz, J. C. (1994). Interpersonal psychotherapy. *Archives of General Psychiatry, 51,* 599–606.

Weissman, M. M., & Olfson, M. (1995). Depression in women: Implications for health care research. *Science, 269,* 799–801.

Wells, K. B., Stewart, A., Hays, R. D., Burnam, A., Rogers, W., Daniels, M., Berry, S., Greenfield, S., & Ware, J. (1989). The functioning and well-being of depressed patients. *Journal of the Amercian Medical Association, 262,* 914–919.

Winokur, G., Coryell, W., Keller, M., Endicott, J., & Leon, A. (1995). A family study of manic–depressive (bipolar I) disease: Is it a distinct illness separable from primary unipolar depression? *Archives of General Psychiatry, 52,* 367–373.

Wirz-Justice, A. (1998). Beginning to see the light [comment]. *Archives of General Psychiatry, 55,* 861–862.

Wu, J. C., & Bunny, W. E. (1990). The biological basis of an antidepressant response to sleep deprivation and relapse: Review and hypothesis. *American Journal of Psychiatry, 147,* 14–21.

Zimmerman, M., Coryell, W., Stangl, D., & Pfohl, B. (1987). Validity of an operational definition for neurotic unipolar major depression. *Journal of Affective Disorders, 12,* 29–40.

Zuroff, D. C., Blatt, S. J., Sanislow, C. A., III, Bondi, C. M., & Pilkonis, P. A. (1999). Vulnerability to depression: Reexamining state dependence and relative stability. *Journal of Abnormal Psychology, 108,* 76–89.

Zuroff, D. C., & Mongrain, M. (1987). Dependency and self-criticism: Vulnerability factors for depressive affective states. *Journal of Abnormal Psychology, 96,* 14–22.

10

Vulnerability to Depression across the Lifespan

CONSTANCE HAMMEN
JUDY GARBER

For the most part, investigators of child/adolescent depression and adult depression have pursued separate tasks. Research on childhood depression has commonly been guided by models and definitions of adult depression, with relatively little independent development of theories unique to youngsters (although see Cole, 1991, for an exception). Both research traditions have largely focused on cross-sectional and static attributes and correlates of depression. It seems apparent in reading Chapters 8 (Garber & Flynn, this volume) and 9 (Hammen, this volume) that there are critical gaps in both fields that are in part attributable to the typical age-related division of labor and its usual designs and methods. In this brief chapter, we note several of these issues and make recommendations for further study.

DIAGNOSTIC AND DEFINITIONAL ISSUES

One critical concern is whether childhood, adolescent, and adult depressions are the same thing; that is, does the application of common diagnostic criteria identify the same underlying disorder that has fundamentally the same etiological and vulnerability factors? As the literatures reviewed in Chapters 8 and 9 indicate, there is an implicit assumption that "depression" is the same disorder across the lifespan, with similar genetic and neuroendocrine precursors and cognitive/personality vulnerabilities possibly triggered by stressful life events. Earlier age of onset, as in childhood, is often regarded as a more severe form of the disorder, and adolescent onset is viewed as the fairly typical origin of "adult" depression. Although it is recognized that there may be variations in the manifestations of depression at different ages, there has been relatively little questioning of the assumption of continuity.

One important aspect of the continuity issue is whether childhood onset of depression predicts depression in adulthood. In one of the longest prospective studies to date, Weissman et al. (1999a) followed 83 prepubertal-onset depressive children into young adulthood and found that there was no specificity for depressive disorder in adulthood. The formerly depressed youngsters had poor outcomes in terms of substance abuse/dependence and conduct disorder/antisocial personality disorder, as well as impaired functioning in important roles. However, for the most part they did not have depressive episodes. Harrington, Fudge, Rutter, Pickles, and Hill (1990) similarly reported that children with prepubertal onset of depression were at significantly lower risk of having major depression as adults compared to postpubertal depressed patients. Harrington et al. (1990), however, suggested that this finding could have been due to artifacts of their methodology such as poor measurement of prepubertal depression or the inaccurate documentation of the onset of puberty. Nevertheless, these findings are consistent with the view that prepubertal-onset depressions might differ from adolescent- and adult-onset depressions in several important ways, including phenomenology and outcome.

The Weissman et al. (1999a) study did identify a subgroup of children with early-onset and recurrent depressions with a familial concentration of depression in first-degree relatives. These findings are consistent with other studies that have suggested that early-onset mood disorders are a more severe and recurrent form of the disorder and are associated with increased familial loading of depression (e.g., Weissman, Warner, Wickramaratne, & Prusoff, 1988). Thus, it is likely that childhood-onset depressions are heterogeneous with respect to long-term outcome and might include both a highly impairing multiproblem symptom picture as well as a group of more "pure" depressions. Numerous studies of extremely high rates of comorbidity in childhood depression (Angold & Costello, 1993) suggest the need for further studies to determine which cases of childhood-onset depression reflect a nonspecific distress reaction that is developmentally an expression of emotional and behavioral dysregulation, and which are the more specific disorder of depression.

In contrast to the findings with regard to the continuity of childhood-onset depression, Weissman et al. (1999b) found substantial specificity for depression in adulthood among those with adolescent onset, which is consistent with other studies of adolescent-onset depression (e.g., Garber, Kriss, Koch, & Lindholm, 1988; Harrington et al., 1990). Nevertheless, the meaning of adolescent depression is not without questions. The noteworthy findings of apparent birth cohort increases in youth depression in recent years (Burke, Burke, Rae, & Regier, 1991; Klerman & Weissman, 1989), along with the accelerating rates of depression for girls when they enter early adolescence (Hankin et al., 1998), suggest developmentally significant challenges at that age along with culturally influenced patterns of reaction that permit females to express depressive symptoms more than males. An important question is what differentiates the more normative and transient experience of depression among young women (e.g., Rao, Hammen, & Daley, 1999; Hankin et al., 1998) from depressions that become recurrent and debilitating during adulthood?

On the other side of the coin, research conducted with adult samples rarely identifies the sample by age of onset. This leaves the impression that they had their onset during adulthood, although it is likely in many cases that the first episodes or significant symptoms occurred in adolescence. Would there be a difference in the features and correlates of the depressive disorder if groups were characterized by age of onset?

Embedded in these queries are a number of issues for further study. Is there commonality among depressions that commence at different ages? If not, are the differences due to developmental forces shaping the same underlying disorder, or are they actually different forms of depression? Should recurrence be a critically defining feature of "depression" that can help make subtype distinctions among the highly heterogeneous phenomena of depressive disorders? What developmental factors influence the differential experience and expression of depressive disorders over time? Do the same processes underlie first-onset, maintenance, and recurrence of depression across the lifespan? These and related definitional issues are far from resolved, and require developmentally informed models to be hypothesized and tested in longitudinal designs.

MODELS OF VULNERABILITY

The problems of definitions and potential phenotypical heterogeneity not only are interesting and critical in their own right but also affect our ability to evaluate the evidence for vulnerability factors and etiological processes that are derived from samples of different ages. These latter issues are further obscured by the relative neglect of developmental perspectives in the models themselves, as noted in the following topics.

Genetic Studies

The rapidly developing technologies for identifying appropriate samples and testing biometric models have resulted in twin studies that are far superior to family pedigree studies in partitioning the relative contributions of heritability and environmental factors. Hammen's review indicated that adult studies are generally consistent in finding moderate genetic factors and strong individual-specific (nonshared environment) factors. Garber and Flynn (Chapter 8, this volume) noted, however, that both twin and adoption studies present a far more inconsistent picture, depending on the age of the child and the source of the data. The inconsistencies raise questions not only of defining and diagnosing depression but also of considering comorbidity and modeling of family (shared) environmental factors. Methodological limitations may make it difficult to know whether the genetic patterns are in fact unknown or simply muddied by neglect of definitional and developmental considerations.

Brain and Neurochemical Studies

Adult studies implicating disordered markers of neuroendocrine functioning such as sleep architecture and cortisol regulation have not translated particularly well to youth samples (Dahl & Ryan, 1996). Several inconsistent or nonsignificant findings in child or adolescent samples seemed eventually to prod investigators to consider that such parameters might not be appropriately measured in youngsters in the same ways as adults due to the developmental differences (Dahl et al., 1992). On the positive side, new research considering the influence of negative experiences on the developing brain represents an exciting and potentially highly significant focus of research on vulnerability. Several intriguing findings highlight important directions for future research on biological vulnerability. These include the influence of maternal depression on the quality of infant–parent relationships potentially affecting brain functioning, genetically transmitted patterns of electrophysiological emotion-related responding (Dawson, Klinger, Panagiotides, Hill, & Spieker, 1992; Dawson, Frey, Panagiotides, Osterling, & Hessl, 1997), and the role of traumatic exposure in childhood sensitizing the child to future experiences with stressors. Such studies may increasingly provide understanding of how depression vulnerabilities operate and how they may affect the further development of at-risk children and adolescents. Such information also may provide fruitful glimpses into potential mechanisms behind recurrent depression in adults and the processes by which critical experiences alter the person's vulnerability to react with depression to provoking situations and stressors.

Cognitive and Social Factors

Among the most extensively developed hypotheses about depression vulnerability in adults, cognitive and life-stress approaches have increasingly been applied to young samples. The cognitive perspective argues not only that individuals become depressed following stress exposure if they interpret the event to reflect badly on their current or future worth or competence, but also that tendencies to interpret events in such negative ways may be acquired and serve as a latent vulnerability for depression. As Chapters 8 and 9 pointed out, however, the vulnerability portion of this model has not been unequivocally supported. Part of the problem has been difficulty in accessing vulnerability markers when the person is not depressed. Turning to paradigms that include activation of proposed negative schemas or induction of depressed mood, adult depression researchers have embarked on a new generation of vulnerability studies (Ingram, Miranda, & Segal, 1998). Childhood depression research has been somewhat slower to embrace such paradigms; it would be highly productive to learn more about depressed children's information processing of schematic information. Moreover, adult depression models generally have predicted that vulnerability schemas are acquired in childhood (e.g., Kovacs & Beck, 1978). There has been some research exploring possible processes by which negative cognitions are acquired (e.g., Garber & Flynn, in press; Jaenicke et al., 1987), although it would be fruitful both for depression models specifically and social cognition research more generally to learn more about children's formation and use of schemas about the self and others.

Similarly, ample evidence attests to the role of stressful life events as triggers for depressive reactions among those who may be vulnerable to respond with significant and enduring depression. Chapters 8 and 9, respectively, note that the evidence of the stress–depression link is strongest in adult samples but appears to be growing in studies of children and adolescents. Developmental issues profoundly affect children's exposure to stressors as well as their resources for coping with them. The problem-solving techniques and coping strategies that children use may greatly affect their reactions to negative events as well as predict their capacity to deal with stressors and challenging situations as adults.

One of the most important predictors of depressive reactions appears to be negative social events, especially if they match underlying interpersonal needs and vulnerabilities. Although the interpersonal perspective is attracting increasing attention in the adult depression field, especially for its role in explicating negative social interactions that often follow from depression (Gotlib & Hammen, 1992), this line of investigation in children is relatively new (Rudolph, Hammen, & Burge, 1997). It would be useful to more directly study the social skills and schemas of depressed youngsters, especially those behaviors and cognitions that may affect the quality of their interpersonal relationships both within and outside the family. At the same time, credit is due to the large number of investigators who have studied family processes among high-risk families in which a parent suffers from depression (reviewed in Goodman & Gotlib, 1999). Such studies have been innovative in the methods of studying dysfunctional transactions between depressed parents and their children and the role of such interactions in the transmission of depression from parent to child. Further studies of the continuities across development of dysfunctional interpersonal styles may help to shed light on an important mechanism of depression and its intergenerational transmission.

INTERVENTION

Whereas there is considerable evidence of the efficacy of psychopharmacological and psychosocial interventions for the treatment of mood disorders in adults, these interventions have only been systematically studied in children and adolescents during the last decade. The different kinds of treatments basically map on to the main kinds of vulnerability factors that have been discussed in both Chapters 8 and 9. That is, controlled treatment studies have tested the efficacy of pharmacological, cognitive, and interpersonal therapies.

Tricyclic antidepressant (TCA) medications have been effective in treating depression in adults but not in children and adolescents (Hazell, O'Connell, Heathcote, Robertson, & Henry, 1995). Because the noradrenergic system presumably does not develop fully until early adulthood (Ryan, 1990), and depressed and nondepressed adolescents differ on external endocrine measures that are more influenced by serotonin central nervous system activity (Kutcher et al., 1991), serotonergic agents are expected to be more effective than noradrenergic agents in youth. Indeed, in a double-blind, randomized, placebo-controlled trial in children between 7 and 17 years old, Emslie et al. (1997) found that 56% receiving the selective serotonin reuptake inhibitor (SSRI) fluoxetine clinically improved compared to 33% receiving placebo. Thus, the use of SSRIs for treating depression in children and adolescents looks promising. More studies are needed that explore the developmental factors that contribute to the differential effectiveness of medications in youth.

Cognitive therapy, which has been found to effectively treat depression in adults (Hollon, Shelton, & Davis, 1993), has been modified to make it developmentally appropriate for youth (Belsher & Wilkes, 1994; Lewinsohn, Clarke, Rohde, Hops, & Seeley, 1996; Stark, 1990). Treatment studies have demonstrated both short- and long-term effectiveness of cognitive therapy in reducing depressive symptoms in adolescents (Reinecke, Ryan, & DuBois, 1998), although more cognitive therapy studies need to be conducted with clinically depressed patients in individual therapy. In one such study, Brent et al. (1997) found that there was a significantly higher rate of remission among adolescents receiving cognitive therapy compared to those receiving either family or supportive therapy. The utility of such cognitive-behavioral approaches with depressed preadolescent children still needs to be examined. Although it is possible that the behavioral components of the therapy might be applicable to younger children, it is less likely that young children will be able to comprehend and use many of the more abstract cognitive procedures due to their still developing cognitive abilities.

A second psychosocial intervention effective in the treatment of depression in adults is interpersonal psychotherapy (IPT) (e.g., Klerman, Weissman, Rounsaville, & Chevron, 1984). Mufson, Moreau, Weissman, and Klerman (1993) modified IPT procedures to make them more appropriate for teens, and in a randomized treatment study, Rossello and Bernal (1999) found that cognitive-behavioral therapy and IPT significantly reduced depressive symptoms compared to a waitlist condition.

Thus, there is growing evidence of the efficacy of different kinds of treatments with depressed adolescents as well as adults. Controlled treatment studies also need to be conducted with younger depressed children. It is likely that interventions with younger children will need to include parents (Mendlowitz et al., 1999) and to emphasize behavioral strategies over cognitive techniques (Kendall, 1993). The presence of marital, parental, and social functioning difficulties in the families and children require multifaceted interventions (Hammen, Rudolph, Weisz, Rao, & Burge, 1999). Finally, treatment studies in both adults and youth should more explicitly explore the mechanisms of change because this could be informative about the processes that maintain and possibly produce depressive symptoms. Identification of such mechanisms would facilitate the development of much needed programs for preventing depression.

CONCLUSIONS

Chapters 8 and 9 noted the burgeoning of research on depression in recent years, contributing to much richer understanding of the phenomenon of depression than in prior eras. We expect that this level of research activity will continue in order to address the many unresolved questions, but we caution that new paradigms are needed for the more mature state of this field. Although cross-sectional studies and single-construct approaches were appropriate to early investigations, there now is a need for integrative, longitudinal, and intervention studies to address the complexities of the topic. Integrations of biological and psychosocial approaches are clearly called for but difficult to accomplish. Yet, it is apparent that such developments are under way and additions will be most welcome. Similarly, static, linear models must yield to more complex models involving transactions among variables. The influence of earlier experiences on later behavior and the mutual influences of the person and environment on each other are some of the obvious dynamic processes that must be captured by a developmental psychopathology of depression at any age. We look forward to many more achievements in the field of depression and predict that increasingly the barriers between child and adult research will disappear in order to address some of the unresolved issues.

REFERENCES

Angold, A., & Costello, E. J. (1993). Depressive comorbidity in children and adolescents: Empirical, theoretical, and methodological issues. *American Journal of Psychiatry, 150,* 1779–1791.

Belsher, G., & Wilkes, T. C. R. (1994). Ten key principles of adolescent cognitive therapy. In T. C. R. Wilkes, G. Belsher, A. J. Rush, E. Frank, & Associates, *Cognitive therapy for depressed adolescents* (pp. 22–44). New York: Guilford Press.

Brent, D., Holder, D., Kolko, D., Birmaher, B., Baugher, M., Roth, C., Iyengar, S., & Johnson, B. (1997). A clinical psychotherapy trial for adolescent depression comparing cognitive, family, and supportive therapy. *Archives of General Psychiatry, 54,* 877–885.

Burke, K. C., Burke, J. D., Rae, D., & Regier, D. A. (1991). Comparing age at onset of major depression and other psychiatric disorders by birth cohorts in five U.S. community populations. *Archives of General Psychiatry, 48,* 789–795.

Cole, D. A. (1991). Preliminary support for a competency-based model of depression in children. *Journal of Abnormal Psychology, 100,* 181–190.

Dahl, R. E., & Ryan, N. D. (1996). The psychobiology of adolescent depression. In D. Cicchetti & S. L. Toth (Eds.), *Adolescence: Opportunities and challenges* (pp. 197–232). Rochester, NY: University of Rochester Press.

Dahl, R. E., Ryan, N. D., Williamson, D. E., Ambrosini, P. J., Rabinovich, H., Novacenko, H., Nelson, B., & Puig-Antich, J. (1992). The regulation of sleep and growth hormone in adolescent depression. *Journal of the American Academy of Child and Adolescent Psychiatry, 31,* 615–621.

Dawson, G., Frey, K., Panagiotides, H., Osterling, J., & Hessl, D. (1997). Infants of depressed mothers exhibit atypical frontal brain activity: A replication and extension of previous findings. *Journal of Child Psychology and Psychiatry, 38,* 179–186.

Dawson, G., Klinger, L. G., Panagiotides, H., Hill, D., & Spieker, S. (1992). Frontal lobe activity and affective behavior of infants of mothers with depressive symptoms. *Child Development, 63,* 725–737.

Emslie, G. J., Rush, A. J., Weinberg, W. A., Kowatch, R. A., Hughes, C. W., Carnody, T., & Rintelmann, J. (1997). A double-blind, randomized, placebo-controlled trial of Fluoxetine in children and adolescents with depression. *Archives of General Psychiatry, 54,* 1031–1037.

Garber, J., & Flynn, C. (in press). Predictors of depressive cognitions in young adolescents. *Cognitive Therapy and Research.*

Garber, J., Kriss, M. R., Koch, M., & Lindholm, L. (1988). Recurrent depression in adolescents: A follow-up study. *Journal of the American Academy of Child and Adolescent Psychiatry, 27,* 49–54.

Goodman, S. H., & Gotlib, I. H. (1999). Risk for psychopathology in the children of depressed mothers: A developmental model for understanding mechanisms of transmission. *Psychological Review, 106,* 458–490.

Gotlib, I. H., & Hammen, C. L. (1992). *Psychological aspects of depression: Toward a cognitive-interpersonal integration.* Chichester, UK: Wiley.

Hammen, C., Rudolph, K., Weisz, J., Rao, U., & Burge, D. (1999). The context of depression in clinic-referred youth: Neglected areas in treatment. *Journal of the American Academy of Child and Adolescent Psychiatry, 38,* 64–71.

Hankin, B. L., Abramson, L. Y., Moffitt, T. E., Silva, P. A., McGee, R., & Angell, K. E. (1998). Development of depression from preadolescence to young adulthood: Emerging gender differences in a 10-year longitudinal study. *Journal of Abnormal Psychology, 107*, 128–140.

Harrington, R., Fudge, H., Rutter, M., Pickles, A., & Hill, J. (1990). Adult outcomes of childhood and adolescent depression. *Archives of General Psychiatry, 47*, 465–473.

Hazell, P., O'Connell, D., Heathcote, D., Robertson, J., & Henry, D. (1995). Efficacy of tricyclic drugs in treating child and adolescent depression: A metaanalysis. *British Medical Journal, 310*, 897–901.

Hollon, S. D., Shelton, R., & Davis, D. (1993). Cognitive therapy for depression: Conceptual issues and clinical efficacy. *Journal of Consulting and Clinical Psychology, 61*, 270–275.

Ingram, R. E., Miranda, J., & Segal., Z. V. (1998). *Cognitive vulnerability to depression*. New York: Guilford Press.

Jaenicke, C., Hammen, C., Zupan, B., Hiroto, D., Gordon, D., Adrian, C., & Burge, D. (1987). Cognitive vulnerability in children at risk for depression. *Journal of Abnormal Child Psychology, 15*, 559–572.

Kendall, P. C. (1993). Cognitive-behavioral therapies with youth: Guiding theory, current status, and emerging developments. *Journal of Consulting and Clinical Psychology, 61*, 235–247.

Klerman, G. L., & Weissman, M. M. (1989). Increasing rates of depression. *Journal of the American Medical Association, 261*, 2229–2235.

Klerman, G. L., Weissman, M. M., Rounsaville, B. J., & Chevron, E. S. (1984). *Interpersonal psychotherapy of depression*. New York: Basic Books.

Kovacs, M., & Beck, A. T. (1978). Maladaptive cognitive structures in depression. *American Journal of Psychiatry, 135*, 525–533.

Kutcher, S. P., Malkin, D., Silverberg, J., Marton, P., Williamson, P., Malkin, A., Szalai, J., & Katic, M. (1991). Nocturnal cortisol, thyroid stimulating hormone and growth hormone secreting properties in depressed adolescents. *Journal of the American Academy of Child and Adolescent Psychiatry, 30*, 407–414.

Lewinsohn, P. M., Clarke, G., Rohde, P., Hops, H., & Seeley, J. (1996). A course in coping: A cognitive-behavioral approach to the treatment of adolescent depression. In E. Hibbs, & P. Jensen (Eds.), *Psychosocial treatments for child and adolescent disorders: Empirically based strategies for clinical practice* (pp. 109–135). Washington, DC: American Psychological Association.

Mendlowitz, S. L., Manassis, K., Bradley, S., Scapillato, D., Miezitis, S., & Shaw, B. R. (1999). Cognitive-behavioral group treatments in childhood anxiety disorders: The role of parental involvement. *Journal of the American Academy of Child and Adolescent Psychiatry, 38*, 1223–1229.

Mufson, L., Moreau, D., Weissman, M. M., & Klerman, G. L. (1993). *Interpersonal psychotherapy for depressed adolescents*. New York: Guilford Press.

Rao, U., Hammen, C., & Daley, S. (1999). Continuity of depression during the transition to adulthood: A 5-year longitudinal study of young women. *Journal of the American Academy of Child and Adolescent Psychiatry, 38*, 908–915.

Reinecke, M. A., Ryan, N. E., & DuBois, D. L. (1998). Cognitive-behavioral therapy of depression and depressive symptoms during adolescence: A review and meta-analysis. *Journal of the American Academy of Child and Adolescent Psychiatry, 37,* 26–34.

Rossello, J., & Bernal, G. (1999). The efficacy of cognitive-behavioral and interpersonal treatments for depression in Puerto Rican adolescents. *Journal of Consulting and Clinical Psychology, 67,* 734–745.

Rudolph, K. D., Hammen, C., & Burge, D. (1997). A cognitive–interpersonal approach to depressive symptoms in preadolescent children. *Journal of Abnormal Child Psychology, 25,* 33–45.

Ryan, N. D. (1990). Pharmacotherapy of adolescent major depression: Beyond TCAs. *Psychopharmacological Bulletin, 26,* 75–79.

Stark, K. D. (1990). *Childhood depression: School-based intervention.* New York: Guilford Press.

Weissman, M. M., Warner, V., Wickramaratne, P., & Prusoff, B. A. (1988). Early-onset major depression in parents and their children. *Journal of Affective Disorders, 15,* 269–277.

Weissman, M. M., Wolk, S., Goldstein, R. B., Moreau, D., Adams, P., Greenwald, S., Klier, C. M., Ryan, N. D., Dahl, R. E., & Wickramaratne, P. (1999b). Depressed adolescents grown up. *Journal of the American Medical Association, 281,* 1707–1713.

Weissman, M. M., Wolk, S., Wickramaratne, P., Goldstein, R. B., Adams, P., Greenwald, S., Ryan, N. D., Dahl, R. E., & Steinberg, D. (1999a). Children with prepubertal-onset major depressive disorder and anxiety grown up. *Archives of General Psychiatry, 56,* 794–801.

ANXIETY DISORDERS

11

Vulnerability to Anxiety Disorders in Childhood and Adolescence

VANESSA L. MALCARNE
INGUNN HANSDOTTIR

The experience of anxiety is part of a normal course of development for children. Although distinctions have been made between fears and anxiety, with the former seen as more specific and the latter as more anticipatory and diffuse, both share similar cognitive, affective, and physiological response patterns (Campbell, 1986), and both are experienced by virtually all children. An important challenge is to distinguish developmentally appropriate fears/anxiety from those which are inappropriate and/or pathological at different ages and developmental stages.

Although the conceptualization of childhood anxiety disorders has its roots in the 1800s, it was not until much more recently, in the taxonomy of the third edition of the *Diagnostic and Statistical Manual of Mental Disorders* (DSM-III; American Psychiatric Association, 1980), that child and adolescent anxiety disorders were systematically described and differentiated (Hooper & March, 1995). At that time, several anxiety disorders were categorized in a separate section of DSM-III for disorders usually first diagnosed in infancy, childhood, and adolescence, including separation anxiety disorder (SAD), overanxious disorder (OAD), and avoidant disorder of childhood (AVD). Subsequent revisions of the DSM have eliminated most of the distinctions between child and adult anxiety. In DSM-IV, only SAD is still considered a children's disorder. OAD is subsumed under generalized anxiety disorder (GAD), with only one of the central symptoms being required for diagnosis in children. AVD is subsumed by social phobia (SOC), with special considerations included for diagnosis in children. All other variants of anxiety are listed as adult syndromes, in some cases with developmental features delineated (American Psychiatric Association, 1994).[1] For example, for specific phobias, SOC, and obsessive–compulsive disorder (OCD), it is not required that children see their fears as excessive or unreasonable (Craske, 1997).

The constant revision of DSM criteria for anxiety disorders has made it difficult to establish definitive prevalence and incidence data, and the results of research conducted using now outdated criteria may have limited applicability (Majcher & Pollack, 1996). More data are needed, particularly for children 5 and younger (Costello & Angold, 1995). However, evidence to date does point clearly to one general conclusion: Considered broadly, anxiety disorders are common in childhood.

EPIDEMIOLOGY

As a group, anxiety disorders represent the most prevalent form of childhood psychopathology (Pollock, Rosenbaum, Marrs, Miller, & Biederman, 1995). Popper (1993) has suggested that anxiety disorders are twice as common as attention deficit disorder (ADD) in children. In a review of recent community-based studies, Costello and Angold (1995) reported that estimates for the presence in children of any anxiety disorder ranged from 5.7 to 17.7%, with half of study estimates falling above 10%. Lower estimates typically reflect studies in which more stringent diagnostic criteria are applied (Bell-Dolan, Last, & Strauss, 1990; Bernstein & Borchardt, 1991). For example, Kashani and Orvaschel (1988) found that 17.3% of their adolescent sample met criteria for at least one anxiety disorder; however, this dropped to 8.7% if clinical impairment was required for classification (Bernstein & Borchardt, 1991).

Prevalence rates vary for specific anxiety disorders in children and adolescents. SAD, specific phobia (SP; previously called simple phobia and renamed for compatibility with the tenth edition of the *International Classification of Diseases* [ICD-10; World Health Organization, 1988]), and OAD appear to be the most common. Estimates of the prevalence of SAD in nonpsychiatric child samples generally range from 3 to 5% (Anderson, Williams, McGee, & Silva, 1987; Benjamin, Costello, & Warren, 1990; Bird et al., 1988; Costello et al., 1996; McGee et al. 1990), although some estimates are much higher (Gurley, Cohen, Pine, & Brook, 1996). Prevalence estimates for SP are generally 6% or less (Anderson et al., 1987; Bird et al., 1988; Fergusson, Horwood, & Lynskey, 1993; McGee et al., 1990), al-

---

[1]Because overanxious disorder and avoidant disorder of childhood were considered separate disorders of childhood until they were subsumed under adult disorders in DSM-IV, much of the research on childhood anxiety disorders has used these diagnostic categories. In this review, the original category names are used when appropriate to reflect the categories utilized in research studies.

though some studies have shown rates above 9% (Benjamin et al., 1990; Costello et al., 1988; Gurley et al., 1996; Kessler et al., 1994). Prevalence estimates for OAD range more broadly, from 1.7 to 14.3% across studies (Anderson et al., 1987; Benjamin et al., 1990; Costello et al., 1996; Fergusson et al., 1993; Gurley et al., 1996; McGee et al., 1990; Whitaker et al., 1990).

Other anxiety disorders appear to be less common in children. Estimates of prevalence rates for AVD are low, ranging from 1 to 2% (Anderson et al., 1987; Benjamin et al., 1990; Costello et al., 1996; Fergusson et al., 1993; Gurley et al., 1996; McGee et al., 1990). OCD estimates fall mostly in the 0–2% range (Benjamin et al., 1990; Costello et al., 1996; Douglass, Moffitt, Dar, McGee, & Silva, 1995; Flament et al., 1988; Whitaker et al., 1990).

There are few epidemiological studies of other anxiety disorders in children. Panic disorder (PD), and agoraphobia (AG) are both rare in children (Bernstein & Borchardt, 1991; Pine, 1997). Posttraumatic stress disorder (PTSD) has not been assessed in many of the epidemiological studies of anxiety disorders in children (Bernstein & Borchardt, 1991; Pine, 1997), and its prevalence is unknown, although it may be fairly common in abused children (McLeer, Deblinger, Hendry, & Orvaschel, 1992).

DEVELOPMENTAL COURSE AND STABILITY

Infancy/Preschool

Anxiety disorders are rarely diagnosed in children at very young ages. However, the experience of anxiety related to specific objects and situations is common in young children. In her review of developmental aspects of children's fears, Campbell (1986) reported that during infancy, children show developmentally appropriate fears of loud and sudden stimuli, loss of support, and heights. By the second half of their first year of life they display fear of strangers and novel objects. Similarly, Morris and Kratochwill (1983) listed loss of support and loud noises as common fears of infants in their first 6 months of life; infants ages 7 to 12 months feared strangers and sudden, unexpected, and looming objects. Children who are 1 to 4 years old commonly fear separation from parents (Dashiff, 1995). This separation anxiety usually appears during the latter 6 months of the first year of life, peaks at around 18 months or after, and is fairly common through age 4 (Dashiff, 1995; Popper, 1993). Animals, darkness, and monsters also constitute common fears of toddlers and preschoolers (Campbell, 1986).

Middle Childhood

Anxiety is a common experience of middle childhood, especially at subclinical levels and when individual symptoms rather than syndromes are assessed. Bell-Dolan et al. (1990) found 9.8 to 30.6% of 62 nonreferred children reported subclinical levels of individual OAD symptoms; 10.7 to 22.6% endorsed subclinical phobias. The most common symptoms were excessive concern about competence, excessive need for reassurance, fear of the dark, fear of harm to an attachment figure, and somatic complaints. Campbell's (1986) review reports that fears of dreams, imaginary creatures, and animals decline dramatically between early and middle childhood, as fears of bodily injury, physical danger, and natural disasters increase. These changes may be due to older children's greater ability to differentiate reality from fantasy (Campbell, 1986).

The anxiety disorder most commonly diagnosed in middle childhood is SAD (Anderson et al., 1987; Bernstein & Borchardt, 1991; Last, Perrin, Hersen, & Kazdin, 1992). Last et al. (1992) found that of 188 clinic-referred children with anxiety disorders, SAD was the most frequent anxiety diagnosis and had the earliest age at intake (mean = 10.3 years) and age at onset (mean = 7.5 years). Francis, Last, and Strauss (1987) found developmental changes in SAD symptom expression, with younger children (ages 5–8) more likely to be concerned about harm to attachment figures, to engage in school refusal, and to report nightmares about separation. In contrast, older children (ages 9–12) were particularly distressed at time of separation and rarely reported nightmares. Younger children endorsed a greater number of symptoms overall. Interestingly, Bell-Dolan et al. (1990) found that separation anxiety fears may be relatively common in nonreferred children as well. The proportion of these children that would meet diagnostic criteria for SAD has not been established.

SP is also diagnosed in middle childhood (Bernstein & Borchardt, 1991). Last et al. (1992) found an average age at onset of 8.4 years and average age at intake of 12.1 years in their clinic sample. Unfortunately, little description of childhood SP exists (Silverman & Ginsburg, 1995), although there is literature on childhood fears, which are quite common in normal children (Ollendick & Francis, 1988; Silverman & Nelles, 1990). Interestingly, Ollendick, King, and Frary (1989), in a study exploring the psychometric properties of the Fear Survey Scale for Children—Revised in large samples of normal children from the United States and Australia, found that specific fears varied little by age, sex, or nationality for children ages 7 to 16. For all ages, the most commonly endorsed fears were "being hit by a car/truck" and "not being able to breathe."

As noted previously, OAD has now been subsumed under GAD, due to problems with the OAD category (notably the lack of specificity; Werry, 1991). Thus, there is little information on GAD in children, and the limited data on OAD must be interpreted with caution. However, there is evidence that OAD first appears in middle childhood, although perhaps in a less severe form. Last et al. (1992) found an average age at intake of 13.6 years for OAD, with average age at onset of 8.8 years. Strauss, Lease, Last, and Francis (1988) found that referred children 12 years of age and younger who met criteria for OAD tended to endorse fewer symptoms than did older children.

Adolescence

The same anxiety disorders seen in middle childhood are also seen in adolescence (Bernstein, Borchardt, & Perwien, 1996), although SAD in particular appears to become less common (Dashiff, 1995; Francis et al., 1987). Also, adolescents diagnosed with SAD appear to show a different pattern of symptom expression than do younger children. Francis et al. (1987) found that adolescents were most likely to refuse to attend school or be away from home overnight and to report physical symptoms, in contrast to their younger counterparts who primarily expressed fears about attachment figures or distress at separation. Francis et al. (1987) also noted that younger children were more likely to meet criteria for a greater number of symptoms. The opposite pattern is seen for OAD, with older children endorsing a greater number of symptoms, especially worries about the future (Strauss, Lease, et al., 1988). For SP, prevalence rates are stable from childhood to adolescence. Although it has been suggested that there may be age variations in the focus of specific phobias, this has not been addressed empirically. And, as noted previously, specific fears seem to change little from middle childhood to adolescence (Ollendick et al., 1989).

OCD is most commonly diagnosed in early to mid-adolescence. Flament et al. (1988) reported a mean age at onset of 12.8 years and age at diagnosis of 16.2 years. Last et al. (1992) found a mean age at onset of 10.8 years and mean age at intake of 12.8 years. Flament et al. (1988) reported that the most common obsessions were fear of contamination (35%) and thoughts of harm to self and familiar figures (30%); the most common compulsion was washing and cleaning (75%). Adolescents also begin to show vulnerability to other anxiety disorders, including AVD and PD, that are rarely seen at earlier ages (Bernstein et al., 1996). AVD (SOC in DSM-IV) does occur before adolescence (e.g., Last et al., 1992 found an age at onset of 8.2 years), but its onset is most common in early to mid-adolescence (Bernstein et al., 1996).

Stability

Few prospective studies have examined the stability of anxiety disorders in children. Existing studies suggest that specific anxiety disorders are not highly stable. Costello and Angold (1995) reviewed five longitudinal studies (Cohen, Cohen, & Brook, 1993; Costello, Stouthamer-Loeber, & DeRosier, 1993; Laucht & Schmidt, 1987; McGee et al., 1990; McGee, Feehan, Williams, & Anderson, 1992; Offord et al., 1992), all of which collected more than one wave of data on children, at intervals ranging from 2 to 5 years. They estimated that, across these studies, approximately 20 to 30% of children with an anxiety disorder at a later time point also had an anxiety disorder at an earlier time point. Costello and Angold interpret these findings as suggesting a moderate level of continuity, exceeding chance levels.

Last, Perrin, Hersen, and Kazdin (1996) identified five prospective studies that have used structured interviews at both baseline and follow-up (Berg et al., 1989; Cantwell & Baker, 1989; Flament et al., 1990; Leonard et al., 1993; Thomsen & Mikkelsen, 1995). Cantwell and Baker's (1989) study focused on linguistically impaired children and examined a variety of anxiety and other psychiatric disorders; the other four studies focused on children diagnosed with OCD. Results of the studies suggest a moderate degree of continuity. For example, across the OCD studies, one- to two-thirds of subjects still met criteria for OCD at follow-up. However, it is notable that many children in these studies no longer met criteria for their initial diagnosis at follow-up, although they often met criteria for other psychiatric disorders, primarily other anxiety disorders and affective disorders.

In the methodologically strongest prospective study completed to date, Last et al. (1996) followed 84 children with anxiety disorders, 50 children with ADHD, and 83 never diagnosed children every year over a 3- to 4-year period. Diagnoses were made using structured interviews, and follow-up interviews were conducted blindly. Results showed that 82% of referred children and adolescents diagnosed with anxiety disorders no longer met criteria for their disorder at final follow-up, and two-thirds went into remission within the first year. SAD had the highest recovery rate (96%); SP had the lowest (69%). At follow-up, one-third of the children had developed new disorders—mostly new anxiety disorders. Children with OAD were the most likely to show new disorders at follow-up (35%); children with SP were the least likely (15%).

Most of the previous studies prospectively examined children who initially met criteria for a DSM anxiety disorder. In contrast, studies that have focused instead on specific anxiety symptoms and/or subclinical levels of anxiety have found evidence of stability throughout childhood and adolescence. Ialongo and colleagues followed a large group of first-graders for several years. They found that self-reported anxiety symptoms were moderately stable over a 4-month period in first grade (Ialongo, Edelsohn, Werthamer-Larsson, Crockett, & Kellam, 1994). Further, they found that anxiety in first grade was a significant predictor of anxiety and adaptive functioning in fifth grade (Ialongo, Edelsohn, Werthamer-Larsson, Crockett, & Kellam, 1995).

No methodologically strong studies have followed children diagnosed with anxiety disorders into adulthood. Instead, studies have relied on the retrospective report of adults diagnosed with anxiety disorders (Majcher & Pollack, 1996) and have found that many adults with anxiety disorders recall having anxious symptoms or disorders as children. For example, Pollack et al. (1996) found that of 194 adults with PD, 54% retrospectively reported a history of childhood anxiety. Of adults with a history of anxiety disorders, 64.8% reported having two or more anxiety disorders as children. However, although retrospective studies provide evidence that a substantial proportion of adults with diagnosed anxiety disorders may have experienced long-standing symptoms, they reveal little about the stability of symptoms in diagnosed children.

There has been particular interest in a hypothesized relationship between SAD in childhood and AG or PD in adulthood, suggested in DSM-III-R (American Psychiatric Association, 1987). Studies investigating this relationship have primarily used retrospective methodology, and findings are mixed (e.g., Gittelman & Klein, 1985, found support; Thyer, Himle, & Fischer, 1988, did not). OAD in children has also been hypothesized to be a precursor of GAD in adulthood. Because these two disorders have now been combined, it is perhaps particularly interesting that there was little evidence found for continuity of OAD (Werry, 1991).

Given the paucity of longitudinal research, and the reliance on retrospective studies, firm conclusions about relationships between childhood and adult anxiety disorders cannot be reached (Klein & Last, 1989; Majcher & Pollack, 1996). The literature does suggest that symptoms of anxiety are more stable throughout childhood than specific syndromes or diagnoses.

COMORBIDITY

Comorbidity is common for childhood anxiety disorders. In their review of epidemiological studies, Costello and Angold (1995) report that many children meet criteria for multiple DSM anxiety diagnoses. However, which anxiety disorders are most likely to co-occur is not yet clear, although some patterns are emerging. For example, Costello and colleagues have found that phobic disorders are not associated or negatively associated with other anxiety disorders (Costello & Angold, 1995; Costello et al., 1988). Last et al. (1992), in their study of 188 children diagnosed with a variety of anxiety disorders, found evidence of extensive comordibity of anxiety diagnoses, with most children meeting current or lifetime criteria for at least two anxiety disorders. In particular, children with OAD were most likely to show a pattern of comorbidity; almost 100% of these children met criteria for an additional current or past anxiety disorder. Last et al. caution that their findings of extensive "overlap" among anxiety disorders may be a function of the referred nature of their sample; that is, it may be that having a history of multiple anxiety disorders is related to severity of disturbance and thus referral status.

Depression has been found to be commonly comorbid with anxiety diagnoses, in both clinic (e.g., Strauss, Last, et al., 1988) and nonclinic samples (e.g., Anderson et al., 1987; Kashani & Orvaschel, 1988). Brady and Kendall (1992) reported that estimates of comorbidity for anxiety and depression among children range from 15.9 to 61.9%. There is some evidence that comorbidity may be higher in more severely disturbed samples (Bernstein & Borchardt, 1991; Kendall, Kortlander, Chansky, & Brady, 1992). Anxiety disorders have also been found to be comorbid with ADD (Anderson et al., 1987; Bird et al., 1988; Last, Strauss, & Francis, 1987; Strauss, Last et al., 1988) and with oppositional disorder (Last et al., 1987). Further study is needed, especially given the recent modifications to DSM diagnostic criteria. However, evidence to date that suggests that comorbidity is widespread complicates the identification of risk factors specific to anxiety, versus those general to child psychopathology.

GENERAL RISK FACTORS

Demographics

Age

Age may not be particularly important as a risk factor. Although, as noted earlier, the prevalence of some anxiety disorders appear to decrease or increase with age, these changes are relatively modest. The decrease of SAD with increasing age of the child is perhaps the most well documented (Costello & Angold, 1995; Bernstein & Borchardt, 1991), although even this finding is not consistent across all studies, and reasons for any age-related changes are unclear.

Perhaps the most interesting age trend concerns the rarity of certain anxiety disorders (e.g., PD and AG) prior to adolescence. Changes associated with puberty may represent risk factors for the development of these disorders. Hayward et al. (1992) studied the relationship between panic attacks and pubertal (Tanner) stage in 754 sixth- and seventh-grade girls and found that rates of panic attacks increased with sexual maturity. Last and Strauss (1989) also found that the vast majority of children (boys and girls) with PD in their clinic sample were postpubertal. Bernstein and Borchardt (1991) have hypothesized that structural and neuroendocrine changes in the brain at puberty may account for changes in prevalence rates for some anxiety disorders, but as yet the nature of these changes and associated mechanisms have not been identified. Developmental changes in cognitions have also been implicated (see section "Cognitive Processes").

Gender

Although it has been generally accepted that girls have higher rates of anxiety disorders than do boys, Costello and Angold (1995) caution that this conclusion is premature, being largely based on studies of adults, referred children, and individuals classified as having "any anxiety disorder." When nonreferred children are studied and specific anxiety disorders are considered, gender ratios for specific anxiety disorders may appear more equal. In their review of recent epidemiological studies of community samples, Costello and Angold (1995) report little evidence of gender differences, with the exception of OAD, which is more common in girls.

Last et al. (1992), in one of the most comprehensive studies of clinic-referred children, also found relatively equal gender ratios across a variety of different anxiety disorders. However, other studies of both referred and nonreferred children have reported evidence for gender differences, and typically these findings suggest a higher prevalence of anxiety disorders in girls. For example, Anderson et al. (1987) found a higher prevalence for SAD and SP in girls, and some studies have found that girls report more nonphobic fears than do boys (Silverman & Nelles, 1990). In a review, Ollendick, Mattis, and King (1994) reported that adolescent girls, like their adult counterparts, are more likely than boys to be diagnosed with PD.

Other studies have found equal prevalence across genders but differences in symptom expression or developmental progression. For example, Flament and colleagues found no gender differences in proportions of boys and girls diagnosed with OCD but reported that boys may have an earlier age of onset and suffer more severe symptoms (Flament et al., 1988; Flament et al., 1990). Swedo, Rapoport, Leonard, Lenane, and Cheslow (1989) also reported more boys in an early-onset group, versus more girls experiencing onset in adolescence.

In sum, at present the most that can be stated is that gender *may* be a risk factor for the presence of some types of anxiety, with girls more at risk than boys. Determination of whether and under what circumstances gender constitutes a risk factor for various anxiety disorders in childhood, and why, will require further study.

Ethnicity

Few studies have examined the relationship between ethnicity and anxiety in children, and of the studies that exist, many have methodological shortcomings that make conclusions difficult. For example, Kashani and Orvaschel (1988) presented some evidence that anxiety disorders are more prevalent in "nonwhite" children, but their sample was extremely small ($n = 8$) and of mixed ethnicity. Strauss and Last (1993) reported that 86% of the children in their clinic sample diagnosed with SOC were Caucasian, and Last et al. (1987) reported that all the children in their sample with OAD were Caucasian, even though 35% of the referred children were African American. However, in Beidel, Turner, and Trager's (1994) study of 8- to 11-year-old children selected for test anxiety, 55% of the children who met criteria for

SOC were African American and 45% were Caucasian. When OAD and SOC were combined, 59% of diagnosed children were African American and 41% Caucasian. Beidel et al. (1994) suggest that differences in methodologies are yielding selection biases that affect results. Consistent with this, Benjamin et al. (1990) found that African American boys who met criteria for only one anxiety disorder were much less likely to have contact with a formal treatment setting, in contrast to African American girls and Caucasian boys and girls.

Last and Perrin (1993), in a study comparing clinic-referred African American and Caucasian American children with anxiety disorders, found similarities on most dimensions. There was an interesting difference in school refusal, with Caucasian American children from lower socioeconomic backgrounds showing a trend toward higher rates of school refusal in comparison with African American children from similar backgrounds. Consistent with that finding, Neal, Lilly, and Zakis (1993) compared the factor structure of self-reported fears in African American versus Caucasian American children, and found a school fear factor that was present only for Caucasian Americans.

Clearly, more research is needed on the role of ethnicity in childhood anxiety disorders. Also, given the potential confound, studies are needed that simultaneously consider ethnic and socioeconomic factors.

Socioeconomic Status

The relationship between socioeconomic status and anxiety disorders is unclear. Adverse socioeconomic conditions may put children at risk for certain anxiety disorders and also will likely influence who seeks treatment. Last et al. (1992) found that most of the clinic-referred children with anxiety disorders in her sample were from middle- to upper-middle-class backgrounds, with the exception of children diagnosed with SAD, who were more commonly from single-parent homes and of low socioeconomic status. Velez, Johnson, and Cohen (1989) and Bird et al. (1988) also found that lower socioeconomic status (SES) was a risk factor for development of SAD. Although no clear conclusions can be drawn, there is at least preliminary evidence that disadvantaged SES may put children at risk for SAD.

VULNERABILITY PROCESSES

Biological Processes

Temperament

Kagan and colleagues (Kagan, 1989; Kagan, Reznick, & Snidman, 1988) defined the temperamental construct of "behavioral inhibition to the unfamiliar" (BI). BI is characterized by an initial reaction to encounters with unfamiliar stimuli that includes withdrawal, inhibition, and seeking the comfort of a parent or caretaker. Developmentally, BI is expressed as irritability in infancy; shy, fearful behavior in early childhood; and cautious introversion in middle childhood (Pollock et al., 1995). BI is hypothesized to be a heritable trait.

Findings from studies conducted by Kagan and colleagues on a sample of Caucasian children recruited through birth registries suggest that approximately 10 to 15% of these children can be classified as BI. In contrast, as many as 30% of these children may show an opposite profile, termed "behaviorally uninhibited" (BUI) and characterized by a sociable, minimally fearful approach to novel situations, people, and objects (Kagan, 1989; Kagan et al., 1988). Kagan's research group followed two independent cohorts of infants from age 21 or 31 months who were categorized as either BI or BUI based on their responses when exposed to unfamiliar rooms, people, or objects. A majority of children in both categories maintained their behavioral style from infancy to later assessments at 4, 5, and 7.5 years, suggesting that the tendency to approach or withdraw from novelty is relatively stable (Kagan, 1989; Kagan et al., 1988).

Kagan et al.'s (1988) findings were based on children at two behavioral extremes. When studying children not at the extreme on either of the two behavioral profiles, inhibition at 14 or 20 months did not predict differences in behavior at 4 years of age (Kagan, 1989). This suggests that the constructs of BI and BUI may refer to qualitatively distinct categories of children.

BI has been hypothesized as a risk factor for the later development of anxiety disorders in children. Caspi, Henry, McGee, Moffitt, and Silva (1995) explored the relationship between early temperament and externalizing/internalizing symptoms in more than 800 children over a 12-year period. They found that boys who at ages 3 and 5 were confident and eager to explore novel situations (termed "approach behavior") were less likely to manifest anxiety in later childhood and adolescence; boys' approach behavior in early childhood was unrelated to indices of other behavior problems. In contrast, girls' approach behavior at ages 3 and 5 was generally unrelated to problems in later childhood and adolescence. However, girls' tendency to react passively and withdraw from novelty (termed "sluggishness") at ages 3 and 5 was predictive of anxiety problems in adolescence; the relationship of sluggishness to later anxiety for boys was less clear. So, for both boys and girls, Caspi et al. (1995) provided evidence of continuity from BI-like characteristics in early childhood to anxiety problems in middle childhood and adolescence. Biederman and colleagues (Biederman et al., 1990; Biederman et al., 1993) further established the relationship between BI and anxiety disorders, finding that BI was associated with higher risk for anxiety disorders in children of parents both with and without psychiatric disorders. Biederman et al. studied two independent samples of children. One sample was derived from Kagan's cohort (described previously), the other was children of outpatient parents treated at Massachusetts General Hospital (MGH) for PD and AG. Children in Kagan's sample had been classified as BI or BUI; children in the MGH sample were classified as either BI or not inhibited (NI). Relying on longitudinal data collected by Kagan et al. (1988) and reassessing the at-risk MGH sample 3 years after baseline, Biederman et al. were able to examine the prospective relationship between BI and the development of anxiety disorders. Children were assessed for psychiatric disorders using structured interviews for DSM-III, and data from both samples were combined to increase statistical power. The results showed significant differences between BI and non-BI in the rates of various anxiety disorders at follow-up. At follow-up, BI children had significantly higher rates of multiple anxiety disorders, AD, and SAD (but not phobic disorders), compared to children who were not BI. Also, the rates of anxiety disorders increased significantly from baseline to follow-up among the behaviorally inhibited children. These findings support the hypothesis that BI constitutes a risk factor for the development of childhood anxiety disorders.

Hirshfeld et al. (1992) hypothesized that if BI increases a child's risk for anxiety disorders, then children who display this temperamental tendency in a stable and consistent way should be more vulnerable to such disorders than those who are not consistently inhibited. To investigate this, Hirschfeld et al. classified children from Kagan et al.'s (1988) study according to the stability or unstability of their BI or BUI. BI was considered stable if children were above the mean BI score at all four assessments (21 months, 4, 5½, and 7½ years). Children in the unstable BI group were originally classified as BI at 21 months but not at one or more subsequent assessments. Children who were originally classified as BUI at 21 months and remained in that category at all subsequent assessments were classified as stable BUI, and those who did not remain in that category were classified as unstable BUI. At the 7½-year follow-up, the stable BI children were significantly more likely than unstable BI children, as well as stable and unstable BUI children, to be diagnosed with any anxiety disorder, multiple (two or more) anxiety disorders, or phobic disorders. These results suggest that children who are consistently inhibited may be at greatest risk of developing later anxiety disorders.

The research on BI does not support the possibility that BI and anxiety disorders are simply variations on a theme. BI is not necessarily associated with dysfunction. For example, in Biederman et al.'s (1990) study, approximately two-thirds of inhibited children did not develop an anxiety disorder. Indeed, BI is much more prevalent than anxiety disorders, suggesting that only a subgroup of inhibited children will develop disorders.

Genetics

Indirect evidence of a genetic contribution has been provided by findings that children of parents with anxiety disorders are at higher risk than children of parents without such disorders (e.g., Turner, Beidel, & Costello,

1987), but of course such findings do not rule out environmental explanations of etiology. Twin, adoptive, and genetic linkage studies more directly examine the role of genetics in childhood anxiety disorders. Unfortunately, only a small number of studies using these methods have been conducted, and some have focused on general or outdated anxiety constructs, such as neurosis (Rabian & Silverman, 1995).

Most of the genetic literature relevant to children's anxiety has focused on the transmission of a BI temperament. BI has been hypothesized to be an expression of a familial anxiety diathesis (Biederman, Rosenbaum, Chaloff, & Kagan, 1995). To test this hypothesis, Rosenbaum et al. (1991) studied the families of children in the Kagan et al. (1988) longitudinal cohort of children selected at 21 months for BI. They found that parents (but not siblings) of BI children had increased risks for anxiety disorders as compared to parents and siblings of BUI and control children. In particular, parents of BI children had significantly higher rates of social phobia, childhood anxiety (avoidant, overanxious), and continuing anxiety disorders. In another study of children from the Kagan cohort, Hirshfeld et al. (1992) found that parents of stable BI children had significantly greater rates of AD and multiple anxiety disorders and were more likely to have received an anxiety disorder diagnosis in both childhood and adulthood than were parents of children classified as unstable BI. Rosenbaum et al. (1988), in a study of 56 children ages 2–7 years, found that children of parents with PD and AG, with or without major depressive disorder, were more likely to be BI than were the offspring of parents without these anxiety disorders. Taken together, these findings suggest the possibility of genetic transmission of BI.

Torgersen (1993) has reviewed the role of genetic factors in the transmission of anxiety disorders, and concluded that evidence supports a genetic role for some disorders (e.g., PD) but not others (e.g., PTSD). However, it may be that genetic heritability is best understood as a predisposition to anxiety disorders in general rather than for a specific disorder (Turner et al., 1987). For example, in one of Torgersen's own studies (1983), concordance rates for the presence of any anxiety disorder was higher for monozygotic than same-sex dyzygotic twins, certainly suggesting a genetic contribution; however, no monozygotic twin had the same anxiety disorder as the proband. Kendler, Neale, Kessler, Heath, and Eaves (1992) used a twin design to examine genetic risk for anxiety and depression in adult women and found an overlapping genetic risk for GAD and major depression but not for environmental risk factors. They suggested that the general expression may result from genetic risk, and the specific expression may result from environmental exposure.

Neurobiology/Neuropsychology

In their recent and comprehensive review, Sallee and Greenawald (1995) describe progress made in identifying possible neurobiological bases of childhood anxiety, and this section draws heavily from their review. Sallee and Greenawald (1995) note that most of the progress to date derives from studies of adults. They argue that if childhood anxiety exists as a risk factor or prodromal condition for adult anxiety, then drawing conclusions from the adult literature may be warranted. However, because the relationship of child to adult anxiety is not well understood, as was pointed out earlier, it remains unclear how relevant studies of adults are to the understanding of children's anxiety.

A number of studies have attempted to explicate the neural structures and pathways underlying behavioral inhibition. Focus has been on the locus ceruleus/sympathetic system and the hypothalamic–pituitary–adrenal (HPA) axis. Studies have shown elevated cortisol levels in normal children under stress (Tennes, Downey, & Vernadakis, 1977; Tennes & Kreye, 1985) and in BI versus uninhibited children (Kagan et al., 1988), suggesting that the HPA axis is at a high level of activity. Interestingly, Nachmias, Gunnar, Mangelsdorf, Parritz, and Buss (1996) found that only insecurely attached BI children showed elevated cortisol change when exposed to novel stimuli; securely attached children responded in a manner similar to that of non-BI children. This underscores the importance of considering the interplay among psychosocial and biological variables.

High-heart-rate and low-heart-rate variability have both been found to correlate with behavioral inhibition; also, heart rates of anxious children appear to habituate less to stress (Kagan et al., 1988). BI children's consistent tendency to show cardiac acceleration to mild cognitive stress may suggest greater sympathetic influence on cardiovascular function. Rosenberg and Kagan (1987) have suggested that these differences may reflect lower reactivity thresholds in the limbic system, with the likely involvement of the amygdala and hypothalamus.

Hooper and March (1995), in their review of the neuropsychology of childhood anxiety disorders, also note that there has been little research on children. However, they describe several comprehensive and potentially important etiological models for anxiety that have been proposed. Gray (1982) has hypothesized a separate subsystem in the brain for mediation of anxiety. This subsystem consists of two behavioral systems. The first mediates behavioral inhibition and is tied to the limbic system, with emphasis on the septohippocampal neural connections. The second mediates fight–flight responses; Gray has emphasized the roles of the amygdala, ventromedial hypothalamus, and midbrain central gray matter. In another model, Tucker (1989) implicates the cognitive functional systems of the right hemisphere as providing control for perceptual arousal, and he deemphasizes the role of the left hemisphere. His model proposes a complex interplay of several systems (including the cortex, subcortex, and neurotransmitters) in the regulation of arousal. Finally, Rourke's (1989) nonverbal learning disability model hypothesizes that abnormalities in the white matter of the right hemisphere, in interaction with developmental experiences, produce a distinct pattern of learning disabilities. Associated with these difficulties are social, emotional, and behavioral deficits, including difficulties in adapting to novel situations and poor social interaction skills, which over time can put children at risk for internalizing problems (e.g., anxiety). Further research is needed to understand the applicability of these models to childhood anxiety disorders.

Cognitive Processes

Cognitive–Developmental Changes

The low prevalence of AVD and PD prior to adolescence may be explained by the development in adolescence of cognitive abilities necessary for the presence of the disorders. For example, Beidel and Morris (1995) have argued that AVD's later onset does not mean that social and performance anxiety are not experienced by preadolescents, and indeed there is evidence that shyness may be quite stable. They suggest instead that preadolescents "may lack the metacognitive and verbal skills to ground description of their fears in a social context" (Beidel & Morris, 1995, p. 187). Similar factors may explain why PD is rarely seen before adolescence (Bernstein & Borchardt, 1991; Black & Robbins, 1990; Craske, 1997; Ollendick et al., 1994). Barlow and colleagues (Chorpita, Albano, & Barlow, 1996a; Nelles & Barlow, 1988) have suggested that prepubertal children may attribute panic symptoms to external events, because they lack sufficient abstract abilities to understand internal causation. Due to their concrete–operational level of cognitive development, these younger children are unable to associate internal sensations with abstract threat cognitions such as fears of going crazy. In contrast, adolescents may be able to make internal attributions necessary to experience spontaneous, uncued panic. Similarly, Vasey (1993) has argued that as children age, the development of relevant cognitive structures, processes, and operations allows them to experience increasingly generalized anxiety.

Perceived Control

Chorpita and Barlow (1998) have proposed a complex model that hypothesizes a pivotal role of control in the development of anxiety in children. Based on an integrative review of literatures on anxiety, depression, helplessness, control, attributions, learning, biology, parenting, attachment theory and vulnerability/resilience, they assert that early experience with reduced control may foster a psychological diathesis that may put children at risk for anxiety and perhaps depression. Specifically, they propose a model in which early experiences with uncontrollable and/or unpredictable stimuli generate perceptions of low perceived control. These experiences lead to increases in the activity of the behavioral inhibition system (BIS), a functional brain system described by Gray (1982; Gray & McNaughton, 1996) and ultimately to the perceptual and somatic experiences described by Kagan and colleagues in their research on behavioral inhibition. As development proceeds and an individual accumulates a history of low-control experiences, cognitive schemas may become rigid and resist new information such as evidence of control; also, they may bias processing of later input. Chorpita and Barlow (1998) suggest that the long-term influence of perceptions of low control would be to intensify BIS activation, which would ultimately lead to the experience of generalized anxiety.

Costanzo, Miller-Johnson, and Wencel (1995), in their review of social development and childhood anxiety, also suggest that low self-perceived control and self-efficacy in children may constitute risk factors for both anxiety and depression. They propose a central etiological role of excessive caregiver control, suggesting that such control will undermine independence and intrinsic motivation in the child while increasing dependence on others for control and mastery. Ultimately, perceptions of personal control and self-efficacy fail to develop fully, and anxiety and depression will result as children encounter life situations for which they feel unprepared and helpless (for a further discussion of this issue, see section "Parent–Child Relationships").

Negative Cognitions

In addition to control, other cognitive variables may be relevant to children's anxiety (for reviews, see Malcarne & Ingram, 1994; Silverman & Ginsburg, 1995). Overall, studies have found that anxious children engage in more negative self-statements, more negative cognitive errors, and more off-task thoughts than do nonanxious children. For example, Zatz and Chassin (1983) found that highly test anxious children endorsed more negative evaluations and off-task thoughts and less positive evaluations than did children who were less test anxious. Zatz and Chassin (1985) found similar results when studying high versus low test-anxious children under naturalistic test-taking conditions.

Although the findings described previously suggest that cognitive processes may play an important role in childhood anxiety, the absence of prospective studies makes it impossible to draw firm conclusions about the role of cognition as a risk factor for the development of anxiety disorders in children. Further, whether or not particular cognitive processes are specific to anxiety is unclear (Malcarne & Ingram, 1994). Beck and colleagues have hypothesized that depression is characterized by cognitions that are more past-focused and concerned with perceived loss and failure, whereas anxiety is characterized by threat cognitions, based on fear of future loss (e.g., Beck, Epstein, & Harrison, 1983; Beck, Brown, Steer, Eidelson, & Riskind, 1987). Unfortunately, only a few studies of cognitive processes have used clinical samples, or have compared anxious children to other relevant comparison groups, such as depressed children or normal controls.

In one such study, Leitenberg, Yost, and Carroll-Wilson (1986) found that negative cognitive errors in children with evaluation anxiety were similar in type and frequency to those found in depressed children and children with low self-esteem. Similarly, Laurent and Stark (1993) found similar frequencies of anxious self-talk in anxious, anxious-depressed, and depressed children. In a study examining ratios of positive to negative cognitions (states-of-mind [SOM] ratios), Treadwell and Kendall (1996) compared negative self-statements of children (ages 8 to 13) with anxiety disorders versus normal controls. Negative self-statements were related to level of anxiety and, for children with anxiety disorders, response to a cognitive-behavioral therapy (CBT) intervention. However, both anxious and depressive self-talk were present at higher rates in anxious children than in normal controls, suggesting a more general negative affectivity rather than content-specific cognitions. Ronan and Kendall (1997) extended this study, examining SOM ratios and specificity of cognitions in anxious-only, depressed-only, mixed anxious-depressed, or normal children. Again, while distressed children's SOM ratios suggested an emphasis on negative cognitions, relative to nondistressed children, there was limited support for content specificity of cognitions between anxious-only and depressed-only children. Ambrose and Rholes (1993), in their study of a nonclinical sample of 5th-, 8th-, and 11th-graders, found some support for content specificity of loss versus threat cognitions, but only at lower levels of perceived threat; as perceptions of threat increased, so did the relationship of these cognitions to depression. Finally, Lerner et al. (1999) factor-analyzed data from 306 children's responses to the Negative Affect Self-Statement Questionnaire. All children in the sample had been referred to an anxiety disorders clinic, and 252 met criteria for a primary diagnosis of an anxiety disorder. The factor analysis yielded distinct anxious and depressive factors, as well as general negative and positive affect factors, consistent with Beck's conceptualization and Clark and Watson's (1991) tripartite model. Examinations of the relationships among self-statements and children's self-reports of trait anxiety and depression yielded mixed results, with strongest support for a specific relationship between depressive cognitive content and depression and less clear findings for cognitive content specific to anxiety. Thus, findings to date have not provided consistent support for specific cognitions as a risk factor for anxiety. Additional studies making direct comparisons between anxious and other children in order to reveal common versus specific cognitive factors are needed (Malcarne & Ingram, 1994).

Social Processes

Parent–Child Relationships

While Kagan and colleagues have emphasized temperament in the development of childhood anxiety disorders, others have pointed out that BI cannot be a complete explanation, because not all BI children share similar outcomes (Manassis & Bradley, 1994). For example, in Kagan's studies, one-quarter of the BI children did not stay inhibited as they aged, and a substantial proportion never developed anxiety disorders (Biederman et al., 1990). Such findings underscore the importance of also considering interactions between the child and his or her environment (Manassis & Bradley, 1994). Most efforts in this area have focused on interpersonal aspects of the parent–child relationship.

Most studies examining quality of parent–child relationships as a risk factor for childhood anxiety have taken either a top-down or bottom-up approach. In the bottom-up approach, studies have typically investigated whether psychopathology is present in parents of children with known anxiety disorders (Klein & Last, 1989). In perhaps the only large-scale bottom-up family study of childhood anxiety disorders, Last, Hersen, Kazdin, Orvaschel, and Perrin (1991) compared mothers, fathers, and siblings of children with anxiety disorders to those of children with attention-deficit/hyperactivity disorder and normal controls. Relatives of anxious children showed a very high morbidity risk for anxiety disorders, compared to relatives of children in the other two groups. This was particularly true for first-degree male relatives of anxious children whose rate of anxiety disorders was twice that of the comparison groups. Results of other bottom-up studies that have examined psychopathology in parents of children with anxiety disorders are mixed in their support of parental disturbance as a risk factor for childhood anxiety (see Klein & Last, 1989, for a review). Although some studies have found that parents (primarily mothers have been studied) of children diagnosed with anxiety disorders are themselves more likely to meet criteria for anxiety disorders, other studies have not found this relationship or have provided mixed support.

In contrast to the bottom-up approach, top-down studies have focused on children of parents with known disorders (Klein & Last, 1989). An assumption of these studies is that the presence of psychopathology in parents can serve as a proxy for disturbance in parenting behavior and attachment relationships. Turner et al. (1987) compared children of parents with anxiety disorders to children whose parents had dysthymic disorders, or who did not meet criteria for any disorder. A comparison group of normal schoolchildren was also included. Turner et al. (1987) found that children of anxious parents were seven times more likely than children of nondiagnosed parents to meet criteria for anxiety disorders, and twice as likely to meet criteria compared to children of dysthymic parents. Weissman, Leckman, Merikangas, Gammon, and Prusoff (1984) compared children of women with major depression with or without a history of anxiety disorders to children of matched normal controls. They found some evidence for increased rate of SAD in children of parents with depression and panic disorder but not of parents with depression and agoraphobia, depression and GAD, depression alone, or normal controls. Because anxiety was only examined with comorbid depression, its effect cannot be isolated. Taken together, these studies suggest that parental anxiety and/or depression may be a risk factor for childhood anxiety and may provide possible support for a genetic contributions, but questions about specificity, or the actual mechanisms involved, remain unanswered.

A few (mostly bottom-up) studies have directly assessed either actual parenting behavior or the quality of the parent–child attachment. Dumas, LaFreniere, and Serketich (1995) classified preschoolers as competent, aggressive, and anxious based on teachers' ratings, then taped and coded their interactions with their mothers. Mothers of anxious children showed the highest levels of aversive control and the lowest levels of compliance and responsivity. Siqueland, Kendall, and Steinberg (1996) compared children with anxiety disorders and their parents to control families on parenting variables of warmth, autonomy granting, and control. Observation ratings found parents of anxious children allowed less autonomy in their children, and anxious children rated their parents as less accepting. Chorpita, Albano, and Barlow (1996b) compared four children (ages 9 to 13) with anxiety disorders to age-matched nondiagnosed children and their parents. Children's cognitive responses to ambiguous situations, which were related to trait anxiety, were affected by an intervening family discussion, suggesting a possible role for parental verbal behavior in influencing children's anxiety-related cognitions. Barrett, Rapee, Dadds, and Ryan (1996) also investigated the impact of family discussion on responses to ambiguous situations in children with anxiety disorders, oppositional defiant disorder, or no disorders. Anxious and oppositional children and their parents were more likely than nondiagnosed children and their parents to view situations as threatening; anxious children were more likely to choose avoidant solutions whereas oppositional children were more likely to choose aggressive solutions. After participating in family discussions, these tendencies increased in the children. A follow-up study (Dadds, Barrett, Rapee, & Ryan, 1996) attempted to identify specific family communication patterns that might be contributing to these exacerbations of children's approaches. Although there were many similarities across the groups, there was evidence that parents (especially mothers) of anxious children may be less likely to listen to and agree with their children and more likely to respond to avoidant communications from their children, especially with their own avoidant communications. Dadds et al. (1996) interpreted their findings as consistent with models suggesting that children are put at risk for anxiety by parental behaviors that inhibit development of autonomy and perceived control. Finally, in a top-down study, Manassis, Bradley, Goldberg, Hood, and Swinson (1994, 1995) studied quality of attachment in mothers with anxiety disorders and their preschool children (ages 18 months to 5 years). Two-thirds of the children were classified as BI based on Kagan's assessment procedures, 80% were insecurely attached, and three children already met criteria for an anxiety disorder.

Manassis and Bradley (1994) have proposed a model for vulnerability to anxiety disorders in children that integrates the constructs of temperament (specifically BI) and the quality of parent–child attachment. In their model, extremes of either BI or insecure attachment may constitute sufficient conditions for the development of certain forms of anxiety. However, they assert that an interaction between BI and insecure attachment would put children at greatest risk.

At present, it remains unclear whether temperament and parent–child relationship variables represent specific risk factors for anxiety or rather for general distress and psychopathology. The effect of disturbed parent–child relationships may be to create general risk for negative affect via impact on cognition, especially perceptions of internal control. A series of studies by Parker and colleagues have related adults' current anxiety to their retrospective reports on the parenting they received as children. Their studies have shown that both overprotection and insufficient care experienced in childhood are associated with anxiety in adulthood. For example, Silove, Parker, Hadzi-Pavlovic, Manicavasagar, and Blaszczynski (1991) obtained retrospective reports of parenting style from adults diagnosed with PD or GAD and from matched controls. They found that overprotection was associated with both PD and GAD, whereas insufficient care was associated with PD. Consistent with Chorpita and Barlow's (1998) model, Parker and colleagues (Parker, 1979a, 1979b, 1981, 1983; Silove et al., 1991) have hypothesized that the parenting combination of too much protection and too little care leaves children vulnerable to anxiety because it creates a childhood experience in which options for children's exercise of control are limited. They suggest that it is this early experience with lack of control that may create risk for the development of anxiety and mood disorders. Unfortunately, all their findings are based on adults' retrospective reports of childhood experiences with parenting, and no research to date has prospectively examined actual parenting behavior as a risk factor for the development of anxiety disorders in childhood or adulthood.

Life Events

Stressful life events have been clearly implicated as a risk factor for anxiety disorders in adults (Monroe & Wade, 1988) but have rarely been studied in children. In their review, Klein and Last (1989) suggest that both clinical experience and empirical data suggest that these events may also play an important role as risk factors for childhood anxiety. They note that studies of children's reactions to major traumatic events such as wars, severe weather, and violence have supported a link between such events and anxiety.

There is also evidence that children with more anxiety report more stressful life events. Kashani and Orvaschel (1990) found that children classified as higher on anxiety reported more stressful life events; Bernstein and

Hoberman (1989) found this same pattern in adolescents. However, life events may be specific risk factors for certain types of anxiety and not others. In their Pittsburgh study, Costello et al. (1988) found that in adolescents, stressful life events and ongoing adversity predicted a variety of anxiety disorders but not phobias. These findings suggest that environmental events may influence the development of some types of anxiety disorders more than others. More research is needed to fully understand the contribution of stressful life events to the development of anxiety in children. It is possible that stressful life events create a sense of lack of personal control, and, as described previously, low perceptions of control have been postulated to constitute a risk factor for anxiety disorders.

IMPLICATIONS FOR PREVENTION AND TREATMENT

Controlled empirical investigations of (1) primary prevention efforts to decrease the incidence of anxiety disorders in children and/or (2) intervention efforts to ameliorate or diminish the impact of such disorders when they occur are scarce in the literature. Controlled clinical trials are needed both to evaluate the efficacy of proposed prevention and intervention approaches and to further understand vulnerability factors.

Although there is much more research to be done, the existing literature points to a variety of potential targets for intervention, including parenting behavior (especially overprotection and failure to promote autonomy) and children's cognitions (most notably perceptions of control and negative thoughts/self-statements). Controlled investigations of efforts to manipulate these variables and the outcome of such manipulations will shed further light on their importance, or lack thereof. Such investigations should carefully delineate components of interventions and whenever possible test their relative efficacy. Although there is general agreement that multimodal treatment approaches will probably be the most effective, studies demonstrating the superiority of multiple-component interventions over waiting-list control conditions often fail to identify which components may be more or less essential to the success of the intervention. A variety of components have comprised interventions, including systematic desensitization (typically *in vivo*), flooding, response prevention (for OCD), coping self-statements training, modeling, social skills training, relaxation training, cognitive restructuring, and parent training, often in combination with one another or with pharmacological agents. As Kendall (1994) has noted, additional research is needed to address the issue of the relative contribution of specific treatment components.

Dadds, Spence, Holland, Barrett, and Laurens (1997), through their Queensland (Australia) Early Intervention and Prevention of Anxiety Project, have published results of what may be the only controlled trial of a prevention program completed to date. Close to 2,000 nonreferred schoolchildren

(7 to 14 years old) were screened for anxiety problems based on teacher- and self-report. Screening resulted in a final sample of 128 children, approximately three-quarters of whom met criteria for at least one DSM-IV anxiety disorder. The children were then randomly assigned to a 10-week school-based group intervention, based on Kendall's (1990; Kendall, Kane, Howard, & Siqueland, 1990) CBT intervention, or to an assessment-only group. Parents of children in the intervention group also participated in group sessions, focusing on child management and management of their own anxiety. At posttreatment both groups had improved, but at 6-month follow-up only the intervention group had maintained their gains. Notably, children who received the intervention were much less likely than children in the assessment-only group to have progressed to a diagnosable anxiety disorder at 6-month follow-up. At 1-year follow-up, the group outcomes again appeared to be similar, but at 2-year follow-up the intervention group looked better on outcomes such as parent and clinician ratings of change and percentage of children meeting criteria for an anxiety disorder (Dadds et al., 1999). Regression analysis showed that initial level of anxiety predicted both short- and long-term response to the intervention. Dadds et al. (1999) interpret their results as suggesting natural improvement over time in anxious children but that children who are initially more anxious are less likely to improve over both the short and long term.

Several controlled trials of interventions for anxious children have been published in recent years. Kendall and colleagues have presented results from two randomized trials evaluating manualized cognitive-behavioral treatment for anxiety disorders in children and young adults. In the first study (Kendall, 1994), 47 children (ages 9–13 years) with a variety of anxiety disorders (OAD, SAD, or AVD) were randomly assigned to 16-session individual CBT or to a waiting list. Children in the waiting-list group also received CBT after 8 weeks. CBT was multicomponent and included training in recognizing anxious feelings, identifying anxious cognitions, and coping skills, as well as such strategies as modeling, *in vivo* exposure, relaxation training, and contingent social reinforcement. There were clear treatment benefits, which were maintained at 1-year follow-up. Also, Kendall and Southam-Gerow (1996) revisited these children 2 to 5 years later and found evidence that treatment gains were maintained, although the authors note that because all children received treatment, it is impossible to rule out alternative explanations for the observed improvement, including maturation. However, research suggesting that childhood anxiety is at least moderately stable over time (described earlier) makes this explanation unlikely.

In a second randomized clinical trial (Kendall et al., 1997), 94 9- to 13-year-olds with anxiety disorders were randomly assigned to CBT or waiting list. This study, which used the same CBT approach as did Kendall (1994), was intended to serve as a replication and extension of the previous study, as well as an initial attempt to identify active treatment components. Again, outcomes for CBT versus waiting-list outcomes were evaluated at posttreat-

ment. Waiting-list children received treatment after 8 weeks, and maintenance of gains for all subjects was examined at 1-year follow-up. Kendall et
al. (1997) again found significant improvements resulting from CBT, which
were sustained at follow-up. Results suggested a particularly important role
for exposure, versus education, in effecting change.

Another randomized clinical trial examined the role of family intervention as a component of therapy for anxious children. Barrett, Dadds, and
Rapee (1996) compared CBT alone and CBT plus family anxiety management training to a waiting-list control condition. CBT was an adaptation of
Kendall's (1990; Kendall et al., 1990) CBT treatment program. Subjects
were 79 children ages 7 to 14 who met diagnostic criteria for SAD, OAD, or
SOC. At posttreatment, children in both the CBT and combined conditions
showed improvement relative to controls. The combination of CBT plus
family therapy seemed to yield the greatest benefits; this was especially true
for younger children. Gains were maintained at 6- and 12-month follow-
ups. Howard and Kendall (1996) also recently evaluated a family-based
CBT intervention for children with anxiety disorders (six children, ages 9 to
13) using a multiple-baseline rather than a randomized controlled design.
They found positive effects of the intervention on children's anxiety levels,
but family characteristics such as conflict and other indices of functioning
were generally unrelated to treatment or outcome.

The potential for benefit from including the family in treatment is intriguing and underscores the potential importance of family factors in the
etiology or maintenance of anxiety disorders. Unfortunately, interventions
have not been tested that focus specifically on parenting variables that have
been identified as possible risk factors, such as overprotection and insufficient care. The family intervention evaluated by Barrett, Dadds, et al. (1996)
was multicomponent, and it is unclear which specific components were more
or less important. Also, it is unclear whether the family focus of the intervention was essential; as Barrett, Dadds, et al. (1996) suggest, it is possible
that the additional benefits found in the combined condition were simply
due to any adjunctive treatment, not specifically to a family-focused approach. In a follow-up study, Cobham, Dadds, and Spence (1998) narrowed
the focus of their family intervention to a single component (parental anxiety management [PAM]) and compared child-focused CBT plus PAM to
child-focused CBT alone. Further, they investigated whether differential response to treatment would be found in anxious children with at least one
anxious parent versus anxious children whose parents were not anxious.
Cobham et al. (1998) found that anxious children with nonanxious parents
responded equally well to either treatment condition, but anxious children
with anxious parents responded more positively to CBT plus PAM.

Controlled studies of pharmacological treatment for anxiety disorders
in children are also limited. Typically, medications found to be effective in
the treatment of adult anxiety disorders are then tested on children. Medications that have attracted recent interest for treating children include tricy-

clic antidepressants (e.g., imipramine) and benzodiazepines (e.g., alprazolam). To date, support for the efficacy of these medications in treating childhood anxiety has been limited (Allen, Leonard, & Swedo, 1995; Pine, 1997). A small literature supports the use of medications with effects on serotonin reuptake for OCD (e.g., clomipramine and fluoxetine; Klein & Last, 1989; Quintana & Birmaher, 1995; Pine, 1997), suggesting a serotonergic mechanism.

FUTURE DIRECTIONS FOR RESEARCH

Sound epidemiological data are needed on both referred and nonreferred children. The profound changes in the classification of childhood anxiety represented by DSM-IV necessitate a new wave of studies of prevalence and incidence rates of these disorders in children. Fortunately, Kendall and Warman's (1996) study of diagnostic consistency between DSM-III-R and DSM-IV found a high level of agreement for 40 referred children diagnosed under both systems, suggesting that generalizations from past research can continue to be made. However, many studies of anxiety symptoms in nonreferred children are decades old and should be updated using improved assessment technologies available today. An up-to-date, comprehensive, and detailed picture of the presence and natural history of anxiety in nonreferred children will serve as the cornerstone for efforts to more fully understand clinically relevant deviations and disturbances in anxiety during childhood.

It is important to continue to improve methodologies employed in studies of childhood anxiety. Studies must include children at a variety of ages, of both genders, and from different cultural backgrounds. Demographic characteristics of samples should be carefully measured, described, and considered. Also, anxiety parameters need to be carefully assessed and described. Children have been identified as anxious based on meeting full DSM criteria for a particular disorder, and based on the self-reported presence of a single symptom of anxiety. Unfortunately, there is no agreement on a "best" approach to identifying anxiety in children. For investigations and trials intending to target children who have an identifiable anxiety disorder, well-validated structured interviews, updated to reflect DSM-IV criteria, should be employed. The practice of grouping children with different anxiety disorders together is generally ill advised because the literature suggests that vulnerability factors and effective intervention agents differ among disorders and these distinctions will be obfuscated. For studies concerned with subclinical anxiety, myriad ways exist to assess symptoms of anxiety, ranging from self-report to teacher nomination to objective evaluation. Multimodal assessment, using the most psychometrically sound and well-established instruments and approaches, is essential to the identification and quantification of symptoms and syndromes of anxiety in children.

In addition, the identification of specific vulnerability processes contributing to the origination and/or maintenance of childhood anxiety disorders is essential to the development of efficacious prevention and intervention approaches. Clearly, prospective studies are needed. Large-scale longitudinal investigations should follow children identified as "at risk" for anxiety disorders, based on biological, cognitive, and/or social vulnerabilities suggested, theoretically or empirically, in the current literature. The largely descriptive literature to date constitutes an important first step in identifying potential vulnerability factors, but cross-sectional and retrospective studies cannot reveal information on cause–effect relationships, necessary to understanding etiology and maintenance of anxiety disorders, and to prevention and intervention efforts.

Finally, as noted previously, controlled clinical trials of both prevention and intervention approaches are essential. In addition to establishing the most efficacious treatment approaches, controlled investigations systematically manipulate potential vulnerability factors identified through descriptive research. Although not definitive, studies reporting positive outcomes (i.e., prevention, reduction or alleviation of anxiety) provide further evidence for the importance of the targeted variables.

REFERENCES

Allen, A. J., Leonard, H. L., & Swedo, S. E. (1995). Current knowledge of medications for the treatment of childhood anxiety disorders. *Journal of the American Academy of Child and Adolescent Psychiatry, 52,* 53–60.

Ambrose, B., & Rholes, W. S. (1993). Automatic cognitions and the symptoms of depression and anxiety in children and adolescents: An examination of the content-specificity hypothesis. *Cognitive Therapy and Research, 17,* 153–171.

American Psychiatric Association. (1980). *Diagnostic and statistical manual of mental disorders* (3rd ed.). Washington, DC: Author.

American Psychiatric Association. (1987). *Diagnostic and statistical manual of mental disorders* (3rd ed., rev.). Washington, DC: Author.

American Psychiatric Association. (1994). *Diagnostic and statistical manual of mental disorders* (4th ed.). Washington, DC: Author.

Anderson, J. C., Williams, S., McGee, R., & Silva, P. A. (1987). DSM-III disorders in preadolescent children: Prevalence in a large sample from the general population. *Archives of General Psychiatry, 44,* 69–76.

Barrett, P. M., Dadds, M. R., & Rapee, R. M. (1996). Family treatment of childhood anxiety disorders: A controlled trial. *Journal of Consulting and Clinical Psychology, 64,* 333–342.

Barrett, P. M., Rapee, R. M., Dadds, M. R., & Ryan, S. (1996). Family enhancement of cognitive style in anxious and aggressive children. *Journal of Abnormal Child Psychology, 24,* 187–203.

Beck, A. T., Brown, G., Steer, R. A., Eidelson, J. I., & Riskind, J. H. (1987). Differentiating anxiety and depression: A test of the cognitive content-specificity hypothesis. *Journal of Abnormal Psychology, 96,* 179–183.

Beck, A. T., Epstein, N., & Harrison, R. (1983). Cognitions, attitudes and personality dimensions in depression. *British Journal of Cognitive Psychotherapy*, *1*, 1–16.

Beidel, D. C., & Morris, T. L. (1995). Social phobia. In J. S. March (Ed.), *Anxiety disorders in children and adolescents* (pp. 181–211). New York: Guilford Press.

Beidel, D. C., Turner, M. W., & Trager, K. N. (1994). Test anxiety and childhood anxiety disorders in African American and White school children. *Journal of Anxiety Disorders, 8*, 169–179.

Bell-Dolan, D. J., Last, C. G., & Strauss, C. C. (1990). Symptoms of anxiety disorders in normal children. *Journal of the American Academy of Child and Adolescent Psychiatry, 29*, 759–765.

Benjamin, R. S., Costello, E. J., & Warren, M. (1990). Anxiety disorders in a pediatric sample. *Journal of the Anxiety Disorders, 4*, 293–316.

Berg, C. Z., Rapoport, J. L., Whitaker, A., Davies, M., Leonard, H., Swedo, S. E., Braiman, S., & Lenane, M. (1989). Childhood obsessive–compulsive disorder: A two-year prospective study of a community sample. *Journal of the American Academy of Child and Adolescent Psychiatry, 28*, 528–533.

Bernstein, G. A., & Borchardt, C. M. (1991). Anxiety disorders of childhood and adolescents: A critical review. *Journal of the American Academy of Child and Adolescent Psychiatry, 30*, 519–532.

Bernstein, G. A., Borchardt, C. M., & Perwien, A. R. (1996). Anxiety disorders in children and adolescents: A review of the past 10 years. *Journal of the American Academy of Child and Adolescent Psychiatry, 35*, 1110–1119.

Bernstein, G. A., & Hoberman, H. M. (1989). Self-reported anxiety in adolescents. *American Journal of Psychiatry, 146*, 384–386.

Biederman, J., Rosenbaum, J. F., Bolduc-Murphy, E. A., Faraone, S. V., Chaloff, J., Hirshfeld, D. R., & Kagan, J. (1993). A three-year follow-up of children with and without behavioral inhibition. *Journal of the American Academy of Child and Adolescent Psychiatry, 32*, 814–821.

Biederman, J., Rosenbaum, J. F., Chaloff, J., & Kagan, J. (1995). Behavioral inhibition as a risk factor for anxiety disorders. In J. S. March (Ed.), *Anxiety disorders in children and adolescents* (pp. 61–81). New York: Guilford Press.

Biederman, J., Rosenbaum, J. F., Hirshfeld, D. R., Faraone, S. V., Bolduc, E. A., Gersten, M., Meminger, S. R., Kagan, J., Snidman, N., & Reznick, J. S. (1990). Psychiatric correlates of behavioral inhibition in young children of parents with and without psychiatric disorders. *Archives of General Psychiatry, 47*, 21–26.

Bird, H. R., Canino, G., Rubio-Stipec, M., Gould, M. S., Ribera, J., Sesman, M., Woodbury, M., Huertas-Goldman, S., Pagan, A., Sanchez-Lacay, A., & Moscoso, M. (1988). Estimates of the prevalence of childhood maladjustment in a community survey in Puerto Rico. *Archives of General Psychiatry, 45*, 1120–1126.

Black, B., & Robbins, D. R. (1990). Panic disorder in children and adolescents. *Journal of the American Academy of Child and Adolescent Psychiatry, 29*, 36–44.

Brady, E. U., & Kendall, P. C. (1992). Comorbidity of anxiety and depression in children and adolescents. *Psychological Bulletin, 111*, 244–255.

Campbell, S. B. (1986). Developmental issues in childhood anxiety. In R. Gittleman (Ed.), *Anxiety disorders of childhood* (pp. 24–57). New York: Guilford Press.

Cantwell, D. P., & Baker, L. (1989). Stability and natural history of DSM-III child-hood diagnoses. *Journal of the American Academy of Child and Adolescent Psychiatry, 30,* 519–532.

Caspi, A., Henry, B., McGee, R. O., Moffitt, T. E., & Silva, P. A. (1995). Tempera-mental origins of child and adolescent behavior problems: From age three to age fifteen. *Child Development, 66,* 55–68.

Chorpita, B. F., Albano, A. M., & Barlow, D. H. (1996a). Child anxiety sensitivity index: Considerations for children with anxiety disorders. *Journal of Clini-cal Child Psychology, 25,* 77–82.

Chorpita, B. F., Albano, A. M., & Barlow, D. H. (1996b). Cognitive processing in children: Relation to anxiety and family influences. *Journal of Clinical Child Psychology, 25,* 170–176.

Chorpita, B. F., & Barlow, D. H. (1998). The development of anxiety: The role of control in the early environment. *Psychological Bulletin, 124,* 3–21.

Clark, L. A., & Watson, D. (1991). Tripartite model of anxiety and depression: Psychometric evidence and taxonomic implications. *Journal of Abnormal Psychology, 100,* 316–336.

Cobham, V. E., Dadds, M. R., & Spence, S. H. (1998). The role of parental anxiety in the treatment of childhood anxiety. *Journal of Consulting and Clinical Psychology, 66,* 893–905.

Cohen, P., Cohen, J., & Brook, J. (1993). An epidemiological study of disorders in late childhood and adolescence: II. Persistence of disorders. *Journal of Child Psychology and Psychiatry, 34,* 869–877.

Costanzo, P., Miller-Johnson, S., & Wencel, H. (1995). Social development. In J. S. March (Ed.), *Anxiety disorders in children and adolescents* (pp. 82–108). New York: Guilford Press.

Costello, E. J., & Angold, A. (1995). Epidemiology. In J. S. March (Ed.), *Anxiety disorders in children and adolescents* (pp. 109–124). New York: Guilford Press.

Costello, E. J., Angold, A., Burns, B. J., Stangl, D. K., Tweed, D. L., Erkanli, A., & Worthman, C. M. (1996). The Great Smoky Mountains Study of Youth: Prevalence and correlates of DSM-III-R disorders. *Archives of General Psy-chiatry, 53,* 1129–1136.

Costello, E. J., Costello, A., Edelbrock, C., Burns, B. J., Dulcan, M. K., Brent, D., & Janiszewski, S. (1988). Psychiatric disorders in pediatric primary care: Preva-lence and risk factors. *Archives of General Psychiatry, 45,* 1107–1116.

Costello, E. J., Stouthamer-Loeber, M., & DeRosier, M. (1993). *Continuity and change in psychopathology from childhood to adolescence.* Paper presented at the annual meeting of the Society for Research in Child and Adolescent Psychopathology, Santa Fe, NM.

Craske, M. (1997). Fear and anxiety in children and adolescents. *Bulletin of the Menninger Clinic, 61*(Suppl.), A4–A36.

Dadds, M. R., Barrett, P. M., Rapee, R. M., & Ryan, S. (1996). Family process and child anxiety and aggression: An observational analysis. *Journal of Abnor-mal Child Psychology, 24,* 715–734.

Dadds, M. R., Holland, D. E., Laurens, K. R., Mullins, M., Barrett, P. M., & Spence, S. H. (1999). Early intervention and prevention of anxiety disorders in chil-dren: Results at 2-year follow-up. *Journal of Consulting and Clinical Psy-chology, 67,* 145–150.

Dadds, M. R., Spence, S. H., Holland, D. E., Barrett, P. M., & Laurens, K. R. (1997). Prevention and early intervention for anxiety disorders: A controlled trial. *Journal of Consulting and Clinical Psychology, 65*, 627–635.

Dashiff, C. J. (1995). Understanding separation anxiety disorder. *Journal of Child and Adolescent Psychiatric Nursing, 8*, 27–38.

Douglass, H. M., Moffitt, T. E., Dar, R., McGee, R., & Silva, P. (1995). Obsessive–compulsive disorder in a birth cohort of 18-year-olds: Prevalence and predictors. *Journal of the American Academy of Child and Adolescent Psychiatry, 34*, 1424–1431.

Dumas, J. E., LaFreniere, P. J., & Serketich, W. J. (1995). "Balance of power": A transactional analysis of control in mother–child dyads involving socially competent, aggressive, and anxious children. *Journal of Abnormal Psychology, 104*, 104–113.

Fergusson, D. M., Horwood, L. J., & Lynskey, M. T. (1993). Prevalence and comorbidity of DSM-III-R diagnoses in a birth cohort of 15 year olds. *Journal of the American Academy of Child and Adolescent Psychiatry, 32*, 1127–1134.

Flament, M. F., Koby, E., Rapoport, J. L., Berg, C. J., Zahn, T., Cox, C., Denckla, M., & Lenane, M. (1990). Childhood obsessive-compulsive disorder: A prospective follow-up study. *Journal of Child Psychology and Psychiatry and Allied Disciplines, 31*, 363–380.

Flament, M. F., Whitaker, A., Rapoport, J. L., Davies, M., Berg, C. Z., Kalikow, K., Sceery, W., & Shaffer, D. (1988). Obsessive compulsive disorder in adolescence: An epidemiological study. *Journal of the American Academy of Child and Adolescent Psychiatry, 27*, 764–771.

Francis, G., Last, C. G., & Strauss, C. C. (1987). Expression of separation anxiety disorder: The roles of age and gender. *Child Psychiatry and Human Development, 18*, 82–89.

Gittelman, R., & Klein, D. F. (1985). Childhood separation anxiety and adult agoraphobia. In A. H. Tuma & J. D. Maser (Eds.), *Anxiety and the anxiety disorders* (pp. 389–402). Hillsdale, NJ: Erlbaum.

Gray, J. A. (1982). *The neuropsychology of anxiety*. New York: Oxford University Press.

Gray, J. A., & McNaughton, N. (1996). The neuropsychology of anxiety: A reprise. In D. A. Hope (Ed.), *Nebraska Symposium on Motivation: Perspectives on anxiety, panic and fear* (pp. 61–134). Lincoln: University of Nebraska Press.

Gurley, D., Cohen, P., Pine, D. S., & Brook, J. (1996). Discriminating depression and anxiety in youth: A role of diagnostic criteria. *Journal of Affective Disorders, 29*, 191–200.

Hayward, C., Killen, J. D., Hammer L. D., Litt, I. F., Wilson, D. M., Simmonds, B., & Taylor, C. B. (1992). Pubertal stage and panic attack history in sixth- and seventh-grade girls. *American Journal of Psychiatry, 49*, 1239–1243.

Hirshfeld, D. R., Rosenbaum, J. F., Biederman, J., Bolduc, E. A., Faraone, S. V., Snidman, N., Reznick, J. S., & Kagan, J. (1992). Stable behavioral inhibition and its association with anxiety disorder. *Journal of the American Academy of Child and Adolescent Psychiatry, 31*, 103-111.

Hooper, S. R., & March, J. S. (1995). Neuropsychology. In J. S. March (Ed.), *Anxiety disorders in children and adolescents* (pp. 35–60). New York: Guilford Press.

Howard, B. L., & Kendall, P. C. (1996). Cognitive-behavioral family therapy for anxiety-disordered children: A multiple-baseline evaluation. *Cognitive Therapy and Research, 20,* 423–443.

Ialongo, N., Edelsohn, G., Werthamer-Larsson, L., Crockett, L., & Kellam, S. (1994). The significance of self-reported anxious symptoms in first-grade children. *Journal of Abnormal Child Psychology, 22,* 441–455.

Ialongo, N., Edelsohn, G., Werthamer-Larsson, L., Crockett, L., & Kellam, S. (1995). The significance of self-reported anxious symptoms in first grade children: Prediction to anxious symptoms and adaptive functioning in fifth grade. *Journal of Child Psychology and Psychiatry, 36,* 427–437.

Kagan, J. (1989). Temperamental contributions to social behavior. *American Psychologist, 44,* 668–674.

Kagan, J., Reznick, J. S., & Snidman, N. (1988). Biological basis of childhood shyness. *Science, 240,* 167–171.

Kashani, J. H., & Orvaschel, H. (1988). Anxiety disorders in midadolescence: A community sample. *American Journal of Psychiatry, 145,* 960–964.

Kashani, J. H., & Orvaschel, H. (1990). A community study of anxiety in children and adolescents. *American Journal of Psychiatry, 147,* 313–318.

Kendall, P. C. (1990). *The coping cat workbook.* Ardmore, PA: Workbook.

Kendall, P. C. (1994). Treating anxiety disorders in children: Results of a randomized clinical trial. *Journal of Consulting and Clinical Psychology, 62,* 100–110.

Kendall, P. C., Flannery-Schroeder, E., Panichelli-Mindel, S. M., Southam-Gerow, M., Henin, A., & Warman, M. (1997). Therapy for youths with anxiety disorders: A second randomized clinical trial. *Journal of Consulting and Clinical Psychology, 65,* 366–380.

Kendall, P. C., Kane, M., Howard, B., & Siqueland, L. (1990). *Cognitive-behavioral therapy for anxious children: Treatment manual* [Available from the first author, Department of Psychology, Temple University, Philadelphia, PA 19122].

Kendall, P. C., Kortlander, E., Chansky, T. E., & Brady, E. U. (1992). Comorbidity of anxiety and depression in youth: Treatment implications. *Journal of Consulting and Clinical Psychology, 60,* 869–880.

Kendall, P. C., & Southam-Gerow, M. A. (1996). Long-term follow-up of a cognitive-behavioral therapy for anxiety-disordered youth. *Journal of Consulting and Clinical Psychology, 64,* 724–730.

Kendall, P. C., & Warman, M. J. (1996). Anxiety disorders in youth: Diagnostic consistency across DSM-III-R and DSM-IV. *Journal of Anxiety Disorders, 10,* 453–463.

Kendler, K. S., Neale, M. C., Kessler, R. C., Heath, A. C., & Eaves, L. J. (1992). Major depression and generalized anxiety disorder: Same genes, (partly) different environments? *Archives of General Psychiatry, 49,* 716–722.

Kessler, R. C., McGonagle, K. A., Zhao, S., Nelson, C. B., Hughes, M., Eshleman, S., Wittchen, H. U., & Kendler, K. S. (1994). Lifetime and 12-month prevalence of DSM-III-R psychiatric disorders in the United States: Results from the National Comorbidity study. *Archives of General Psychiatry, 51,* 8–19.

Klein, R. G., & Last, C. G. (1989). *Anxiety disorders in children.* Newbury Park, CA: Sage.

Last, C. G., Hersen, M., Kazdin, A., Orvaschel, H., & Perrin, S. (1991). Anxiety disorders in children and their families. *Archives of General Psychiatry, 48,* 928–934.

Last, C. G., & Perrin, S. (1993). Anxiety disorders in African-American and white children. *Journal of Abnormal Child Psychology, 21,* 153–164.

Last, C. G., Perrin, S., Hersen, M., & Kazdin, A. E. (1992). DSM-III-R anxiety disorders in children: Sociodemographic and clinical characteristics. *Journal of the American Academy of Child and Adolescent Psychiatry, 31,* 1070–1076.

Last, C. G., Perrin, S., Hersen, M., & Kazdin, A. E. (1996). A prospective study of childhood anxiety disorders. *Journal of the American Academy of Child and Adolescent Psychiatry, 35,* 1502–1510.

Last, C. G., & Strauss, C. C. (1989). Panic disorder in children and adolescents. *Journal of Anxiety Disorders, 3,* 87–95.

Last, C. G., Strauss, C. C., & Francis, G. (1987). Comorbidity among childhood anxiety disorders. *Journal of Nervous and Mental Disease, 175,* 726–730.

Laucht, M., & Schmidt, M. H. (1987). Psychiatric disorders at the age of 13: Results and problems of a long-term study. In B. Cooper (Ed.), *Psychiatric epidemiology: Progress and prospects* (pp. 212–224). London: Croom Helm.

Laurent, J., & Stark, K. D. (1993). Testing the cognitive content-specificity hypothesis with anxious and depressed youngsters. *Journal of Abnormal Psychology, 102,* 226–237.

Leitenberg, H., Yost, L. W., & Carroll-Wilson, M. (1986). Negative cognitive errors in children: Questionnaire development, normative data and comparisons between children with and without self-reported symptoms of depression, low self-esteem, and evaluation anxiety. *Journal of Consulting and Clinical Psychology, 54,* 528-536.

Leonard, H. L., Swedo, S. E., Lenane, M. C., Rettew, D. C., Hamburger, S. D., Bartko, J. J., & Rapoport, J. L. (1993). A 2- to 7-year follow-up study of 54 obsessive–compulsive children and adolescents. *Archives of General Psychiatry, 50,* 429-439.

Lerner, J., Safren, S., Henin, A., Warman, M., Heimberg, R. G., & Kendall, P. C. (1999). Differentiating anxious and depressive self-statements in youth: Factor structure of the Negative Affect Self-Statement Questionnaire among youth referred to an anxiety disorders clinic. *Journal of Clinical Child Psychology, 28,* 82–93.

Majcher, D., & Pollack, M. H. (1996). Childhood anxiety disorders. In L. Hechtman (Ed.), *Do they grow out of it?* (pp. 139–169). Washington, DC: American Psychiatric Press.

Malcarne, V. L., & Ingram, R. E. (1994). Cognition and negative affectivity. In T. H. Ollendick & R. J. Prinz (Eds.), *Advances in clinical child psychology* (pp. 141–176). New York: Plenum.

Manassis, K., & Bradley, S. (1994). The development of childhood anxiety disorders: Toward an integrated model. *Journal of Applied Developmental Psychology, 15,* 345–366.

Manassis, K., Bradley, S., Goldberg, S., Hood, J., & Swinson, R. P. (1994). Attachment in mothers with anxiety disorders and their children. *Journal of the American Academy of Child and Adolescent Psychiatry, 33,* 1106–1113.

Manassis, K., Bradley, S., Goldberg, S., Hood, J., & Swinson, R. P. (1995). Behavioral inhibition, attachment and anxiety in children of mothers with anxiety disorders. *Canadian Journal of Psychiatry, 40,* 87–92.

McGee, R., Feehan, M., Williams, S., & Anderson, J. (1992). DSM-III disorders from age 11 to age 15 years. *Journal of the American Academy of Child and Adolescent Psychiatry, 31,* 51–59.

McGee, R., Feehan, M., Williams, S., Partridge, F., Silva, P. A., & Kelly, J. (1990). DSM-III disorders in a large sample of adolescents. *Journal of the American Academy of Child and Adolescent Psychiatry, 29,* 611–619.

McLeer, S. V., Deblinger, E., Hendry, D., & Orvaschel, H. (1992). Sexually abused children at risk for post-traumatic stress disorder. *Journal of the American Academy of Child and Adolescent Psychiatry, 31,* 875–879.

Monroe, S. M., & Wade, S. L. (1988). Life events. In C. G. Last & M. Hersen (Eds.), *Handbook of anxiety disorders* (pp. 293–305). New York: Pergamon Press.

Morris, R. J., & Kratochwill, T. R. (1983). *Treating children's fears and phobias.* New York: Pergamon Press.

Nachmias, M., Gunnar, M., Mangelsdorf, S., Parritz, R. H., & Buss, K. (1996). Behavioral inhibition and stress reactivity: The moderating role of attachment security. *Child Development, 67,* 508–522.

Neal, A. M., Lilly, R. S., & Zakis, S. (1993). What are African American children afraid of? A preliminary study. *Journal of Anxiety Disorders, 7,* 129–139.

Nelles, W. B., & Barlow, D. H. (1988). Do children panic? *Clinical Psychology Review, 12,* 121–139.

Offord, D. R., Boyle, M. H., Racine, Y. A., Fleming, J. E., Cadman, D. T., Blum, H. M., Byrne, C., Links, P. S., Lipman, E. L., & MacMillan, H. L. (1992). Outcome, prognosis, and risk in a longitudinal follow-up study. *Journal of the American Academy of Child and Adolescent Psychiatry, 31,* 916–923.

Ollendick, T. H., & Francis, G. (1988). Behavioral assessment and treatment of childhood phobias. *Behavior Modification, 12,* 165–204.

Ollendick, T. H., King, N. J., & Frary, R. B. (1989). Fears in children and adolescents: Reliability and generalizability across gender, age and nationality. *Behavior Research and Therapy, 27,* 19–26.

Ollendick, T. H., Mattis, S. G., & King, N. J. (1994). Panic in children and adolescents: A review. *Journal of Child Psychology and Psychiatry and Allied Disciplines, 35,* 113–134.

Parker, G. (1979a). Reported parental characteristics of agoraphobics and social phobics. *British Journal of Psychiatry, 135,* 555–560.

Parker, G. (1979b). Reported parental characteristics in relation to trait depression and anxiety levels in a non-clinical group. *Australian and New Zealand Journal of Psychiatry, 13,* 260–264.

Parker, G. (1981). Parental representation of patients with anxiety neurosis. *Acta Psychiatrica Scandinavica, 63,* 33–36.

Parker, G. (1983). *Parental overprotection: A risk factor in psychosocial development.* New York: Grune & Stratton.

Pine, D. S. (1997). Childhood anxiety disorders. *Current Opinion in Pediatrics, 9,* 329–338.

Pollack, M. H., Otto, M. W., Sabatino, S., Majcher, D., Worthington, J. J., McArdle, E. T., & Rosenbaum, J. F. (1996). Relationship of childhood anxiety to adult panic disorder: Correlates and influence on course. *American Journal of Psychiatry, 153,* 376–381.

Pollock, R. A., Rosenbaum, J. F., Marrs, A., Miller, B. S., & Biederman, J. (1995).

Anxiety disorders of childhood: Implications for adult psychopathology. *Psychiatric Clinics of North America, 18,* 745–766.

Popper, C. W. (1993). Psychopharmacologic treatment of anxiety disorders in adolescents and children. *Journal of Clinical Psychiatry, 54,* 52–63.

Quintana, H., & Birmaher, B. (1995). Pharmacological treatment. In M. Hersen & R. T. Ammerman (Eds.), *Advanced abnormal child psychology* (pp. 189–212). Hillsdale, NJ: Erlbaum.

Rabian, B., & Silverman, W. K. (1995). Anxiety disorders. In M. Hersen & R. T. Ammerman (Eds.), *Advanced abnormal child psychology* (pp. 235–252). Hillsdale, NJ: Erlbaum.

Ronan, K. R., & Kendall, P. C. (1997). Self-talk in distressed youth: States-of-mind and content specificity. *Journal of Clinical Child Psychology, 26,* 330–337.

Rosenbaum, J. F., Biederman, J., Gersten, M., Hirshfeld, D. R., Meminger, S. R., Herman, J. B., Kagan, J., Reznick, J. S., & Snidman, N. (1988). Behavioral inhibition in children of parents with panic disorder and agoraphobia. *Archives of General Psychiatry, 45,* 463–470.

Rosenbaum, J. F., Biederman, J., Hirshfeld, D. R., Bolduc, E. A., Faraone, S. V., Kagan, J., Snidman, N., & Reznick, J. S. (1991). Further evidence of an association between behavioral inhibition and anxiety disorders: Results from a family study of children from a non-clinical sample. *Journal of Psychiatric Research, 25,* 49–65.

Rosenberg, A., & Kagan, J. (1987). Iris pigmentation and behavioral inhibition. *Developmental Psychobiology, 20,* 377–392.

Rourke, B. P. (1989). *Nonverbal learning disabilities: The syndrome and the model.* New York: Guilford Press.

Sallee, R., & Greenawald, J. (1995). Neurobiology. In J. S. March (Ed.), *Anxiety disorders in children and adolescents* (pp. 3–34). New York: Guilford Press.

Silove, D., Parker, G., Hadzi-Pavlovic, D., Manicavasagar, V., & Blaszczynski, A. (1991). Parental representations of patients with panic disorder and generalised anxiety disorder. *British Journal of Psychiatry, 159,* 835–841.

Silverman, W. K., & Ginsburg, G. S. (1995). Specific phobias and generalized anxiety disorder. In J. S. March (Ed.), *Anxiety disorders in children and adolescents* (pp. 151–180). New York: Guilford Press.

Silverman, W. K., & Nelles, W. B. (1990). Simple phobia in childhood. In M. Hersen & C. G. Last (Eds.), *Handbook of child and adult psychopathology: A longitudinal perspective* (pp. 183–195). New York: Pergamon Press.

Siqueland, L., Kendall, P. C., & Steinberg, L. (1996). Anxiety in children: Perceived family environments and observed family interactions. *Journal of Clinical Child Psychology, 25,* 225–237.

Strauss, C. C., & Last, C. G. (1993). Social and simple phobias in children. *Journal of Anxiety Disorders, 7,* 141–152.

Strauss, C. C., Last, C. G., Hersen, M., & Kazdin, A. E. (1988). Association between anxiety and depression in children and adolescents with anxiety disorders. *Journal of Abnormal Child Psychology, 16,* 57–68.

Strauss, C. C., Lease, C. A., Last, C. G., & Francis, G. (1988). Overanxious disorder: An examination of developmental differences. *Journal of Abnormal Child Psychology, 16,* 433–443.

Swedo, S. E., Rapoport, J. L., Leonard, H., Lenane, M., & Cheslow, D. (1989). Obsessive–compulsive disorder in children and adolescents: Clinical phenomenology of 70 consecutive cases. *Archives of General Psychiatry, 46,* 335–341.

Tennes, K., Downey, K., & Vernadakis, A. (1977). Urinary cortisol excretion rates and anxiety in normal 1-year-old infants. *Psychosomatic Medicine, 39,* 178–187.

Tennes, K., & Kreye, M. (1985). Children's adrenocortical responses to classroom activities and tests in elementary school. *Psychosomatic Medicine, 47,* 451–460.

Thomsen, P. H., & Mikkelsen, H. U. (1995). Course of obsessive–compulsive disorder in children and adolescents: A prospective follow-up study of 23 Danish cases. *Journal of the American Academy of Child and Adolescent Psychiatry, 34,* 1432–1440.

Thyer, B. A., Himle, J., & Fischer, D. (1988). Is parental death a selective precursor to either panic disorder or agoraphobia?: A test of the separation anxiety hypothesis. *Journal of Anxiety Disorders, 2,* 333–338.

Torgersen, S. (1983). Genetic factors in anxiety disorders. *Archives of General Psychiatry, 40,* 1085–1089.

Torgersen, S. (1993). Relationship between adult and childhood anxiety disorders: Genetic hypothesis. In C. G. Last (Ed.), *Anxiety across the lifespan: A developmental perspective* (pp. 113–127). New York: Springer.

Treadwell, K. R. H., & Kendall, P. C. (1996). Self-talk in youth with anxiety disorders: States of mind, content specificity, and treatment outcome. *Journal of Consulting and Clinical Psychology, 64,* 941–950.

Tucker, D. M. (1989). Neural and psychological maturation in a social context. In D. Cicchetti (Ed.), *The emergence of a discipline: Rochester Symposium on Developmental Psychopathology* (Vol. 1, pp. 69–88). Hillsdale, NJ: Erlbaum.

Turner, S. M., Beidel, D. C., & Costello, A. (1987). Psychopathology in the offspring of anxiety disorders patients. *Journal of Consulting and Clinical Psychology, 55,* 229–235.

Vasey, M. W. (1993). Development and cognition in childhood anxiety: The example of worry. *Advances in Clinical Child Psychology, 15,* 1–39.

Velez, C. N., Johnson, J., & Cohen, P. (1989). A longitudinal analysis of selected risk factors of childhood psychopathology. *Journal of the American Academy of Child and Adolescent Psychiatry, 28,* 861–864.

Weissman, M. M., Leckman, J. R., Merikangas, K. R., Gammon, G. D., & Prusoff, B. A. (1984). Depression and anxiety disorders in parents and children: Results from the Yale Family Study. *Archives of General Psychiatry, 41,* 845–852.

Werry, J. S. (1991). Overanxious disorder: A review of taxonomic properties. *Journal of the American Academy of Child and Adolescent Psychiatry, 30,* 533–544.

Whitaker, A., Johnson, J., Shaffer, D., Rapoport, J. L., Kalikow, K., Walsh, B. T., Davies, M., Braiman, S., & Dolinsky, A. (1990). Uncommon troubles in young people: Prevalence estimates of selected psychiatric disorders in a nonreferred adolescent population. *Archives of General Psychiatry, 47,* 487–496.

World Health Organization. (1988). *International classification of diseases* (10th ed.). Geneva: Author.

Zatz, S., & Chassin, L. (1983). Cognitions of test-anxious children. *Journal of Consulting and Clinical Psychology, 51,* 524–534.

Zatz, S., & Chassin, L. (1985). Cognitions of test-anxious children under naturalistic test-taking conditions. *Journal of Consulting and Clinical Psychology, 53,* 393–401.

12

Vulnerability to Anxiety Disorders in Adulthood

RICHARD J. McNALLY

Most clinicians believe that people vary in their proneness for developing anxiety disorders. Certain psychobiological characteristics presumably render some individuals more likely than others to fall ill. Despite widespread endorsement of such bromidic assumptions, knowledge about vulnerability is scarce. There are several reasons for this. First, the base rate for many risk factors is so high relative to disorder prevalence that their presence is not especially informative. For example, being female is associated with increased risk—relative to being male—for panic disorder. Because few women develop panic disorder, knowing that someone is female affords little in the way of predictive power. Second, many risk factors only indirectly reflect the causal processes underlying disorder emergence. Because not all statistical risk factors are causal vulnerability factors, identifying what predicts the development of a disorder need not reveal what causes it. Predicting disorder emergence does not necessarily mean that something participates in the causal chain. Third, inferences about causation are hampered because experimental manipulation of putative vulnerability factors is neither feasible nor ethical. Prospective longitudinal studies may be the best we can do with regard to identifying vulnerabilities. Fourth, conducting prospective, longitudinal studies is both expensive and difficult. One must have some sense about what populations are at risk and some sense about what variables ought to be measured over time. These limitations notwithstanding, researchers have at least some clues about factors that render some people prone to develop pathological anxiety.

The purpose of this chapter is to review what is known about vulnerability for developing anxiety disorders in adulthood. Restricting coverage to adulthood eliminates from consideration several syndromes that usually emerge in childhood and adolescence. Thus, most specific phobias have their origins in childhood (Öst, 1987), and social phobia rarely begins after adolescence (Rapee, 1995). Likewise, many people who suffer from generalized anxiety disorder claim that they have been anxious throughout their entire life (Rapee, 1991). Accordingly, these disorders are discussed elsewhere in this volume. Panic disorder, posttraumatic stress disorder (PTSD), and obsessive–compulsive disorder (OCD) are the foci of this chapter. Panic disorder rarely begins before puberty, PTSD can occur at any age, and many people develop OCD in adulthood.

HISTORICAL PROLOGUE

Clinicians have long speculated about vulnerability factors for what are now called panic disorder, OCD, and PTSD. Although two-factor learning theorists emphasized Pavlovian and instrumental conditioning episodes as etiologically significant events, they also assumed that not all people were equally conditionable (Eysenck & Rachman, 1965, pp. 24, 58). They cited laboratory studies showing that individuals scoring high on self-report measures of introversion developed more robust and reliable conditioned eyeblink responses to air puffs than did those scoring high on measures of extraversion (Eysenck & Rachman, 1965, p. 36). Extrapolating from these experiments, they assumed that neurotic problems would be acquired as easily as conditioned responses in the laboratory. They also hypothesized that people scoring high on questionnaires of neuroticism were characterized by a labile autonomic nervous system that enhanced susceptibility for developing anxiety problems. Behavior theorists, such as Eysenck and Rachman, were disinclined to interpret these problems in terms of risk for specific syndromes; they favored a dimensional approach whereby people scoring high on introversion and neuroticism were rendered vulnerable to develop a range of related conditioned anxiety reactions (e.g., fears, obsessions, and panic). The notion that there might be risk factors for specific nosological entities was not part of this framework.

Theoretical emphasis on vulnerability factors for PTSD has waxed and waned throughout psychiatric history (McNally, 1999a; Young, 1995). Prevailing opinion at the time PTSD was formally ratified as a syndrome in the third edition of the *Diagnostic and Statistical Manual of Mental Disorders* (DSM-III; American Psychiatric Association, 1980) awarded causal priority to the traumatic event itself, thereby downplaying vulnerability factors. Indeed, the definition of a traumatic stressor was one "that would evoke significant symptoms of distress in almost everyone" (American Psychiatric Association, 1980, p. 238). The emphasis on the traumatic event itself may have reflected a desire to avoid "blaming the victim." But in recent years, clinical scholars have increasingly addressed vulnerability factors, in part because most people exposed to these stressors do not develop chronic PTSD (e.g., Bowman, 1999; Yehuda & McFarlane, 1995). Moreover, identifying predictors of PTSD no more assigns "blame" to the patient than doing so does for other diseases (e.g., cancer). Causal discourse and moral discourse are entirely separate domains.

PANIC DISORDER AND AGORAPHOBIA

A panic attack is characterized by the sudden onset of intense fear accompanied by physiological symptoms and thoughts that one is about to die, go crazy, or lose self-control. Common symptoms include rapid heart rate, difficulty breathing, dizziness, and trembling. Classic, unexpected panic attacks seem to emerge "out of the blue," untriggered by any obvious precipitant. Although panic attacks rarely last for more than a few minutes, people can develop disabling dread of their recurrence. Individuals who experience repeated, unexpected attacks and report at least 1 month of persistent concern about their recurrence qualify for a diagnosis of panic disorder. They may begin to avoid activities and situations in which panic attacks would be especially unwelcome (e.g., driving a car and shopping). If avoidance becomes widespread, panic disorder with agoraphobia is diagnosed.

According to the National Comorbidity Study (NCS), 7% of adults have experienced a panic attack at some point in their lives, and lifetime prevalence rates of panic disorder and panic disorder with agoraphobia are 3.5% and 1.5%, respectively (Eaton, Kessler, Wittchen, & Magee, 1994). Fifty percent of those with panic disorder reported no agoraphobic symptoms. People ranging from 15 to 24 years of age are at highest risk for developing panic attacks and panic disorder, and women are about twice as likely as men to have panic disorder (1-month prevalence rate: 2.0% vs. 0.8%). Individuals with less than a high school education are 10 times more likely to develop panic disorder than are people who have completed college. Risk for panic disorder, however, is unrelated to annual income.

The diagnosis of panic disorder jointly requires recurrent unexpected attacks and persistent dread of their recurrence. Therefore, vulnerability for panic may consist of proneness to experience eruptions of intense physiological sensations, a fear of these sensations, or both.

Anxiety Sensitivity

One psychological variable that has received considerable attention as a possible vulnerability factor for panic disorder is *anxiety sensitivity*. Anxiety sensitivity refers to fears of anxiety symptoms that are based on beliefs about their possible harmfulness (Reiss & McNally, 1985). Thus, a person with high anxiety sensitivity may fear that heart palpitations signify an impending heart attack, whereas a person with low anxiety sensitivity is likely to regard these sensations as merely unpleasant. Thus, just as people vary in their proneness to experience anxiety symptoms (i.e., trait anxiety), so do they vary in their proneness to react fearfully to these symptoms (i.e., anxiety sensitivity). People with high anxiety sensitivity are likely to report episodes of anticipatory anxiety about the possible recurrence of panic attacks.

Several lines of evidence point to anxiety sensitivity as a vulnerability factor for panic disorder. Patients with panic disorder score higher than do either those with other anxiety disorders or no disorder on the Anxiety Sensitivity Index (ASI), a 16-item self-report measure tapping concerns about anxiety symptoms (McNally & Lorenz, 1987; Reiss, Peterson, Gursky, & McNally, 1986; Taylor, Koch, & McNally, 1992). Elevated ASI scores in panic patients do not, of course, confirm anxiety sensitivity as a vulnerability factor for panic; high anxiety sensitivity might result from having experienced panic attacks. At the very least, elevated ASI scores must occur in people who have never had a panic attack.

Several surveys have confirmed that this is, indeed, the case. Donnell and McNally (1990) found that 67% of 425 college students whose ASI scores were at least one standard deviation higher than the normative mean had never experienced a spontaneous panic attack. Another survey revealed that 70% of high-ASI students had never had a spontaneous panic, and that 50% had had neither a spontaneous nor a cued panic attack (Cox, Endler, Norton, & Swinson, 1991). Of their high-ASI students, Asmundson and Norton (1993) found that 77% had never had a spontaneous panic and 42% had never had a cued panic. Taken together, these surveys indicate that concerns about the harmful implications of anxiety symptoms can emerge prior to the eruption of panic attacks.

Relevant to anxiety sensitivity's possible status as a vulnerability factor are biological challenge studies involving provocation of feared sensations in people varying in their levels of anxiety sensitivity. Rapee, Brown, Antony, and Barlow (1992) found that the ASI was the only significant predictor of fear triggered by either inhalation of 5.5% carbon dioxide or voluntary hyperventilation in patients with a range of anxiety disorders. If anxiety sensitivity is crucial for challenge-induced anxiety and panic, then psychiatrically healthy people who score high on the ASI should respond like panic patients to challenges that provoke intense bodily sensations.

Applying this strategy, Holloway and McNally (1987) had college students with either high or low ASI scores to hyperventilate for 5 minutes. They found that those with high ASI scores reported more intense physical symptoms and more subjective anxiety than did those with low ASI scores. In a subsequent study, Donnell and McNally (1989) found that a history of spontaneous panic was not associated with an enhanced emotional response to hyperventilation unless the participant also had high anxiety sensitivity. Studies involving carbon dioxide (Eke & McNally, 1996; McNally & Eke, 1996) and caffeine (Telch, Silverman, & Schmidt, 1996) challenges have yielded similar findings.

Scores on the ASI are better predictors of response to challenge than are scores on measures of general trait anxiety (e.g., Eke & McNally, 1996). Rapee and Medoro (1994) conducted three studies showing that the ASI is a better predictor of an anxious response to challenge than is a measure of trait anxiety. That is, knowing that someone has a specific tendency to fear bodily sensations is more valuable in predicting his or her response to challenge than is knowing that he or she has a general proneness to experience anxiety (McNally, 1989).

Showing that high-ASI nonclinical participants respond more fearfully to biological challenges than do their low-ASI counterparts is consistent with the hypothesis that elevated anxiety sensitivity is a risk factor for panic attacks. But to clinch this assertion, investigators must use prospective longitudinal methods. In an early study, Maller and Reiss (1992) interviewed college graduates who had scored either high ($n = 23$) or low ($n = 25$) on the ASI 3 years previously. Three out of the four participants who experienced panic attacks for the first time during the follow-up period were from the high-ASI group.

Subsequent prospective studies have provided results consistent with those of Maller and Reiss (1992). Thus, the German translation of the ASI predicted the emergence of spontaneous panics among a group of nonclinical participants and patients with simple phobias in a 1-year follow-up study, whereas a measure of trait anxiety did not (Ehlers, 1995). In another study, four of six students who experienced spontaneous panics during the year following their participation in a challenge experiment had preexisting high ASI scores (Harrington, Schmidt, & Telch, 1996).

In a landmark study in psychopathology, Schmidt, Lerew, and Jackson (1997) assessed more than 1,000 cadets at the U.S. Air Force Academy before and after their highly stressful 5-week basic training program. Approximately 6% ($n = 74$) of the cadets reported a spontaneous panic during basic training, and of these cases, 34 had never experienced panic before. Schmidt et al. (1997) found that the ASI predicted panic even after they controlled for trait anxiety and a history of panic. Those subjects in the upper quartile of the ASI were twice as likely to experience a panic during basic training than were all other subjects. This research team has since replicated these findings in another cohort of more than 1,000 cadets (Schmidt, Lerew, & Jackson, 1999). ASI scores again predicted the incidence of spontaneous panic during basic training even after Schmidt et al. (1997) controlled for trait anxiety and a history of panic. Cadets scoring above the group median on the ASI were about three times as likely to experience panic as were those scoring below the median.

In summary, the studies by Schmidt et al. (1997, 1999) indicate that anxiety sensitivity is a vulnerability factor for the development of spontaneous panic attacks. It remains to be seen whether elevated ASI scores will predict the development of panic *disorder* as well (Schmidt, 1999).

In addition to studying aberrant cognition via self-report questionnaires, such as the ASI, researchers have increasingly applied the methods of cognitive psychology to elucidate information-processing abnormalities in panic and other anxiety disorders (McNally, 1994, pp. 123–136; McNally, 1996; Williams, Watts, MacLeod, & Mathews, 1997). Most experiments identifying attentional, memory, and interpretive biases favoring the processing of threatening information in people with high anxiety sensitivity have been done on patients with panic disorder (McNally, 1999b). Are such biases evident in people at risk for panic disorder? To address this issue, Stewart, Conrod, Gignac, and Pihl (1998) conducted two emotional Stroop experiments involving nonclinical subjects who scored either low or high on the ASI. In their first experiment, male high-ASI subjects exhibited enhanced Stroop interference only for words related to social threat (e.g., *embarrass*), whereas female high-ASI subjects exhibited interference only for words related to physical threat (e.g., *suffocated*). However, many of Stewart et al.'s (1998) high-ASI subjects had experienced panic attacks before, and therefore it is unclear whether they would have obtained similar results with high-ASI subjects with no experience with panic. Using regression analyses on nonclinical subjects who had never panicked, McNally, Hornig, Hoffman, and Han (1999) found scant evidence that ASI scores predicted interpretive bias favoring threat and no evidence of any attentional or memory biases favoring threat. In summary, it is possible that cognitive risk for panic is expressed only on self-report measures, such as the ASI, that tap explicit concerns about anxiety symptoms, whereas relatively automatic biases as studied in the laboratory may only emerge concurrent with the disorder itself.

Genetics

Several lines of evidence suggest a genetic vulnerability for panic disorder. Reviewing this literature, Smoller and Tsuang (1998) cite eight studies indicating that panic disorder runs in families (e.g., Crowe, Noyes, Pauls, & Slymen, 1983; Fyer et al., 1996; Noyes et al., 1986). First-degree relatives of a proband with panic disorder are 3 to 21 times more likely to develop the disorder than are first-degree relatives of healthy probands (Smoller & Tsuang, 1998). For example, one research group reported morbidity risks for panic disorder and probable panic disorder of 17.3% and 7.4%, respectively, among the first-degree relatives of 41 panic disorder probands (Crowe et al., 1983). The morbidity risks for panic disorder and probable panic disorder were only 1.8% and 0.4%, respectively, among the first-degree relatives of 41 healthy probands. These data strongly implicate genetic transmission of vulnerability to panic.

Twin studies can provide further evidence of genetic influence. Studying psychiatric patients, Torgersen (1983) interviewed 32 monozygotic (MZ) and 53 same-sex dizygotic (DZ) twin pairs in Norway. When he collapsed cases of infrequent panic, panic disorder, and agoraphobia with panic attacks into a single category, Torgersen (1983) found significantly higher concordance rates for MZ twins than for DZ twins (31% vs. 0%). In an attempt to disentangle the influence of shared rearing environment from shared genes, he examined the relation between concordance and subject-rated similarity in childhood environment. There was no relation between similarity in childhood environment and concordance for panic. This suggests that psychiatric similarity between cotwins was a function of shared genes not shared environments.

More recently, Perna, Caldirola, Arancio, and Bellodi (1997) reported a much higher concordance rate for panic disorder in MZ cotwins relative to DZ cotwins (73% vs. 0%) in participants recruited from the community. Perna et al. (1997), however, reported no difference in concordance rates for sporadic panic attacks (MZ: 57% vs. DZ: 43%). These data suggest possibility genetic heterogeneity in the panic attack phenotype.

Kendler, Neale, Kessler, Heath, and Eaves (1993) conducted a population-based study of 2,163 women from a Virginia twin registry. Social workers interviewed the participants, and Kendler blindly reviewed the structured interview data and assigned his "clinician diagnosis." The same data were submitted to a DSM-III-R computer algorithm, yielding a "computer diagnosis."

Kendler et al. (1993) found that probandwise concordance rates for definite and definite plus probable panic disorder differed for the clinician versus computer diagnoses. When Kendler made the diagnoses, the concordance rate for MZ twins was about twice as great as that for DZ twins (23.9% vs. 10.9%). When the computer made the diagnoses, the concordance rates were nearly identical (MZ: 15.5% vs. DZ: 14.6%). The reason for this discrepancy is not entirely clear, but it appears that concordance rates seem higher when twins are drawn from the general population rather than from the clinic (but see Perna et al., 1997).

In addition to computing concordance rates, Kendler et al. (1993) parsed the variance in panic disorder liability into that attributed to genetic variance (i.e., heritability), to shared nongenetic (i.e., environmental) variance, and to nonshared nongenetic variance (i.e., specific environmental events experienced by one twin but not by her cotwin). Again, the results varied depending on whether diagnoses were based on Kendler's judgment or on the computer algorithm. The model that best fit the clinician diagnoses indicated that liability for panic disorder was attributable solely to genetic variance (46%) plus nonshared nongenetic variance (54%). In striking contrast, the model that best fit the computer diagnoses indicated that liability was attributable solely to shared (32%) and nonshared (68%) nongenetic variance. Therefore, estimates of the heritability of panic disorder ranged from 46% to 0% depending on whether diagnoses relied on the clinician or computer.

Although the data have sometimes been mixed, most studies point to a heritable contribution to vulnerability for panic disorder. Recent innovative studies have clarified this further. Inspired by Klein's (1993) suffocation false alarm theory of panic disorder, Perna and his colleagues have used carbon dioxide challenges to test hypotheses about genetically transmitted abnormalities in respiratory function that may constitute vulnerability for panic. They found that rates of panic provoked by inhalation of 35% carbon dioxide are higher in healthy first-degree relatives of probands with panic disorder (22%) than in first-degree relatives of healthy controls (2%) (Perna, Cocchi, Bertani, Arancio, & Bellodi, 1995) and that the morbidity risk for panic disorder is higher in families whose panic proband panicked in response to carbon dioxide inhalation than in families whose panic proband did not panic in response to carbon dioxide challenge (Perna, Bertani, Caldirola, & Bellodi, 1996). Studying 90 twins recruited from the general population, Bellodi et al. (1998) reported higher probandwise concordance rates for carbon-dioxide-induced panic in MZ than in DZ twins (55.6% vs. 12.5%).

Bellodi et al. (1998) speculated about the possible genetic basis for vulnerability to carbon-dioxide-induced panic. They noted that there is evidence for genetic influence on carbon dioxide chemosensitivity, emphasizing that panic might arise because of respiratory dysfunction traceable to genetic influence. Another possibility is that genetic influences on vulnerability to panic are mediated by anxiety sensitivity (Stein, Jang, & Livesley, 1999). Although familial vulnerability to panic has most often been interpreted as inheritance of a physiological risk factor (e.g., abnormality in the respiratory system), it is possible that heritable influence on anxiety sensitivity may be relevant. Stein et al. (1999) had 179 MZ and 158 DZ twin pairs complete the ASI. Their model-fitting analyses yielded a heritability of 45% for the total ASI score, and heritabilities of 35%, 0%, and 22% for the physical, psychological, and social factors of the ASI, respectively. The remaining variance was attributable to nonshared environmental variance (55%) for the total ASI, for the physical factor (65%), and for the social factor (78%). Variance on the psychological factor was attributable to common environmental variance (11%) and nonshared environmental variance (89%).

In a subsequent analysis of this data set, these researchers tested for gender differences in the heritability of anxiety sensitivity (Jang, Stein, Taylor, & Livesley, 1999). Strikingly, they found that ASI scores were heritable in women but not in men. In women, the heritabilities of the ASI total score, physical concerns, psychological concerns, and social concerns were 49%, 48%, 33%, and 37%, respectively. Nonshared environment accounted for the remaining variance among female subjects. In men, slightly under half the variance was attributable to shared environment, whereas unshared environment accounted for the rest for the total ASI score and the three factor scores. Thus, the heritability of anxiety sensitivity in men was estimated at zero.

Summary

Research on vulnerability for panic disorder suggests several conclusions. First, studies on anxiety sensitivity implicate the fear of bodily sensations as a risk factor for panic attacks and perhaps panic disorder. Second, evidence for other cognitive risk factors is scant and mixed. Third, panic disorder is heritable. Both physiological and cognitive variables are characterized by impressive estimates of heritability.

POSTTRAUMATIC STRESS DISORDER

PTSD follows exposure to (typically) a horrific, life-threatening event (e.g., combat and rape). Its characteristic symptoms comprise reexperiencing the traumatic event (rather than merely remembering it) in the form of nightmares, intrusive thoughts, and physiological reactions to reminders of the trauma. PTSD sufferers will report avoidance of stimuli associated with event and report emotional numbing. They will experience symptoms of hyperarousal such as enhanced startle, irritability, and sleep disturbance.

Exposure to traumatic events is required for a diagnosis of PTSD. Accordingly, vulnerability for PTSD would be increased in people who are prone to get in harm's way, thereby sustaining exposure to events that can incite the syndrome. Studying community participants in metropolitan Detroit, Breslau, Davis, Andreski, and Peterson (1991) found that (retrospectively identified) risk factors for exposure to such events included male sex, extraversion, neuroticism, having less than a college education, a history of childhood conduct problems, and a family history of psychiatric disorder (Breslau et al., 1991). In a subsequent 3-year prospective study, this research team found that extraversion and neuroticism predicted exposure to traumatic events, whereas childhood history of conduct disorder and family history of psychiatric disorder did not (Breslau, Davis, & Andreski, 1995). Blacks had a higher rate of exposure than whites, and being male and having less than a college education marginally predicted exposure.

High-magnitude stressors vary in their capacity to produce PTSD. Epidemiological data indicate that rape is the most consistently traumatogenic high-magnitude stressor. In Breslau et al.'s (1991) study, 1.6% of the women had been raped, and 80% of them qualified for a lifetime diagnosis of PTSD. Other high-magnitude events produced PTSD at much lower rates. For example, only 22.6% of those who had been nonsexually assaulted developed PTSD, and only 24% of those who had been exposed to other life-threatening events did so.

The NCS also confirmed rape as the most consistently traumatic stressor (Kessler et al., 1995). Both men and women who had been raped cited it as the most distressing thing that had ever happened to them; 9.2% of the women and 0.7% of the men had suffered this trauma. Among rape victims, 65% of the men and 45.9% of the women had developed PTSD. Among people diagnosed with PTSD, the NCS researchers determined what traumatic events were most often responsible. For women with PTSD, 29.9% developed it after rape, and for men with PTSD, 28.8% developed it after combat.

Contrary to DSM-III's implication that highly traumatic stressors are rare events that occur outside the bounds of ordinary experience, recent epidemiological studies indicate the opposite. Nearly 40% of Breslau et al.'s (1991) sample had been exposed to highly traumatic events, and 60.7% of the men and 51.2% of the women in the NCS study had been similarly exposed (Kessler et al., 1995), as were 93% of the community sample in the DSM-IV PTSD field trial (Kilpatrick et al., 1991). Although these data strongly indicate that extreme stressors are far from rare, they also indicate that traumatic exposure is insufficient to produce PTSD. Indeed, the percentages of trauma-exposed people who developed the disorder are not especially high. Thus, among trauma-exposed people in Breslau et al.'s (1991) study, only 23.6% developed PTSD. Likewise, rates of PTSD in trauma-exposed men and women in the NCS were only 8.2% and 20.4%, respectively (Kessler et al., 1995). Only 10.3% of the community respondents in the DSM-IV field trial developed the disorder (Kilpatrick et al., 1991). These findings strongly indicate that individual difference variables strongly influence which trauma-exposed people develop PTSD.

Most recently, Breslau et al. (1998) surveyed Detroit-area community participants about their history of exposure to traumatic events and about any PTSD symptoms in response to them. They found that the conditional risk of developing PTSD given exposure to a qualifying traumatic event was only 9.2% The conditional probability of developing PTSD was highest after exposure to assaultive violence (20.9%). However, the largest proportion of PTSD cases in the community (31% of the total) followed the unexpected death of a loved one, an event experienced by 60% of the sample.

The realization that only a minority of people exposed to extreme stressors develop PTSD has prompted research into risk factors among those who have been exposed to high-magnitude stressors. Risk factors include female sex (e.g., Breslau et al., 1991; Kessler et al., 1995); neuroticism (e.g., Breslau et al., 1991); low social support (e.g., Boscarino, 1995); lower IQ (Macklin et al., 1998; McNally & Shin, 1995); preexisting psychiatric illness, especially mood and anxiety disorders (e.g., Breslau et al., 1991; Smith, North, McCool, & Shea, 1990); having a parent who survived the Holocaust (Solomon, Kotler, & Mikulincer, 1988; Yehuda, Schmeidler, Wainberg, Binder-Brynes, & Duvdevani, 1998); childhood physical (Bremner, Southwick, Johnson, Yehuda, & Charney, 1993) or sexual (Engel et al., 1993) abuse; childhood separation from parents (Breslau et al., 1991); a family history of mood, anxiety, or substance abuse disorders (Breslau et al., 1991); premilitary traumatic events (King, King, Foy, & Gudanowski, 1996); and family instability (King et al., 1996).

A different approach to identifying vulnerability is to examine what immediate and short-term responses to traumatic events predict subsequent PTSD. Retrospective studies suggest that peritraumatic dissociation (i.e., occurring at the time of the event) predicts later PTSD (Bremner et al., 1992; Marmar et al., 1994). That is, people who felt disconnected from their bodies, felt that events were happening in slow motion, and so on were especially likely to develop PTSD later. A prospective study of civilian trauma survivors of car accidents, terrorist attacks, and similar events in Israel confirmed these results (Shalev, Peri, Canetti, & Schreiber, 1996). Peritraumatic dissociation, mainly time distortion and derealization, predicted PTSD onset 6 months posttrauma even when Shalev et al. (1996) controlled for the intensity of other peritraumatic responses.

Studying car accident survivors, Harvey and Bryant (1998) found that 78% of participants who met criteria for acute stress disorder (ASD) subsequently developed PTSD. Item analyses of ASD symptoms indicated that acute numbing, depersonalization, a sense of reliving the event, and motor restlessness were strong predictors of PTSD 6 months postaccident.

Studying civilian trauma survivors, Shalev et al. (1998) reported that elevated heart rate shortly after the traumatic event predicted subsequent development of PTSD. The patients who later developed PTSD had a mean heart rate of 95.5 beats per minute, whereas those who did not develop PTSD had a mean heart rate of 83.3 beats per minute.

True et al. (1993) studied 4,042 Vietnam-era veteran MZ and DZ twin pairs to ascertain the contribution of genetic and environmental variance on liability for 15 PTSD symptoms. They found that heritabilities ranged from 13% to 30% for symptoms in the reexperiencing cluster, from 30% to 34% for symptoms in the avoidance cluster, and from 28% to 32% in the arousal cluster. There was no evidence that shared environment contributed to cotwin similarity in PTSD symptoms.

Summary

Vulnerability research on PTSD suggests several conclusions. First, scholars have separately identified risk factors for exposure to traumatic events and risk factors for developing PTSD in those so exposed. Second, identification of risk factors in most studies has been retrospective, although prospective studies have finally begun to appear. Third, trauma studies are currently undergoing a major shift in emphasis from investigation of the pathogenic properties of events themselves to investigation of vulnerability factors that render some people more susceptible than others to develop PTSD.

OBSESSIVE–COMPULSIVE DISORDER

People with OCD experience recurrent, intrusive thoughts, images, or impulses that increase anxiety or distress (i.e., obsessions), and they perform repetitive thoughts or actions to attenuate the distress associated with the obsessions (i.e., compulsions). The disorder usually begins gradually with modal age of onset between the ages of 6 and 15 years for males and between the ages 20 and 29 for females (American Psychiatric Association, 1994, p. 420). Men and women are affected equally. Estimates of prevalence vary. The Epidemiologic Catchment Area (ECA) survey revealed a lifetime prevalence rate of 2.6% (Karno & Golding, 1991). Oddly, 53% of those with OCD reported only compulsions, whereas only 9% reported both obsessions and compulsions as is typical in most clinical samples. The 1-month prevalence rate for OCD in the ECA survey was 1.33%. In an epidemiological study in Canada (Stein, Forde, Anderson, & Walker, 1997), the 1-month prevalence rate was 3.1% when assessed by lay interviewers (as was done in the ECA study) but only 0.6% when clinical interviewers reassessed these respondents. OCD was not assessed in the NCS.

Data relevant to vulnerability are chiefly confined to genetics. Reviewing the literature on twins with OCD, Tallis (1995, pp. 39–41) concluded that concordance rates for MZ twins are higher than for DZ twins. For example, Carey and Gottesman (1981) reported concordance rates of 87% and 47% for MZ and DZ twin pairs, respectively, drawn from the Maudsley twin register.

It is unclear, however, whether a specific vulnerability for OCD is transmitted or whether a general proneness for anxiety disorders constitutes the vulnerability. Black and his colleagues blindly interviewed first-degree relatives of 32 probands with OCD and first-degree relatives of 33 healthy controls (Black, Noyes, Goldstein, & Blum, 1992). They found that the morbidity risk for anxiety disorders in general was elevated among the relatives of OCD probands relative to the relatives of control probands, but the specific risk for OCD was not. The only evidence pointing to transmission of OCD per se was that parents of OCD probands were more likely than parents of controls (16% vs. 3%) to exhibit either OCD or subclinical OCD.

Clinicians have speculated about possible psychological vulnerability factors for OCD. Most of this theorizing has been based on observations of people who already have the disorder; prospective longitudinal studies on the development of OCD in adulthood are nonexistent. Rachman (1997), for example, has suggested that premorbid high moral standards, tendencies to misinterpret the significance of one's thoughts as in thought/action fusion (i.e., thinking a bad thought is morally equivalent to bad action), depressed mood (e.g., Ricciardi & McNally, 1995), and exaggerated sense of personal responsibility (e.g., Salkovskis, 1985, 1999) may render people vulnerable to OCD.

Summary

Few firm conclusions can be culled from OCD vulnerability research. First, it is unclear whether genetic factors increase specific risk for OCD or whether they predispose people to develop anxiety syndromes in general. Second, an upsurge in theoretical work on pathogenic beliefs linked to OCD promises to provide clues to cognitive risk factors.

CONCLUSIONS

The search for vulnerability factors for adult anxiety disorders is likely to continue to occur at multiple levels of analysis: genetic, cognitive, and social. Students of panic disorder, OCD, and PTSD will further explore the possibility that certain cognitive factors, especially pathogenic beliefs, may predispose people to develop specific syndromes. Some variables, such as anxiety sensitivity, may be relatively specific for panic disorder, whereas others, such as excessive responsibility, may be relatively specific for OCD. Further work will clarify these matters. The chief challenge will be to identify relevant participants premorbidly and to test hypotheses about risk prospectively.

A major shift in genetic vulnerability research is likely to occur within the next few years. Most extant studies have tested for a heritable component to liability. But merely demonstrating that a condition is heritable provides no clues as to the location of "aberrant" alleles associated with disorder liability. Advances in basic science will prompt a shift from mathematical to molecular methods, thereby enabling scientists to identify risk factors at the level of DNA (Faraone, Tsuang, & Tsuang, 1999).

The study of vulnerability has both honorable and ominous aspects. In addition to deepening our understanding regarding causation, such knowledge satisfies our scientific curiosity. Moreover, to the extent that we can identify people at risk, we may be able to take steps to prevent the full-blown emergence of these syndromes. But there are ominous implications, too (Hubbard & Wald, 1993). Employers, insurance companies, and other third parties have a vested interest in identifying people who may be vulnerable to developing anxiety disorders. For example, might employers insist on obtaining information about risk factors for psychopathology (e.g., having a parent with panic disorder) before interviewing job applicants? Might insurance companies use such information to exclude individuals from coverage?

Events of the summer of 1999 have revealed yet another ominous twist to the study of vulnerability. In a historically unprecedented move, the U.S. Congress voted unanimously 355 to 0 (13 abstentions) to condemn and denounce conclusions expressed by the authors of a meta-analysis published in *Psychological Bulletin* (Rind, Tromovitch, & Bauserman, 1998). The purpose of this meta-analysis was to test whether a self-reported history of childhood sexual abuse (CSA) constituted a vulnerability factor for subsequent psychopathology among college students. The authors reported that less than 1% of the variance in mental health outcomes was attributable to a self-reported history of CSA. They concluded that clinicians have overestimated the traumatogenic impact of CSA, thereby inciting Congress to condemn their study as "severely flawed" and as providing "information endangering children" (U.S. House of Representatives, 1999). In response to the congressional uproar, the American Psychological Association for the first time sought an independent critique of an article published in one of its journals, conceding that "we must take into account not only the scientific merit of articles but also their implications for public policy."

It remains to be seen whether scientists will be able to publish findings concerning vulnerability for psychiatric disorder if the data run counter to prevailing public opinion.

REFERENCES

American Psychiatric Association. (1980). *Diagnostic and statistical manual of mental disorders* (3rd ed.). Washington, DC: Author.

American Psychiatric Association. (1994). *Diagnostic and statistical manual of mental disorders* (4th ed.). Washington, DC: Author.

Asmundson, G. J. G., & Norton, G. R. (1993). Anxiety sensitivity and its relationship to spontaneous and cued panic attacks in college students. *Behaviour Research and Therapy, 31,* 199–201.

Bellodi, L., Perna, G., Caldirola, D., Arancio, C., Bertani, A., & Di Bella, D. (1998). CO_2-induced panic attacks: A twin study. *American Journal of Psychiatry, 155,* 1184–1188.

Black, D. W., Noyes, R., Jr., Goldstein, R. B., & Blum, N. (1992). A family study of obsessive–compulsive disorder. *Archives of General Psychiatry, 49,* 362–368.

Boscarino, J. A. (1995). Post-traumatic stress and associated disorders among Vietnam veterans: The significance of combat exposure and social support. *Journal of Traumatic Stress, 8,* 317–336.

Bowman, M. L. (1999). Individual differences in posttraumatic distress: Problems with the DSM-IV model. *Canadian Journal of Psychiatry, 44,* 21–33.

Bremner, J. D., Southwick, S. M., Brett, E., Fontana, A., Rosenheck, R., & Charney, D. S. (1992). Dissociation and posttraumatic stress disorder in Vietnam combat veterans. *American Journal of Psychiatry, 149,* 328–332.

Bremner, J. D., Southwick, S. M., Johnson, D. R., Yehuda, R., & Charney, D. S. (1993). Childhood physical abuse and combat-related posttraumatic stress disorder in Vietnam veterans. *American Journal of Psychiatry, 150,* 235–239.

Breslau, N., Davis, G. C., & Andreski, P. (1995). Risk factors for PTSD-related traumatic events: A prospective analysis. *American Journal of Psychiatry, 152,* 529–535.

Breslau, N., Davis, G. C., Andreski, P., & Peterson, E. (1991). Traumatic events and posttraumatic stress disorder in an urban population of young adults. *Archives of General Psychiatry, 48,* 216–222.

Breslau, N., Kessler, R. C., Chilcoat, H. D., Schultz, L. R., Davis, G. C., & Andreski, P. (1998). Trauma and posttraumatic stress disorder in the community: The 1996 Detroit Area Survey of Trauma. *Archives of General Psychiatry, 55,* 626–632.

Carey, G., & Gottesman, I. I. (1981). Twin and family studies of anxiety, phobic, and obsessive disorders. In D. F. Klein & J. G. Rabkin (Eds.), *Anxiety: New research and changing concepts* (pp. 117–136). New York: Raven Press.

Cox, B. J., Endler, N. S., Norton, G. R., & Swinson, R. P. (1991). Anxiety sensitivity and nonclinical panic attacks. *Behaviour Research and Therapy, 29,* 367–369.

Crowe, R. R., Noyes, R., Pauls, D. L., & Slymen, D. (1983). A family study of panic disorder. *Archives of General Psychiatry, 40,* 1065–1069.

Donnell, C. D., & McNally, R. J. (1989). Anxiety sensitivity and history of panic as predictors of response to hyperventilation. *Behaviour Research and Therapy, 27,* 325–332.

Donnell, C. D., & McNally, R. J. (1990). Anxiety sensitivity and panic attacks in a nonclinical population. *Behaviour Research and Therapy, 28,* 83–85.

Eaton, W. W., Kessler, R. C., Wittchen, H. U., & Magee, W. J. (1994). Panic and panic disorder in the United States. *American Journal of Psychiatry, 151,* 413–420.

Ehlers, A. (1995). A 1-year prospective study of panic attacks: Clinical course and factors associated with maintenance. *Journal of Abnormal Psychology, 104,* 164–172.

Eke, M., & McNally, R. J. (1996). Anxiety sensitivity, suffocation fear, trait anxiety, and breath-holding duration as predictors of response to carbon dioxide challenge. *Behaviour Research and Therapy, 34,* 603–607.

Engel, C. C., Jr., Engel, A. L., Campbell, S. J., McFall, M. E., Russo, J., & Katon, W. (1993). Posttraumatic stress disorder symptoms and precombat sexual and physical abuse in Desert Storm veterans. *Journal of Nervous and Mental Disease, 181,* 683–688.

Eysenck, H. J., & Rachman, S. (1965). *The causes and cures of neurosis.* San Diego, CA: Knapp.

Faraone, S. V., Tsuang, M. T., & Tsuang, D. W. (1999). *Genetics of mental disorders: A guide for students, clinicians, and researchers.* New York: Guilford Press.

Fyer, A., Mannuzza, S., Chapman, T., Lipsitz, J., Martin, L. Y., & Klein, D. F. (1996). Panic disorder and social phobia: Effects of comorbidity on the familial transmission. *Anxiety, 2,* 173–178.

Harrington, P. H., Schmidt, N. B., & Telch, M. J. (1996). Prospective evaluation of panic potentiation following 35% CO_2 challenge in a nonclinical sample. *American Journal of Psychiatry, 153,* 823–825.

Harvey, A. G., & Bryant, R. A. (1998). The relationship between acute stress disorder and posttraumatic stress disorder: A prospective evaluation of motor vehicle accident survivors. *Journal of Consulting and Clinical Psychology, 66,* 507–512.

Holloway, W., & McNally, R. J. (1987). Effects of anxiety sensitivity on the response to hyperventilation. *Journal of Abnormal Psychology, 96,* 330–334.

Hubbard, R., & Wald, E. (1993). *Exploding the gene myth.* Boston: Beacon Press.

Jang, K. L., Stein, M. B., Taylor, S., & Livesley, W. J. (1999). Gender differences in the etiology of anxiety sensitivity: A twin study. *Journal of Gender-Specific Medicine, 2,* 39–44.

Karno, M., & Golding, J. M. (1991). Obsessive compulsive disorder. In L. N. Robins & D. A. Regier (Eds.), *Psychiatric disorders in America* (pp. 204–219). New York: Free Press.

Kendler, K. S., Neale, M. C., Kessler, R. C., Heath, A. C., & Eaves, L. J. (1993).

Panic disorder in women: A population-based twin study. *Psychological Medicine, 23,* 397–406.

Kessler, R. C., Sonnega, A., Bromet, E., Hughes, M., & Nelson, C. B. (1995). Posttraumatic stress disorder in the National Comorbidity Survey. *Archives of General Psychiatry, 52,* 1048–1060.

Kilpatrick, D. G., Resnick, H. S., Freedy, J. R., Pelcovitz, D., Resick, P., Roth, S., & van der Kolk, B. (1991). *Report of findings from the DSM-IV PTSD field trial: Emphasis on Criterion A and overall PTSD diagnosis.* Paper written for the DSM-IV Workgroup on PTSD.

King, D. W., King, L. A., Foy, D. W., & Gudanowski, D. M. (1996). Prewar factors in combat-related posttraumatic stress disorder: Structural equation modeling with a national sample of female and male Vietnam veterans. *Journal of Consulting and Clinical Psychology, 64,* 520–531.

Klein, D. F. (1993). False suffocation alarms, spontaneous panics, and related conditions: An integrative hypothesis. *Archives of General Psychiatry, 50,* 306–317.

Macklin, M. L., Metzger, L. J., Litz, B. T., McNally, R. J., Lasko, N. B., Orr, S. P., & Pitman, R. K. (1998). *Journal of Consulting and Clinical Psychology, 66,* 323–326.

Maller, R. G., & Reiss, S. (1992). Anxiety sensitivity in 1984 and panic attacks in 1987. *Journal of Anxiety Disorders, 6,* 241–247.

Marmar, C. R., Weiss, D. S., Schlenger, W. E., Fairbank, J. A., Jordan, B. K., Kulka, R. A., & Hough, R. L. (1994). Peritraumatic dissociation and posttraumatic stress in male Vietnam theater veterans. *American Journal of Psychiatry, 151,* 902–907.

McNally, R. J. (1989). Is anxiety sensitivity distinguishable from trait anxiety? A reply to Lilienfeld, Jacob, and Turner (1989). *Journal of Abnormal Psychology, 98,* 193–194.

McNally, R. J. (1994). *Panic disorder: A critical analysis.* New York: Guilford Press.

McNally, R. J. (1996). Cognitive bias in the anxiety disorders. *Nebraska Symposium on Motivation, 43,* 211–250.

McNally, R. J. (1999a). Posttraumatic stress disorder. In T. Millon, P. H. Blaney, & R. D. Davis (Eds.), *Oxford textbook of psychopathology* (pp. 144–165). Oxford, UK: Oxford University Press.

McNally, R. J. (1999b). Anxiety sensitivity and information-processing biases for threat. In S. Taylor (Ed.), *Anxiety sensitivity: Theory, research, and treatment of the fear of anxiety* (pp. 183–197). Mahwah, NJ: Erlbaum.

McNally, R. J., & Eke, M. (1996). Anxiety sensitivity, suffocation fear, and breath-holding duration as predictors of response to carbon dioxide challenge. *Journal of Abnormal Psychology, 105,* 146–149.

McNally, R. J., Hornig, C. D., Hoffman, E. C., & Han, E. M. (1999). Anxiety sensitivity and cognitive biases for threat. *Behavior Therapy, 30,* 51–61.

McNally, R. J., & Lorenz, M. (1987). Anxiety sensitivity in agoraphobics. *Journal of Behavior Therapy and Experimental Psychiatry, 18,* 3–11.

McNally, R. J., & Shin, L. M. (1995). Association of intelligence with severity of posttraumatic stress disorder symptoms in Vietnam combat veterans. *American Journal of Psychiatry, 152,* 936–938.

Noyes, R., Jr., Crowe, R. R., Harris, E. L., Hamra, B. J., McChesney, C. M., & Chaudhry, D. R. (1986). Relationship between panic disorder and agoraphobia: A family study. *Archives of General Psychiatry, 43,* 227–232.

Öst, L.-G. (1987). Age of onset in different phobias. *Journal of Abnormal Psychology, 96,* 223–229.

Perna, G., Bertani, A., Caldirola, D., & Bellodi, L. (1996). Family history of panic disorder and hypersensitivity to CO_2 in patients with panic disorder. *American Journal of Psychiatry, 153,* 1060–1064.

Perna, G., Caldirola, D., Arancio, C., & Bellodi, L. (1997). Panic attacks: A twin study. *Psychiatry Research, 66,* 69–71.

Perna, G., Cocchi, S., Bertani, A., Arancio, C., & Bellodi, L. (1995). Sensitivity to 35% CO_2 healthy first-degree relatives of patients with panic disorder. *American Journal of Psychiatry, 152,* 623–625.

Rachman, S. (1997). A cognitive theory of obsessions. *Behaviour Research and Therapy, 35,* 793–802.

Rapee, R. M. (1991). Generalized anxiety disorder: A review of clinical features and theoretical concepts. *Clinical Psychology Review, 11,* 419–440.

Rapee, R. M. (1995). Descriptive psychopathology of social phobia. In R. G. Heimberg, M. R. Liebowitz, D. A. Hope, & F. R. Schneier (Eds.), *Social phobia: Diagnosis, assessment, and treatment* (pp. 41–66). New York: Guilford Press.

Rapee, R. M., Brown, T. A., Antony, M. M., & Barlow, D. H. (1992). Response to hyperventilation and inhalation of 5.5% carbon dioxide-enriched air across the *DSM-III-R* anxiety disorders. *Journal of Abnormal Psychology, 101,* 538–552.

Rapee, R. M., & Medoro, L. (1994). Fear of physical sensations and trait anxiety as mediators of the response to hyperventilation in nonclinical subjects. *Journal of Abnormal Psychology, 103,* 693–699.

Reiss, S., & McNally, R. J. (1985). Expectancy model of fear. In S. Reiss & R. R. Bootzin (Eds.), *Theoretical issues in behavior therapy* (pp. 107–121). San Diego, CA: Academic Press.

Reiss, S., Peterson, R. A., Gursky, D. M., & McNally, R. J. (1986). Anxiety sensitivity, anxiety frequency and the prediction of fearfulness. *Behaviour Research and Therapy, 24,* 1–8.

Ricciardi, J. N., & McNally, R. J. (1995). Depression is related to obsessions, not to compulsions, in obsessive–compulsive disorder. *Journal of Anxiety Disorders, 9,* 249–256.

Rind, B., Tromovitch, P., & Bauserman, R. (1998). A meta-analytic examination of assumed properties of child sexual abuse using college samples. *Psychological Bulletin, 124,* 22–53.

Salkovskis, P. M. (1985). Obsessional–compulsive problems: A cognitive-behavioural analysis. *Behaviour Research and Therapy, 25,* 571–583.

Salkovskis, P. M. (1999). Understanding and treating obsessive–compulsive disorder. *Behaviour Research and Therapy, 37*(Suppl. 1), S29–S52.

Schmidt, N. B. (1999). Prospective evaluations of anxiety sensitivity. In S. Taylor (Ed.), *Anxiety sensitivity: Theory, research, and treatment of the fear of anxiety* (pp. 217–235). Mahwah, NJ: Erlbaum.

Schmidt, N. B., Lerew, D. R., & Jackson, R. J. (1997). The role of anxiety sensitivity in the pathogenesis of panic: Prospective evaluation of spontaneous panic attacks during acute stress. *Journal of Abnormal Psychology, 106,* 355–364.

Schmidt, N. B., Lerew, D. R., & Jackson, R. J. (1999). Prospective evaluation of anxiety sensitivity in the pathogenesis of panic: Replication and extension. *Journal of Abnormal Psychology, 108,* 532–537.

Shalev, A. Y., Peri, T., Canetti, L., & Schreiber, S. (1996). Predictors of PTSD in injured trauma survivors: A prospective study. *American Journal of Psychiatry, 153,* 219–225.

Shalev, A. Y., Sahar, T., Freedman, S., Peri, T., Glick, N., Brandes, D., Orr, S. P., & Pitman, R. K. (1998). A prospective study of heart rate response following trauma and the subsequent development of posttraumatic stress disorder. *Archives of General Psychiatry, 55,* 553–559.

Smith, E. M., North, C. S., McCool, R. E., & Shea, J. M. (1990). Acute postdisaster psychiatric disorders: Identification of persons at risk. *American Journal of Psychiatry, 147,* 202–206.

Smoller, J. W., & Tsuang, M. T. (1998). Panic and phobic anxiety: Defining phenotypes for genetic studies. *American Journal of Psychiatry, 155,* 1152–1162.

Solomon, Z., Kotler, M., & Mikulincer, M. (1988). Combat-related posttraumatic stress disorder among second-generation Holocaust survivors: Preliminary findings. *American Journal of Psychiatry, 145,* 865–868.

Stein, M. B., Forde, D. R., Anderson, G., & Walker, J. R. (1997). Obsessive–compulsive disorder in the community: An epidemiologic survey with clinical reappraisal. *American Journal of Psychiatry, 154,* 1120–1126.

Stein, M. B., Jang, K. L., & Livesley, W. J. (1999). Heritability of anxiety sensitivity: A twin study. *American Journal of Psychiatry, 156,* 246–251.

Stewart, S. H., Conrod, P. J., Gignac, M. L., & Pihl, R. O. (1998). Selective processing biases in anxiety-sensitive men and women. *Cognition and Emotion, 12,* 105–133.

Tallis, F. (1995). *Obsessive–compulsive disorder: A cognitive and neuropsychological perspective.* Chichester, UK: Wiley.

Taylor, S., Koch, W. J., & McNally, R. J. (1992). How does anxiety sensitivity vary across the anxiety disorders? *Journal of Anxiety Disorders, 6,* 249–259.

Telch, M. J., Silverman, A., & Schmidt, N. B. (1996). Effects of anxiety sensitivity and perceived control on emotional responding to caffeine challenge. *Journal of Anxiety Disorders, 10,* 21–35.

Torgersen, S. (1983). Genetic factors in anxiety disorders. *Archives of General Psychiatry, 40,* 1085–1089.

True, W. R., Rice, J., Eisen, S. A., Heath, A. C., Goldberg, J., Lyons, M. J., & Nowak, J. (1993). A twin study of genetic and environmental contributions to liability for posttraumatic stress symptoms. *Archives of General Psychiatry, 50,* 257-264.

U.S. House of Representatives. (1999, July 12). *Concurrent resolution 107 of the 106th Congress.*

Williams, J. M. G., Watts, F. N., MacLeod, C., & Mathews, A. (1997). *Cognitive psychology and emotional disorders* (2nd ed.). Chichester, UK: Wiley.

Yehuda, R., & McFarlane, A. C. (1995). Conflict between current knowledge about posttraumatic stress disorder and its original conceptual basis. *American Journal of Psychiatry, 152,* 1705–1713.

Yehuda, R., Schmeidler, J., Wainberg, M., Binder-Brynes, K., & Duvdevani, T. (1998). Vulnerability to posttraumatic stress disorder in adult offspring of Holocaust survivors. *American Journal of Psychiatry, 155,* 1163–1171.

Young, A. (1995). *The harmony of illusions: Inventing post-traumatic stress disorder.* Princeton, NJ: Princeton University Press.

13

Vulnerability to Anxiety Disorders across the Lifespan

RICHARD J. McNALLY
VANESSA L. MALCARNE
INGUNN HANSDOTTIR

Kuhn (1962) famously proclaimed that a discipline must become paradigmatic if it is to enjoy normal scientific progress. Although this assertion has often been interpreted as a call for unification by those who bemoan psychology's fractured diversity (e.g., Staats, 1991), Kuhn's (1991) later work suggests another interpretation (McNally, 1992). Progress in any cultural endeavor, including science, reflects a process akin to biological speciation (Kuhn, 1991). Species that share a recent ancestor have more in common than those that share a distant ancestor. Likewise, as the tree of science branches outward, new limbs share increasingly fewer features, despite their arising from a common trunk. Progress means specialization, and specialization means that increasingly larger fragments of the field will become unfamiliar to its practitioners.

This has certainly happened in the field of psychopathology, whose conceptual and empirical terrain has become dauntingly vast. Even the most ambitious polymath would be incapable of mastering its plenitude today. Echoing the rest of abnormal psychology, the subfield of vulnerability studies has branched into two parallel tracks that rarely intersect: childhood and adulthood. Increased cross-fertilization between these two areas is needed for a more comprehensive and integrated perspective on vulnerability to psychopathology.

ESTABLISHING COMMON GROUND

In this brief chapter, we underscore several points that occurred to us after having read each other's individual contributions. First, vulnerability issues differ drastically across various syndromes. Some conditions rarely emerge in childhood (e.g., schizophrenia), others rarely emerge in adulthood (e.g., pervasive developmental disorders), and still others can emerge during any phase of life (e.g., major depressive disorder). So, whereas it makes sense to consider how the vulnerability picture changes as a function of development for depression, it does not hold for autistic disorder. Anxiety disorders are a mixed bag. For example, panic disorder rarely develops in children, animal phobias rarely begin in adulthood, but obsessive–compulsive disorder (OCD) can emerge in either childhood or adulthood. Questions of vulnerability for the anxiety disorders, then, partly depend on the particular anxiety syndrome under consideration.

Second, and closely related, questions of vulnerability for the anxiety disorders partly depend on what vulnerability processes or risk factors are being considered. For example, parenting behavior is almost exclusively studied as a risk factor for the development of anxiety disorders in childhood. Research on genetic factors has mostly focused on transmission of a behaviorally inhibited temperament; this may have greater relevance for anxiety disorders emerging early in childhood than for ones that largely appear in adolescence or adulthood. Suggestions that genetic heritability may represent a general diathesis for anxiety, with environmental risk factors (such as life events) representing the stress that activates a specific anxiety disorder, are sensible and suggest greater applicability to understanding anxiety disorders across the lifespan. However, these environmental risk factors have not been clearly identified, and their possible interactions with genetic predispositions are poorly understood. Moreover, genetically influenced personality variables may themselves affect exposure to these environmental stressors.

Third, some childhood syndromes may themselves constitute vulnerability conditions for adult syndromes. The suggestion that separation anxiety disorder increases risk for later panic disorder and agoraphobia would constitute such an example. Also, some childhood syndromes may be developmental variants of adult syndromes. Overanxious disorder of childhood appears to be an age variant of generalized anxiety disorder rather than a separate disorder and thus is now appropriately subsumed under generalized anxiety disorder in the fourth edition of the *Diagnostic and Statistical Manual of Mental Disorders* (DSM IV; American Psychiatric Association, 1994). Alternatively, some syndromes in adults, such as blood or animal phobia, may merely constitute a chronic condition that has never waned as the patient has grown into adulthood. Assuming discontinuity or dissimilarity between child and adult syndromes, based on what may be developmentally based or environmentally influenced variations in symptom expression, may obscure essential similarities in vulnerability processes.

Therefore, perhaps the most important lesson is that the childhood–adulthood distinction is arbitrary and unhelpful for understanding vulnerability for most anxiety disorders. Although there is tremendous overlap in many of the vulnerability processes considered in the adult and child anxiety literatures, these literatures seem to exist quite separately. This separation is no longer justified and, indeed, may impede progress in understanding vulnerability. It is likely more useful to ask, "What are the vulnerability factors for Syndrome X?" than to presuppose that different vulnerability factors account for its emergence in childhood and others for its emergence in adulthood. Overall, there may be more similarities than differences.

FUTURE DIRECTIONS FOR RESEARCH

Our reviews of the adult and child anxiety literatures underscore the need for lifespan research. The artificial separation between child and adult research investigating vulnerability to anxiety is no longer useful, if it ever was. A more sophisticated lifespan developmental perspective on the anxiety disorders is needed, one not limited to differentiating "child" versus "adult" risk factors. In addition to identifying risk factors for anxiety, research from such a perspective would include (1) consideration of when risk factors emerge, and within what biopsychosocial and developmental contexts, as well as (2) developmental variations and similarities in symptom expression.

Research to date has suggested a variety of potentially important risk factors for anxiety disorders, applicable throughout the lifespan. These can be broadly categorized as genetic, cognitive, and social/environmental. Research into genetic vulnerability has to date focused on uncovering evidence of heritability. Future research in genetic transmission needs to advance in two related directions. First, specific alleles associated with vulnerability to anxiety must be identified. Then, persons identified as genetically "at risk" for development of anxiety problems must be followed over time, from infancy to adulthood. This prospective longitudinal approach, although expensive and time-consuming, is essential if we are to understand how genetic risk is expressed throughout development. This approach is also essential to understanding how interactions of genetic risk with environmental exposure result in the development and expression of anxiety disorders.

A similar prospective longitudinal approach is needed for elucidating the role of cognitive and social/environmental variables in the development and maintenance of anxiety. Studies to date examining cognitive contributors to anxiety have suggested important roles of perceptions of control and a variety of negative cognitions including cognitive errors and pathogenic beliefs. These same variables have been identified as risk factors in both the child and adult literatures, although there may be developmental variations in their expression. However, whether these cognitions increase vulnerability to anxiety disorders or instead constitute emerging symptoms of those disorders remains unclear due to the paucity of prospective longitudinal studies.

Research on social/environmental risk factors for anxiety has focused on life events as risk factors for adult anxiety and parenting behavior and parent–child relationships as risk factors for child anxiety. Although this research has been successful in establishing the presence of adverse life events and disturbed parenting in the histories of a significant proportion of individuals with certain anxiety disorders, much of this research is retrospective. It is also problematic that in their studies on parental rearing practices, psychosocial researchers have rarely distinguished between shared environmental and shared genetic influences on childhood psychopathology. Also, findings to date, although limited, suggest that only a small proportion of individuals exposed to adverse life events or disturbed parenting actually develop anxiety disorders. Future research needs to expand beyond its current focus on risk factors to include identification and examination of protective factors as well.

Overall, it is clear that, despite the inherent difficulties in reconciling specialized research tracks, progress in understanding vulnerability to anxiety will be facilitated by a reintegration of child- and adult-oriented perspectives into a truly lifespan perspective on anxiety. Such a reintegration underscores the necessity of prospective long-term longitudinal research, following from childhood through adulthood persons determined to be "at risk" due to their exposure to identified risk factors. Only in this way can we characterize short- and long-term general and specific anxiety-related outcomes, and identify important interactions contributing to the emergency of anxiety disorders.

REFERENCES

American Psychiatric Association. (1994). *Diagnostic and statistical manual of mental disorders* (4th ed.). Washington, DC: Author.

Kuhn, T. S. (1962). *The structure of scientific revolutions*. Chicago: University of Chicago Press.

Kuhn, T. S. (1991, November). *The problem with the historical philosophy of science* (The Robert and Maurine Rothschild Distinguished Lecture). Address delivered in the History of Science Department, Harvard University, Cambridge, MA.

McNally, R. J. (1992). Disunity in psychology: Chaos or speciation? *American Psychologist, 47*, 1054.

Staats, A. W. (1991). Unified positivism and unification psychology: Fad or new field? *American Psychologist, 46*, 899–912.

SCHIZOPHRENIA

14

Vulnerability to Schizophrenia
*Risk Factors in Childhood
and Adolescence*

PATRICIA A. BRENNAN
ELAINE F. WALKER

Schizophrenia is a debilitating mental disorder that has posed formidable challenges to researchers. Despite decades of investigation, we have not yet identified any specific causal agent or pathophysiological process. Nonetheless, as empirical findings have accumulated, our conceptual framework about the etiology of schizophrenia has been modified to accommodate the data. As a result, contemporary theoretical models have become more complex and sophisticated and, it is hoped, more accurate.

In recent years, what has come to be known as the "neurodevelopmental" perspective has played a central role in theorizing about the etiology of schizophrenia (Waddington & Buckley, 1996). Historical roots for contemporary neurodevelopmental models can be found in Meehl's (1962) diathesis–stress model, which suggested an interaction between genetically based brain aberrations and noxious environmental events as the basis for the eventual outcome of schizophrenia. The accumulation of empirical data linking obstetrical complications with schizophrenia narrowed the focus on early brain development as a critical period. The central premise of current neurodevelopmental theories is that vulnerability for schizophrenia is acquired early in life and involves an aberration in the development of the central nervous system (Mednick & Hollister, 1995; Walker & Neumann, 1996). The neurodevelopmental abnormalities are assumed to arise from obstetrical complications and/or genetic predispositions. It is also assumed that the brain abnormalities observed in patients with schizophrenia reflect these early developmental deviations.

The neurodevelopmental perspective is often contrasted with Kraepelin's (1919) notion of schizophrenia as a degenerative brain pathology, similar to dementia. The degenerative model implies that the neuropathology underlying schizophrenia arises in the prodromal period, usually late adolescence or early adulthood. In fact, however, the two perspectives, neurodevelopmental and degenerative, are not incompatible. It is possible that schizophrenia involves an abnormality in the embryogenesis of the central nervous system *and* that there is a subsequent neurodegenerative process prior to and/or following the onset of the clinical symptoms.

Normal maturational processes also have potential relevance for understanding the development of schizophrenia (Walker & Neumann, 1996). The human brain undergoes a protracted period of postnatal maturation. Changes in brain morphology and physiology have been documented into early adulthood, and these changes are presumed to give rise to the more complex cognitive abilities displayed by young adults. It is likely that these normal maturational processes "moderate" the expression of any preexisting brain abnormalities. The notion of "developmental moderation" thus implies that behavioral manifestations of a static, congenital neuropathology will vary across the lifespan.

In this chapter, we examine some of the research evidence that lends support to a neurodevelopmental model of schizophrenia. Specifically, we posit a model that assumes that (1) schizophrenia involves a congenital neural abnormality, (2) the expression of this abnormality is moderated by ongoing brain maturation and experience, and (3) a neurodegenerative process can ensue as a consequence of the illness. We begin by discussing some key areas of evidence supporting a congenital brain abnormality in schizophrenia, including data on genetic and prenatal factors. We then explore the potential role of hormonal factors, including adrenal hormones, in triggering the expression of vulnerability for schizophrenia. In this connection, the effects of hormones on gene expression may prove to be important in the etiology of schizophrenia. Finally, we conclude with a discussion of the implications of neurodevelopmental theories for early identification and intervention with schizophrenia. (For a broader overview of vulnerability for schizophrenia outside the context of neurodevelopmental theory, see Harvey, Chapter 15, this volume).

EVIDENCE OF CONGENITAL VULNERABILITY TO SCHIZOPHRENIA

The clinical onset of schizophrenia typically occurs in early adulthood; after the individual has passed through the first two decades of life, usually with no previous psychiatric diagnosis. It is theoretically plausible that the onset of the underlying neuropathology coincides with the onset of the clinical syndrome. For example, a gene or polygene that leads to defective brain function may only be biologically expressed when the individual passes through a specific developmental stage. But several strands of empirical data have converged, instead, on the notion that the biological vulnerability to schizophrenia is present at birth. Thus, the behavioral expression of the vulnerability may change in response to maturational processes, but it involves a brain abnormality that is congenital. Here we offer an overview of some of the findings that support this assumption.

Physical Signs of Vulnerability

Assuming a biological basis for schizophrenia, investigators have searched for physical correlates of the illness for over seven decades. Postmortem studies of brain structure and electroencephalographic studies of brain function were initiated in the 1920s. But the introduction of modern neuroimaging techniques marked the beginning of the most rapid progress in reliably identifying the presence of brain abnormalities in schizophrenia and other mental disorders. Nonetheless, the question of temporal onset cannot be answered with these sophisticated techniques. But other physical indicators, most notably dysmorphic features of the body, have provided more convincing evidence about the congenital nature of the biological vulnerability.

Structural Brain Abnormalities

The most replicated structural brain deficit in patients with schizophrenia is lateral ventricular enlargement. This finding has been noted in both computed tomography (CT) studies (e.g., Andreasen et al., 1990) and magnetic resonance imaging (MRI) studies (e.g., Zipursky, Lim, Sullivan, Brown, & Pfefferbaum, 1992). A reduction in gray matter volume in the hippocampus, amygdala, thalamus, and temporal cortex has also been noted (Cannon, 1998). Over the years, investigators have noted that postmortem studies do not reveal an excess of gliosis in the brains of patients with schizophrenia, suggesting that the structural abnormalities are not a consequence of a degenerative process.

Several studies have examined the brain structure of adults with schizophrenia early in their illness and have noted that structural anomalies are apparent at the onset of the disorder (Cecil, Lenkinski, Gur, & Gur, 1999; Velakoulis et al., 1999; Whitworth et al., 1998). Among the brain abnormalities observed in first-episode patients are ventricular enlargement and reductions in hippocampal and temporal volume. Structural brain abnormalities, such as smaller amygdala and temporal cortex volumes, are also present in children with schizophrenia (Jacobson et al., 1998; Yeo et al., 1997). A recent study of children ages 8 to 12 with schizophrenia spectrum symptoms revealed increased metabolic abnormalities in the frontal lobe in comparison to controls (Brooks et al., 1998). Taken together, these findings indicate that the brain abnormalities observed in patients with schizophrenia are not solely attributable to treatment or chronic illness.

But more direct evidence of the congenital nature of neuroanatomical abnormality in schizophrenia is the relation between early events or behavioral phenomena and adult brain morphology. In a longitudinal study of the Danish high-risk sample, Cannon and his colleagues linked exposure to delivery complications with ventricular enlargement in adult patients with schizophrenia (Cannon et al., 1993). In a subsequent study, Walker, Lewine, and Neumann (1996) examined the relation between childhood behavioral phenomena and adult brain morphology on MRI among patients with schizophrenia. Using childhood home movies as a source of data on early behavior, they found that neuromotor deficits and negative affect during infancy were linked with greater ventricular enlargement in adulthood. Also, parental ratings of the severity of "externalized" childhood behavior problems showed an inverse relation with adult cortical volume. These associations are consistent with neurodevelopmental theories of schizophrenia; they suggest that obstetrical factors contribute to brain abnormalities in schizophrenia, *and* that these abnormalities can influence behavior. Of course, the neuroimaging results were obtained after the onset of schizophrenia, so a causal chain from prenatal risk to early brain abnormalities to later schizophrenia can only be inferred with these findings. But the evidence is persuasive and lends support to the assumption that the origins of schizophrenia lay in the early development of the central nervous system.

At the same time, however, there is some evidence that a degenerative process characterizes in at least some cases of schizophrenia. Several investigations involving repeated measures of brain structure have revealed increasing abnormalities over time (DeLisi, 1999; DeLisi et al., 1997; Rapoport et al., 1997), although others have not provided evidence for degeneration over the course of the illness (Cannon, 1991; Keshavan, Schooler, Sweeney, Haas, & Pettegrew, 1998). Rapoport et al. (1997) found an increase in ventricular volume in the brains of children with onset of schizophrenia before age 12; during the course of adolescence, these young patients showed a measurable ventricular enlargement. Rapoport et al. (1999) also found that children with schizophrenia showed a decrease in the volume of temporal gray matter greater than that of healthy controls over a 4-year follow-up in adolescence. Along these same lines, a study of patients with chronic schizophrenia revealed that the volume of the hippocampus was correlated with age and illness duration (Velakoulis et al., 1999). Although the evidence of a degenerative brain process is suggestive, we must await the results of future research aimed at replicating these findings. Ultimately, our understanding of the developmental course of brain morphology in schizophrenia may rely on advances in imaging technology that afford greater resolution and reliability of measurement. The advent of more powerful MRI structural and functional imaging procedures should pave the way for more prospective, longitudinal studies of children at risk for schizophrenia, early brain pathology, and eventual schizophrenic outcomes.

Dysmorphic Features: Minor Physical Anomalies and Dermatoglyphic Abnormalities

Minor physical anomalies (MPAs) are irregularities in the structure of the face, head, hands, and feet. The most widely used measure of MPAs, the Waldrop scale (Waldrop & Halverson, 1971), indexes anomalies such as steepled palate, asymmetric ears, and hyperteliorism. Research has provided evidence that MPAs are a consequence of fetal exposure to prenatal insult as well as genetic factors (Smith, 1982). The ectoderm, from which these external features of the head and extremities originate, undergoes rapid development during the first and second trimesters—the same periods when the central nervous system (CNS) undergoes significant development. Therefore, abnormalities in the morphological characteristics derived from the ectoderm are considered indirect markers of nonoptimal fetal neurodevelopment.

MPAs have been found to occur at an elevated rate in individuals with a variety of disorders, including autism (Gualtieri, Adams, Chen, & Loiselle, 1982), attention-deficit disorder (Deutsch, Matthysse, Swanson, & Farkas, 1990), childhood adjustment disorder (Fogel, Mednick, & Michelsen, 1985; Halverson & Victor, 1976; Pomeroy, Sprafkin, & Gadow, 1988), aggressive behavior (Kandel, Brennan, Mednick, & Michelson, 1989), schizophrenia (Griffiths et al., 1998), and schizotypal personality disorder (Davis-Weinstein, Diforio, Schiffman, Walker, & Bonsall, 1999). In a recent family study, MPAs were found to be more pronounced in patients with schizophrenia without a family history of schizophrenia when compared to those with a family history (Griffiths et al. 1998). This finding suggests that MPAs reflect early (prenatal) environmental events as opposed to a genetically determined sensitivity to prenatal insult.

Taken together, the research findings suggest that MPAs are nonspecific indicators of abnormalities in fetal CNS development that compromise postnatal CNS function, thereby conferring an increased risk for a variety of behavioral abnormalities. It has been suggested that the nonspecificity of the relationship between MPAs and schizophrenia may be a result of methodological weaknesses of research in this area (Buckley, 1998). As stated previously, the Waldrop scale is the one most commonly used to measure MPAs. Evidence for test–retest reliability with this measure is lacking, and ethnic differences are confounded with several items on the scale. Moreover, the Waldrop scale includes a wide variety of MPAs, some of which are not relevant to schizophrenia. The most current research in this area is attempting to focus on craniofacial features that are both easier to quantify, and also more relevant to the development of schizophrenia. For example, a narrowing and heightening of the palate has been noted to be one of the most prominent MPAs related to schizophrenia (Lane, Larkin, Waddington, & O'Callaghan, 1996). Moreover, craniofacial abnormalities have been found to be related to ventricular surface in schizophrenia (Dequardo, Bookstein, Green, & Tandon, 1996), suggesting an important link between these features and neurological vulnerability for this disorder. The continued use of these refined measures may result in findings of specificity in the relationship between particular types of MPAs and schizophrenia. In addition, these craniofacial measures may provide useful information about critical periods for prenatal damage that might be a source of vulnerability for schizophrenia. As described later, this issue of critical periods has arisen from work linking prenatal viral infection in the second trimester to schizophrenic outcomes.

Irregularities in palm and fingerprints are another dysmorphic sign associated with behavioral dysfunction (Schaumann & Alter, 1976). Among the most commonly measured aspects are differences in finger ridge counts between corresponding digits on the right and left hands ("fluctuating asymmetries" or FAs), total finger ridge counts, and palmar a–b ridge count. Like MPAs, these irregularities have their origins in prenatal development and appear to be a consequence of both genetic factors and prenatal insult (Cummins & Midlow, 1961; Mellor, 1968). In addition, a causal effect of prenatal stress is indicated by findings that exposure of pregnant monkeys to stress results in an increase in dermatoglyphic abnormalities (DAs) in offspring (Newell-Morris, Fahrenbruch, & Sackett, 1989). The timing of dermatoglyphic formation in the upper limbs is primarily the 14th through the 22nd week of gestation, the first part of the second trimester. As with MPAs, it is assumed that DAs predict behavioral dysfunction because they are a nonspecific marker of neurodevelopmental abnormalities that compromise CNS structure (Schaumann & Alter, 1976).

DAs occur at an elevated rate in several mental disorders, including affective disorders (Balgir, 1982), autism and developmental disorders (Hartin & Barry, 1979), and schizophrenia (Bracha, Torrey, Bigelow, Lohr, & Livingston, 1991; Lohr & Flynn, 1993; Mellor, 1968). The prenatal environmental origin of at least some DAs is suggested by findings that in comparison with their nonaffected twin controls, the affected twins in monozygotic pairs discordant for schizophrenia show reduced dermal ridges (Davis & Bracha, 1996).

Although it is assumed that the presence of dysmorphic features is an indirect indicator of abnormalities in CNS development, little research has been conducted on the relation between brain morphology and either MPAs or dermal abnormalities. The one reported study of which we are aware indicated no correlation between MPAs and ventricular volume in patients with schizophrenia, although the three subjects with the most pronounced MPAs also had notable ventricular abnormality (O'Callaghan, Buckley, Madigan, & Redmond, 1995). Clearly, this an important issue for further investigation. To understand the significance of dysmorphic features, it is important to determine their relation with brain morphology in both disturbed and nondisturbed populations.

Behavioral Markers of Vulnerability

The research findings reviewed previously offer persuasive evidence that some patients with schizophrenia have a congenital brain abnormality. But does this have any behavioral implications prior to the clinical onset of symptoms? The literature on premorbid behavior in schizophrenia suggests that the answer to this question is "yes." In addition, the findings lend further support to the neurodevelopmental model.

Neuromotor Abnormalities

Childhood neuromotor abnormalities are a consequence of both obstetrical complications (El-DeFrawi, Hirsch, Jurkowicz, & Craig, 1996; Hadders-Algra, Huisjes, & Touwen, 1988; Walker, 1994) and hereditary factors (Fouad, Servidei, Durcan, Bertini, & Ptacek, 1996). An extensive body of literature has also documented deficits in motor function among childhood psychiatric and learning disorders (Neumann & Walker, 1996). Gross motor and visual–motor deficits have been noted in infants and children with parents with schizophrenia (Fish, Marcus, Hans, Auerbach, & Perdue, 1992; Marcus, Hans, Auerbach, & Auerbach, 1993; McNeil, Harty, Blennow, & Cantor-Graae, 1993; Mednick, Mura, Schulsinger, & Mednick, 1971). Similarly, numerous studies have shown that motor abnormalities are associated with psychoses and affective disorder in adulthood (for reviews, see Neumann & Walker, 1996; Swerdlow & Koob, 1987; Walker, 1994).

Consistent with neurodevelopmental theory, recent investigations have documented that childhood motor abnormality precedes the onset of major psychiatric disorder. For example, delays in reaching motor milestones were associated with schizophrenia in a British cohort follow-back study, although, in the absence of a psychiatric control group the authors could not conclude that such motor delays are specific to schizophrenic outcomes (Davies, Russell, Jones, & Murray, 1998). Investigations that have compared children at risk for schizophrenia with those at risk for other psychiatric disorders have shown that motor deficits are more pronounced in those who subsequently develop schizophrenia (Fish et al., 1992; McNeil et al., 1993; Walker, Savoie, & Davis, 1994). Thus, there appears to be some specificity of neuromotor dysfunction to schizophrenia.

There is evidence suggesting that one subtype of motor abnormality, excessive involuntary movements (clinical and subclinical hyperkinesias or "dyskinesias"), may be uniquely linked with schizophrenia and spectrum disorders (e.g., schizotypal personality disorder). Elevated rates of involuntary movements are observed in treatment-naive and medicated patients with schizophrenia (Khot & Wyatt, 1991). Further, it has been shown that ratings of dyskinetic movements in adult patients with schizophrenia are positively correlated with the severity of childhood premorbid deficits (Chakos et al., 1996). Like adult patients with schizophrenia, children who subsequently manifest the disorder show heightened involuntary movements (e.g., hand posturing, and irregular, writhing movements of the hands) as observed in home movies of children from birth to 2 years of age who are preschizophrenic (Walker et al., 1994). Further, the severity of premorbid dyskinesia is predictive of the severity of psychiatric symptoms in adulthood (Neumann & Walker, 1996). Two recent reports also document an excess of involuntary movements in children (Walker, Lewis, Loewy, & Palyo, 1999) and adults (Cassady, Asami, Moran, Kunkel, & Thaker, 1998) with schizotypal personality disorder.

Observations of significant associations between childhood motor abnormalities and schizophrenia spectrum outcomes lend support to neurodevelopmental models of schizophrenia. The CNS abnormality associated with hyperkinesias (e g., associated, choreoathetoid and ballistic movements) have been localized to particular brain regions. Hyperkinesias are due to abnormalities in the striatum which, in interaction with dopamine (DA) activity, disrupt motor circuitry (Walker, 1994). Specifically, theories of the neural circuitry of movement disorders assume that hyperkinetic syndromes are due to overactivation of compromised DA pathways in the striatum, particularly the pathway mediated by the DA D2 receptor subtype (Alexander, Crutcher, & Delong, 1990; Gerfen, 1992; Smith, Bevan, Shink, & Bolam, 1998).

It has been proposed that DA overactivity in proximal striatal regions contributes to psychotic symptoms, and some authors have postulated neural mechanisms through which DA receptor abnormalities disrupt the striatal–cortical neural circuitry to produce both movement disorder and psychotic symptoms (Swerdlow & Koob, 1990; Walker, 1994). Thus, based on contemporary neural circuitry models, the presence of hyperkinesia in children at risk for schizophrenia is consistent with neurodevelopmental etiologic theories of schizophrenia.

Sustained Attention

Attentional deficits have also been documented in patients with schizophrenia and in children at high risk for schizophrenia (Cornblatt, Obuchowski, Schnur, & O'Brien, 1998; Nuechterlein, 1983). Adults with schizophrenia, children of parents with schizophrenia, and premorbid individuals with schizophrenia have been found to evidence deficits in sustained attention on a variety of measures, most notably the continuous performance task (CPT).

In this task, subjects are asked to attend to a series of letters or numbers and to detect an intermittently presented target stimulus. Individuals at risk for schizophrenia and those that have schizophrenia show poor detection of this target stimulus. This deficit is thought to reflect fragmented and inefficient attentional mechanisms. A deficit in working memory has also been hypothesized as the cause of this attentional difficulty (Nuechterlein et al., 1998).

Longitudinal analyses from the New York High-Risk Project suggest that sustained attention deficits that appear early in development are relatively stable over time and may be specific to risk for schizophrenia in individuals at genetic risk for this disorder (Winters, Cornblatt, & Erlenmeyer-Kimling, 1991). A subgroup of the offspring of parents with schizophrenia has been found to be attentionally deviant, and this subgroup is more likely to manifest adjustment problems in adolescence and schizophrenia in adulthood. This subgroup has been hypothesized to represent the 35–45% of adult patients with schizophrenia who also have significant attentional deficits.

The presence of attentional deficits in children at risk for schizophrenia suggests that brain dysfunction precedes the onset of clinical symptoms. Again, this points to the likelihood of a congenital brain impairment.

Smooth-Pursuit Eye Movements

Abnormalities in smooth-pursuit eye movement (SPEM) have also been found consistently in patients with schizophrenia and individuals at risk for the illness (Iacono & Clementz, 1993). SPEM are elicited in normal individuals by a continuously moving stimulus such as a target on a screen or a swinging pendulum. In eye tracking, the eye velocity matches the target velocity within a specified range of movement. If eye tracking fails, then saccadic eye movements are observed rather than smooth tracking of the stimulus. The neural mechanisms that underlie SPEM have not been fully determined; however, there is evidence for frontal lobe involvement in this process (Katsanis & Iacono, 1991). A recent study also suggests that medication induced hypodopaminergia in the cortex might directly disrupt SPEM in normal individuals (Malaspina et al., 1994). In this study, haloperidol disrupted eye tracking in healthy subjects and created saccadic movements similar to those noted in schizophrenics. It is assumed that haloperidol administration to healthy individuals results in reduced dopamine release in cortical but not subcortical brain regions (Lambert et al., 1995). Thus, haloperidol disruption of eye tracking may suggest a link between cortical hypodopaminergia and disruptions in SPEM.

SPEM deficits have been found in patients with schizophrenia (e.g., Mialet & Pichot, 1981), their unaffected relatives (e.g., Holzman & Levy, 1977), and children at high genetic risk for schizophrenia (Mather, 1985).

A recent study of children of patients with schizophrenia has noted deficits in anticipatory saccades in offspring as young as 6 years of age (Ross, Hommer, Radant, Roath, & Freedman, 1996). To date, however, no study has been able to test for the link between premorbid SPEM deficits and eventual schizophrenic outcomes.

Overall, the research on eye tracking has provided compelling evidence that SPEM deficits qualify as a risk marker for schizophrenia (Iacono & Ficken, 1989; Iacono, Moreau, Beiser, Fleming, & Lin, 1992). These deficits have been found to be stable over time, to be present in patients under remission, to be present in first-degree relatives of persons with schizophrenias, to have higher concordance in monozygotic versus dizygotic twins, and to be relatively rare in normal individuals.

Prenatal and Perinatal Factors as a Source of Vulnerability

There is now compelling evidence that obstetrical complications are linked with schizophrenia (Cannon, 1997; Dalman, Allebeck, Cullberg, Grunewald, & Koester, 1999; Jones, Rantakallio, Hartikainen, Isohanni, & Sipila, 1998). Included among the factors that have been identified in multiple studies are preeclampsia, maternal bleeding, toxemia, and prolonged labor. The consequences of these complications for neural development are not known, but it is assumed that they compromise regions of the brain that are implicated in schizophrenia.

In winter and spring, there is also an increase in births of babies who later develop schizophrenia (Hare, 1988). One plausible explanation for this epidemiological finding is that schizophrenia is caused by exposure to viral infections during gestation. There have been numerous reports of a significant association between second trimester exposure to influenza and increased schizophrenic outcomes (e.g. Mednick, Machon, Huttunen, & Bonet, 1988, Sham et al., 1992), although this finding has not always been replicated (e.g., Crow, Done, & Johnstone, 1992). Influenza exposure has also been linked to the outcome of major affective disorders, suggesting that the effect may not be specific to schizophrenia (Machon, Mednick, & Huttunen, 1992). Mednick et al. (1998) have proposed that the timing of the prenatal insult is critically important in that exposure during one window of fetal development may lead to schizophrenia whereas exposure during another window of fetal development may lead to affective disorder.

In a sample of patients with schizophrenia, a correlation has been reported between increased sylvan fissure volume and risk of influenza exposure during the second trimester (Takei, Lewis, Jones, Harvey, & Murray, 1994). This finding provides preliminary evidence for the hypothesized pathway from flu exposure *in utero*, to neurodevelopmental damage to schizophrenia. Several hypotheses exist for the mechanisms by which flu exposure during a critical period of fetal development might lead to brain damage.

These include increased risk for associated obstetrical complications, exposure to maternal antibodies, heat shock, and stress. As described later, the literature on the relationship between stress and schizophrenia suggests that this factor, in particular, is a viable candidate as a neurodevelopmental factor in schizophrenia.

Genetics as a Source of Vulnerability

There is no disputing the evidence that hereditary factors are involved in the etiology of schizophrenia; behavior genetic paradigms have elegantly demonstrated this point (Gottesman, 1991). A review of the evidence is beyond the scope of this chapter; it is sufficient to say that the findings provide convincing support that at least some persons who succumb to schizophrenia are born with predisposition to the disorder. But subsequent paradigms aimed at identifying the specific nature of the genotype have not met with comparable success. Sophisticated quantitative (linkage and association) and molecular genetic procedures have failed to yield replicable findings (Gothelf, Munitz, & Weizman, 1997; Rall, 1998; Yee & Yolken, 1997).

In part, the failure of these new techniques to identify etiologically relevant genotypes may indicate that there is more than one genetic pathway to schizophrenia. For example, not all families of schizophrenics show SPEM deficits, and it has been suggested that those who do might reflect a particular genetic subtype of schizophrenia (Clementz, Grove, Iacono, & Sweeney, 1992). It may be that there are a variety of genetic markers of schizophrenia, with each being useful for the identification of a specific genetic liability (Grove et al., 1991).

The failure to obtain replicable findings may also be attributable to the complex role of environmental factors in triggering the expression of genetic liabilities that confer vulnerability. This is particularly true if the vulnerability involves a polygenotype, as opposed to a single gene. Studies of monozygotic twins that are discordant for schizophrenia have illustrated the extent to which relatively subtle environmental factors can produce pronounced biological and behavioral differences (Stassen et al., 1999). Some of these environmental effects may be independent of the genotype, whereas others may reflect the impact of environmental factors on gene expression. For example, some prenatal insults may have a direct "mechanical" impact on the fetal brain that results in compromised function. Other prenatal events may affect the biochemical milieu which, in turn, can alter gene expression (Schulkin, Gold, & McEwan, 1998). In either case, the end result is environmentally induced biological and behavioral changes that add complexity to the measurement of the phenotype.

In the remainder of this chapter, we focus on the conceptualization of the neurodevelopmental processes involved in schizophrenia, with a special emphasis on developmental aspects of the expression of genotypes. In the past decade, neuroscience has illuminated the mechanisms involved in gene expression, as well as the potential role these processes can play in biological adaptation and maladaptation (Schulkin et al., 1998). To date, the issue of gene expression is one that has been given little attention in neurodevelopmental accounts of schizophrenia and other major mental disorders. In the following discussion, we explore the potential relevance of maturational processes and environmental factors on the behavioral expression of genetic liabilities.

INTERACTIONAL PROCESSES
IN THE NEURODEVELOPMENT OF SCHIZOPHRENIA

We have reviewed findings from several key areas that converge on two general conclusions: (1) that a substantial proportion of those at risk for schizophrenia have a congenital central nervous system vulnerability and (2) that subclinical manifestations of the vulnerability are measurable prior to the onset of clinical symptoms. The abnormalities in brain structure and the dysmorphic features observed in patients with schizophrenia point to fetal origins, in at least some cases. The cognitive and behavioral abnormalities manifested by children who are preschizophrenic indicate that the congenital liability is behaviorally expressed before the clinical syndrome arises.

Although it is clear that congenital vulnerability to schizophrenia can be conferred through heredity, it also appears that its behavioral expression is often contingent upon environmental events. For example, the Finnish adoption study showed that only those biological offspring of parents with schizophrenia who were exposed to an unstable family environment had an elevated rate of schizophrenia (Tienari et al., 1994). Such interactional processes have been the core assumption of the *diathesis–stress model*; a central framework in theorizing about the etiology of schizophrenia for decades. Its basic assumption is that schizophrenia is the consequence of interactions among multiple factors, in particular, biological vulnerability and environmental stress. As our understanding of the neural mechanism mediating the effects of stress has increased in recent years, so has the heuristic value of the diathesis–stress model (Walker & Diforio, 1997).

The Role of Stress in the Etiology of Schizophrenia

The notion that psychosocial stress can trigger or exacerbate psychopathology has received support from a substantial body of literature. Because a chief goal of much of this research has been to determine whether stress contributes to symptoms, the primary focus has been on stressful events that are *not* attributable to the individual's behavior. Recent articles have reviewed the behavioral evidence for psychosocial stress effects on schizophrenia and spectrum disorders (Fowles, 1992; Norman & Malla, 1993). They conclude that the occurrence of stressors predicts subsequent worsening of symptoms. As noted previously, deleterious effects of stress in the premorbid period are suggested by findings that children at genetic high risk for mental illness (i.e., offspring of parents with major psychiatric disorders) show greater behavioral dysfunction if they are exposed to nonoptimal caregiving such as a disturbed adoptive parent or institutional child care (Tienari, 1991; Valone, Norton, Goldstein, & Doane, 1983; Walker, Cudek, Mednick, & Schulsinger, 1981; Walker, Downey, & Bergman, 1989).

Extending this to the biological level, preliminary findings from our longitudinal study of adolescents with schizotypal personality disorder show an interactive effect of dysmorphic signs and secretion of the stress hormone cortisol. Specifically, schizotypal adolescents with high rates of dysmorphic signs are more likely to manifest an increase in subsequent adjustment problems if they also manifest elevated cortisol release. This effect appears to be generalized across several behavioral dimensions. In contrast, there appears to be an interactive effect of movement abnormality and cortisol level that is specific to the development of schizophrenia-spectrum symptoms. These findings suggest that morphological and movement abnormalities may be indicators of "biobehavioral" stress sensitivity.

It now appears likely that the role of stress in the etiology of psychopathology extends to the prenatal period. At least two studies have demonstrated that the rate of psychiatric disorder, including major mental illness, is increased in the offspring of pregnant women exposed to stress. One of these studies focused on the children of women whose spouses died during their pregnancy (Huttunen, 1989) and the other on women who experienced a major natural disaster while pregnant (Watson & Mednick, 1998).

Laboratory studies of animals indicate that the effect of prenatal stress (restraint of the dam) on postnatal functioning is mediated by the hippocampal and hypothalamic–pituitary–adrenal (HPA) systems. When exposed to prenatal stress of sufficient magnitude, not only do they manifest short-term behavioral changes and increases in corticosterone, but they also show an augmentation of subsequent behavioral and biological responses to stress (Levine, 1993; Plotsky & Meaney, 1993). Further, prenatal stress can produce hippocampal structural and cellular abnormalities in offspring (Maccari et al., 1995). Such hippocampal abnormalities have been observed in adult patients with schizophrenia (Bogerts, Meertz, & Schonfeldt-Bausch, 1985; Breier & Buchanan, 1992; Jeste & Lohr, 1989; Suddath, Christison, Torrey, Casanova, & Weinberger, 1990; Waldo et al., 1994), and they are associated with younger age at onset of illness (Nasrallah & Olson, 1996).

Developmental Moderation of Vulnerability

The pubertal period has been of intense interest to researchers in the field of psychopathology because it is during this period that the prodromal signs of schizophrenia and affective disorder typically emerge (Tyrka et al., 1995; Walker, Baum, & Diforio, 1998; Wolfradt & Straube, 1998). Contemporary models of the neurodevelopmental processes involved in schizophrenia have attempted to account for this.

For example, Walker (1994) proposed that normal maturational changes in the circuitry linking cortical and subcortical regions may influence the behavioral expression of the brain abnormality underlying schizophrenia. In this model it is assumed that the congenital diathesis involves an abnormality in striatal dopamine activity and that functionally specialized striatal–cortical circuits come "on line" during different developmental periods. Striatal neuropathology can produce disruptions in the "late maturing" circuits, such as the frontal and limbic circuits, that play a key role in higher-level cognitive functions. Thus, Walker theorizes that striatal dopaminergic abnormality manifests itself in distinct patterns of behavioral dysfunction during the course of development—pronounced neuromotor abnormalities early and late in life and psychotic symptoms in late adolescence/early adulthood.

Weinberger (1987) also posits a developmental moderation model, suggesting that a congenital lesion in the dorsolateral prefrontal cortex may be the initial etiological factor in schizophrenia. The lesion is hypothesized to result in schizophrenic symptoms at the time of functional maturation of the dorsolateral prefrontal cortex; namely, late adolescence/early adulthood. Before full maturation, the lesion is hypothesized to cause more subtle behavioral and emotional abnormalities—the types of deficits noted in premorbid histories of individuals with schizophrenia. Weinberger theorizes that the dorsolateral prefrontal lesion compromises the mesocortical dopamine system projecting from prefrontal cortex to the midbrain. Hypodopaminergia in the cortex results in defect symptoms of schizophrenia (e.g., cognitive defects). Concomitant hyperdopaminergia in subcortical (mesolimbic) regions is assumed to result in positive symptoms of schizophrenia. Further, it is assumed the symptoms of schizophrenia arise in early adulthood because this is the time of maximum dopaminergic activity in the brain.

To date, hormonal factors have been given relatively little attention in neurodevelopmental models of schizophrenia. Of course, adolescence is characterized by a dramatic change in the level of gonadol hormones (O'Leary, 1997; Susman, Worrall, Murowchick, Frobrose, & Schwab, 1996). In addition, adolescence may be associated with a normative increase in biobehavioral sensitivity to stress. Our research and some other studies suggest that adolescence is associated with an increase in cortisol secretion (Walker et al., 1998). It is therefore possible that maturational increases in HPA activity are one of the neurodevelopmental processes that potentiate symptom expression in vulnerable youth.

The incorporation of the HPA system into neurodevelopmental models of developmental psychopathology yields a framework for explaining several key findings (Walker & Diforio, 1997). First, it suggests a biological mechanism for explaining the relation between psychosocial stress and psychopathology. Second, the demonstrated effect of persistent HPA over-activation on hippocampal morphology provides an explanation for the apparent worsening of the prognosis for schizophrenia when episodes recur or go untreated (Wyatt, 1995), and for the degenerative brain changes observed in some longitudinal studies of young patients with schizophrenia (DeLisi et al., 1997; Rapoport et al., 1997). Third, the apparent sensitivity of the HPA axis to prenatal events helps to explain the association between prenatal complications and risk for mental illness (Cantor-Graae et al., 1994; Cantor-Graae, McNeil, Sjostrom, Nordstrom, & Rosenlund, 1995; Eyler-Zorilla & Cannon, 1995; Guth, Jones, & Murray, 1993). Finally, neuro-maturational changes in HPA function may be implicated in the gradually escalating behavioral problems observed in adolescents who subsequently show serious psychopathology (Neumann, Grimes, Walker, & Baum, 1995). Maturational changes could be a critical factor in triggering the expression of premorbid behavioral deficits, making adolescence/early adulthood the peak risk period for illness onset. This may be especially true of individuals with preexisting hippocampal abnormality and thus may explain the association between reduced hippocampal volume and earlier age at onset of psychotic symptoms (Nasrallah, Skinner, Schmalbrock, & Robitaille, 1994).

Our understanding of the role of hormones in brain function has increased dramatically in recent years (Meyer et al., 1999; Schulkin et al., 1998). It has been demonstrated that gonadal and adrenal hormones influence brain function through a variety of mechanisms. Some of the effects are nongenomic, whereas others are mediated by genomic mechanisms (Picard, 1998). For example, in the realm of nongenomic effects, estrogen and progesterone can affect neurotransmitter activity by altering receptor sensitivity, neurotransmitter synthesis, and neurotransmitter release. Glucocorticoids can have similar effects. When the effects are genomic, they operate through intracellular mRNA transcription; thus the message from the genotype, in the form of protein synthesis, is moderated. Future research will undoubtedly unlock more of the mysteries of how the organism's hormonal milieu influences the expression of genes.

What these and related findings clearly indicate is that the hormonal changes produced by both normal maturation *and* environmental factors can play a significant role in determining how an inherited genetic vulnerability for a major mental illness is biologically and, therefore, behaviorally expressed. Figure 14.1 illustrates a hypothetical model of these causal pathways.

The association between pubertal maturation and onset of psychiatric symptoms may be due to hormonal influences on the expression of genes. These effects could be a consequence of genetically programmed gonadal

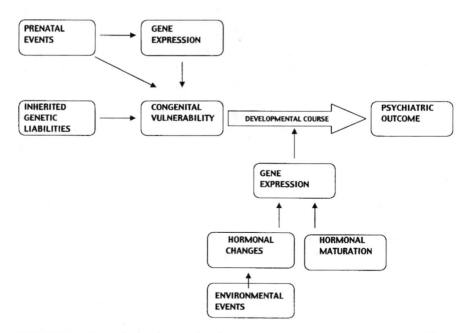

FIGURE 14.1. Hypothesized neurodevelopmental influences on the course of schizophrenia.

and/or adrenal hormone changes. In addition, the individual's environment has the potential for modulating adrenal hormone release across the lifespan. Thus fluctuating levels of glucocorticoids might act in concert with gonadal hormones to determine the expression of genetic vulnerabilities.

The genomic effects of hormones are, of course, not restricted to the peripubertal period. They are operative during fetal development and undoubtedly play a role in the effects of hormones on fetal brain development. One component or "subtype" of the inherited vulnerability for schizophrenia may be a heightened sensitivity to the deleterious effects of glucocorticoids on neurodevelopment.

On the other hand, the diathesis for schizophrenia and other major mental disorders need not be inherited in order to be influenced by hormonal factors. A congenital brain abnormality produced by prenatal events could also be moderated in its expression by hormonal factors. Our findings, mentioned earlier, of an interactive effect of dysmorphic signs and cortisol secretion are consistent with this assumption.

IMPLICATIONS FOR INTERVENTION

At the present time, there are several ongoing studies of early intervention strategies under way in the United States and elsewhere (McGlashan &

Johannessen, 1996). These studies have typically employed psycho-educational approaches with families in combination with medication trials immediately following the onset of psychotic symptoms. Preliminary results of these early intervention programs indicate that early beneficial effects on psychotic relapse may not last over longer periods of follow-up (Linszen, Lenior, De Haan, Dingemans, & Gersons, 1998).

Our model suggests that primary prevention might be a more useful strategy than early intervention with schizophrenia. To date, there are no systematic efforts under way to implement primary prevention programs for serious mental disorders. But it is likely that such programs will be formulated by clinical researchers in the near future, *and* that they will draw on neurodevelopmental models of etiology as a basis for generating hypotheses about the critical periods and strategies for intervention.

For example, the model presented in this chapter suggests several potential strategies for prevention. First, the assumption that prenatal insults are involved in the etiological process implies the option of intervening to reduce fetal exposure to such complications. If it is the case that the genetic liability for schizophrenia confers a heightened sensitivity to factors that perturb fetal neurodevelopment, then the presence of a family history of schizophrenia might serve as one indicator for preventive intervention. Further, if heightened maternal steroids potentiate neurodevelopmental abnormalities, then pharmacological interventions aimed at buffering the fetus from the effects of steroid elevations might be plausible. Adolescence may be another key period for preventive intervention. Again, if hormonal changes are playing a role in triggering the expression of vulnerabilities during this period, the options for preventive intervention may entail modulating pubertal changes in adrenal and gonadal hormones. Psychosocial interventions that are effective in modulating stress reactivity may also be beneficial to adolescents at risk.

DIRECTIONS FOR FUTURE RESEARCH

Although we have presented evidence that is consistent with a neurodevelopmental perspective on schizophrenia, there are many specific questions that remain unanswered in this area of research. Studies employing MRI technologies in high-risk groups, before and after the onset of schizophrenia, are necessary to determine the complex role of preexisting neuropathology and neurodegenerative processes in this disorder. The use of more refined measures of MPAs and the assessment of prenatal stressors that can be linked to specific prenatal stages of development will help to determine whether critical risk periods exist for the development of schizophrenia. We would also argue that more research is necessary on the potential role of the HPA axis in the diathesis–stress model of schizophrenia. Attention to the developmental phase of adolescence in terms of hormonal changes and stress responsivity would be a particularly fertile area of research and potentially could be linked with early-intervention programs designed to reduce the occurrence and severity of schizophrenia. Finally, the expanding area of gene expression research will have a significant impact on our conceptualization of the development of schizophrenia and all disorders with significant heritable components. We now recognize that genetic and environmental factors are in complex interaction from the very earliest stages of development. Separating out genetic from environmental causes and determining which is "more important" becomes nonsensical in light of this realization. A more productive strategy of research will be to examine the interactions of genetic and environmental effects (at molecular, cellular, neurological, hormonal, behavioral, familial, community, and societal levels) as they unfold over the process of development and culminate in the onset and course of schizophrenia.

REFERENCES

Alexander, G. E., Crutcher, M. D., & DeLong, M. R. (1990). Basal ganglia–thalamo-cortical circuits: Parallel substrates for motor, oculomotor, "prefrontal" and "limbic" functions. *Progress in Brain Research, 85,* 119–145.

Andreasen, N. C., Swayze, V. W., Flaum, M., Yates, W. R., Arndt, S., & McChesney, C. (1990). Ventricular enlargement in schizophrenia evaluated with computed tomographic scanning. *Archives of General Psychiatry, 47,* 1008–1015.

Balgir, R. S. (1982). Dermatoglyphic studies in affective disorders: An appraisal. *Biological Psychiatry, 17,* 69–82.

Bogerts, B., Meertz, E., & Schonfeldt-Bausch, R. (1985). Basal ganglia and limbic system pathology in schizophrenia. *Archives of General Psychiatry, 42,* 784–791.

Bracha, H. S., Torrey, E. F., Bigelow, L. B., Lohr, J. B., & Linington, B. B. (1991). Subtle signs of prenatal maldevelopment of the hand ectoderm in schizophrenia: A preliminary monozygotic twin study. *Biological Psychiatry, 30,* 719–725.

Breier, A., & Buchanan, R. W. (1992). The effects of metabolic stress on plasma progesterone in healthy volunteers and schizophrenic patients. *Life Sciences, 51,* 1527–1534.

Brooks, W. M., Hodde-Vargas, J., Vargas, L. A., Yeo, R. A., Ford, G. C., & Hendren, R. L. (1998). Frontal lobe of children with schizophrenia spectrum disorders: A proton magnetic resonance spectroscopic study. *Biological Psychiatry, 43,* 263–269.

Buckley, P. F. (1998). The clinical stigmata of aberrant neurodevelopment in schizophrenia. *Journal of Nervous and Mental Disease, 186,* 79–86.

Cannon, T. D. (1991). Genetic and perinatal sources of structural brain abnormalities in schizophrenia. In S. A. Mednick, T. D. Cannon, C. E. Barr, & M. Lyon (Eds.), *Fetal neurodevelopment and adult schizophrenia* (pp. 174–198). Cambridge, UK: Cambridge University Presss.

Cannon, T. D. (1997). On the nature and mechanisms of obstetric influences in schizophrenia: A review and synthesis of epidemiologic studies. *International Review of Psychiatry, 9,* 387–397.

Cannon, T. D. (1998). Genetic and perinatal influences in the etiology of schizophrenia: A neurodevelopmental model. In M. Lenzenweger & B. Dworkin (Eds.), *Origins and development of schizophrenia* (pp. 67–92). Washington, DC: American Psychological Association.

Cannon, T. D., Mednick, S. A., Parnas, J., Schulsinger, F., Praestholm, J., & Aage, V. (1993). Developmental brain abnormalities in the offspring of schizophrenic mothers: I. Contributions of genetic and perinatal factors. *Archives of General Psychiatry, 50,* 551–564.

Cantor-Graae, E., McNeil, T. F., Sjostrom, K., Nordstrom, L. G., & Rosenlund, T. (1995). Obstetric complications and their relationship to other etiological risk factors in schizophrenia: A case-control study. *Journal of Nervous and Mental Disease, 182,* 645–650.

Cantor-Graae, E., McNeil, T. F., Torrey, E. F., Quinn, P., Bowies, A., Sjostrom, K., & Rawlings, R. (1994). Link between pregnancy complications and minor physical anomalies in MZ twins discordant for schizophrenia. *American Journal of Psychiatry, 151,* 1188–1193.

Cassady, S. L., Adami, H., Moran, M., Kunkel, R., & Thaker, G. K. (1998). Spontaneous dyskinesia in subjects with schizophrenia spectrum personality. *American Journal of Psychiatry, 155,* 70–75.

Cecil, K. M., Lenkinski, R. E., Gur, R. E., & Gur, R. C. (1999). Proton magnetic resonance spectroscopy in the frontal and temporal lobes of neuroleptic naive patients with schizophrenia. *Neuropsychopharmacology, 20,* 131–140.

Chakos, M. H., Alvir, J. M. J., Woerner, M., Koreen, A., Geisler, S., Mayerhoff, D., Sobel, S., Kane, J. M., Borenstein, M., & Leiberman, J. A. (1996). Incidents and correlates of tardive dyskinesia in first episode of schizophrenia. *Archives of General Psychiatry, 53,* 313–319.

Clementz, B. A., Grove, W. M., Iacono, W. G., & Sweeney, J. A. (1992). Smooth-pursuit eye movement dysfunction and liability for schizophrenia: Implications for genetic modeling. *Journal of Abnormal Psychology, 101,* 117–129.

Cornblatt, B., Obuchowski, M., Schnur, D., & O'Brien, J. D. (1998). Hillside study of risk and early detection in schizophrenia. *British Journal of Psychiatry. 172,* 26–32.

Crow, T. J., Done, D. J., & Johnstone, E. C. (1992). Schizophrenia is not due to maternal influenza in the second (or other) trimester of pregnancy. *Schizophrenia Research, 6,* 99–100.

Cummins, H., & Midlow, C. (1961). *Finger-prints, palms and soles: An introduction to dermatoglyphics.* New York: Dover.

Dalman, C., Allebeck, P., Cullberg, J., Grunewald, C., & Koester, M. (1999). Obstetric complications and the risk of schizophrenia: A longitudinal study of a national birth cohort. *Archives of General Psychiatry, 56,* 234–240.

Davies, N., Russell, A., Jones, P., & Murray, R. M. (1998). Which characteristics of schizophrenia predate psychosis? *Journal of Psychiatric Research, 32,* 121–131.

Davis, J. O., & Bracha, H. S. (1996). Prenatal growth markers in schizophrenia: A monozygotic co-twin control study. *American Journal of Psychiatry, 153,* 1166–1172.

Davis-Weinstein, D., Diforio, D., Schiffman, J., Walker, E., & Bonsall, B. (1999). Minor physical anomalies, dermatoglyphic abnormalities and cortisol levels in adolescents with schizotypal personality disorder. *American Journal of Psychiatry, 156,* 617–623.

DeLisi, L. E. (1999). Regional brain volume change over the life-time course of schizophrenia. *Journal of Psychiatric Research, 33,* 535–541.

DeLisi, L. E., Sakuma, M., Tew, W., Kushner, M., Hoff, A. L., & Grimson, R. (1997). Schizophrenia as a chronic active brain process: A study of progressive brain structural change subsequent to the onset of schizophrenia. *Psychiatry Research: Neuroimaging, 34,* 129–140.

Dequardo, J. R., Bookstein, F. L., Green, W. D., & Tandon, R. (1996). Spatial relationships of neuroanatomical landmarks in schizophrenia. *Psychiatric Research, 67,* 81–95.

Deutsch, C. K., Matthysse, S., Swanson, J. M., & Farkas, L. G. (1990). Genetic latent structure analysis of dysmorphology in attention deficit disorder. *Journal of the American Academy of Child and Adolescent Psychiatry, 29,* 189–194.

El-DeFrawi, M. H., Hirsch, G., Jurkowicz, A., & Craig, T. J. (1996). Tardive dyskinesia and pregnancy and delivery complications. *Child Psychiatry and Human Development, 26,* 151–157.

Eyler-Zorrilla, L. T., & Cannon, T. D. (1995). Structural brain abnormalities in schizophrenia: Distribution, etiology, and implications. In S. A. Mednick & J. M. Hollister (Eds.), *Neural development and schizophrenia* (pp. 57–69). New York: Plenum.

Fish, B., Marcus, J., Hans, S. L., Auerbach, J. G., & Perdue, S. (1992). Infants at risk for schizophrenia: Sequelae of a genetic neurointegrative defect. *Archives of General Psychiatry, 49,* 221–235.

Fogel, C. A., Mednick, S. A., & Michelsen, N. (1985). Hyperactive behavior and minor physical anomalies. *Acta Psychiatrica Scandinavica, 72,* 551–556.

Fouad, G. T., Servidei, S., Durcan, S., Bertini, E., & Ptacek, L. J. (1996). A gene for familial paroxysmal dyskinesia (FPD1) maps to chromosome 2q. *American Journal of Human Genetics, 59,* 135–139.

Fowles, D. C. (1992). Schizophrenia: Diathesis–stress revisited. *Annual Review of Psychology, 43,* 303–336.

Gerfen, C. R. (1992). The neostriatal mosaic: Multiple levels of compartmental organization in the basal ganglia. *Annual Review of Neuroscience, 15,* 285–320.

Gothelf, D., Munitz, H., & Weizman, A. (1997). The complexity of molecular genetic research in psychiatric disorders: Advances and pitfalls. *Israel Journal of Psychiatry and Related Sciences, 34,* 254–269.

Gottesman, I. I. (1991). *Schizophrenia genesis: The origins of madness.* New York: W. H. Freeman.

Griffiths, T. D., Sigmundsson, T., Takei, N., Frangou, S., Birkett, P. B., Sharma, T., Reveley, A. M., & Murray, R. M. (1998). Minor physical anomalies in familial and sporadic schizophrenia: The Maudsley family study. *Journal of Neurology, Neurosurgery, and Psychiatry, 65,* 56–60.

Grove, W. M., Lebow, B. S., Clementz, B. A., Cerri, A., Medus, C., & Iacono, W. G. (1991). Familial prevalence and co-aggregation of schizotypy indicators: A multitrait family study. *Journal of Abnormal Psychology, 100,* 115–121.

Gualtieri, C. T., Adams, A., Chen, C. D., & Loiselle, D. (1982). Minor physical anomalies in alcoholic and schizophrenic adults and hyperactive and autistic children. *American Journal of Psychiatry, 139,* 640–643.

Guth, C. W., Jones, P., & Murray, R. (1993). Familial psychiatric illness and obstetric complications in early-onset affective disorder: A case-control study. *British Journal of Psychiatry, 163,* 492–498.

Hadders-Algra, M., Huisjes, H. J., & Touwen, B. C. (1988). Perinatal risk factors and minor neurological dysfunction: Significance for behavior and school achievement at nine years. *Developmental Medicine and Child Neurology, 30,* 482–491.

Halverson, C., & Victor, J. B. (1976). Minor physical anomalies and problem behavior in elementary school children. *Child Development, 47,* 281–285.

Hare, E. (1988). Temporal factors and trends, including birth seasonality and the viral hypothesis. In H. A. Nasrallah (Ed.), *Handbook of schizophrenia* (pp. 345–377). Amsterdam: Elsevier.

Hartin, P. J., & Barry, R. J. (1979). A comparative dermatoglyphic study of autistic, retarded, and normal children. *Journal of Autism and Developmental Disorders, 9,* 233–246.

Holzman, P. S., & Levy, D. L. (1977). Smooth pursuit eye movements and functional psychoses: A review. *Schizophrenia Bulletin, 3,* 15–27.

Huttunen, M. O. (1989). Maternal stress during pregnancy and the behavior of the offspring. In S. Doxiadis (Ed.), *Early influences shaping the individual* (pp. 175–182). New York: Plenum.

Iacono, W. G., & Clementz, B. A. (1993). A strategy for elucidating genetic influence on complex psychopathological syndromes. *Progress in Experimental Psychopathology Research, 16,* 11–65.

Iacono, W. G., & Ficken, J. W. (1989). Research strategies employing psychophysiological measures: Identifying and using psychophysiological markers. In G. Turpin (Ed.), *Handbook of clinical psychophysiology* (pp. 45–70). Chichester, UK: Wiley.

Iacono, W. G., Moreau, M., Beiser, M., Fleming, J. A., & Lin, T. (1992). Smooth-pursuit eye tracking in first-episode psychotic patients and their relatives. *Journal of Abnormal Psychology, 101,* 104–116.

Jacobsen, L. K., Giedd, J. N., Castellanos, F. X., Vaituzis, C. A., Hamburger, S. D., Kumra, S., Lenane, M. C., & Rapoport, J. L. (1998). Progressive reduction of temporal lobe structures in childhood-onset schizophrenia. *American Journal of Psychiatry, 155,* 678–685.

Jeste, D. V., & Lohr, J. B. (1989). Hippocampal pathologic findings in schizophrenia. *Archives of General Psychiatry, 46,* 1019–1024.

Jones, P. B., Rantakallio, P., Hartikainen, A., Isohanni, M., & Sipila, P. (1998). Schizophrenia as a long-term outcome of pregnancy, delivery, and perinatal complications: A 28-year follow-up of the 1966 North Finland general population birth cohort. *American Journal of Psychiatry, 155,* 355–364.

Kandel, E., Brennan, P. A., Mednick, S. A., & Michelson, N. M. (1989). Minor physical anomalies and recidivistic adult violent criminal behavior. *Acta Psychiatrica Scandinavica, 79,* 103–107.

Katsanis, J., & Iacono, W. G. (1991). Clinical, neuropsychological, and brain structural correlates of smooth-pursuit eye tracking performance in chronic schizophrenia. *Journal of Abnormal Psychology, 100,* 526–534.

Keshavan, M. S., Schooler, N. R., Sweeney, J. A., Haas, G. L., & Pettegrew, J. W. (1998). Research and treatment strategies in first-episode psychosis. *British Journal of Psychiatry, 172,* 60–65.

Khot, V., & Wyatt, R. J. (1991). Not all that moves is tardive dyskinesia. *American Journal of Psychiatry, 148,* 661–666.

Kraeplin, E. (1919). *Dementia praecox and paraphrenia.* New York: Kreiger.

Lambert, G. W., Horne, M., Kalff, V., Kelly, M. J., Turner, A. G., Cox, H. S., Jennings, G. L., & Esler, M. D. (1995). Central nervous system noradrenergic and dopaminergic turnover in response to acute neuroleptic challenge. *Life Sciences, 56,* 1545–1555.

Lane, A., Larkin, C., Waddington, J. L., & O'Callaghan, E. (1996). Dysmorphic features in schizophrenia. In J. L. Waddington & P. F. Buckley (Eds.), *The neurodevelopmental basis of schizophrenia* (pp. 79–93). Austin, TX: R. G. Landes.

Levine, S. (1993). Psychosocial factors in the regulation of the stress response during infancy. *Biological Psychiatry, 33,* 38–39.

Linszen, D., Lenior, M., De Haan, L., Dingemans, P., & Gersons, B. (1998). Early intervention, untreated psychosis and the course of early schizophrenia. *British Journal of Psychiatry, 172,* 84–89.

Lohr, J. B., & Flynn, K. (1993). Minor physical anomalies in schizophrenia and mood disorders. *Schizophrenia Bulletin, 19,* 551–556.

Maccari, S., Piazza, P. V., Kabbaj, M., Barbazanges, A., Simon, H., & Maol, M. L. (1995). Adoption reverses the long-term impairment in glucocorticoid feedback induced by prenatal stress. *Journal of Neuroscience, 15,* 110–116.

Machon, R. A., Mednick, S. A., & Huttunen, M. O. (1997). Adult major affective disorder after prenatal exposure to an influenza epidemic. *Archives of General Psychiatry, 54,* 322–328.

Malaspina, D., Coleman, E. A., Quitkin, M., Amador, X. F., Kaufmann, C. A., Gorman, J. M., & Sackheim, H. A. (1994). Effects of pharmacologic catecholamine manipulation on smooth pursuit eye movement in normals. *Schizophrenia Research, 13,* 151–160.

Marcus, J., Hans, S. L., Auerbach, J. G., & Auerbach, A. G. (1993). Children at risk for schizophrenia: The Jerusalem Infant Development Study: II. Neurobehavioral deficits at school age. *Archives of General Psychiatry, 50,* 797–809.

Mather, J. A. (1985). Eye movements of teenage children of schizophrenics: A possible inherited marker of susceptibility to the disease. *Journal of Psychiatric Research, 19,* 523–532.

McGlashan, T. H., & Johanessen, J. O. (1996). Early detection and intervention with schizophrenia. *Schizophrenia Bulletin, 22,* 201–217.

McNeil, T. F., Harty, B., Blennow, G., & Cantor-Graae, E. (1993). Neuromotor deviation in offspring of psychotic mothers: A selective developmental deficiency in two groups of children at heightened psychiatric risk? *Journal of Psychiatric Research, 27,* 39-54.

Mednick, S. A., & Hollister, J. M. (1995). *Neural development and schizophrenia: Theory and research.* New York: Plenum.

Mednick, S. A., Machon, R. A., Huttunen, M. O., & Bonet, D. (1988). Adult schizophrenia following prenatal exposure to an influenza epidemic. *Archives of General Psychiatry, 45,* 189–192.

Mednick, S. A., Mura, E., Schulsinger, F., & Mednick, B. (1971). Perinatal conditions and infant development in children with schizophrenic parents. *Social Biology, 18,* S103–S113.

Mednick, S. A., Watson, J. B., Huttunen, M., Cannon, T. D., Katila, H., Machon, R., Mednick, B., Hollister, M., Parnas, J., Schulsinger, F., Sajaniemi, N., Voldsgaard, P., Reijo, P., Gutkind, D., & Wang, X. (1998). A two-hit working model of the etiology of schizophrenia. In M. F. Lenzenweger & R. H. Dworkin (Eds.), *Origins and development of schizophrenia: Advances in experimental psychopathology* (pp. 27–66). Washington, DC: American Psychological Association.

Meehl, P. E. (1962). Schizotaxia, schizotypy, schizophrenia. *American Psychologist, 17,* 827–838.

Mellor, C. S. (1968). Dermatoglyphics in schizophrenia: I. Qualitative aspects. *British Journal of Psychiatry, 114,* 1387–1397.

Meyer, J. M., Silberg, J. L., Eaves, L. J., Maes, H. H., Simonoff, E., Pickles, A., Rutter, M. L., & Hewitt, J. K. (1999). Variable age of gene expression: Implications for developmental genetic models. In M. C. LaBuda, & E. L. Grigorenko (Eds.), *On the way to individuality: Current methodological issues in behavioral genetics* (pp. 23–52). Commack, NY: Nova Science.

Mialet, J. P., & Pichot, P. (1981). Eye-tracking patterns in schizophrenia: An analysis based on the incidence of saccades. *Archives of General Psychiatry, 38,* 183–186.

Nasrallah, H. A., & Olson, S. C. (1996). Hippocampal and entorhinal hypoplasia in schizophrenia is associated with early onset. *Biological Psychiatry, 39,* 597.

Nasrallah, H. A., Skinner, T. E., Schmalbrock, P., & Robitaille, P. (1994). Proton magnetic resonance spectroscopy (-1H MRS) of the hippocampal formation in schizophrenia: A pilot study. *British Journal of Psychiatry, 165,* 481–485.

Neumann, C. S., Grimes, K., Walker, E. F., & Baum, K. (1995). Developmental pathways to schizophrenia: Behavioral subtypes. *Journal of Abnormal Psychology, 104,* 1–9.

Neumann, C. S., & Walker, E. F. (1996). Childhood neuromotor soft-signs, behavior problems and adult psychopathology. In T. Ollendick & R. Prinz (Eds.), *Advances in clinical child psychology* (pp. 173–203). New York: Plenum.

Newell-Morris, L. L., Fahrenbruch, C. E., & Sackett, G. P. (1989). Prenatal psychological stress, dermatoglyphic asymmetry and pregnancy outcome in the pigtailed macaque (Macaca nemestrina). *Biology of the Neonate, 56,* 61–75.

Norman, R. M., & Malla, A. K. (1993). Stressful life events and schizophrenia: II. Conceptual and methodological issues. *British Journal of Psychiatry, 162,* 166–174.

Nuechterlein, K. H. (1983). Signal detection in vigilance tasks and behavioral attributes among offspring of schizophrenic mothers and among hyperactive children. *Journal of Abnormal Psychology, 92,* 4–28.

Nuechterlein, K. H., Asarnow, R. F., Subotnik, K. L., Fogelson, D. L., Ventura, J., Torquato, R. D., & Dawson, M. E. (1998). Neurocognitive vulnerability factors for schizophrenia: Convergence across genetic risk studies and longitudinal trait-state studies. In M. F. Lenzenweger & R. H. Dworkin (Eds.), *Origins and development of schizophrenia: Advances in experimental psychopathology* (pp. 299–327). Washington, DC: American Psychological Association.

O'Callaghan, E., Buckley, P., Madigan, C., & Redmond, O. (1995). The relationship of minor physical anomalies and other putative indices of developmental disturbance in schizophrenia to abnormalities of cerebral structure on magnetic resonance imaging. *Biological Psychiatry, 38,* 516–524.

O'Leary, D. D. M. (1997). A real specialization of the developing neocortex: Differentiation, developmental plasticity and genetic specification. In D. Magnusson, T. Greitz, T. Hokfelt, L. Nilsson, L. Terenius, & B. Winblad (Eds.), *The lifespan development of individuals: Behavioral, neurobiological, and psychosocial perspectives: A synthesis* (pp. 23–37). New York: Cambridge University Press.

Picard, D. (1998). Molecular endocrinology: Steroids tickle cells inside and out. *Nature, 369,* 437–438.

Plotsky, P. M., & Meaney, M. J. (1993). Early postnatal experience alters hypothalamic corticotrophin releasing factor (CRF) mRNA, median eminence CRF content, and stress-induced release in adult rats. *Molecular Brain Research, 18,* 195–200.

Pomeroy, J. C., Sprafkin, J., & Gadow, K. D. (1988). Minor physical anomalies as a biological marker for behavior disorders. *Journal of the American Academy of Child and Adolescent Psychiatry, 27,* 466–473.

Rall, J. E. (1998). Where are the genes specifying mental illness? *Journal of Nervous and Mental Disease, 186,* 722–723.

Rapoport, J. L., Giedd, J. N., Blumenthal, J., Hamburger, S., Jeffries, N., Fernandez, T., Nicolson, R., Bedwell, J., Lenane, M., Zijdenbos, A., Paus, T., & Evans, A. (1999). Progressive cortical change during adolescence in childhood-onset schizophrenia: A longitudinal magnetic resonance imaging study. *Archives of General Psychiatry, 56,* 649–654.

Rapoport, J. L., Giedd, J., Kumra, S., Jacobsen, L., Smith, A., Lee, P., Nelson, J., & Hamburger, S. (1997). Childhood-onset schizophrenia: Progressive ventricular change during adolescence. *Archives of General Psychiatry, 54,* 897–903.

Ross, R. G., Hommer, D., Radant, A., Roath, M., & Freedman, D. (1996). Early expression of smooth-pursuit eye movement abnormalities in children of schizophrenic parents. *Journal of the American Academy of Child and Adolescent Psychiatry, 35,* 941–949.

Schaumann, B., & Alter, M. (1976). *Dermatoglyphics in medical disorders.* New York: Springer-Verlag.

Schulkin, J., Gold, P. W., & McEwen, B. S. (1998). Induction of corticotropin-releasing hormone gene expression by glucocorticoids: Implication for understanding the states of fear and anxiety and allostatic load. *Psychoneuroendocrinology, 23,* 219–243.

Sham, P., O'Callaghan, E., Takei, N., Murray, G., Hare, E., & Murray, R. M. (1992). Schizophrenia following prenatal exposure to influenza epidemics between 1939–1960. *British Journal of Psychiatry, 160,* 461–466.

Smith, D. (1982). *Recognizable patterns of human malformation.* London: W. B. Saunders.

Smith, Y., Bevan, M. D., Shink, E., & Bolam, P. (1998). Microcircuitry of the direct and indirect pathways of the basal ganglia. *Neuroscience, 86,* 353–387.

Stassen, H. H., Coppola, R., Gottesman, I. I., Torrey, E. F., Kuny, S., Rickler, K. C., & Hell, D. (1999). EEG differences in monozygotic twins discordant and concordant for schizophrenia. *Psychophysiology, 36,* 109–117.

Suddath, R. L., Christison, G. W., Torrey, E. F., Casanova, M. F., & Weinberger, D. R. (1990). Anatomical abnormalities in the brains of monozygotic twins discordant for schizophrenia. *New England Journal of Medicine, 322,* 789–794.

Susman, E. J., Worrall, B. K., Murowchick, E., Frobose, C. A., & Schwab, J. E.

(1996). Experience and neuroendocrine parameters of development: Aggressive behavior and competencies. In D. M. Stoff & R. B. Cairns (Eds.), *Aggression and violence: Genetic, neurobiological, and biosocial perspectives* (pp. 267–289). Mahwah, NJ: Erlbaum.

Swerdlow, N. R., & Koob, G. F. (1987). Dopamine, schizophrenia, mania and depression: Toward a unified hypothesis of cortico–striato–pallido–thalamic function. *Behavioral and Brain Sciences, 10,* 197–245.

Swerdlow, N. R., & Koob, G. F. (1990). Toward a unified hypothesis of cortico–striato–pallido-thalamus function? *Behavioral and Brain Sciences, 13,* 172–177.

Takei, N., Lewis, S., Jones, P., Harvey, I., & Murray, R. M. (1994). Is prenatal exposure to influenza epidemics associated with increased cerebrospinal fluid spaces in schizophrenia. *Schizophrenia Bulletin, 22,* 521–534.

Tienari, P. (1991). Interaction between genetic vulnerability and family environment. *Acta Psychiatrica Scandinavica, 84,* 460–465.

Tienari, P., Wynne, L. C., Moring, J., Lahti, I., Naarala, M., Sorri, A., Wahlberg, K., Saarento, O., Seitamaa, M., Kaleva, M., & Laksy, K. (1994). The Finnish adoptive family study of schizophrenia: Implications for family research. *British Journal of Psychiatry, 164*(Supp. 23), 20–26.

Tyrka, A. R., Cannon, T. D., Haslam, N., Mednick, S. A., Schulsinger, F., Schulsinger, H., & Parnas, J. (1995). The latent structure of schizotypy: I. Premorbid indicators of a taxon of individuals at risk for schizophrenia-spectrum disorders. *Journal of Abnormal Psychology, 104,* 173–183.

Valone, K., Norton, J. P., Goldstein, M. J., & Doane, J. A. (1983). Parental expressed emotion and affective style in an adolescent sample at risk for schizophrenia spectrum disorders. *Journal of Abnormal Psychology, 92,* 399–407.

Velakoulis, D., Pantelis, C., McGorry, P. D., Dudgeon, P., Brewer, W., Cook, M., Desmond, P., Bridle, N., Tierney, P., Murrie, V., Singh, B., & Copolov, D. (1999). Hippocampal volume in first-episode psychoses and chronic schizophrenia: A high resolution magnetic resonance imaging study. *Archives of General Psychiatry, 56,* 133–141.

Waddington, J., & Buckley, P. (1996). *The neurodevelopmental basis of schizophrenia.* Austin, TX: R. G. Landes.

Waldo, M. C., Cawthra, E., Adler, L. E., Dubester, S., Staunton, M., Nagamoto, H., Baker, N., Madison, A., Simon, J., Scherzinger, A., Drebing, C., Gerhardt, G., & Freedman, R. (1994). Auditory sensory gaiting, hippocampal volume, and catecholamine metabolism in schizophrenics and their siblings. *Schizophrenia Research, 12,* 93–106.

Waldrop, M. F., & Halverson, C. F. (1971). Minor physical anomalies and hyperactive behavior in young children. In J. Helmuth (Ed.), *Exceptional infant: Studies in abnormalities* (pp. 343–380). New York: Brunner/Mazel.

Walker, E. (1994). The developmentally moderated expression of the neuropathology underlying schizophrenia. *Schizophrenia Bulletin, 20,* 453–480.

Walker, E., Baum, K., & Diforio, D. (1998). Developmental changes in the behavioral expression of vulnerability for schizophrenia. In M. Lenzenweger & B. Dworkin (Eds.), *Origins and development of schizophrenia* (pp. 469–492). Washington, DC: American Psychological Association.

Walker, E., Cudek, R., Mednick, S. A., & Schulsinger, F. (1981). The effects of parental absence and institutionalization on the development of clinical symptoms in high-risk children. *Acta Psychiatrica Scandinavica, 63,* 95–109.

Walker, E., & Diforio, D. (1997). Schizophrenia: A neural diathesis–stress model. *Psychological Review, 104,* 1–19.

Walker, E. F., Downey, G., & Bergman, A. (1989). The effects of parental psychopathology and maltreatment on child behavior: A test of the diathesis–stress model. *Child Development, 60,* 15–24.

Walker, E. F., Lewine, R. R., & J. Neumann, C. (1996). Childhood behavioral characteristics and adult brain morphology in schizophrenia. *Schizophrenia Research, 22,* 93–101.

Walker, E. F., Lewis, N., Loewy, R., & Palyo, S. (1999). Motor dysfuntion and risk for schizophrenia. *Development and Psychopathology, 11,* 509–523.

Walker, E., & Neumann, C. (1996). Neuordevelopmental models of schizophreina. In J. Waddington & P. Buckley (Eds.), *The neurodevelopmental basis of schizophrenia* (pp. 1–12). Austin, TX: R.G. Landes.

Walker, E. F., Savoie, T., & Davis, D. (1994). Neuromotor precursors of schizophrenia. *Schizophrenia Bulletin, 20,* 453–480.

Watson, J., & Mednick S. A. (1998). *Depressive symptoms in offspring following severe prenatal stress.* Proceedings of the annual meeting of the Society for Research in Psychopathology, Boston.

Weinberger, D. R. (1987). Implications of normal brain development for the pathogenisis of schizophrenia. *Archives of General Psychiatry, 44,* 660–669.

Whitworth, A. B., Honeder, M., Kremser, C., Kemmler, G., Felber, S., Hausmann, A., Wanko, C., Wechdorn, H., Aichner, F., Stuppaeck, C. H., & Fleischhacker, W. W. (1998). Hippocampal volume reduction in male schizophrenic patients. *Schizophrenia Research, 31,* 73–81.

Winters, L., Cornblatt, B. A., & Erlenmeyer-Kimling, L. (1991). The prediction of psychiatric disorders in late adolescence. In E. F. Walker (Ed.), *Schizophrenia: A life-course developmental perspective* (pp. 123–137). San Diego, CA: Academic Press.

Wolfradt, U., & Straube, E. R. (1998). Factor structure of schizotypal traits among adolescents. *Personality and Individual Differences, 24,* 201–206.

Wyatt, R. J. (1995). Antipsychotic medication and the long-term course of schizophrenia. In C. L. Shriqui & H. A. Nasrallah (Eds.), *Contemporary issues in the treatment of schizophrenia* (pp. 385–410). Washington, DC: American Psychiatric Association.

Yee, F., & Yolken, R. H. (1997). Identification of differentially expressed RNA transcripts in neuropsychiatric disorders. *Biological Psychiatry, 41,* 759–761.

Yeo, R. A., Hodde-Vargas, J., Hendren, R. L., Vargas, L. A., Brooks, W. M., Ford, C. C., Gangestad, S. W., & Hart, B. L. (1997). Brain abnormalities in schizophrenia-spectrum children: Implications for a neurodevelopmental perspective. *Psychiatry Research: Neuroimaging, 76,* 1–13.

Zipursky, R. B., Lim, K. O., Sullivan, E. V., Brown B. W., & Pfefferbaum, A. (1992). Widespread cerebral gray matter volume deficits in schizophrenia. *Archives of General Psychiatry, 49,* 195–205.

15

Vulnerability to Schizophrenia in Adulthood

PHILIP D. HARVEY

Schizophrenia is a devastating mental illness that has multiple direct and indirect costs to the individuals afflicted and to society in general. This illness has been a puzzle to researchers and clinicians because of the difficulty in its treatment and the long-standing problems in identifying even basic components of the causes of the disorder. Whereas the study of some aspects of the disorder such as the prevalence, symptoms, course, and the outcome of the illness has lead to a comprehensive knowledge base, other aspects of the illness have remained illusive. Most illusive is the cause of the illness, including genetic and environmental factors. This chapter presents information about the factors that influence vulnerability to the development of this disorder, with a focus on onset of the illness during the adult years.

Schizophrenia in its current conception is a disorder defined with a polythetic structure. Polythetic means that the signs of illness are variable across individuals and some combination of these signs is required to identify the presence of the illness, with no single "pathognomic" indicator. To meet current U.S. or worldwide criteria, an individual must show two different symptoms, including delusions (fixed false beliefs), hallucinations (aberrant perceptual experiences in any sensory modality), impairments in communication or affect, or bizarre behavior. If the delusions or hallucinations are "characteristic," they can be the only active sign. Patients must also have signs of a 6-month or greater decline in their overall level of functioning and the symptoms cannot be due to alcohol or drug abuse or to the presence of a brain disease or injury or affective disorder. This conception of schizophrenia has its basis in the illness "dementia praecox," defined by Kraepelin (1896). There are several aspects of schizophrenia outside the

355

diagnostic criteria that merit additional attention. Extreme functional deficit is common in schizophrenia and only 30% of patients with schizophrenia are ever able to live independent lives, with this level of functional deficit not changing markedly over the last 100 years (Hegarty, Baldessarino, & Tohen, 1994). The vast majority of patients with schizophrenia also have significant cognitive impairments and most have lives that are marked by social isolation, poverty, and ostracism by the community as a whole.

When Kraepelin (1896) defined dementia praecox over 100 years ago, incorporated into the term was his idea about the prototypical onset age. Praecox denotes "late-adolescent/ early adult," and his belief was that this illness, characterized by a deteriorating course, cognitive and functional impairment, and a wide array of other symptoms, had its typical onset during these years. Although later clinicians such as Bleuler (1911) disagreed with Kraepelin about the absoluteness of the onset age for the illness, considerable research has indicated that the majority of cases of schizophrenia have an onset age during the early adult years.

Schizophrenia can have an onset age, according to current criteria, that ranges from early childhood to the end of life. The "typical" onset age of schizophrenia, as marked by the greatest new incidence of cases with the illness, is late adolescence or early adulthood. Individuals who develop schizophrenia during this period have a number of characteristics that separate them from individuals with other illnesses and from the normal populations. These characteristics are described in the next section.

GENERAL CHARACTERISTICS
OF ADULT-ONSET SCHIZOPHRENIA

Prevalence

Although it is difficult to make absolute statements about the prevalence of many less severe disorders, the disabling nature of schizophrenia as it is currently defined means that most cases can be identified. Worldwide estimates of the prevalence of schizophrenia generally cite an overall prevalence of about 1% of the population or slightly less. Prevalence estimates and symptomatic presentation do not vary markedly across different countries (World Health Organization, 1972). This prevalence has been reported to be slightly increased in isolated areas where the genetic pool is compacted because of geographic isolation (Kendler et al., 1993). About 0.87% of the population of the world will meet criteria for schizophrenia at some time in their lives.

Incidence

Prevalence data do not necessarily link directly to the incidence rates of new cases because of factors affecting the number of cases such as differential mortality across genders with the illness. The "typical" age of onset for schizophrenia is in the early 20s for males and the early 30s for females. Thus, the average age of onset for schizophrenia is in the adult years. Population-based incidence studies suggest that the new-case rates of schizophrenia are slightly higher in males than in females. They also suggest that the peak age of onset is shifted across the genders. In a large-scale study of the development of schizophrenia in a London Borough, Castle and Murray (1993) reported average age of onset for males (31.2) was 10 years younger than that of females (41.1). The male/female ratio changed as a function of age of onset, with the ratio at 1.6 to 1 for onset from age 16 to 25 and 0.2 to 1 for onset age in late life. The later the age of onset, the greater the bias toward females being the newly incident cases. Median age of onset was actually considerably lower than mean age of onset because some cases were seen to have their first schizophrenia symptoms after the age of 65. Thus, gender appears to be a vulnerability factor for schizophrenia and to affects its clinical characteristics as well.

This study had the benefit of being a door-to-door epidemiological study in contrast to a first-admission study. Ascertainment bias is a major factor when first admission is used as the criterion to estimate onset age. Referral to treatment is often associated with behavioral disturbances, which are more common in male patients who are therefore more difficult to manage at home.

Factors Associated with Age of Onset

Particularly early-onset age, although still during the adult years, has been known for years to be associated with a more adverse lifetime course, a poorer functional outcome, and a reduced likelihood of positive response to treatment. Patients with early (i.e., late adolescent to very early adult) onset are more likely to have reduced academic and social achievement and to have relatives with schizophrenia-spectrum conditions (Keefe et al., 1987; Zigler, Glick, & Marsh, 1979). Earlier age of onset for males is found even if cases with relatively poor lifetime outcome are compared across the genders (Davidson et al., 1995). At the same time, in patients with a positive family history of schizophrenia, female patients are reported to have the same age at onset as males (Albus & Maier, 1995), suggesting that family history of the illness may exert a stronger influence on onset age than gender.

VULNERABILITY TO SCHIZOPHRENIA

The distribution of cases of schizophrenia is not consistent with any well-understood pattern of genetic inheritance. Searches for a uniform environmental factor have proven equivalently unsuccessful. Schizophrenia also appears to occur in several variants that describe a "spectrum" of related conditions. The fact that there is a group of related conditions and a number of indicators of risk for the illness has been understood since Kraepelin. These other conditions appear to occur more frequently in relatives of patients with schizophrenia than in relatives of individuals without the illness, but these disorders are not limited in their occurrence to relatives (see Kety & Ingraham, 1992, for a review of this concept). Furthermore, individuals who are destined to develop schizophrenia have been shown to manifest a number of cognitive and behavioral abnormalities before the development of the illness, but these abnormalities have not been found to form a pattern that is specific to schizophrenia. Finally, the combination of multiple cognitive or behavioral abnormalities appears to be associated with an increased risk for developing the illness.

The Concept

The concept of vulnerability to schizophrenia has been described by several different researchers as far back as Kraepelin. Meehl (1962) provided the earliest clear scientifically oriented description of this model. He described a genetically inherited predisposition to the illness he called schizotaxia. This predisposition was seen to be multiufactorial and probably transmitted across several different genetic loci (polygenic). The observable behavioral signs of the predisposition were referred to as "schizotypy," which itself was seen to be a condition related to and similar to schizophrenia. Further experiential factors were then seen to lead schizotypes down the etiological path to schizophrenia. For the past 35 years, research on the development of schizophrenia has largely been informed by a vulnerability approach.

Because it has proven possible to retrospectively identify several potential risk factors for the development of schizophrenia, and because no single factor appears to be a necessary and sufficient cause of the disorder, research has been oriented at explanation and prediction of the factors that are associated with vulnerability to the development of schizophrenia. One of the most commonly applied models is the diathesis–stress model (Zubin & Spring, 1977). The overall framework of this model suggests that there is a necessary but not sufficient predisposing factor for the illness, combined with a similarly necessary but not sufficient stressor that interacts with the diathesis to cause the development of the illness. Such a predisposition could be genetically transmitted or acquired environmentally, whereas the stressor could be psychological or physiological (Harvey, Walker, & Wielgus, 1986). Predispositions could have measurable psychological or physiological correlates, with the psychological correlates being in the domains of cognitive deficits, personality traits, or behavioral tendencies. Biological correlates of the predisposition could be found in the domains of abnormal brain structure or activity, abnormal patterns of physiological reactivity to environmental stimuli, or genetic markers.

Strengths of the Model

The strengths of this model are clear in that schizophrenia appears to have multiple domains of potential cause and to consist of several unique but similar entities. This model helps to structure research and direct attention to the fact that the symptomatic diversity in schizophrenia may be associated with diversity in etiological factors. The evidence regarding the etiology of schizophrenia has indicated that it is unlikely that a single factor is the root cause of all cases of the illness. For example, individuals who share similar potential predispositions (e.g., an identical twin with the illness) vary in the extent to which they express the full syndrome (Gottesman & Shields, 1982). Thus, research using this perspective might study individuals who shared a common predisposing factor and relate variation in their outcome to differences in their life experiences (or stressors). A similar approach could be applied to individuals who were exposed to similar stressors (e.g., maternal exposure to influenza or famine) in order to relate variations in their outcomes to variations in potential predisposing factors.

Weaknesses of the Model

The principal weakness in this model is that little is known precisely about either potential predispositions to schizophrenia or stressors that could activate these predispositions. Often this approach is applied post hoc. As a result, this framework is often used for explanatory purposes more than for predictive ones. It is possible that there is a biological factor, as yet undiscovered, that fully accounts for many cases of schizophrenia regardless of environmental experience. Similarly, certain experiential factors might cause schizophrenia in anyone exposed. A rigid application of the diathesis–stress model may suppress research on factors that might prove to be necessary and sufficient to cause some cases of the illness.

Heterogeneity and Vulnerability

Schizophrenia may be several different diseases that share behavioral features. There is enormous heterogeneity in this illness, in terms of symptom presentation, clinical course, response to available treatments, family history of the illness, age at onset, type of onset (rapid vs. insidious), premorbid adjustment, and other factors. If schizophrenia was actually eight different illnesses of equal prevalence (Ciompi, 1980), identification of a single necessary and sufficient vulnerability factor that was present in all cases with one of the variants might still lead to negative results in studies in which that illness variant was present in only one-eighth of the cases. In fact, schizophrenia may be eight different disorders of different prevalence. As a result, the search for vulnerability factors in schizophrenia is complicated by the heterogeneity of the illness, while some failures to replicate previous findings may be due to this heterogeneity.

DOMAINS OF VULNERABILITY FACTORS

Factors that increase risk for schizophrenia arise from several different domains. These include factors that appear to be genetic, prenatal, but not genetic, and postnatal experiential factors. The postnatal experiential factors include both general social experiences (e.g., social class) and specific environmental events (e.g., poor nutrition and possible family interaction variables). Each of these domains has received considerable research attention, and there is reason to believe that they may be important factors in the development of some cases of schizophrenia.

Genetic Factors

Schizophrenia has been known to be familial since its definition. Although familial does not necessarily mean genetic, studies of adopted-away children of parents with schizophrenia have suggested that their risk for illness is the same as the risk for those children of parents with schizophrenia who were reared at home (Heston, 1966; Kety, Rosenthal, Wender, & Schulsinger, 1968). Comprehensive studies of the risk for schizophrenia in the relatives of affected individuals suggests a pattern of inheritance that is incompatible with a single-gene model with full penetrance or expressivity or a simple polygenic model. As Table 15.1, based on Gottesman and Shields (1982), illustrates, even monozygotic twins are concordant for the illness at levels much greater than would be expected from a typical genetic inheritance model. In fact, the concordance ratio for schizophrenia is less than half that which would be expected from any genetic transmission model that does not posit reductions in penetrance. At the same time, twin studies that examined differences in the concordance rates of monozygotic (MZ) and dizygotic (DZ) twins have suggested estimates of heritability of the illness in the range of 80%. Although relatives of individuals with schizophrenia are more than 10 times as likely to develop the illness as individuals without such relatives, only about 30% of patients with schizophrenia have a relative who has the illness or some agreed-on variant of the illness. Furthermore, an average concordance rate of 50% for MZ twins for schizophrenia could also be produced by some variants of the illness being determined com-

TABLE 15.1. Risks for Schizophrenia in Relatives of Patients with Schizophrenia

Relationship	Risk[a]
MZ cotwin	44.30
DZ cotwin	12.08
Sibling	7.30
Child	9.35
Grandchild	2.85
Spouse	1.00
General population	0.87

Note. Data from Gottesman and Shields (1982).
[a]Expressed as percentage of individuals with this type of relation who have the illness.

pletely by genetic factors and other variants having a small or negligible genetic component.

Current genetic results have not advanced consistently beyond population genetic findings. There have been huge numbers of reports of linkage markers that focus on many different chromosomes. In fact, the summer 1998 issue of the *American Journal of Medical Genetics* was devoted in large part to a review of workshops on nine different chromosomes that may be potential linkage sites for schizophrenia. A recent genome-wide survey (Shaw et al., 1998) found 12 different chromosomes that had statistically significant potential linkage for schizophrenia.

In contrast to the increased replicability of other findings in schizophrenia, linkage studies are routinely not replicated. In fact, there are no published linkage studies of schizophrenia that have not had at least one published failure to replicate. Given the heterogeneity of schizophrenia, failures in replication of linkage results are not necessarily definitive. Because schizophrenia may constitute a set of related disorders, there may be multiple genetic sites in which predispositions are transmitted. Predispositions may be multifactorial in that the convergence of multiple genetically transmitted vulnerabilities may be required before the illness is fully expressed.

Related to this point, alternative variants of schizophrenia, referred to as schizophrenia-spectrum conditions (Kety, 1985), may reflect the incomplete expression of the predispositions for schizophrenia. For example, some individuals with flat affect and social anhedonia may possess some of the genetically transmitted vulnerabilities to the illness without ever developing the full condition because they did not inherit other required traits. As described later, some of these traits may be measurable, such as attentional abnormalities, whereas others, such as subtle alterations in neurotransmission or cerebral structure, may be more difficult to detect. There are many cases of schizophrenia in which no relatives at all appear affected with any of the schizophrenia-spectrum conditions, with these cases referred to as sporadic cases. These sporadic cases may actually be cases in which a critical number of relatives possessed some combination of the traits associated with schizophrenia. On the other hand, these cases may well be phenocopies produced by some of the environmental factors described later. All in all, the level of complexity of the inheritance pattern for schizophrenia has led to slower progress in the area of identification of genetic factors in schizophrenia than in some of the other areas of the illness.

Experiential Factors

Experience can include exposure to both physiological factors (toxins, deprivation states) and psychological events. Psychological events could be discrete traumata or they can be constant and cumulative, such as those associated with daily experience to a stressful environment. These events can occur between conception and birth or between birth and the development of schizophrenia.

Prenatal Factors

Prenatal factors have been studied in detail as risk factors for the development of schizophrenia. Maternal exposure to influenza (Takei et al., 1996) as well as famine (Susser et al., 1996) has been shown in some studies to increase risk for schizophrenia. Specifically, having a mother who contracts the flu during her second trimester of gestation appears to be a risk factor that increases the likelihood of developing schizophrenia. In the Takei study, for every 100,000 cases of influenza during the second trimester there was a 12% increase in the rates of schizophrenia. Furthermore, the incidence of schizophrenia in the general population is also increased during other disasters, such as the "Dutch Hunger Winter" of 1944–1945 (Susser et al., 1996). Although an increase in population incidence of schizophrenia associated with a famine or a pandemic may appear to suggest that stress alone increases risk for the development of the illness, it cannot be determined whether genetic diatheses are also involved. Because not every child who was born to a mother who was experiencing starvation or influenza developed schizophrenia, this stressor alone could not be adequate to be a necessary and sufficient cause of schizophrenia. In fact, the Takei study reported that only 1.4% of the total cases of schizophrenia could be attributed to possible influenza-related causes. Furthermore, a recent study reported that affective disorder also increased in prevalence among individuals exposed to influenza *in utero* in the second trimester (Machon, Mednick, & Huttunen, 1997). Finally, stress alone, including exposure to national disasters (e.g., the Nazi invasion of the Netherlands), has also been found to be associated with increased risk for the development of schizophrenia (van Os & Selten, 1998). Thus, both biological and psychological experiences of the mother appear to have the potential to lead to the changes in fetal development that are associated with increased risk for the development of schizophrenia.

A number of indicators have suggested that the second trimester is the critical stage for the occurrence of prenatal incidents that influence the development of schizophrenia. For example, brain regions that develop rapidly during this trimester and require appropriate cell migration (e.g., corpus callosum) are found to be abnormal in schizophrenia (Bunney, Potkin, & Bunney, 1995). In addition, evidence of abnormalities in body regions other than the brain that develop in the second trimester (dermatoglyphic symmetry) is found to be correlated with the presence of other minor physical anomalies and to be elevated in patients with schizophrenia (Fananas et al., 1996). Because some studies failed to replicate findings of second-trimester influenza and schizophrenia (Morgan et al., 1997) and the number of patients in whom the occurrence of influenza can be demonstrated is quite small, caution needs to be applied before any clinical use can be made of second-trimester maternal stress or illness as an intervention point for the primary prevention of schizophrenia.

Postnatal Factors

Postnatal environmental factors influencing the development of schizophrenia have proven difficult to identify. Toxic exposure, head trauma, and drug use and other causes of psychotic conditions appear remarkably unassociated with increased risk for enduring schizophrenia. Exposure to some drugs, especially drugs that have effects on the glutamatergic system, appears to have the potential to cause states that resemble schizophrenia (Abi-Saab, D'Souza, Moghaddam, & Krystal, 1998). Phencyclidine (PCP; "Angel dust") and ketamine ("Special K"), for example, have been drugs of abuse for years and have been shown in experimental studies to exacerbate symptoms of schizophrenia and to cause transitory psychotic experiences in normal individuals (Krystal et al., 1994). The rate of exposure to these drugs is so low in the population as a whole and in individuals who develop schizophrenia that it cannot be considered a general risk factor for the illness.

Despite the early primacy of psychological theories of the etiology of schizophrenia, including theories focusing on interpersonal interaction and communication, there is little evidence of general or specific postnatal psychological experience factors associated with the initial development of schizophrenia. Early theories focused on patterns of familial interaction. These theories included ideas such as the influence of a "schizophrenogenic" mother (Fromm-Reichman, 1948), whose interaction with the child caused schizophrenia. Later theories more clearly specified the characteristics of the potentially problematic interactions, including communications that implied a "double bind" (Bateson, Jackson, Haley, & Weakland, 1956). Such a communication would have the form of "I order you to disobey me" or "I'll only love you if you hate me." Other theories specified aberrant patterns of family organization or attributed certain personality character-istics to parents (i.e., "battle-axe mother") that then led their offspring to develop schizophrenia.

Theories such as these have never been well-supported empirically. Much the same as such grossly invasive surgical procedures as frontal lobotomies were applied to patients with schizophrenia as a "desperate cure" for schizo-phrenia, such theories appear now to be the product of a desperate search for any idea that could explain the cause of the illness and lead to an inter-vention. Their effect on families was certainly pernicious, whereby parents who were already devastated by the horrible illness affecting their children were also told that they had in some way caused it. In fact, not a single psychological factor has been found to be associated with the development of schizophrenia, even those with powerful face validity. As noted earlier, being reared by a schizophrenic parent has no apparent impact on risk for the illness, in that children of parents with schizophrenia who are reared separately from their parents have essentially identical risk to children whose parents with schizophrenia are their caregivers (Heston, 1966). Being reared by an adoptive parent with schizophrenia without having a biological par-ent with schizophrenia also apparently does not increase the risk for the illness either.

There are some well-replicated environmental predictors of relapse in schizophrenia. Most prominently, the level of expressed emotion (EE) on the part of family members who directly interact with community dwelling patients who have recovered from an acute exacerbation of schizophrenia predicts risk of later worsening of symptoms (Leff, 1976; Vaughn & Leff, 1976). This risk factor has also been shown to be even more important in other illnesses, such as depression and eating disorders (Miklowitz, Goldstein, Nuechterlein, Snyder, & Mintz, 1988). This factor has not been shown to be a predictor of risk for the development of the illness, however, as families of patients with schizophrenia can be discriminated into those who do and do not express high levels of EE. The low level of specificity of EE to schizo-phrenia, with high levels of EE detected in subsets of relatives of patients with depression, bipolar disorder, eating disorders, and traumatic brain in-juries (Butzlaff & Hooley, 1998), also argues against its importance as a specific etiological factor.

Neurodevelopmental Factors and the Timing of Onset of Schizophrenia

As seen from the sections immediately preceding this one, no environmental factors that reliably occur between gestation and the onset of illness have been identified. This situation has led to the popularity of "neuro-developmental" models of the origin of the illness. These models, as convincingly articulated by Weinberger (1987), suggest that one or more neurobiological insults, occurring at an early stage of fetal development, lead to the abnormal development of the central nervous system and eventually to the development of schizophrenia. These insults can be genetic predispositions, developmental insults, or most likely some combination of the two. Early neurodevelopmental abnormalities may have various behavioral manifestations at different stages of development, as shown by Hyde, Ziegler, and Weinberger's (1992) elegant comparison of the symptomatic course of progressive metachromatic leukodystrophy, a neurodegenerative disease caused by an early brain lesion, to the course of schizophrenia. Thus, a single neurodevelopmental lesion can cause variable symptomatic manifestations depending on the state of development and age of the brain. In addition, early neurodevelopmental problems may lead to a lifelong pattern of behavioral and cerebral change, as evidenced by recent studies finding progressive enlargement of the cerebral ventricles in a subset of patients with both adult- and childhood-onset schizophrenia (Davis et al., 1998; DeLisi et al., 1997; Rapoport et al., 1997).

Thus, by the time of identification of potential indicators of vulnerability to schizophrenia, both the diathesis and the stress may have already had their effect. It is possible that all the factors associated with the development of schizophrenia are already in place by the time a child is born, including genetically transmitted factors predisposing the individual to develop schizophrenia when exposed to intrauterine events and the occurrence of the events themselves. Regardless of whether or not this theoretical scenario is correct, there would be no difference in the research on behavioral, physiological, and biological indicators of vulnerability to schizophrenia, because the timing of the insult is not intrinsically related to the measurement of its correlates.

MARKERS OF VULNERABILITY

Markers of vulnerability to schizophrenia are measurable indicators of increased risk for the development of the illness (Zubin & Spring, 1977). In terms of the logic of identifying increased risk for the illness, it would not matter what the domain of predisposition was, biological, psychological, or physiological, as long as measurable indicators could be identified. This review focuses on previous research on putative psychological and psychophysiological markers of vulnerability rather than attempting to focus on specific genetic markers or other biological traits.

Identification

The ideal process of identification of a marker of vulnerability would be a predictive validity study. A putative marker is identified early in life, the child is followed until adulthood, and the outcome of the child is related to the presence/absence or severity level of the indicator. In reality, such studies are difficult to complete because of the long follow-up period required. If the wrong marker was tested, many years would pass before the results of the study were in. The domains of vulnerability markers must first be narrowed through the use of concurrent validity studies. In these studies, aspects of cognitive or physiological abnormalities that are present in individuals with schizophrenia are evaluated for their potential as vulnerability markers and then procedures measuring these markers are administered to potentially vulnerable individuals.

One of the limitations of this approach for the identification of markers of vulnerability is that aspects of schizophrenia other than the causes of the illness may influence performance on cognitive and psychophysiological measures. For example, aspects of the treatment of schizophrenia, symptomatic features that develop over time with chronic illness, poor health care and diet, and the lengthy inpatient stays or chronic social isolation experienced by some patients could influence performance on these measures. Because most patients with schizophrenia have cognitive deficits that are greater than would be expected from their premorbid intelligence (Gold, Randolph, Carpenter, Goldberg, & Weinberg, 1992), tests on which patients with schizophrenia perform quite poorly might still be quite easy for individuals who have not yet developed the full syndrome of illness. Thus, it is important to identify whether aspects of the cognitive and behavioral abnormalities of patients with schizophrenia are consequences of the illness and not potential precursor signs.

Who should be examined for vulnerability? For years research on vulnerability markers has focused on individuals who are at extra high risk for the development of the illness—individuals who have a first-degree relative with the illness. Many of these studies have employed a longitudinal prospective methodology (Mednick & McNeil, 1968). Such a method allows for the selection of the specific indicators to be examined, rather than relying on the contents of an archive. Prospective studies of high-risk children have the advantage of identifying of individuals at risk before they have had a wide array of environmental experiences, but they necessitate a long follow-up period. Studies of adult relatives are not complicated by the need to carefully consider developmental factors, but they may be hampered by selection bias. The easy-to-locate adult relatives of patients with schizophrenia may well be the ones with minimal psychopathology and minimal vulnerability to the illness. Studying these cases may lead to a bias toward negative findings.

Whole population studies are essentially impossible for a single investigator because of logistical factors related to the low prevalence rate of schizophrenia. Any selected population study also runs the risk of bias, because early-onset cases of schizophrenia will be selectively eliminated from any subpopulation. Several population-based studies have been completed, all of which have relied on archival data. The government of the United Kingdom initiated two child development studies, one in 1946 and another in 1958. Children born in specific periods in these 2 years were followed over early childhood and into adult life. Of those children, approximately 0.63% developed schizophrenia (Jones, Rodgers, Murray, & Marmot, 1994). Their characteristics in early childhood, as long as 20 years before the onset of their other symptoms of schizophrenia, could then be related to their eventual outcome. In both these studies, children destined to develop schizophrenia manifested patterns of deficits in academic skills that discriminated them from children who grew up without developing schizophrenia (Crow, Done, & Sacker, 1995; Jones et al., 1994). These children demonstrated deficits in math and reading skills that were about 1.5 standard deviations below those seen in children who developed normally. Social deficits were also seen in these children, with the children characterized by teachers as having few friends and being asocial. In addition, cognitive deficits were reported several years before social deficits in one sample (Jones et al., 1994) and concurrently to social deficits in another (Done, Crow, Johnstone, & Sacker, 1994). These data indicate that the developmental progression of schizophrenia may include cognitive impairments and social deficits in those individuals who develop schizophrenia later in life, with the exact pattern of occurrence of these deficits not yet clearly determined.

Similar studies have been performed in countries with universal military service. These countries routinely evaluate large numbers of potential conscripts before their induction. Often these evaluations are quite comprehensive and include assessments of psychological and social functioning. In countries such as Sweden (David, Malmberg, Brandt, Allebeck, & Lewis, 1997) and Israel (Davidson et al., 1999), where there are also detailed mental health records on the country as a whole, the entire population of early adolescents can be examined for their outcome and its relationship to characteristics that were present before the onset of other signs of the illness.

Two studies have generated similar results. In the first, David et al. (1997) found that lower performance on aspects of verbal and mechanical abilities predicted risk for developing schizophrenia in a Swedish conscript cohort, with the relationship relatively linear. Patients at risk for affective disorders had higher IQs and the relationship between IQ performance and risk for illness was nonlinear. Both verbal and constructional skills were related to risk. In a study of Israeli conscripts that included comprehensive assessments of cognitive and personality factors, Davidson et al. (1999) reported that the combination of specific personality deficits and cognitive impairments was highly sensitive and specific to identify risk for schizophrenia. Specifically, a pattern of social aversiveness, lack of close friends, and impairments in attentional and motor skills was more than 90% likely to identify individuals at the time of their conscription exam who later developed schizophrenia.

Cognitive Impairments

As just described, patterns of cognitive deficits can be proven to have been present in individuals who later develop schizophrenia. In addition, patterns of cognitive impairments can be detected in individuals who are empirically at high risk for schizophrenia. For example, residual performance deficits in individuals who have had a previous psychotic episode have been reported for years (Asarnow & MacCrimmon, 1978). These deficits are primarily in the areas of attention, vigilance, and accurate perception of rapidly presented information, especially under distracting conditions. These same deficits have been reported in children of parents with schizophrenia and in the adult relatives of individuals who have schizophrenia (Harvey et al., 1986).

Vigilance or Sustained Attention

Deficits in the ability to process a rapidly presented series of visual stimuli and to correctly identify a predetermined target stimulus have been reported in potentially vulnerable individuals for years. Individuals who have recovered from schizophrenic episodes manifest these deficits (Asarnow & MacCrimmon, 1978), as do children of parents with schizophrenia (Cornblatt & Erlenmeyer-Kimling, 1985) and the first-degree relatives of patients with schizophrenia (Keefe et al., 1997). These deficits have typically been detected with the continuous performance test (CPT). The CPT has been used in several forms and it has been noted that vulnerable individuals have deficits on many different versions of the CPT. These findings suggest that vigilance deficits are one of the most consistently detected cognitive impairments in individuals who are potentially vulnerable to schizophrenia.

Recent research has indicated that deficits in vigilance may also be correlated with the presence of other potential markers of vulnerability to schizophrenia or membership in the schizophrenia spectrum. In a recent study, Keefe et al. (1997) found that adult first-degree relatives of patients with schizophrenia who manifested performance deficits on the CPT were also likely to manifest symptoms of schizotypal personality disorder. In contrast, deficient eye-tracking performance, a putative vulnerability marker, was found to be uncorrelated with behavioral symptoms of schizotypal personality.

The most exciting study to date in the area of vulnerability to schizophrenia has found that CPT deficits detected in early adolescence are powerful predictors of vulnerability to the development of adult-onset schizophrenia. Cornblatt, Obuchowski, Roberts, Pollack, and Erlenmeyer-Kimling (1999) found that deficits on the CPT at age 12 identified those children of parents with schizophrenia who developed schizophrenia or schizophrenia spectrum conditions by the age of 26 with sensitivity and specificity levels over 85%. Children of parents with schizophrenia without attentional deficits at age 12 were no more likely to develop schizophrenia than were the children of parents with no evidence of mental illness.

This study is the first study of vulnerability processes in schizophrenia that used longitudinal methodology to demonstrate that a putative marker was actually associated with vulnerability to schizophrenia. Pending replication, this study also indicates that vigilance deficit is a crucial feature of the individual vulnerable to the development of schizophrenia in adulthood and that this deficit in cognitive functioning and the underlying biological processes it reflects are central to the development of the illness in individuals who have a relative with schizophrenia.

Rapid Visual Processing

Deficits in the ability to identify rapidly presented visual information have been reported in schizophrenia for over 30 years (Neale, McIntyre, Fox, & Cromwell, 1969). Remitted patients with schizophrenia (Asarnow & MacCrimmon, 1978) and children of patients with schizophrenia (Asarnow, Steffy, Cleghorn, & MacCrimmon, 1977) have also been reported to manifest these deficits as well. For example, using the Span of Apprehension Test (SOA), remitted patients with schizophrenia were found to have deficits in their performance, as were children of parents with schizophrenia. These deficits are limited to conditions in which the subject is required to process target information in the presence of irrelevant information. Although these findings have not always been replicated (Harvey, Weintraub, & Neale, 1985), methodological differences between studies may be responsible for the variation in findings. Although there have been extensive debates about the underlying mechanism of these deficits, their relationship to vulnerability to schizophrenia appears clear. Likewise, poor performance on tests of vulnerability to the effects of backward masking appears linked to vulnerability to schizophrenia (Green, Nuechterlein, & Mintz, 1994). Deficits are seen on the part of patients with schizophrenia (Rund, 1993) and patients without schizophrenia with schizophrenia-spectrum disorders (Braff, 1981). Some studies have not found a strong relationship between poor performance schizophrenia (Green et al., 1994), so this potential marker may be more limited in its predictive value than are other aspects of attention and rapid visual processing.

Selective Attention and Distractibility

Excessive vulnerability to the effects of irrelevant distracting information during information processing appears to be related to vulnerability to schizophrenia. Psychotic (Oltmanns, 1978) and remitted (Harvey, Docherty, Serper,

& Rasmussen, 1990) patients with schizophrenia appear to be excessively distractible, as are children of parents with schizophrenia (Harvey, Winters, Weintraub, & Neale, 1981). Distractibility appears to be stable over time within patients with schizophrenia (Harvey et al., 1990), across variations in clinical state, and patients who respond better to treatment with conventional antipsychotic medications appear to respond in their level of distractibility as well (Serper, Davidson, & Harvey, 1994).

Behavior and Personality

The occurrence of certain behavioral symptoms and syndromes in the relatives of patients with schizophrenia was the original defining feature of the schizophrenia spectrum. Reductions in emotional response, odd behavior, and interpersonal deficits were delineated for decades by researchers studying the relatives of patients with schizophrenia (Siever, Kalus, & Keefe, 1993). When these symptoms were also noted in the relatives of patients with schizophrenia who did not live with the proband and could not have been influenced by their behavior, the importance of these symptoms as markers of vulnerability (Kety, 1985) was underscored.

It has been reported that the frequency of several different psychopathological symptoms were elevated in relatives of individuals with schizophrenia. Most notably, these symptoms were in the domains of affective response, perceptual aberrations, communication abnormalities, and interpersonal isolation and aloofness (Kety, 1985). Whereas the presence of diagnosable schizotypal personality disorder is markedly elevated in relatives of patients with schizophrenia, the presence of these other symptoms is even higher (Siever et al., 1993).

As noted previously, there is some evidence for the convergence of schizotypal symptoms and certain types of attentional abnormalities in relatives of patients with schizophrenia. One fact that suggests that these symptoms may be nonspecific as far as the prediction of risk for the full syndrome of schizophrenia is the high rate of occurrence of these symptoms in the general population. Multiple studies based on college undergraduate populations have found that the prevalence of these same symptoms is considerably higher than the lifetime risk of schizophrenia in the college population (Chapman, Edell, & Chapman, 1980). Similarly, follow-up studies of individuals with these behavioral traits have found that the risk for the development of schizophrenia in these individuals is quite low (Chapman, Chapman, Kwapil, Eckblad, & Zinser, 1994). The individuals who manifest these "schizotypal" symptoms also often manifest cognitive impairments that are qualitatively similar to those seen in patients with schizotypal personality disorder and schizophrenia (Lenzenweger, Cornblatt, & Putnick, 1991; Merritt & Balogh, 1989), although the magnitude of impairment is often considerably less than that seen in these clinical populations. Thus, there appears to be a behavioral syndrome that shares some symptoms with relatives of patients with schizophrenia but where there is little, if any, risk for the development of schizophrenia. These individuals may share some genes with individuals who are vulnerable to schizophrenia, but apparently either they did not experience events that led to the expression of schizophrenia or these genetic predispositions may themselves be only weakly related to the development of schizophrenia. Some of these problematic issues are addressed in later sections of this chapter.

Psychophysiological Abnormalities

Individuals with schizophrenia manifest a number of psychophysiological abnormalities, including reduced habituation of startle responses, reduced evidence of appropriate sensory gating, changes in the evoked potentials and psychophysiological reactivity to environmental events, and changes in smooth-pursuit eye tracking.

Although many of these impairments in psychophysiological functioning have been confirmed in patients with schizophrenia, the aspect of psychophysiological functioning most consistently studied in individuals without clinical schizophrenia is eye tracking (Levy, Holzman, Mathysse, & Mendell, 1994). For the past 25 years, it has been known that patients with schizophrenia (Holzman, Proctor, & Hughes, 1973) and about 60% of their first-degree relatives (Holzman et al., 1974) manifest abnormalities in smooth-pursuit eye movements (SPEM). These deficits are found when an individual is asked to follow the movement of an object with his or her eyes, with the object moving at either a consistent or an accelerating rate. There are several different eye-movement abnormalities that are noted, including slow pursuit, irregular catchup saccades, and generally irregular movements. Analyses of these data using genetic models have been consistent with the presence of a single dominant gene that predicts eye-tracking deficits in both schizophrenic patients and their first-degree relatives (Holzman et al., 1988). This gene could not be a necessary and sufficient cause of schizophrenia, because many relatives of patients with schizophrenia who do not meet diagnostic criteria have evidence of eye-tracking problems.

Although multiple theoretical models have been proposed to explain the reasons for the eye-tracking deficits in relatives of patients with schizophrenia, an important finding to keep in mind is that eye-tracking deficit is not specific to patients with schizophrenia or vulnerability to the development of schizophrenia. In fact, eye-tracking deficits are uncorrelated with the severity of schizotypal symptoms in the first-degree relatives of patients with schizophrenia (Keefe et al., 1997). Thus, eye-tracking abnormalities are most likely related to some genetic features that are necessary but not sufficient for the development of schizophrenia. Our finding that eye-tracking problems were unrelated to schizotypal symptom severity likely reflects the multiple paths to the development of schizophrenia. For example, eye-tracking impairments are reliably found in individuals with the illness and some number of their relatives, but not necessarily those relatives who manifest the putative behavioral symptoms associated with membership in the schizophrenia spectrum.

PREVENTION OF SCHIZOPHRENIA

Prevention of schizophrenia would free millions of people worldwide from lives of isolation, terror, and poverty and would result in a huge boost to the world economy. Estimates of the indirect costs of schizophrenia in the United States alone are approximately $25 billion per year. Yet, prevention of schizophrenia has been a low priority until the recent past. The identification of points of intervention has been a major roadblock because of the paucity of indicators of vulnerability with any predictive validity. Essentially no psychological factors have proven related to the development of the illness, limiting interventions in this area. Recent developments in the study of attentional deficits have indicated that in children whose parents have schizophrenia, manifesting deficits in sustained attention is a powerful indicator of vulnerability and indicates that interventions should capitalize on this finding.

This recent finding leads to several critical questions in the domain of interventions. Should the interventions be psychological, aimed at improvement of sustained attention and vigilance? This would presuppose that deficits in vigilance have some etiological role and are not simply a behavioral reflection of underlying functional or structural brain deficits. Should the interventions be biological, assuming that these attentional impairments are simply an indicator of brain dysfunction? This intervention would make the assumption, possibly unsubstantiated, that brain dysfunction requires a biological intervention.

Both biological and psychological interventions have demonstrated prophylactic value for relapse prevention in schizophrenia. Should these interventions be directly adapted for primary prevention? In the case of psychological relapse prevention, all effective interventions have involved reduction of EE or have focused on medication compliance. Both these factors are not particularly relevant to prevention of the first episode of illness in schizophrenia. As noted previously, EE on the part of relatives is predictive of relapse but not predictive of the occurrence of a first episode. Medication compliance is not an issue in the case of an individual who has never received medication for a first episode.

Recently, primary prevention of the first episode of schizophrenia in the form of medication-based interventions for the illness has received increased attention. These interventions have relied on the use of "novel" antipsychotic medications. Novel medications differ from older "conventional" medications in several ways, the most important being that these medications have greatly reduced risk for permanent neurological side effects such as tardive dyskinesia (TD). Previously, the risk of TD would have precluded the use of medication-based interventions, even if the information from studies such as those conducted by Cornblatt et al. (1999) and Davidson et al. (1999) had been available. Currently, with the results of independent studies indicating that prediction of risk for schizophrenia, at least in certain subpopulations (children of individuals with schizophrenia), can be accomplished with high accuracy, the use of medication-based primary-prevention interventions has been attempted.

Although primary-prevention studies using antipsychotic medications are in the pilot stage, these studies have produced no efficacy information. As a result, these studies should be carefully monitored for their results, so that both early primary-prevention intervention results can be capitalized upon and unjustified optimism does not result.

DIFFICULT DATA TO RECONCILE

If schizophrenia was not a puzzle, the number of articles and books about the illness would be greatly reduced. One of the major problems in the study of the development of schizophrenia is the fact that many of the results do not add up. Factors that should be associated with risk for schizophrenia are entirely too common in population as a whole. Illnesses that were identified as being common in relatives of patients with schizophrenia and hence were labeled "schizophrenia-spectrum conditions" are also common in individuals who have no relatives with the illness. The occurrence of "markers of vulnerability" is much more common than could possibly be the case in an illness that influences only 1% of the population. Several of these issues are discussed next.

Low Risk for Schizophrenia in "Schizotypes"

In 1962, Meehl delineated his model of the behavioral and cognitive factors that are present in individuals who are vulnerable to the development of schizophrenia. Since that time, there has been considerable research on the identification of these individuals and the description of their characteristics. These individuals have been identified in general population samples, largely from universities but also from other sources such as personnel agencies. The identification of these individuals often comes from their responses on questionnaires examining perceptual aberration, magical thinking, anhedonic experiences (Chapman et al., 1980), and other similar features. Individuals with these behavioral and personality features have also been reported to manifest a number of cognitive and psychophysiological abnormalities. Thus, this group has behavioral symptoms that are similar to those seen in the relatives of individuals with schizophrenia and also has cognitive deficits similar to those seen in schizophrenia and in individuals with diagnosable schizophrenia-spectrum conditions.

Follow-up studies of these individuals ascertained independently from any information about their relatives have found, however, that their risk of developing schizophrenia is quite low (Chapman et al., 1994). The prevalence of these individuals alone precludes the possibility that the majority could be vulnerable to schizophrenia, because some studies include as many as 3% of college undergraduates in the high-scoring range on the indicators used to select the subjects (Lenzenweger et al., 1991). Because the lifetime risk of schizophrenia in college undergraduates is likely to be considerably lower than the overall population risk of slightly less than 1%, the behavioral and cognitive indicators detected in these individuals must also be nonspecific to vulnerability to the development of schizophrenia. As with eye-tracking abnormalities, these impairments could very well be linked to some component of the overall profile of vulnerability to schizophrenia, but they are clearly not a specific indicator of vulnerability to the illness.

Cognitive Impairments in Relatives without Other Symptoms of the Illness

A related issue has arisen from the results of research on the characteristics of adult first-degree relatives of patients with schizophrenia. Although these relatives are at higher risk than the general population for the development of schizophrenia, only a minority of these individuals are actually at risk. In the case of older relatives, even fewer are at risk because of the reduction in risk with increasing age. Despite their low risk, many of these relatives manifest the same types of attentional and cognitive abnormalities that are present in children who later go on to develop schizophrenia (Keefe et al., 1994). The presence of these cognitive and attentional abnormalities in individuals who are related to patients with schizophrenia suggests that these attentional abnormalities are again likely to be linked to some component of the predisposition for schizophrenia, but are clearly not specific indicators of vulnerability.

Common Occurrence of Schizophrenia-Spectrum Conditions Unrelated to Schizophrenic Index Cases

A final, and also related, issue is that of the occurrence of schizophrenia-spectrum conditions in individuals who have no relatives with a diagnosis of schizophrenia. Although the initial definition of the schizophrenia spectrum was the disorders that occurred with elevated frequency in the relatives of patients with schizophrenia, fewer than 15% of individuals with these "spectrum" disorders have an identifiable schizophrenic relative. As a result, these disorders are actually more common in individuals with no observable predisposing factors than in persons who are related to patients with schizophrenia. Thus, they cannot be seen to be specific to individuals with a relative with clearly diagnosable schizophrenia.

Summary of the Difficult Data

Although many different genetic models can explain the reasons that schizophrenia-spectrum conditions can occur in individuals with no obvious predispositions to schizophrenia, the result is that individual behavioral and cognitive "markers of vulnerability" to schizophrenia does not provide specific information about which individuals will actually develop the illness. Whether or not these indicators should actually be seen as markers at all could be questioned, although advances in genetic methodology will improve the specificity of these findings in the future.

CONCLUSIONS

The study of vulnerability processes in adult-onset schizophrenia has yielded some consistent results and a large number of inconsistencies. Inconsistencies in schizophrenia research have the potential to be related to the heterogeneity of the illness itself. Diathesis–stress models of the development of schizophrenia have shaped research for the past 30 years, although it could currently be concluded that there is inadequate consistent evidence to support any single factor as either a predisposition or a stressor/releasing factor. Clearly deficits in attention are found in children and adolescents who develop schizophrenia later, but the specificity of these deficits is in question. Likewise, the pattern of deficits in smooth-pursuit eye tracking appears to follow a distribution associated with a single-gene mode of inheritance, but it is not clear that this is the gene responsible for the symptomatic features of schizophrenia. The closest to a set of research findings that accounts for a reasonable amount of variable in risk for schizophrenia are those of Davidson et al. (1999), but even those findings may apply only to males and only to individuals with a relatively late onset and relatively better premorbid functioning. Data on viral and other prenatal etiological factors provide a possible model to explain why only some predisposed cases may develop the illness, but many individuals with schizophrenia can easily be demonstrated to have been exposed to no such identifiable prenatal stressor.

The results coming from the New York High Risk Project have suggested the first prospectively identified marker of vulnerability that has received validation in a longitudinal study. These compelling results, suggesting that attentional impairment identified before age 15 is reliable predictor of risk for schizophrenia in offspring of schizophrenic parents, is the first concrete lead as to the identification of truly vulnerable individuals. This finding provides a hard lead for interventions in the children of people with schizophrenia. Similarly promising results come from the results of the Davidson (1999) follow-up studies. The fact that a profile of behavioral and cognitive abnormalities can be found to have major longitudinal predictive power may lead to future intervention possibilities as well.

This research could be advanced in the area of determining the breadth of indicators of risk for schizophrenia. Are there additional attentional factors, other than the CPT, that predict risk for the development of schizophrenia and are not simply more likely to be abnormal in relatives of patients with schizophrenia? Are CPT deficits a predictor of risk for the development of schizophrenia in individuals without a relative with schizophrenia? These are critical questions if populationwide screening and risk reduction are to be considered.

Later research in this area will benefit from the application of neuroimaging and neuropharmacological strategies to these problems. Randomized clinical intervention trials, using newer lower-risk treatments, may tell us whether these vulnerability factors are truly predictive of schizophrenia. Although these studies carry risk, schizophrenia is an illness with high mortality and morbidity.

Future research aimed at the identification of vulnerability factors in schizophrenia will be enhanced by studies aimed at reduction of the heterogeneity of schizophrenia, through identification of more meaningful subtypes. The classical Kraepelinian subtypes maintained in the fourth edition of the *Diagnostic and Statistical Manual of Mental Disorders* (DSM-IV; American Psychiatric Association, 1994) are clearly not the way to achieve this end. Subtypes based on other factors such as level of functional impairment, variations in cerebral structure, or other biological factors may allow more clearly for the separation of individuals with schizophrenia who have a genetic predisposition from those who are "phenocopies." When the true subtypes are identified, the processes of vulnerability to the illness and their related markers of vulnerability may be easier to identify and disentangle.

REFERENCES

Abi-Saab, W. M., D'Souza, D. C., Moghaddam, B., & Krystal, J. H. (1998). The NMDA antagonist model for schizophrenia: Promise and pitfalls. *Pharmacopsychiatry, 31*(Suppl. 2), 104–109.

Albus, M., & Maier, W. (1995). Lack of gender differences at age of onset in familial schizophrenia. *Schizophrenia Research, 18,* 51–57.

American Psychiatric Association. (1994). *Diagnostic and statistical manual of mental disorders* (4th ed.). Washington, DC: Author.

Asarnow, R. F., & MacCrimmon D. (1978). Residual performance deficit in clinically remitted schizophrenics: A marker of schizophrenia? *Journal of Abnormal Psychology, 87,* 597–608.

Asarnow, R. F., Steffy, R., Cleghorn, J. M., & MacCrimmon, D. J. (1977). Attentional assessment of foster children vulnerable to schizophrenia. *Journal of Abnormal Psychology, 86,* 267–275.

Bateson, G., Jackson, D. D., Haley, J., & Weakland, J. (1956). Toward a theory of schizophrenia. *Behavioral Science, 1,* 251–264.

Bleuler, E. (1911). *Dementia praecox; or the group of schizophrenias.* New York: International Universities Press.

Braff, D. L. (1981). Impaired speed of information processing in unmedicated schizotypal patients. *Schizophrenia Bulletin, 7,* 499–508.

Bunney, S. G., Potkin, S., & Bunney, W. E., Jr. (1995). New morphological and neuropathological findings in schizophrenia: A neurodevelopmental perspective. *Clinical Neuroscience, 3,* 381–388.

Butzlaff, R. L., & Hooley, J. M. (1998). Expressed emotion and psychiatric relapse: A meta-analysis. *Archives of General Psychiatry, 55,* 547–552.

Castle, D. J., & Murray, R. M. (1993). The epidemiology of late-onset schizophrenia. *Schizophrenia Bulletin, 19,* 691–700.

Chapman, L. J., Chapman, J. M., Kwapil, T. R., Eckblad, M., & Zinser, M. C. (1994). Putatively psychosis-prone subjects 10 years later. *Journal of Abnormal Psychology 103,* 171–183.

Chapman, L. J., Edell, W., & Chapman, J. M. (1980). Physical anhedonia, perceptual aberration, and psychosis proneness. *Journal of Abnormal Psychology, 89,* 639–653.

Ciompi, L. (1980). Catamnestic long-term study on the course of life and aging of schizophrenics. *Schizophrenia Bulletin, 6,* 606–618.

Cornblatt, B. A., & Erlenmeyer-Kimling, L. (1985). Global attentional deviance as a marker of risk for schizophrenia: Specificity and predictive validity. *Journal of Abnormal Psychology, 94,* 470–486.

Cornblatt, B. A., Obuchowski, M., Roberts, S., Pollack, S., & Erlenmeyer-Kimling, L. (1999). Cognitive and behavioral precursors of schizophrenia. *Development and Psychopathology, 11,* 487–508.

Crow, T. J., Done, D. J., & Sacker, A. (1995). Childhood precursors of psychosis as clues to its evolutionary origins. *European Archives of Psychiatry and Clinical Neuroscience, 245,* 61–69.

David, A. S., Malmberg, A., Brandt, L., Allebeck, P., & Lewis, G. (1997). IQ and risk for schizophrenia: A population-based cohort study. *Psychological Medicine, 27,* 1311–1323.

Davidson, M., Harvey, P. D., Powchik, P., Parrella, M., White, L., Knobler, H. Y., Losonczy, M., Keefe, R. S. E., Katz, S., & Frecksa, E. (1995). Severity of symptoms in geriatric chronic schizophrenic patients. *American Journal of Psychiatry, 152,* 197–207.

Davidson, M., Reichenberg, A., Rabinowitz, J., Weiser, M., Kaplan, Z., & Mark, M. (1999). Behavioral and intellectual markers for schizophrenia in apparently healthy male adolescents. *American Journal of Psychiatry, 156,* 1328–1335.

Davis, K. L., Buchsbaum, M. S., Shihabuddin, L., Spiegel-Cohen, J., Metzger, M., Frecska, E., Keefe, R. S., & Powchik, P. (1998). Ventricular enlargement in poor outcome schizophreia. *Biological Psychiatry, 43,* 783–793.

Delisi, L., Sakuma, M., Tew, W., Kushner, M., Hoff, A. L., & Grimson, R. (1997). Schizophrenia as a chronic active brain process: A study of progressive brain structural change subsequent to the onset of psychosis. *Psychiatry Research: Brain Imaging, 74,* 129–140.

Done, D. J., Crow, T. J., Johnstone, E. C., & Sacker, A. (1994). Childhood antecedents of schizophrenia and affective illness: Social adjustment at ages 7 and 11. *British Medical Journal, 309,* 699–703.

Fananas, L., van Os, J., Hoyos, C., McGrath, J., Mellor, C. S., & Murray, R. (1996). Dermatoglyphic a–b ridge count as a possible marker for developmental disturbance in schizophrenia: Replication in two samples. *Schizophrenia Research, 20,* 307–314.

Fromm-Reichman, F. (1948). Notes on the development of treatment of schizophrenics by psychoanalytic therapy. *Psychiatry, 11,* 263–273.

Gold, J. M., Randolph, C., Carpenter, C. J., Goldberg, T. E., & Weinberger D. R. (1992). Forms of memory failure in schizophrenia. *Journal of Abnormal Psychology, 101,* 487–494.

Gottesman, I. I., & Shields, J. (1982). *Schizophrenia: The epigenetic puzzle.* New York: Oxford University Press.

Green, M. F., Nuechterlein, K. H., & Mintz, J. (1994). Backward masking in schizophrenia and mania: I. Specifying a mechanism. *Archives of General Psychiatry, 51,* 939–944.

Harvey, P. D., Docherty, N., Serper, M. R., & Rasmussen, M. (1990). Cognitive deficits and thought disorder: II. An eight-month followup study. *Schizophrenia Bulletin, 16,* 147–156.

Harvey, P. D., Walker, E., & Wielgus, M. S. (1986). Psychological markers of vulnerability to schizophrenia. In B. Maher & W. Maher (Eds.), *Progress in experimental personality research* (Vol. 14, pp. 231–268). New York: Academic Press.

Harvey, P. D., Weintraub, S., & Neale, J. M. (1985). Span of apprehension deficits in children vulnerable to psychopathology: A failure to replicate. *Journal of Abnormal Psychology, 94,* 410–413.

Harvey, P., Winters, K., Weintraub, S., & Neale, J. M. (1981). Distractibility in children vulnerable to psychopathology. *Journal of Abnormal Psychology, 90,* 298–304.

Hegarty, J. D., Baldessarini, R. J., & Tohen, M. (1994). One hundred years of schizophrenia: A meta-analysis of the outcome literature. *American Journal of Psychiatry, 151,* 1409–1416.

Heston, L. L. (1966). Psychiatric disorders in foster home reared children of schizophrenic parents. *British Journal of Psychiatry, 112,* 819–825.

Holzman, P. S., Kringlen, E., Matthysse, S., Flanagan, S. D., Lipton, R. B., Cramer, G., Levin, S., Lange, K., & Levy, D. L. (1988). A single dominant gene can account for eye-tracking dysfunctions and schizophrenia in offspring of discordant twins. *Archives of General Psychiatry, 45,* 641–647.

Holzman, P. S., Proctor, L. R., & Hughes, D. W. (1973). Eye-tracking patterns in schizophrenia. *Science, 181,* 179–181.

Holzman, P. S., Proctor, L. R., Levy, D. L., Yasillo, N. J., Meltzer, H. Y., & Hurt, S. W. (1974). Eye-tracking dysfunctions in schizophrenic patients and their relatives. *Archives of General Psychiatry, 31,* 143–151.

Hyde, T. M., Ziegler, J. C., & Weinberger, D. R. (1992). Psychiatric disturbances in metachromatic leukodystrophy: Insights into the neurobiology of psychosis. *Archives of Neurology, 49,* 401–406.

Jones, P., Rodgers, B., Murray, R., & Marmot, M. (1994). Child development risk factors for adult schizophrenia in the British 1946 birth cohort. *Lancet, 344,* 1398–1402.

Keefe, R. S., Mohs, R. C., Losonczy, M. F., Davidson, M., Silverman, J. M., Kendler, K. S., Horvath, T. B., Nora, R., & Davis, K. L. (1987). Characteristics of very poor outcome schizophrenia. *American Journal of Psychiatry, 144,* 889–895.

Keefe, R. S. E., Silverman, J. M., Lees Roitman, S. E., Harvey, P. D., Duncan, A., Alroy, D., Siever, L. J., Davis, K. L., & Mohs, R. C. (1994). Performance of nonpsychotic first degree relatives of schizophrenic patients on cognitive tests. *Psychiatry Research, 53,* 1–12.

Keefe, R. S. E., Silverman, J. M., Mohs, R. C., Siever, L. J., Harvey, P. D., Friedman, L., Lees Roitman, S., DuPre, R., Smith, C. J., Schmeidler, J., & Davis, K. L. (1997). Eye-tracking, attention, and schizotypal personality symptoms in nonpsychotic relatives of schizophrenic patients. *Archives of General Psychiatry, 54,* 169–177.

Kendler, K. S., McGuire, M., Gruenberg, A. M., O'Hare, A., Spellman, M., &Walsh, D. (1993). The Roscommon Family Study: I. Methods, diagnosis of probands, and risk of schizophrenia in relatives. *Archives of General Psychiatry, 50,* 527–540.

Kety, S. S. (1985). Schizotypal personality disorder: An operationaliztion of Beluer's latent schizophrenia. *Schizophrenia Bulletin, 11,* 590–594.

Kety, S. S., & Ingraham, L. J. (1992). Genetic transmission and improved diagnosis of schizophrenia from pedigrees of adoptees. *Journal of Psychiatric Research, 26,* 247–255.

Kety, S. S., Rosenthal, D., Wender, P. H., & Schulsinger, F. (1968). The types and prevalance of mental illness in the biological and adoptive relatives of adopted schizophrenics. In D. Rosenthal & S. S. Kety (Eds.), *The transmission of schizophrenia* (pp. 86–101). Oxford, England: Pergamon Press.

Kraepelin, E. (1896). *Psychiatrie* (5th ed.). Leipzig: Barth.

Krystal, J. H., Karper, L. P., Seibyl, J. P., Freeman, G. K., Delaney, R., Bremner, J. D., Heninger, G. R., Bowers, M. B., Jr., & Charney, D. S. (1994). Subanesthetic effects of the noncompetitive NMDA antagonist, ketamine, in humans. Psychotomimetic, perceptual, cognitive, and neuroendocrine responses. *Archives of General Psychiatry, 51,* 199–214.

Leff, J. (1976). Schizophrenia and sensitivity to the family environment. *Schizophrenia Bulletin, 2,* 566–574.

Lenzenweger, M. S., Cornblatt, B. A., & Putnick, M. (1991) Schizotypy and sustained attention. *Journal of Abnormal Psychology, 100,* 84–89.

Levy, D. L., Holzman, P. S., Mathysse, S., & Mendell, N. R. (1994). Eye tracking and schizophrenia: A critical review. *Schizophrenia Bulletin, 20,* 47–62.

Machon, R. A., Mednick, S. A., & Huttunen, M. O. (1997). Adult major affective disorder after prenatal exposure to an influenza epidemic. *Archives of General Psychiatry, 54,* 322–328.

Mednick, S. A., & McNeil, T. (1968). Current methodology in research on the etiology of schizophrenia: Serious methodological difficulties which suggest the use of the high-risk group method. *Psychological Bulletin, 70,* 681–693.

Meehl, P. E. (1962). Schizotaxia, schizotypy, schizophrenia. *American Psychologist, 17,* 827–838.

Merritt, R. D., & Balogh, D. W. (1989). Backward masking spatial frequency effects among hypothetically schizotypal individuals. *Schizophrenia Bulletin, 15,* 573–583.

Miklowitz, D. J., Goldstein, M. J., Nuechterlein, K. H., Snyder, K. S., & Mintz, J. (1988). Family factors and the course of bipolar affective disorder. *Archives of General Psychiatry, 45,* 225–231.

Morgan, V., Castle, D., Page, A., Fazio, S., Gurrin, L., Burton, P., Montgomery P., & Jablensky, A. (1997). Influenza epidemics and incidence of schizophrenia, affective disorders and mental retardation in Western Australia: No evidence of a major effect. *Schizophrenia Research, 26,* 25–39.

Neale, J. M., McIntyre, C. W., Fox, R., & Cromwell, R. L. (1969). Span of apprehension in acute schizophrenics. *Journal of Abnormal Psychology, 74,* 593–596.

Oltmanns, T. F. (1978). Selective attention in manic and schizophrenic psychoses: The effect of distraction on information processing. *Journal of Abnormal Psychology, 87,* 212–225.

Rapoport, J. L., Giedd, J., Kumra, S., Jacobsen, L., Smith, A., Lee, P., Nelson, J., & Hamburger, S. (1997). Childhood onset schizophrenia: Progressive ventricular change during adolescence. *Archives of General Psychiatry, 54,* 897–903.

Rund, B. R. (1993). Backward masking performance in chronic and nonchronic schizophrenics, affectively disturbed patients, and normal control subjects. *Journal of Abnormal Psychology, 102,* 74–81.

Serper, M. R., Davidson, M., & Harvey, P. D. (1994). Attentional predictors of clinical change during neuroleptic treatment. *Schizophrenia Research, 13,* 65–71.

Shaw, S. H., Kelly, M., Smith, A. B., Shields, G., Hopkins, P. J., Loftus, J., Laval, S. H., Vita, A., De Hert, M., Cardon, L. R., Crow, T. J., Sherrington, R., & DeLisi, L. E. (1998). A genome-wide search for schizophrenia susceptibility genes. *American Journal of Medical Genetics, 81,* 364–376.

Siever, L. J., Kalus, O. F., & Keefe, R. S. (1993). The boundaries of schizophrenia. *Psychiatric Clinics of North America, 16,* 217–244.

Susser, E., Neugebauer, R., Hoek, H. W., Brown, A. S., Lin, S., Labovitz, D., & Gorman, J. M. (1996). Schizophrenia after prenatal famine: Further evidence. *Archives of General Psychiatry, 53,* 25–31.

Takei, N., Mortensen, P. B., Klaening, U., Murray, R. M., Sham, P. C., O'Callaghan, E., & Munk-Jorgensen, P. (1996). Relationship between in utero exposure to influenza epidemics and risk of schizophrenia in Denmark. *Biological Psychiatry, 40,* 817–824.

van Os, J., & Selten, J. P. (1998). Prenatal exposure to maternal stress and subsequent schizophrenia: The May 1940 invasion of The Netherlands. *British Journal of Psychiatry, 172,* 324–326.

Vaughn, C. E., & Leff, J. P. (1976). The influence of family and social factors on the course of psychiatric illness: A comparison of schizophrenic and depressed neurotic patients. *British Journal of Psychiatry, 129,* 125–137.

Weinberger, D. R. (1987). Implications of normal brain development for the pathogenesis of schizophrenia. *Archives of General Psychiatry, 44,* 660–669.

World Health Organization. (1972). *The international pilot study of schizophrenia.* Geneva: Author.

Zigler, E., Glick, M., & Marsh, A. (1979). Premorbid social competence and outcome among schizophrenia and nonschizophrenic patients. *Journal of Nervous and Mental Disease, 116,* 478–483.

Zubin, J., & Spring, B. (1977). Vulnerability—a new view of schizophrenia. *Journal of Abnormal Psychology, 86,* 103–126.

16

Vulnerability to Schizophrenia across the Lifespan

PATRICIA A. BRENNAN
PHILIP D. HARVEY

We have each contributed to this volume a separate chapter focused on vulnerability to schizophrenia. Our separate chapters did not distinctly focus on child-onset versus adult-onset types of a particular psychiatric disorder. Rather, we focused on developmental versus other types of approaches that have been applied to research and theory concerning schizophrenia. Nevertheless, integration of the material across our chapters highlights the questions that remain regarding vulnerability to schizophrenia and also suggests important and necessary directions for future research. In our view, future research on schizophrenia needs to examine combinations of risk factors, to attend to potential developmental effects, to consider separate etiological pathways for subtypes of schizophrenia, and to use prediction models that test the utility of risk factors in identifying individuals who will eventually develop this disorder.

The vast majority of individuals who are diagnosed with schizophrenia receive this diagnosis in late adolescence or later. Nevertheless, premorbid characteristics suggest that the process that ultimately results in this diagnostic outcome may already be under way in early infancy (e.g., Walker, Savoie, & Davis, 1994). Brennan and Walker (Chapter 14, this volume) argue that by examining the developmental course of schizophrenia carefully, we might be able to discover the causal factors in this process and how they interact with one another to produce this illness. One difficulty with this tactic to date is that the factors associated with the premorbid phase of schizophrenia do not appear to be specific to schizophrenia. Longitudinal and follow-back studies have been able to compare those who develop schizophrenia with those who do not. They typically assess mean differences between these groups and have noted that those who later develop schizophrenia have comparatively worse attentional problems (e.g., Cornblatt, Obuchowski, Roberts, Pollack, & Erlenmeyer-Kimling, 1999), higher levels of motor abnormalities (e.g., Walker et al.,1994), and worse behavioral disturbances (e.g., Amminger et al., 1999). Evidence that any one of these premorbid factors necessarily results in schizophrenia rather than some other psychiatric illness or a relatively normal course of functioning is lacking.

One method of potential discovery in this area is to look for particular combinations of vulnerability factors that occur at a base rate that is commensurate with the base rate of schizophrenia. Testing these particular combinations and their relationship to schizophrenic outcomes might help to determine both the necessary and sufficient causes of this disorder. This approach of focusing on combinations of vulnerability factors might also be helpful in determining the ultimate causes of schizophrenia. Many vulnerability factors are not themselves considered to be causal factors but, rather, markers of causal factors for schizophrenia. Deficits in smooth-pursuit eye movement (SPEM), for example, are thought not to cause schizophrenia but to be markers of a genetic cause for this disorder. Particular combinations of vulnerability factors might suggest a common underlying cause (e.g., neurotransmitter dysfunction) that can then be tested as a necessary and sufficient condition for schizophrenia.

Neurodevelopmental models of schizophrenia suggest that the vulnerability factors associated with schizophrenia might vary in response to the interaction of pathological causal factors with normal maturation processes. As we continue to increase our knowledge base concerning normal neurodevelopmental processes, we should be able to combine it with developmentally specific findings of vulnerability to schizophrenia to better determine the underlying causes of this disorder. A focus on when as well as what vulnerabilities exist will be important in future research on schizophrenia.

As Brennan and Walker suggest, neurodevelopmental and neurodegenerative models of schizophrenia need not be contradictory. It is likely that some deficits in neurological functioning may be apparent before the onset of schizophrenia, whereas others may result from the course of the illness itself. Comparisons of results from studies of adults with schizophrenia with those of children who later develop schizophrenia have been and will continue to be useful in distinguishing neurological precursors from neurological effects of this disorder.

Harvey (Chapter 15, this volume) outlines some of the weaknesses of the diathesis–stress model as it has been applied to the area of schizophrenia research. Current research on gene expression indicates that traditional diathesis–stress models do indeed need to be expanded. The previous notion that a single gene, in combination with an environmental stressor that exceeds a certain threshold, results in schizophrenia does not capture the complexity of gene environment interactions as we now understand them to exist. Not only are genes present or absent, but they are also turned on or off in response to developmental, hormonal, environmental and (other) genetic effects. Of course, the diathesis for schizophrenia need not be only genetic in nature but might be the result of early prenatal or perinatal insults to the central nervous system. Findings from animal research even suggest that an environmental diathesis in one generation might translate into a genetic diathesis in the next. Viral agents have been shown to change the genetic makeup of embryos, with these genetic alterations then being transmitted to the next generation of offspring (e.g., Lin et al., 1994). As gene-expression studies expand, our attention to their results will help us to revise and expand our notions of diathesis–stress as well.

As Harvey points out, one potential downfall of the diathesis–stress model is that if it is adhered to too stringently, the main effects of causal factors on schizophrenia may not be detected even if they do exist. He suggests that the failure to find strong results for individual predictors of schizophrenia to date might be the result of the heterogeneity of schizophrenia rather than the need for interactive models. He argues that if we continue to treat all cases of schizophrenia as the same illness when they are different, we will obtain results that do not replicate and are not valid. The question we then face is how to create meaningful, etiologically distinct, subgroups of individuals with schizophrenia. Several researchers have distinguished between positive symptom and negative symptom types of schizophrenia, with distinct etiologies noted for each of these types (Baron, Gruen, & Romo-Gruen, 1992; Cannon, Mednick, & Parnas, 1990). Other researchers have compared the predictors of childhood-onset to adult-onset schizophrenia and have noted that there are more similarities than differences across these two groups (Nicolson & Rapoport, 1999). However, age of onset has been found to be related to family loading for schizophrenia, suggesting a potentially differential genetic basis for childhood-onset versus adult-onset schizophrenia.

Because family history is related to age of onset (Suvisaari, Haukka, Tanskanen, & Loennqvist, 1998), it might be more parsimonious to compare family history present versus family history absent cases of schizophrenia to assess for potentially distinct etiological pathways to these conditions. This type of study is more rare than one would think. In fact, high-risk research usually focuses exclusively on individuals with a family history for this disorder. Thus, the question is left open concerning the generalizability of high-risk study results to the larger population of individuals with schizophrenia. Attention to family history might help to explain failures of replication in studies of the predictors of schizophrenia.

This type of research design would also address the issue of heterogeneity. If individuals with a positive family history of schizophrenia had, for example, a more homogenous presentation than individuals without such a history, then some ideas about the path from risk factors to clinical presentation could be developed. The study of "phenocopies" in other illnesses has helped to refine ideas about the breadth of genetic predispositions to the illness.

Brennan and Walker present a model suggesting the interactive events and developmental processes that may predict to the outcome of schizophrenia. This and other neurodevelopmental models may apply only to a subset of individuals with schizophrenia rather than all the individuals who evidence this diagnostic condition. It might be potentially useful to examine a subtype of individuals with schizophrenia who evidence particular neurological deficits (such as hippocampal damage) to see whether neurodevelopmental models can explain and predict their pathological outcomes. Such an approach is, of course, constrained by the prevalence of such neurological risk factors.

Brennan and Walker's model suggests that particular biological abnormalities, including hypothalamic–pituitary–adrenal (HPA) overactivation and striatal dopaminergic anomalies, might play a causal role in schizophrenia. Genetic and congenital risk factors are hypothesized to cause neurotransmitter anomalies, which, in turn might be related to the behavioral abnormalities observed in both individuals with schizophrenia and in individuals at high genetic risk for schizophrenia. For example, dopaminergic anomalies might be related to both SPEM deficits and motor abnormalities. Brennan and Walker's model also suggests that perinatal or environmental stressors may increase HPA activation, which, especially when combined with normal increases in gonadal hormone secretion during adolescence, may be related to hippocampal damage. Damage to the hippocampus may underlie some of the cognitive abnormalities noted in individuals with schizophrenia, including poor performance on sustained attention tasks. This neurodevelopmental model clearly requires further empirical support, especially in terms of its predictive utility. As noted previously, most studies examining vulnerability to schizophrenia use post hoc approaches rather than assessing for predictive validity. One exception to this rule is the recent work of Davidson et al. (1999). By combining behavioral and cognitive predictors, they were able to predict well who obtained a diagnosis schizophrenia in their cohort. Replications and extensions of their findings would be valuable and necessary tools for the translation of research on vulnerability into the practice of early intervention.

In summary, success in the identification of vulnerability processes in schizophrenia will be contingent upon several factors. Prospective research designs, despite the difficulty in conducting such studies, are a prerequisite. Comparative studies of as-yet-unaffected individuals who vary in risk factors (e.g., family history and occurrence of neurological events) are required. Finally, researchers must more closely attend to heterogeneity of the illness and its implications. Approaching schizophrenia as a single disease with a single cause, single course, and unitary outcome appears to have been an impediment to success in the past.

The adoption of a lifespan perspective is essential to the future study of schizophrenia. Neurodevelopmental models of schizophrenia are primarily focused on development from prenatal stages through the onset of the symptoms of schizophrenia. Neurodegenerative models focus more on the post-onset and later-life course of schizophrenia. A lifespan perspective suggests that we need to further explore both of these models in the study of schizophrenia. In doing so, we will discover both the complementary and the distinctive roles of these models in determining the causes and the best available treatment of schizophrenia.

REFERENCES

Amminger, G. P., Pape, S., Rock, D., Roberts, S. A., Ott, S. L., Squires-Wheeler, E., Kestenbaum, C., & Erlenmeyer-Kimling, L. (1999). Relationship between childhood behavioral disturbance and later schizophrenia in the New York High-Risk Project. *American Journal of Psychiatry, 156,* 525–530.

Baron, M., Gruen, R. S., & Romo-Gruen, J. M. (1992). Positive and negative symptoms: Relation to familial transmission of schizophrenia. *British Journal of Psychiatry, 161,* 610–614.

Cannon, T. D., Mednick, S. A., & Parnas, J. (1990). Antecedents of predominantly negative- and predominantly positive-symptom schizophrenia in a high-risk population. *Archives of General Psychiatry, 47,* 622–632.

Cornblatt, B., Obuchowski, M., Roberts, S., Pollack, S., & Erlenmeyer-Kimling, L. (1999). Cognitive and behavioral precursors of schizophrenia. *Development and Psychopathology, 11,* 487–508.

Davidson, M., Reichenberg, A., Rabinowitz, J., Weiser, M., Kaplan, Z., & Mark, M. (1999). Behavioral and intellectual markers for schizophrenia in apparently health male adolescents. *American Journal of Psychiatry, 156,* 1328–1335.

Lin, S., Gaiano, N., Culp, P., Burns, J. C., Friedman, T., Yee, J. K., & Hopkins, N. (1994). Integration and germ-line transmission of a pseudotyped retrovial vector in zebrafish. *Science, 265,* 666–669.

Nicolson, R., & Rapoport, J. L. (1999). Childhood-onset schizophrenia: Rare but worth studying. *Biological Psychiatry, 46,* 1418–1428.

Suvisaari, J. M., Haukka, J., Tanskanen, A., & Loennqvist, J. K. (1998). Age at onset and outcome in schizophrenia are related to the degree of familial loading. *British Journal of Psychiatry, 173,* 494–500.

Walker, E. F., Savoie, T., & Davis, D. (1994). Neuromotor precursors of schizophrenia. *Schizophrenia Bulletin, 20,* 441–451.

EATING DISORDERS

17

Vulnerability to Eating Disorders in Childhood and Adolescence

PAMELA K. KEEL
GLORIA R. LEON
JAYNE A. FULKERSON

In this chapter, we present a developmental perspective on eating disorders during childhood and adolescence within a biopsychosocial model. Eating disorders include the formal categories of anorexia nervosa and bulimia nervosa as well as several forms of eating pathology grouped within the classification of eating disorders not otherwise specified. Although anorexia nervosa may be the most easily recognized eating disorder, it is also the least common affecting between 0.5% to 1.0% of the female adolescent population (American Psychiatric Association, 1994). Under criteria according to the fourth edition of the *Diagnostic and Statistical Manual of Mental Disorders* (DSM-IV; American Psychiatric Association, 1994), individuals with anorexia nervosa deliberately starve themselves to weights below 85% of that expected for height. They also fear becoming fat and may think of themselves as being fat. Finally, anorexia nervosa is marked by loss of menstrual function for at least 3 consecutive months. Individuals with anorexia nervosa maintain their state with fasting and excessive exercise (restricting subtype) or recurrent binge eating and purging episodes (binge/purge subtype).

Bulimia nervosa affects between 0.9% to 4.1% of adolescent females (American Psychiatric Association, 1994; Graber, Brooks-Gunn, Paikoff, & Warren, 1994; Killen et al., 1994; Killen et al., 1996; Leon, Fulkerson, Perry, & Cudeck, 1993; Leon, Perry, Mangelsdorf, & Tell, 1989; Patton, 1988; Patton, Johnson-Sabine, Wood, Mann, & Wakeling, 1990; Phelps, Andrea, Rizzo, Johnston, & Main, 1993). The DSM-IV characterizes bulimia nervosa as involving recurrent binge eating episodes coupled with behaviors that compensate for the caloric consumption. Weight and body shape unduly influence self-evaluation. Compensatory behaviors can include either purging (e.g., self-induced vomiting, laxative abuse, or diuretic abuse) or nonpurging (e.g., fasting or excessive exercise) methods. Weight is often normal or slightly above average among individuals with bulimia nervosa. Menstrual irregularities are also common in this disorder (Copeland, Sacks, & Herzog, 1995; Fairburn, Kirk, O'Connor, & Cooper, 1986; Swift, Ritholz, Kalin, & Kaslow, 1987).

A much higher percentage of the population suffers from eating disorders not otherwise specified. Binge-eating disorder (BED) represents one subtype within this heterogeneous classification. Surveys of young adults indicate that BED affects 5.3% of women (Spitzer et al., 1992). Age of onset is often noted in childhood or adolescence (Mussell et al., 1995). Other common forms of subclinical eating disorders include purging in the absence of recurrent binge eating episodes, such as after the consumption of small amounts of food, rumination, chewing and spitting out food without swallowing, and recurrent binge eating and purging episodes at subthreshold frequencies. Taken together, these syndromes affect between 6.5% to 36% of patients seeking treatment for an eating disorder (Ash & Piazza, 1995; Mitrany, 1992). Because many individuals affected by these disorders may not seek treatment, prevalence in the general population is unclear.

Eating disorders are clearly more prevalent among women; however, 5 to 15% of cases of anorexia and bulimia nervosa occur in males (Carlat & Camargo, 1991; Scott, 1986). Disordered-eating behaviors in males appear to be more consistent with BED and bulimia nervosa than with anorexia nervosa (Keel, Klump, Leon, & Fulkerson, 1998). Indeed, BED appears to be almost as common in males as in females (Spitzer et al., 1992).

RISK FACTOR RESEARCH METHODOLOGY

The identification of risk factors for any disorder can be approached using cross-sectional and longitudinal designs. Cross-sectional designs seek to determine whether a given factor is concurrently associated with the presence of disordered-eating behaviors or attitudes. Moreover, if a factor does not distinguish between individuals with disordered eating and individuals without disordered eating, it is unlikely to represent a risk factor for eating disorders. However, a concurrent association between eating pathology and a given factor does not demonstrate that the factor increases risk for developing eating pathology. The factor could be a result of the eating pathology. For example, hormonal imbalances are associated with the presence of anorexia nervosa. However, they appear to be the result of severe food restriction. Alternatively, disordered eating and the associated factor could both result from a common underlying determinant. For example, bulimia nervosa is associated with increased levels of depression. However, both the depression and the bulimic symptoms may be elevated by deficits in interpersonal relationships. Longitudinal research designs seek to identify factors that are present prior to the onset of disordered eating. Employing the logic that cause precedes effect, factors that distinguish between who will and will not develop disordered eating at a later point in time represent risk factors.

Many studies rely on surveys or self-report questionnaires to assess the presence of disordered-eating attitudes and behaviors. However, frequencies of disordered-eating behaviors are often higher in self-report questionnaires than in interviews (French et al., 1998). The increased frequencies may reflect false positives because adolescents misinterpret the intent of particular questions. Alternatively, adolescents may feel reluctant to report certain eating-disordered behaviors during a personal interview (French et al., 1998). Some researchers (e.g., Killen et al., 1996; Leon, Fulkerson, Perry, Keel, & Klump, 1999) sought to maximize the sensitivity (reduction of false negatives) and specificity (reduction of false positives) of assessment by employing both self-report surveys and semistructured interviews. Initial surveys screen for the possible presence of disordered-eating behaviors and interviews confirm their presence.

DEVELOPMENTAL COURSE OF EATING DISORDERS

Our biopsychosocial model of vulnerability to develop eating disorders is conceived within the context of a theory of normal development. The transition periods from childhood to adolescence and adolescence to young adulthood are associated with increased risk for developing eating disorders. Our theory of normal development focuses on the particular intra- and interpersonal demands the individual is required to negotiate at different stages of development. We ascribe to the views of Erikson (1968) and others (Vaillant, 1977) who conceptualized adolescence as the period in which the influence of "society" replaces the childhood milieu. The core issues of interpersonal relationships, intimacy, and autonomy remain salient throughout the transition from childhood to adulthood. The transition from childhood to adolescence is marked by the initiation of pubertal changes that signal sexual maturation, identity formation, transition of intimate relationships from within the family to extrafamily peers, and initiation of dating. The transition from adolescence to young adulthood is marked by choices regarding higher education or employment, living away from home, and the assumption of greater financial responsibility. Issues related to sexual preference and establishing enduring monogamous relationships take on added importance during this transition.

These changing expectations and increasing demands within the individual's life are marked by increased risk for eating disorders. Investigations of age of onset for anorexia nervosa suggest two periods of enhanced risk, ages 14 and 18 (Halmi, Casper, Eckert, Goldberg, & Davies, 1979; Steinhausen, 1994) with a mean age of onset at 17 years (American Psychiatric Association, 1994). Age of onset for bulimia nervosa appears to be concentrated in the transition from adolescence to early adulthood and ranges from 18 to 22 years (Fairburn & Cooper, 1984; Pyle, Mitchell, & Eckert, 1981) with a mean age of onset at 19 years (Steinhausen, 1994). Thus the transition from childhood to adolescence is associated with the onset of anorexia nervosa whereas the transition from adolescence to adulthood is associated with the onset of both anorexia and bulimia nervosa.

Although many of the challenges associated with these developmental transition periods are psychosocial in nature, they occur within a context of biological changes. In addition, biological factors likely influence responses to these challenges. Viewing risk factors in terms of interactions among biological, psychological, and social processes seems most useful because divisions among them can be fairly artificial. Data collected within a predominantly psychosocial paradigm may be reinterpreted according to biological influences, and vice versa. To facilitate discussion of interactions among biological, psychological, and social processes, we review research relevant to each.

BIOLOGICAL CONTRIBUTIONS TO EATING PATHOLOGY

Genetic Factors

Eating disorders appear to be more common among first-degree female relatives of individuals with eating disorders than among females from the general population (Lilenfeld et al., 1998; Treasure & Holland, 1990). Twin research indicates an influence of genetic factors (Fichter & Noegel, 1990; Holland, Hall, Murray, Russell, & Crisp, 1984; Holland, Sicotte, & Treasure, 1988; Hsu, Chesler, & Santhouse, 1990; Kendler et al., 1991). More recently, twin and family studies have begun to look at shared transmission between eating disorders and other forms of psychopathology. Three investigations (Kendler et al., 1995; Klump, Miller, Keel, McGue, & Iacono, 2000; Lilenfeld et al., 1998) support the possibility that eating disorders and anxiety disorders may share a common genetic liability. These data support the role of genetic factors in creating a nonspecific diathesis for the development of eating disorders and anxiety disorders.

Neurophysiological Function

Neurotransmitter function has long been a focus of research attempting to discern the biological underpinnings of psychopathology. Given the association between serotonin (5-HT) function and disturbances in appetite and mood, research has focused attention on 5-HT function as a mechanism for conferring risk for eating pathology (for review, see Kaye, 1997). However, evidence of serotonin dysfunction in anorexia nervosa and bulimia nervosa has been mixed.

Much research has found decreased serotonin function in both disorders. Cerebral spinal fluid 5-HT metabolites (5-HIAA) and urine concentrations of 5-HIAA are decreased in patients with eating disorders compared to normal controls (Jimerson, Lesem, Kaye, & Brewerton, 1992; Kaye, Gwirtsman, George, Jimerson, & Ebert, 1988). Patients with eating disorders also show altered platelet 5-HT receptor function (Hassanyeh & Marshall, 1991; McBride, Anderson, Khait, Sunday, & Halmi, 1991). Finally, patients with eating disorders have demonstrated diminished prolactin release in response to ingestion of a serotonin agonist (Brewerton, Mueller, Lesem, & Brandt, 1992; Golden & Shenker, 1994; McBride et al., 1991). Notably, many indicators of serotonin function normalize upon nutritional rehabilitation suggesting that these findings may reflect a result rather than a cause of eating pathology (Kaye et al., 1988).

Investigators have begun to explore the presence of serotonin dysfunction among weight-recovered anorexic patients as a possible indication of premorbid serotonin function. One such finding indicates the presence of *increased* cerebral spinal fluid concentrations of 5-HIAA after weight recovery in anorexia nervosa (Kaye, 1997; Kaye, Gwirtsman, George, & Ebert, 1991). Some authors (Kaye, 1997) have suggested that this reflects the presence of excessive serotonin function prior to disordered eating. Kaye (1997) has suggested that increased serotonin function may represent a biologically based temperamental predisposition to perfectionism and obsessionality among girls who develop anorexia nervosa. This hypothesis could explain the high comorbidity between eating disorders and anxiety disorders. However, prospective studies to predict the onset of eating disorders are unlikely given the expense and invasiveness of measuring 5-HIAA in cerebral spinal fluid.

Age of onset and gender differences in eating disorder prevalence are also being explored from a biological perspective. Some investigators question whether puberty and its associated hormonal changes may trigger the expression of genes that confer risk for eating pathology during adolescence for females. Both age of onset and gender difference issues have been conceptualized from a psychosocial perspective as well.

Temperament

The biological underpinning we emphasize is temperament, specifically negative affectivity, with high stress reactivity as its major component. Our prospective longitudinal study of the development of disordered eating among adolescents ages 13 to 18 revealed temperament as a significant predictor in both girls and boys (Leon et al., 1999). Specifically, girls and boys characterized by high levels of negative affectivity on the Multidimensional Personality Questionnaire (Tellegen, 1982) were most likely to develop disordered-eating behaviors and attitudes over the course of the longitudinal study. Disordered-eating attitudes and behaviors were assessed using surveys and semistructured interviews. The impact of negative affectivity was demonstrated among students who had no eating pathology at baseline assessment and those with moderate to high levels of disordered eating at initial testing. As a diathesis, negative affectivity is likely to be associated with negative attitudes toward the self, leading to low self-esteem and dissatisfaction with many aspects of the self, including physical appearance. These attitudes are discussed in more detail in a later section of this chapter. Moreover, negative affectivity appears to represent a nonspecific diathesis for the development of psychopathology in general (Clark, Watson, & Mineka, 1994; Watson, Clark, & Harkness, 1994), particularly disorders involving mood and anxiety disturbance. Much research, including our own (Leon et al., 1999), has demonstrated significant comorbidity among eating, mood, anxiety, and substance use disorders in adolescents, a finding that supports the role of temperament as a nonspecific diathesis.

PSYCHOLOGICAL CONTRIBUTIONS TO EATING PATHOLOGY

Several psychological variables have been explored as possible contributants to the development of disordered eating. These factors include personality, learning, and maladaptive responses to stress. Bruch (1978) proposed that the underlying cause of eating disorders is the inability to correctly identify and differentiate the signals of hunger and other bodily and emotional sensations, a condition Sifneos (1972) termed "alexithymia." Bruch (1978) believed that this confusion resulted from early childhood experiences of a mother responding to all her infant's emotional needs with the giving of food, or failing to respond to her infant's hunger with feeding. Work from Chatoor, Egan, Getson, Menvielle, and O'Donnell (1988) supported the thesis of disrupted feeding interactions between mothers and infants who exhibit food refusal. According to Bruch (1978), the mother's inability to appropriately mirror the child's desires results in the child's inability to differentiate between physical and emotional needs and also undermines the child's sense of identity, autonomy, and control. Because the child is unable to secure an appropriate response from her caretaker, she modifies her expectations of her role within the world and attempts to alter her needs to fit the care that is given. This pattern of overcompliance with the expectations of others is radically altered with the onset of disordered eating in which the adolescent attempts to achieve a feeling of autonomy by controlling her food intake and weight (Bruch, 1978). Findings from our 4-year prospective study confirm the importance of poor interoceptive awareness in predicting eating disorder symptoms in adolescents but did not support ineffectiveness as a predictor of disordered eating (Leon et al., 1993; Leon, Fulkerson, Perry, & Early-Zald, 1995; Leon et al., 1999). Other investigators have also found higher alexithymia scores in eating-disordered compared to normal control groups (Bourke, Taylor, Parker, & Bagby, 1992; Schmidt, Jiwany, & Treasure, 1993). Greater problems in interoceptive awareness but not ineffectiveness have been reported for eating-disordered samples compared to psychiatric control samples suffering primarily from depression (Hurley, Palmer, & Stretch, 1990). Thus empirical research supports part but not all of Bruch's (1978) theory.

Some researchers have argued that difficulties labeling hunger and satiation result from chronic dieting (Polivy & Herman, 1985), thus shifting focus from early parent–child relationships to results of denying or ignoring one's own physical needs in attempts to lose weight. Patton et al. (1990) demonstrated that girls with a history of dieting were eight times more likely to develop an eating disorder compared to girls with no history of dieting. The association between dieting and anorexia nervosa is relatively direct— attempts to lose weight through food restriction represent the core behavior of anorexia nervosa.

The association between dieting and bulimia nervosa can be explained by the restraint hypothesis (Polivy & Herman, 1985), which posits that dieting causes binge eating. Polivy and Herman (1985) argue that attempts to control food intake leave an individual vulnerable to disinhibitors that can be cognitive, emotional, or pharmacological in form. For example, a 14-year-old girl may initiate a diet to lose weight. However, her attempts to control her food intake are undermined when she becomes upset after arguing with her older brother (emotional disinhibitor). This event then leads to counterregulation (binge eating). Several laboratory experiments have supported an association between dietary restraint and binge eating in nonclinical populations (Ruderman, 1985). Thus dieting leads indirectly to the core feature of both bulimia nervosa and BED (Polivy & Herman, 1985).

Heatherton and Baumeister (1991) provided a slightly different explanation of the relationship between dieting and binge eating. These authors suggested that individuals with low self-esteem were more likely to diet in an attempt to improve self-worth. However, difficulty losing weight decreased self-esteem and increased feelings of ineffectiveness. The binge eating episode then served to shift attention from aversive self-perceptions to the simple physical act of eating. Thus binge eating was motivated by the desire to escape self-awareness. Anecdotal evidence from women with bulimic episodes suggests that many use binge eating to "zone out." Indeed, Neckowitz and Morrison (1991) found that bulimic women were more likely than normal control females to engage in escape–avoidant coping strategies in response to stressful situations. However, the escape from self-awareness hypothesis would be exceptionally difficult to test experimentally because the very act of asking women to report their levels of self-awareness preceding,

during, and following a binge episode would alter their level of self-awareness.

Although dieting often precedes binge eating in retrospective reports of
individuals with eating disorders, nearly 17% of women with bulimia nervosa
and 48% of individuals with BED report onset of binge eating prior to the
first weight loss diet (Mussell et al., 1997; Spitzer et al., 1992, respectively).
Some authors (Arnow, Kenardy, & Agras, 1992; Ruderman, 1986) have
argued that binge eating can be directly triggered by negative emotions in
the absence of dieting behaviors. Research (Arnow, Kenardy, & Agras, 1995;
Telch, Pratt, & Niego, 1998) supports the theory that binge eating is used
to cope with negative emotional states. Recent research suggests that binge
eating may provide an exchange of less tolerable negative states, such as
anger, for more acceptable negative emotions, such as guilt (Kenardy, Arnow,
& Agras, 1996). Thus negative emotional states precipitate both dieting
and binge eating behaviors. Notably, a temperament marked by negative
affectivity would increase an individual's predisposition to experience such
negative emotional states.

Negative affectivity likely increases negative attitudes toward the self,
such as low self-esteem and body dissatisfaction. A prospective study of the
development of eating pathology in girls linked poor self-esteem to onset of
disordered-eating behaviors (Button, Sonuga-Barke, Davies, & Thompson,
1996). However, other studies (Keel, Fulkerson, & Leon, 1997; Leon et al.,
1999) have not found a significant association between low self-esteem and
development of disordered eating in multivariate analyses. It is likely that
self-esteem is an important factor in determining onset of eating pathology,
but its influence is probably not independent of other factors that would be
strongly related to disordered eating, such as body dissatisfaction.

Killen et al. (1996) found that weight concerns predicted the onset of
partial syndrome eating disorders over a 4-year prospective follow-up study
of 877 high school girls. The overall incidence of partial syndrome eating
disorders was 4%. Among girls in the highest quartile of weight concerns at
baseline assessment, the incidence was 10% for partial syndrome eating
disorders. Among girls in the lowest quartile of weight concerns, the incidence was 0%. Similar results for boys have been found. Keel, Fulkerson, &
Leon (1997) demonstrated that poor body image predicted onset of disordered eating measured by a short form of the Eating Attitudes Test (Garner,
Olmstead, Bohr, & Garfinkel, 1982) in a 1-year prospective follow-up study
of 102 elementary school boys.

Dieting, body dissatisfaction, and unrealistic weight ideals have a high
base rate among girls (Leon, Carroll, Chernyk, & Finn, 1985). According
to the National Centers for Disease Control and Prevention, the point prevalence of dieting among high school girls was 44%. Dieting, body dissatisfaction, and disordered eating are evident even among preadolescent girls
(Keel, Fulkerson, & Leon, 1997; Keel, Heatherton, Harnden, & Hornig,
1997). Among pre- and early adolescents, girls report worse body image,

lower self-esteem, and greater disordered eating compared to boys (Keel, Fulkerson, & Leon, 1997). However, some researchers (Adams, Katz, Beauchamp, Cohen, & Zavis, 1993; Cohn et al., 1987) have found significant gender differences only among older adolescents. The significant gender differences in disordered eating, the presence of these problems at such early ages, and the pervasiveness of related behaviors and attitudes in the general population all point to societal contributions to eating pathology.

SOCIAL CONTRIBUTIONS TO EATING PATHOLOGY

Important societal influences in the development of eating disorders are suggested by three general findings: (1) the relatively recent increase in the prevalence of anorexia nervosa (Hoek, 1995) and bulimia nervosa (Kendler et al., 1991), (2) the increased rate of eating disorders in industrialized nations compared to nonindustrialized nations (Hsu, 1990), and (3) the significant gender difference in who is at risk for eating disorders. Social influences can be viewed as existing at multiple levels (Bronfenbrenner, 1979). At the level of culture, studies (e.g., Garner, Garfinkel, Schwartz, & Thompson, 1980; Wiseman, Gray, Mosimann, & Ahrens, 1992) have demonstrated increasingly thinner beauty ideals during the latter third of this century. Indeed, fashion models such as Kate Moss represent unrealistic weight ideals for the average female. Ironically, as girls enter puberty, body fat composition increases, as does their awareness of these unrealistic societal aesthetic ideals.

The association between societal aesthetic ideals and body dissatisfaction among women has been demonstrated in a number of studies. Tiggeman and Pickering (1996) found a significant association between body dissatisfaction and time spent watching music videos, soap operas, and movies on television among adolescent girls. Two experimental studies have supported a causal relationship between media images and body dissatisfaction (Heinberg & Thompson, 1995; Stice & Shaw, 1994). Heinberg and Thompson (1995) randomly assigned female subjects to view television commercials containing either appearance-related images or nonappearance-related images. Women in the appearance-related condition reported significantly greater body dissatisfaction after exposure compared to women in the nonappearance-related condition (Heinberg & Thompson, 1995). Stice and Shaw (1994) randomly assigned women to view magazine pictures of very thin models, average models, or no models. Women assigned to view pictures of very thin models reported significantly greater body dissatisfaction than did women assigned to the other two conditions (Stice & Shaw, 1994). Thus cultural ideals of beauty can influence levels of body dissatisfaction experienced by girls.

Several explanations exist for the current emphasis on thinness in our culture. Historian Joan Brumberg (1988) followed women's social roles in U.S. society and weight ideals and notes an association between thinness as an aesthetic ideal and periods in which women are encouraged to adopt responsibilities outside the home and outside their roles as wives and mothers. This theory explains changing rates of anorexia nervosa found by Lucas, Beard, O'Fallon, and Kurland (1991) in their review of medical charts in Rochester, Minnesota, from 1935 to 1984. Hsu (1989) argued that financial prosperity following the industrial revolution led to an abundance of food that disrupted the traditional positive correlation between wealth and weight. In societies in which wealth is associated with thinness, beauty is associated with thinness (Hsu, 1989). This theory may explain the increased prevalence of eating disorders in industrialized nations compared to nonindustrialized nations and why rates of eating pathology increase as cultures become more Westernized (for review, see Pate, Pumariega, Hester, & Garner, 1992). Bordo (1990) has argued that industrial societies promote two conflicting ideals: immediate gratification through consumerism and delay of gratification (in order to reinvest profits to produce greater profits). This conflict leads to ideals of self-control competing with attainment of happiness through consumption (Bordo, 1990). A review of these perspectives on societal values suggests that development of eating disorders may be overdetermined within our current cultural climate.

Below the level of cultural influence, there exists the influence of local social networks such as schools, peer groups, and extracurricular activities. Research has demonstrated higher rates of eating disorders among girls enrolled in ballet schools (Garner, Garfinkel, Rockert, & Olmstead, 1987), as well as among adolescents who participate in team activities such as gymnastics and dance (Leon, 1991; Rosen & Hough, 1988). Indeed, eating disorders in adolescent males have been significantly associated with participation in sports with weight limits such as wrestling (Dick, 1991; Garner & Rosen, 1991). For males, sexual preference has been posited as a risk factor for eating pathology (Carlat & Camargo, 1991). An investigation of 135 male patients with eating disorders revealed that 27% endorsed a homosexual orientation compared to a population base rate of 1% to 6% in healthy males (Carlat, Camargo, & Herzog, 1997). Research suggests that homosexual and bisexual males may experience greater pressure to maintain lean and muscular physiques than do heterosexual males (Epel, Spanakos, Kasl-Godley, & Brownell, 1996). In these cases, societal values are reinforced by emphasis placed on weight either for performance or for appearance within local social networks.

A third level of social influences involves the family. Although family factors have already been implicated with biological and psychological aspects of the biopsychosocial model, a family may further reinforce societal ideals of thinness (Garfinkel & Garner, 1982). This reinforcement may occur via modeling or directly encouraging a child to adopt disordered-eating behaviors and attitudes (Pike & Rodin, 1991). Nonorganic failure to thrive in young children has been associated with a history of eating pathology in the mother (van Wezel-Meijler & Wit, 1989). There is evidence of increased eating pathology among mothers of daughters with disordered eating (Pike & Rodin, 1991), as well as significant associations between parents' tendency to comment on their daughter's weight and her tendency to restrict food intake and express body dissatisfaction (Keel, Heatherton, et al., 1997).

Much literature on the development of eating pathology has focused on the role of sexually traumatic experiences; however, less literature has focused on general physical abuse or neglect. Although sexual abuse is associated with increased risk for eating pathology, it does not appear to be a risk factor unique to eating disorders (Finn, Hartman, Leon, & Lawson, 1986). Several studies have demonstrated an increased rate of sexual abuse among women with eating disorders compared to normal controls; however, no significant difference is found between women with eating disorders and women with other forms of psychopathology (Wonderlich, Brewerton, Jocic, Dansky, & Abbott, 1997). Similar to the role of temperament as a nonspecific diathesis, sexual abuse appears to represent a nonspecific stressor in the development of disordered eating.

Eating disorders are precipitated through an interaction at several levels within an individual's culture, mind, and body. At the cultural level, our society values and rewards thinness. This cultural value may be further emphasized within groups, such as athletic teams, or within families. Families may influence a child at several levels in the development of eating pathology. The family may directly convey the importance of thinness or becoming aesthetically pleasing to others. In addition, the family may influence selection of extracurricular activities and thus peer groups. Members of a family also may model disordered eating or contribute to early childhood difficulties in differentiating between physical and emotional needs. Families may engender significant levels of conflict or inhibit an adolescent's quest for autonomy leading to disordered eating as a coping response. Finally, families contribute the genetic material that may form a child's temperament in predisposing their reactions to stress with emotional and behavioral dysregulation. These same biological contributants may shape levels of constraint and perfectionism, which may propel the individual to seek a "perfect body" or to participate in activities that emphasize success through self-denial. These personality features may leave the person ill-equipped to deal with minor setbacks, increasing the likelihood of counterregulation (binge eating) in response to cognitive disinhibitors (such as a minor violation of one's diet). Thus biological, psychological, and social factors require integration for a comprehensive understanding of vulnerability to develop eating pathology during childhood and adolescence.

DEVELOPMENTAL CHANGES IN RISK FACTORS

In this chapter we reviewed factors that act as a diathesis and how these factors interact with one another within the context of stressors brought about by developmental changes. We now turn to a discussion of developmental transitions in risk factors. Specifically, we address how certain factors may increase vulnerability to developing an eating disorder only at younger ages. These factors include pubertal development, actual body weight, and shared family influences. Studies have demonstrated that younger girls are more likely to demonstrate body dissatisfaction (Gralen, Levine, Smolak, & Murnen, 1990) and disordered-eating behaviors (Keel, Fulkerson, & Leon, 1997) if they weigh more for their height than do their peers. Conversely, studies of older adolescents demonstrate no significant relationship between actual body weight and body dissatisfaction, dieting, or disordered eating (Leon et al., 1993, 1995, and 1999). In addition, pubertal development has been uniquely associated with disordered eating in younger girls (Attie & Brooks-Gunn, 1989; Gralen et al., 1990; Keel, Fulkerson, & Leon, 1997; Killen et al., 1992; Koff & Rierdan, 1993) but not older adolescents (Gralen et al., 1990; Leon et al., 1993, 1995, 1999). These findings are consistent with developmental shifts occurring during adolescence. As a child matures, emphasis may shift from concrete aspects of the self, such as actual body size, to abstract aspects of the self, such as body image. As a cohort of children mature, individual differences in pubertal level diminish and thus decrease in their impact on behaviors and attitudes. A study of genetic versus environmental factors associated with disordered eating in twins (Klump, McGue, & Iacono, 2000) demonstrated that shared family environmental factors (e.g., parental styles and socioeconomic status) were a significant predictor of disordered eating for 11-year-old twins but not for 17-year-old twins. As children mature, interpersonal influences on eating behaviors and attitudes expand beyond the family to the peer group and decisions surrounding food and eating are made outside the home more frequently. This increased autonomy may increase the impact of genetically influenced temperamental styles or preferences on decisions surrounding eating and exercise.

THE BIOPSYCHOSOCIAL MODEL OF THE DEVELOPMENT OF EATING PATHOLOGY: INTEGRATION OF BIOLOGICAL, PSYCHOLOGICAL, AND SOCIAL INFLUENCES

Thus far, this chapter has presented an overview of research findings supporting the role of biological, psychological, and social factors in the development of eating pathology among children and adolescents. However, we feel the true strength of this conceptual approach comes from the integration of these various factors in understanding the etiology of eating disorders within the course of normal development. To take advantage of this strength, we now present a case history derived from a composite of patients and explore the congruence of factors leading to this adolescent's eating disorder.

Riley was 17 years old when she began treatment at the eating disorders clinic. Her mother accompanied Riley to her initial assessment. According to her mother, Riley had always been healthy and performed well in sports, academics, and music. Indeed, Riley was an exceptional student and had been selected for a summer program for gifted and talented students over the past summer. Although Riley had attended summer camp since she was 10 years of age, the 8-week summer enrichment program represented the longest period of time that she had been separated from her home, family, and friends. During the first week of the program, Riley reported feeling awkward in her attempts to meet people and make friends. She felt particularly insecure in her interactions with boys and noticed that everyone around her, including her roommate, appeared to have paired off into couples as if they were preparing for "Noah's Ark." Rather than feeling like a "third arm" Riley decided to begin a rigorous exercise program with her free time. She reasoned that she would take advantage of the program's facilities to ensure that she was in especially good shape at the beginning of her school's soccer season. Riley was initially satisfied with her training program of running, swimming, and weight lifting. However, one day on her way from the pool to the women's locker room, she passed by some boys and heard them making derogatory comments about her body. As she entered the locker room, she stopped in front of the mirror and suddenly noticed her thighs. According to Riley, her thighs were "pale and bumpy like cottage cheese." She reported an epiphany at that moment that she was "too fat." She skipped dinner that night and did leg lifts before bed and after getting up the next morning. She decided to limit herself to eating only "healthy foods" such as fruits and vegetables and only in small amounts. When asked how she decided what foods were healthy or how many calories she could eat a day, Riley reported that she occasionally read her mother's magazines and scanned through the "lose 10 pounds in a week!" diets. In fact, for fun, she and her mom had gone on a diet together when Riley was 12 years old. Riley joked that it was not a "real diet" because she and her mother would eat several high-calorie, high-fat foods like peanut butter on celery sticks or ice cream in diet rootbeer floats. Riley reported other short-lived diets that involved eating tuna fish or grapefruit that she and her friends would go on together. However, the summer diet was the first time that Riley followed a rigid program of food and exercise. Riley reported that her program made her feel "great"—she felt "strong and in control" and was frequently complimented by her roommate for how "good" she was. Riley also noticed that if she went long enough without eating, she would stop feeling hungry. When she would eat, she would feel full after very little food. She took this as evidence that her stomach was shrinking. When Riley returned home from the summer program, her mother was dismayed by how much weight her daughter had lost. Riley had gone from weighing 125 lbs. at 5'5" to weighing 105 lbs. Meal times became very stressful as Riley refused to eat anything with her family. However, Riley's mother started noticing certain food items would disappear over night. After 4 months of rigid adherence to her summer program, Riley reported that she "lost control" one night and ate an entire package of cookies. Distraught by her actions, she resolved to eat nothing the next day and doubled her exercise routine. Within a week, Riley had another episode in which she consumed a gallon of ice cream at night when everyone else was asleep. Riley's binge episodes came more frequently, and, despite her frantic efforts to compensate through exercising and fasting, she quickly regained all the weight she had lost. Riley reported feeling "trapped." Every attempt she made to regain control was thwarted with binge eating episodes. By late fall, Riley became increasingly depressed and anxious over her binge eating. As she became more depressed, her binge episodes grew worse and as her binge episodes grew worse, she became more depressed. Her cycle of binge eating/fasting and exercising increased during times of stress such as soccer finals and college interviews. Riley's mother was particularly concerned about the impact the eating disorder was having on Riley's mood and on the family. Riley began talking about "feeling suicidal," and Riley's 10-year-old sister was beginning to talk about "feeling fat" and "needing to lose weight."

This case study illustrates many of the points made earlier in this chapter. Riley's disordered eating occurred during her first significant separation from her home, which may signal the separation associated with going to college. The summer program also presented Riley with a developmental shift from interpersonal affiliations within the family to monogamous dating relationships. These changes represented stressors in her life. With regard to her diathesis or vulnerability for eating pathology, she was exposed to societal idealization of thinness through her mother's magazines. She was also encouraged to engage in dieting by her mother and peers starting at 12 years of age as she was transitioning into puberty. Riley received positive reinforcement for being "good" from her roommate in the summer program. Indeed, the evaluation of Riley's self-denial as being "good" by her roommate represented a culturally embedded moral declaration.

At the level of psychological factors, Riley's exercise program was initiated during a period of feeling insecure in her peer interactions. Her diet program was initiated after feeling self-conscious of her body in front of teenage boys. Riley's epiphany of "being fat" engendered body dissatisfaction that motivated her dieting. Her severe food restriction interfered with her hunger and satiety signals. Later, her dieting seemed to lead to binge eating and the eventual use of binge eating episodes to cope with feelings of depression and anxiety.

For biological risk factors, Riley's case history suggests a temperament marked by high stress reactivity. This temperamental characteristic led Riley to be vulnerable not only to eating disorders but also to significant levels of depression and anxiety. Although her 10-year-old sister's statements about weight and diet may be a result of modeling, they may also reflect a culturally shaped response to a shared genetic vulnerability for high stress reactivity. For Riley, treatment involved antidepressant medication and individual psychotherapy.

TREATMENT AND PREVENTION

Multimodal treatments are employed for both anorexia and bulimia nervosa. Many treatment investigations include combined samples of adolescent and adult subjects. However, most studies indicate that age at treatment is not significantly associated with outcome (Keel & Mitchell, 1997; Steinhausen, 1997), suggesting that conclusions from combined samples validly reflect treatment response among younger patients. Psychotherapy often involves cognitive-behavioral therapy in which associations between cultural ideals of thinness, body dissatisfaction, dieting, and disordered eating are made explicit and challenged. In family therapy, problems with communication and conflict resolution are addressed. Pharmacological treatment often involves antidepressant medications, especially selective serotonin reuptake inhibitors due to their more tolerable side effects. Interestingly, the efficacy of antidepressant medication in reducing binge eating behavior appears to be independent of its impact on levels of depression (Mitchell et al., 1990). The efficacy of each of these treatment modalities further supports the biopsychosocial model in conceptualizing eating disorder vulnerability.

Thus far, prevention programs aimed at children and adolescents have demonstrated limited efficacy (Carter, Stewart, Dunn, & Fairburn, 1997; Paxton, 1993; Smolak, Levine, & Schermer, 1998). Components of these programs have included psychoeducation to increase adolescents' awareness of media influences on "ideal" body types, determinants of body size, nutritional needs, consequences of dieting, and consequences of disordered eating. However, duration of programs has been limited to 5 (Paxton, 1993), 8 (Carter et al., 1997), and 10 lessons (Smolak et al., 1998). There has been some concern that such programs inadvertently encourage the very behaviors they attempt to prevent (Carter et al., 1997; Mann et al., 1997). In one study, intervention participants reported increased levels of dietary restraint following the program (Carter et al., 1997). In a second study, intervention participants reported more symptoms of eating disorders than did control subjects (Mann et al., 1997). Prevention efforts will likely improve with further development and refinement.

FUTURE DIRECTIONS

Future research could benefit from identifying factors that protect against the development of eating pathology in children and adolescents who appear to be at high risk. Such factors may include social support, greater range of qualities influencing self-worth, and greater flexibility in responding to change. Our study found that male and female athletes reported greater body satisfaction (Fulkerson, Keel, Leon, & Dorr, 1999), suggesting that participation in "nonelite" athletics may serve as a protective factor. The identification of protective factors would significantly contribute to the efficacy of prevention programs. Given the confluence of onset of eating pathology with a developmental shift in primary relationships from the nuclear family to peers, research on the influence of peers in the development of eating pathology also seems warranted. Such research may elucidate the transmission of specific behaviors such as fasting and self-induced vomiting that appear to spread within peer groups. In addition, this focus may reveal how membership within certain peer groups may protect girls from the development of eating disorders during adolescence. Because longitudinal studies with frequent follow-up intervals extending throughout the period of risk are labor and time intensive, collaborative studies that evaluate risk and protective factors for several forms of psychopathology may be efficient in terms of costs and range of relevant findings. This approach increases the feasibility of studying a full range of factors in large samples from early childhood to adulthood. Krueger, Caspi, Moffitt, Silva, and McGee (1996) provided a model of this approach with their longitudinal study in New Zealand. This research also provides a model for studying developmental psychopathology within a biopsychosocial model.

CONCLUSIONS

In this chapter, we presented a developmental perspective on eating disorders during childhood and adolescence within a biopsychosocial model. The periods of risk for onset of eating disorders are marked by developmental transitions from childhood to adolescence and from adolescence to adulthood. The changing demands of these developmental transitions provide the context in which various biological, psychological, and social risk factors increase vulnerability to eating pathology.

Temperamental styles marked by negative affectivity, genetic liability to develop eating pathology and anxiety disorders, and serotonin dysregulation have all received empirical support as biological factors that may contribute to the etiology of eating disorders. Psychodynamic, behavioral, and cognitive emotional perspectives have shed light on the role of psychological factors such as alexythymia, dieting, body dissatisfaction, emotion regulation, and self-esteem in the development of disordered eating. We have reviewed levels of social influence spanning cultural ideals of beauty and morality to impact of family and peer groups in the adoption of disordered-eating behaviors and attitudes. Finally, we presented an integration of these various factors into a unified biopsychosocial model tracing the development of an eating disorder within a case study.

Although many risk factors may remain stable in their impact on vulnerability throughout the lifespan, we presented research suggesting developmental changes in risk factors. As more research is conducted from a developmental perspective, we anticipate that more developmental changes in risk factors will be revealed. Attention to this question may improve formation of appropriate intervention and prevention programs. To date, the efficacy of prevention efforts has received mixed support. Continued research is required to develop and validate programs that will alter the tide of young girls developing eating disorders.

REFERENCES

Adams, P. J., Katz, R. C., Beauchamp, K., Cohen, E., & Zavis, D. (1993). Body dissatisfaction, eating disorders, and depression: A developmental perspective. *Journal of Child and Family Studies, 2,* 37–46.

American Psychiatric Association. (1994). *Diagnostic and statistical manual of mental disorders* (4th ed.). Washington, DC: Author.

Arnow, B., Kenardy, J., & Agras, W. S. (1992). Binge eating among the obese: A descriptive study. *Journal of Behavioral Medicine, 15,* 155–170.

Arnow, B., Kenardy, J., & Agras, W. S. (1995). The Emotional Eating Scale: The development of a measure to assess coping with negative affect by eating. *International Journal of Eating Disorders, 18,* 79–90.

Ash, J. B., & Piazza, E. (1995).Changing symptomatology in eating disorders. *International Journal of Eating Disorders, 18,* 27–38.

Attie, I., & Brooks-Gunn, J. (1989). Development of eating problems in adolescent girls: A longitudinal study. *Developmental Psychology, 25,* 70–79.

Bordo, S. (1990). Reading the slender body. In M. Jacobus, E. Fox Keller, & S. Shuttleworth (Eds.), *Body/politics: Women and the discourse of science* (pp. 83–112). New York: Routledge.

Bourke, M. P., Taylor, G. J., Parker, J. D., & Bagby, R. M. (1992). Alexithymia in women with anorexia nervosa: A preliminary investigation. *British Journal of Psychiatry, 161,* 240–243.

Brewerton, T. D., Mueller, E. A., Lesem, M. D., & Brandt, H. A. (1992). Neuroendocrine responses to m-chlorophenylpiperazine and L-tryptophan in bulimia. *Archives of General Psychiatry, 49,* 852–861.

Bronfenbrenner, U. (1979). *The ecology of human development: Experiments by nature and design.* Cambridge, MA: Harvard University Press.

Bruch, H. (1978). *The golden cage.* New York: Vintage Books.

Brumberg, J. J. (1988). *Fasting girls: The emergence of anorexia nervosa as a modern disease.* Cambridge, MA: Harvard University Press.

Button, E. J., Sonuga-Barke, E. J. S., Davies, J., & Thompson, M. (1996). A prospective study of self-esteem in the prediction of eating problems in adolescent schoolgirls: Questionnaire findings. *British Journal of Clinical Psychology, 35,* 193–203.

Carlat, D. J., & Camargo, C. A. (1991). Review of bulimia nervosa in males. *American Journal of Psychiatry, 148,* 831–843.

Carlat, D. J., Camargo, C. A., & Herzog, D. B. (1997). Eating disorders in males: A report on 135 patients. *American Journal of Psychiatry, 154,* 1127–1132.

Carter, J. C., Stewart, D. A., Dunn, V. J., & Fairburn, C. G. (1997). Primary prevention of eating disorders: Might it do more harm than good? *International Journal of Eating Disorders, 22,* 167–172.

Chatoor, I., Egan, J., Getson, P., Menvielle, E., & O'Donnell, R. (1988). Mother–infant interactions in infantile anorexia nervosa. *Journal of the American Academy of Child and Adolescent Psychiatry, 27,* 535–540.

Clark, L. A., Watson, D., & Mineka, S. (1994). Temperament, personality, and the mood and anxiety disorders. *Journal of Abnormal Psychology, 103,* 103–116.

Cohn, L. D., Adler, N. E., Irwin, C. E., Millstein, S. G., Kegeles, S. M., & Stone, G. (1987). Body–figure preferences in male and female adolescents. *Journal of Abnormal Psychology, 96,* 276–279.

Copeland, P. M., Sacks, N. R., & Herzog, D. B. (1995). Longitudinal follow-up of amenorrhea in eating disorders. *Psychosomatic Medicine, 57,* 121–126.

Dick, R.W. (1991). Eating disorders in NCAA athletic programs. *Athletic Training, 26,* 136–140.

Epel, E. S., Spanakos, A., Kasl-Godley, J., & Brownell, K. D. (1996). Body shape ideals across gender, sexual orientation, socioeconomic status, race, and age in personal advertisements. *International Journal of Eating Disorders, 19,* 265–273.

Erikson, E. H. (1968). *Identity, youth, and crisis.* New York: Norton.

Fairburn, C. G., & Cooper, P. J. (1984). The clinical features of bulimia nervosa. *British Journal of Psychiatry, 144,* 238–246.

Fairburn, C. G., Kirk, J., O'Connor, M., & Cooper, P. J. (1986). A comparison of two psychological treatments for bulimia nervosa. *Behaviour Research and Therapy, 24,* 629–643.

Fichter, M. M., & Noegel, R. (1990). Concordance for bulimia nervosa in twins. *International Journal of Eating Disorders, 9,* 255–263.

Finn, S. E., Hartman, M., Leon, G. R., & Lawson, L. (1986). Eating disorders and sexual abuse: Lack of confirmation for a clinical hypothesis. *International Journal of Eating Disorders, 5,* 1051–1060.

French, S. A., Peterson, C. B., Story, M., Anderson, N., Mussell, M. P., & Mitchell, J. E. (1998). Agreement between survey and interview measures of weight control practices in adolescents. *International Journal of Eating Disorders, 23,* 45–56.

Fulkerson, J. A., Keel, P. K., Leon, G. R., & Dorr, T. (1999). Eating disordered behaviors and personality characteristics of high school athletes and nonathletes. *International Journal of Eating Disorders, 26,* 73–79.

Garfinkel, P. E., & Garner, D. M. (1982). *Anorexia nervosa: A multidimensional perspective.* New York: Brunner/Mazel.

Garner, D. M., Garfinkel, P. E., Rockert, W., & Olmstead, M. P. (1987). A prospective study of eating disturbances in the ballet. *Psychotherapy and Psychosomatics, 48,* 170–175.

Garner, D. M., Garfinkel, P. E., Schwartz, D., & Thompson, M. (1980). Cultural expectations of thinness in women. *Psychological Reports, 47,* 483–491.

Garner, D. M., Olmstead, M. P., Bohr, Y., & Garfinkel, P. E. (1982). The Eating Attitudes Test: Psychometric features and clinical correlates. *Psychological Medicine, 12,* 871–878.

Garner, D. M., & Rosen, J. C. (1991). Eating disorders among athletes: Research and recommendations. *Journal of Applied Sport Sciences Research, 5,* 100–107.

Golden, N. H., & Shenker, I. R. (1994). Amenorrhea in anorexia nervosa: Neuroendocrine control of hypothalamic dysfunction. *International Journal of Eating Disorders, 16,* 53–60.

Graber, J. A., Brooks-Gunn, J., Paikoff, R. L., & Warren, M. P. (1994). Prediction of eating problems: An 8-year study of adolescent girls. *Developmental Psychology, 30,* 823–834.

Gralen, S. J., Levine, M. P., Smolak, L., & Murnen, S. K. (1990). Dieting and disordered eating during early and middle adolescence: Do the influences remain the same? *International Journal of Eating Disorders, 9,* 501–512.

Halmi, K. A., Casper, R. C., Eckert, E. D., Goldberg, S. C., & Davis J. M. (1979). Unique features associated with age of onset of anorexia nervosa. *Psychiatry Research, 1,* 209–215.

Hassanyeh, F., & Marshall, E. F. (1991). Measures of serotonin metabolism in anorexia nervosa. *Acta Psychiatrica Scandinavica, 84,* 561–563.

Heatherton, T. F., & Baumeister, R. F. (1991). Binge eating as escape from self-awareness. *Psychological Bulletin, 110,* 86–108.

Heinberg, L. J., & Thompson, J. K. (1995). Body image and televised images of thinness and attractiveness: A controlled laboratory investigation. *Journal of Social and Clinical Psychology, 14,* 325–338.

Hoek, H. W. (1995). The distribution of eating disorders. In K. D. Brownell & C. G. Fairburn (Eds.), *Eating disorders and obesity: A comprehensive handbook* (pp. 207–211). New York: Guilford Press.

Holland, A. J., Hall, A., Murray, R., Russell, G. F. M., & Crisp, A. H. (1984). Anorexia nervosa: A study of 34 twin pairs. *British Journal of Psychiatry, 145,* 414–419.

Holland, A. J., Sicotte, N., & Treasure, J. (1988). Anorexia nervosa: Evidence for a genetic basis. *Journal of Psychosomatic Research, 32,* 561–571.

Hsu, L. K. (1989). The gender gap in eating disorders: Why are the eating disorders more common among women? *Clinical Psychology Review, 9,* 393–407.

Hsu, L. K. (1990). *Eating disorders.* New York: Guilford Press.

Hsu, L. K. G., Chesler, B. E., & Santhouse, R. (1990). Bulimia nervosa in eleven sets of twins: A clinical report. *International Journal of Eating Disorders, 9,* 275–282.

Hurley, J. B., Palmer, R. L., & Stretch, D. (1990). The specificity of the Eating Disorders Inventory: A reappraisal. *International Journal of Eating Disorders, 9,* 419–424.

Jimerson, D. C., Lesem, M. D., Kaye, W. H., & Brewerton, T. D. (1992). Low serotonin and dopamine metabolite concentrations in cerebrospinal fluid from bulimic patients with frequent binge episodes. *Archives of General Psychiatry, 49,* 132–138.

Kaye, W. H. (1997). Anorexia nervosa, obsessional behavior, and serotonin. *Psychopharmacology Bulletin, 33,* 335–344.

Kaye, W. H., Gwirtsman, H. E., George, D. T., & Ebert, M. H. (1991). Altered serotonin activity in anorexia nervosa after long-term weight restoration: Does elevated cerebrospinal fluid 5-hydroxyindoleacetic acid level correlate with rigid and obsessive behavior? *Archives of General Psychiatry, 48,* 556–562.

Kaye, W. H., Gwirtsman, H. E., George, D. T., Jimerson, D. C., & Ebert, M. H. (1988). CSF 5-HIAA concentrations in anorexia nervosa: Reduced values in underweight subjects normalize after weight gain. *Biological Psychiatry, 23,* 102-105.

Keel, P. K., Fulkerson, J. A., & Leon, G. R. (1997). Disordered eating precursors in pre- and early adolescent girls and boys. *Journal of Youth and Adolescence, 26,* 203–216.

Keel, P. K., Heatherton, T. F., Harnden, J. L., & Hornig, C. D. (1997). Mothers, fathers, and daughters: Dieting and disordered eating. *Eating Disorders: The Journal of Treatment and Prevention, 5,* 216–228.

Keel, P. K., Klump, K. L., Leon, G. R., & Fulkerson, J. A. (1998). Disordered eating in adolescent males from a school-based sample. *International Journal of Eating Disorders, 23,* 125–132.

Keel, P. K., & Mitchell, J. E. (1997). Outcome in bulimia nervosa. *American Journal of Psychiatry, 154,* 313–321.

Kenardy, J., Arnow, B., & Agras, W. S. (1996). The aversiveness of specific emotional states associated with binge-eating in obese subjects. *Australian and New Zealand Journal of Psychiatry, 30,* 839–844.

Kendler, K. S., MacLean, C., Neale, M., Kessler, R. C., Heath, A., & Eaves, L. (1991). The genetic epidemiology of bulimia nervosa. *American Journal of Psychiatry, 148,* 1627–1637.

Kendler, K. S., Walters, E. E., Neale, M. C., Kessler, R., Heath, A., & Eaves, L. (1995). The structure of genetic and environmental risk factors for six major psychiatric disorders in women. *Archives of General Psychiatry, 52,* 374–383.

Killen, J. D., Hayward, C., Litt, I., Hammer, L. D., Wilson, D. M., Miner, B., Taylor, C. B., Varady, A., & Shisslak, C. (1992). Is puberty a risk factor for eating disorders? *American Journal of Disorders of Childhood, 146,* 323–325.

Killen, J. D., Taylor, C. B., Hayward, C., Haydel, K. F., Wilson, D. M., Hammer, L., Kraemer, H., Blair-Greiner, A., & Strachowski, D. (1996). Weight concerns influence the development of eating disorders: A 4-year prospective study. *Journal of Consulting and Clinical Psychology, 64,* 936–940.

Killen, J. D., Taylor, C. B., Hayward, C., Wilson, D. M., Haydel, K. F., Robinson, T. N., Litt, I., Simmonds, B. A., Varady, A., & Kraemer, H. (1994). Pursuit of thinness and onset of eating disorder symptoms in a community sample of adolescent girls: A three-year prospective analysis. *International Journal of Eating Disorders, 16,* 227–238.

Klump, K. L., McGue, M., & Iacono, W. G. (2000). Age differences in genetic and environmental influences on eating attitudes and behaviors in preadolescent and adolescent female twins. *Journal of Abnormal Psychology, 109,* 239–251.

Klump, K. L., Miller, K. B., Keel, P. K., McGue, M., & Iacono, W. G. (2000). *A population-based twin study of anorexia and bulimia nervosa: Heritability and shared transmission with anxiety disorders.* Manuscript submitted for publication.

Koff, E., & Rierdan, J. (1993). Advanced pubertal development and eating disturbance in early adolescent girls. *Journal Adolescent Health, 14,* 433–439.

Kruegger, R. F., Caspi, A., Moffitt, T. E., Silva, P. A., & McGee, R. (1996). Personality traits are differentially linked to mental disorders: A multitrait–

multidiagnosis study of an adolescent birth cohort. *Journal of Abnormal Psychology, 105,* 299–312.

Leon, G. R. (1991). Eating disorders in female athletes. *Sports Medicine, 12,* 219–227.

Leon, G. R., Carroll, K., Chernyk, B., & Finn, S. (1985). Binge eating and associated habit patterns within college student and identified bulimic populations. *International Journal of Eating Disorders, 4,* 43–57.

Leon, G. R., Fulkerson, J. A., Perry, C. L., & Cudeck, R. (1993). Personality and behavioral vulnerabilities associated with risk status for eating disorders in adolescent girls. *Journal of Abnormal Psychology, 102,* 438–444.

Leon, G. R., Fulkerson, J. A., Perry, C. L., & Early-Zald, M. B. (1995). Prospective analysis of personality and behavioral vulnerabilities and gender influences in the later development of disordered eating. *Journal of Abnormal Psychology, 104,* 140–149.

Leon, G. R., Fulkerson, J. A., Perry, C. L., Keel, P. K., & Klump, K. L. (1999). Three to four year prospective evaluation of personality and behavioral risk factors for later disordered eating in adolescent girls and boys. *Journal of Youth and Adolescence, 28,* 181–196.

Leon, G. R., Perry, C. L., Mangelsdorf, C., & Tell, G. J. (1989). Adolescent nutritional and psychological patterns and risk for the development of an eating disorder. *Journal of Youth and Adolescence, 18,* 273–282.

Lilenfeld, L. R., Kaye, W. H., Greeno, C. G., Merikangas, K. R., Plotnicov, K., Pollice, C., Rao, R., Strober, M., Bulik, C. M., & Nagy, L. (1998). A controlled family study of anorexia nervosa and bulimia nervosa: Psychiatric disorders in first-degree relatives and effects of proband comorbidity. *Archives of General Psychiatry, 55,* 603–610.

Lucas, A. R., Beard, C. M., O'Fallon, W. M., & Kurland, L. T. (1991). 50-year trends in the incidence of anorexia nervosa in Rochester, Minn.: A population-based study. *American Journal of Psychiatry, 148,* 917–922.

Mann, T., Nolen-Hoeksema, S., Huang, K., Burgard, D., Wright, A., & Hanson, K. (1997). Are two interventions worse than none?: Joint primary and secondary prevention of eating disorders in college females. *Health Psychology, 16,* 215–225.

McBride, P. A., Anderson, G. M., Khait, V. D., Sunday, S. R., & Halmi, K. A. (1991). Serotonergic responsivity in eating disorders. *Psychopharmacology Bulletin, 27,* 365–372.

Mitchell, J. E., Pyle, R. L., Eckert, E. D., Hatsukami, D., Pomeroy, C., & Zimmerman, R. (1990). A comparison study of antidepressants and structured intensive group psychotherapy in the treatment of bulimia nervosa. *Archives of General Psychiatry, 47,* 149–157.

Mitrany, E. (1992). Atypical eating disorders. *Journal of Adolescent Health, 13,* 400–402.

Mussell, M. P., Mitchell, J. E., Fenna, C. J., Crosby, R. D., Miller, J. P., & Hoberman, H. M. (1997). A comparison of onset of binge eating versus dieting in the development of bulimia nervosa. *International Journal of Eating Disorders, 21,* 353–360.

Mussell, M. P., Mitchell, J. E., Weller, C. L., Raymond, N. C., Crow, S. J., & Crosby, R. D. (1995). Onset of binge eating, dieting, obesity, and mood disorders among subjects seeking treatment for binge eating disorder. *International Journal of Eating Disorders, 17,* 395–401.

Neckowitz, P., & Morrison, T. L. (1991). Interactional coping strategies of normal-weight bulimic women in intimate and nonintimate stressful situations. *Psychological Reports, 69,* 1167–1175.

Pate, J. E., Pumariega, A. J., Hester, C., & Garner, D. M. (1992). Cross-cultural patterns in eating disorders: A review. *Journal of the American Academy of Child and Adolescent Psychiatry, 31,* 802–809.

Patton, G. C. (1988). The spectrum of eating disorders in adolescence. *Journal of Psychosomatic Research, 32,* 579–584.

Patton, G. C., Johnson-Sabine, E., Wood, K., Mann, A. H., & Wakeling, A. (1990). Abnormal eating attitudes in London schoolgirls: A prospective epidemiological study—outcome at twelve month follow-up. *Psychological Medicine, 20,* 383–394.

Paxton, S. J. (1993). A prevention program for disturbed eating and body dissatisfaction in adolescent girls: A 1 year follow-up. *Health Education Research, 8,* 43–51.

Phelps, L., Andrea, R., Rizzo, F. G., Johnston, L., & Main, C. M. (1993). Prevalence of self-induced vomiting and laxative/medication abuse among female adolescents: A longitudinal study. *International Journal of Eating Disorders, 14,* 375–378.

Pike, K. M., & Rodin, J. (1991). Mothers, daughters, and disordered eating. *Journal of Abnormal Psychology, 100,* 198–204.

Polivy, J., & Herman, C. P. (1985). Dieting and bingeing: A causal analysis. *American Psychologist, 40,* 193–201.

Pyle, R. L., Mitchell, J. E., & Eckert, E. D. (1981). Bulimia: A report of 34 cases. *Journal of Clinical Psychiatry, 42,* 60–64.

Rosen, L. W., & Hough, D. O. (1988). Pathogenic weight-control behaviors of female college gymnasts. *The Physician and Sports Medicine, 16,* 141–144.

Ruderman, A. J. (1985). Dysphoric mood and overeating: A test of restraint theory's disinhibition hypothesis. *Journal of Abnormal Psychology, 94,* 78–85.

Ruderman, A. J. (1986). Dietary restraint: A theoretical and empirical review. *Psychological Bulletin, 99,* 247–262.

Schmidt, U., Jiwany, A., & Treasure, J. (1993). A controlled study of alexithymia in eating disorders. *Comprehensive Psychiatry, 34,* 54–58.

Scott, D. W. (1986). Anorexia nervosa in the male: A review of clinical, epidemiological and biological findings. *International Journal of Eating Disorders, 5,* 799–819.

Sifneos, P. E. (1972). *Short-term psychotherapy and emotional crises.* Cambridge, MA: Harvard University Press.

Smolak, L., Levine, M. P., & Schermer, F. (1998). A controlled evaluation of an elementary school primary prevention program for eating problems. *Journal of Psychosomatic Research, 44,* 339–353.

Spitzer, R. L., Devlin, M. J., Walsh, B. T., Hasin, D., Wing, R., Marcus, M., Stunkard, A., Wadden, T., Yanovski, S., Agras, S., Mitchell, J., & Nonas, C. (1992). Binge eating disorder: A multisite field trial of the diagnostic criteria. *International Journal of Eating Disorders, 11,* 191–203.

Steinhausen, H. C. (1994). Psychosocial aspects of chronic disease in children and adolescents. *Hormone Research 41,* 36–41.

Steinhausen, H. C. (1997). Outcome of anorexia nervosa in the younger patient.

Journal of Child Psychology and Psychiatry and Allied Disciplines, 38, 271–276.

Stice, E., & Shaw, H. E. (1994). Adverse effects of the media portrayed thin-ideal on women and linkages to bulimic symptom-atology. *Journal of Social and Clinical Psychology, 13,* 288–308.

Swift, W. J., Ritholz, M., Kalin, N. H., & Kaslow, N. (1987). A follow-up study of thirty hospitalized bulimics. *Psychosomatic Medicine, 49,* 45–55.

Telch, C. F., Pratt, E. M., & Niego, S. H. (1998). Obese women with binge eating disorder define the term binge. *International Journal of Eating Disorders, 24,* 313–317.

Tellegen, A. (1982). *Brief manual for the Differential Personality Questionnaire.* Unpublished manuscript, University of Minnesota, Department of Psychology.

Tiggemann, M., & Pickering, A. S. (1996) Role of television in adolescent women's body dissatisfaction and drive for thinness. *International Journal of Eating Disorders, 20,* 199–203.

Treasure, J., & Holland, A. (1990). Genetic vulnerability to eating disorders: Evidence from twin and family studies. In H. Remschmidt & M. H. Schmidt (Eds.), *Child and youth psychiatry: European perspectives* (pp. 59–68). Lewiston, NY: Hogrefe & Huber.

Vaillant, G. E. (1977). *Adaption to life.* Boston: Little, Brown.

van Wezel-Meijler, G., & Wit, J. M.(1989). The offspring of mothers with anorexia nervosa: A high-risk group for undernutrition and stunting? *European Journal of Pediatrics, 149,* 130–135.

Watson, D., Clark, L. A., & Harkness, A. R. (1994). Structures of personality and their relevance to psychopathology. *Journal of Abnormal Psychology, 103,* 18–31.

Wiseman, C. V., Gray, J. J., Mosimann, J. E., & Ahrens, A. H. (1992). Cultural expectations of thinness in women: An update. *International Journal of Eating Disorders, 11,* 85–89.

Wonderlich, S. A., Brewerton, T. D., Jocic, Z., Dansky, B. S., & Abbott, D. W. (1997). Relationship of childhood sexual abuse and eating disorders. *Journal of the American Academy of Child and Adolescent Psychiatry, 36,* 1107–1115.

18

Vulnerability to Eating Disorders in Adulthood

MARLENE B. SCHWARTZ
KELLY D. BROWNELL

The aim of this chapter is to evaluate the research on vulnerability to the development of eating disorders in adulthood. Eating disorders encompass four distinct diagnoses in the fourth edition of the *Diagnostic and Statistical Manual of Mental Disorders* (DSM-IV; American Psychiatric Association, 1994): anorexia nervosa, bulimia nervosa, eating disorder, not otherwise specified, and within that, the research category of binge-eating disorder (BED). Obesity is not considered an eating disorder; however, most individuals who meet criteria for BED are also obese. Both anorexia nervosa and bulimia nervosa typically begin in adolescence, and the vulnerability factors for these two disorders are discussed by Keel, Leon, and Fulkerson (Chapter 17, this volume). In the case of BED, however, data suggest that approximately half of those affected begin binge eating in adulthood (Abbott et al., 1998; Spurrell, Wilfley, Tanofsky, & Brownell, 1997). Although there are individuals who develop anorexia nervosa and bulimia nervosa as adults, it is a rare occurrence; therefore, this chapter focuses primarily on BED. We first present the definition of BED and research on the prevalence of BED in adults, followed by a discussion of the relevant history of approaches to study risk factors and vulnerability. In our discussion of the theory and research on vulnerability to BED in adulthood we include (1) models of the etiology of BED, (2) treatments for BED, (3) biological risk factors, (4) the role of dieting, (5) characteristics of individuals with BED, (6) life events that contribute to vulnerability, and (7) individual difference variables as risk factors. We also have a short section on the research on late-onset bulimia nervosa and the transition from bulimia nervosa to BED. Finally, we address how vulnerability factors may interact, implications of what is known for prevention and treatment, and important research needed in the field.

DEFINITION OF BINGE-EATING DISORDER

The diagnostic features of BED are similar to bulimia nervosa in that both disorders include binge eating episodes. The primary difference is that patients with BED do not engage in any compensatory behaviors (i.e., vomiting, laxative abuse, diuretics, fasting, or excessive exercise). Table 18.1 presents DSM-IV criteria.

PREVALENCE OF BINGE-EATING DISORDER IN ADULTS

Studies have examined the prevalence of BED both in nonpatient community samples and among individuals who are presenting for weight loss treatment. First, within nonpatient community samples, rates of BED range from 2.0 to 4.6% (Spitzer et al., 1992, 1993). Similarly, the prevalence rate among

TABLE 18.1. DSM-IV Criteria for Binge-Eating Disorder

A. Recurrent episodes of binge eating. An episode of binge eating is characterized by both of the following:
   (1) eating, in a discrete period of time (e.g., within any 2-hour period), an amount of food that is definitely larger than most people would eat during a similar period of time in similar circumstances.
   (2) a sense of loss of control during the episode (e.g., a feeling that one cannot stop eating or control what or how much one is eating)

B. The binge-eating episodes are associated with three (or more) of the following:
   (1) eating much more rapidly than normal
   (2) eating until feeling uncomfortably full
   (3) eating large amounts of food when not feeling physically hungry
   (4) eating alone because of being embarrassed by how much one is eating
   (5) feeling disgusted with oneself, depressed, or very guilty after overeating

C. Marked distress regarding binge eating is present.

D. The binge eating occurs, on average, at least 2 days a week for 6 months.

E. The binge eating is not associated with the regular use of inappropriate compensatory behaviors (e.g., purging, fasting, excessive exercise) and does not occur exclusively during the course of Anorexia Nervosa or Bulimia Nervosa.

Note. From American Psychiatric Association (1994). Copyright 1994 by the American Psychiatric Association. Reprinted by permission.

college students is 2.6% (Spitzer et al., 1993). In contrast, the prevalence estimates of BED among individuals seeking weight control are much higher, ranging from 15 to 70% (Schwartz & Brownell, 1998; Spitzer et al., 1992, 1993). Specifically, 30% of individuals seeking treatment at a university clinic (Spitzer et al., 1992, 1993) and 15% of those attending Jenny Craig, a commercial weight loss program, (Schwartz & Brownell, 1998; Spitzer et al., 1993) meet criteria for BED. The highest rates of BED have been reported in the self-help group Overeaters Anonymous, with rates ranging from 50% (Schwartz & Brownell, 1998) to 70% (Spitzer et al., 1993).

In addition to individuals suffering from the full syndrome, a significant minority of obese persons experience some binge eating and loss of control. Robertson and Palmer (1997) found that 24% of a sample of 88 British women with a history of obesity reported binge eating (i.e., eating an unusually large amount of food), and of those, half (i.e., 12%) reported a loss of control while binge eating. Only one subject of the 88 met full criteria for BED.

HISTORY OF APPROACHES
TO STUDY RISK FACTORS
AND VULNERABILITY

In reviewing this literature, we distinguish between risk factors and vulnerability processes in the following way: (1) Risk factors are those characteristics or events that appear empirically to correlate with the incidence of the eating disorder but do not necessarily imply causality (such as being a heterosexual female or a homosexual male); (2) vulnerability refers to factors that might serve as the mechanisms or psychological processes that are causally linked to the disorder (such as low self-esteem or an "all or nothing" cognitive style). Many of the studies reviewed include a combination of these two types of variables.

Demographic Variables

Historically, the risk factors that were identified for eating disorders began with the clear demographic variables of anorexia nervosa and bulimia nervosa patients presenting for treatment (i.e., affluent, Caucasian, adolescent females). Theories about vulnerability tried to answer the question: Why were young Caucasian women developing eating disorders while other people were not? Cultural influence theories suggested that exposure to media messages about women and societal pressure for thinness led to the development of eating disorders (see review by Wilfley & Rodin, 1995). Feminist and developmental theories focused on the adolescent developmental tasks of separation and individuation and the challenge of becoming a woman in our society (e.g., Striegel-Moore, 1993, 1995; Striegel-Moore, Silberstein, & Rodin, 1986).

Although these ideas explained why young women as a group are at risk, the issue of why certain young women develop eating disorders whereas others do not led researchers to look for more specific vulnerability factors. Some empirical work focused on family characteristics that make particular individuals vulnerable to the development of an eating disorder, such as experiencing maternal criticism about their weight (Pike & Rodin, 1991). Other studies identified individual personality characteristics as vulnerability factors, such as negative self-evaluation (Fairburn, Welch, Doll, Davies, & O'Connor, 1997). This body of research primarily focuses on female adolescents; therefore, it does not provide information about vulnerability to the development of eating disorders in adulthood.

It appears that the typical patient with BED is not an adolescent female. Even early clinical descriptions of patients with BED included a case of a middle-age obese man (Stunkard, 1976). Unlike anorexia nervosa and bulimia nervosa, BED appears to affect both men and women, Caucasians and minority groups, and adults throughout the lifespan (Wilfley, Pike, & Striegel-Moore, 1997). Due to the heterogeneous population of individuals with BED, Wilfley, Pike, and Striegel-Moore (1997) propose an expansion of the existing etiological models of eating disorders. Because this new diagnostic group differs so much from the traditional eating-disorder population, past empirical studies examining vulnerability among adolescent girls cannot be assumed to fit for patients with BED.

Study Designs

Two approaches have been used to study risk factors and vulnerability to eating disorders in adults: (1) retrospective self-report and (2) case-control studies. In retrospective self-report studies, individuals are asked to recall relevant life events that preceded their binge eating (e.g., when they began dieting) (see Abbott et al., 1998; Spurrell et al., 1997). In case-control studies, individuals who have the disorder are identified, and for each subject, a control subject with the same demographic profile is identified. This method is used by Fairburn et al. (1998) to compare patients with BED to normal controls matched on age and parental social class.

Longitudinal studies follow participants over time and measure the risk factors as they occur. The primary benefit of this method is that data about relevant factors are collected at the time they occur, but this method is also costly and time-consuming. Using this method, Leon, Keel, and Fulkerson (1997) followed adolescents for 4 years (beginning in grades 7 through 10), assessing a wide range of risk factors for the development of eating disorders. We know of no longitudinal studies examining vulnerability processes for eating disorders in adulthood.

Methods of Assessment

The study of eating disorders uses two primary methods of assessment: questionnaires and interviews. Because the variables of interest are behaviors that individuals often hide due to shame (i.e., binge eating and purging), it is difficult to validate measures by observation or corroborative interviews with family members. The features associated with BED are also difficult to describe; for example, evidence indicates that people do not agree on what constitutes a binge (Belgin & Fairburn, 1992). Although weight and other physiological measures may suggest binge eating or purging, these are typically not used in research as indicators of psychopathology. Sometimes self-monitoring of food intake is used to assess eating behavior. This may be more accurate than retrospective self-report, but it is time-consuming and the process of recording intake may promote change. A few studies have measured binge eating in the laboratory, but these studies are most useful to examine eating in response to specific stimuli rather than indicators of typical eating pathology (Wilson, 1993).

The most common method of assessment of eating pathology is the self-report questionnaire. Commonly used measures include the Binge Eating Scale (BES; Gormally, Black, Dalson, & Rardin, 1982), the Eating Disorder Inventory (EDI; Garner, Olmstead, & Polivy, 1983), the Eating Disorders Examination Questionnaire (EDE-Q; Fairburn & Belgin, 1994), and the Questionnaire on Eating and Weight Patterns (QEWP; Spitzer et al., 1993). Each of these measures has adequate psychometric properties, although due to the secretive nature of the features of eating disorders, validity remains a concern.

The second method of assessment is the interview. The Eating Disorder Examination (EDE; Cooper & Fairburn, 1987) is an investigator-based, semistructured interview that assesses the core psychopathology of eating disorders. This technique is preferred over self-report questionnaires because the interviewer can clarify definitions for the participants and use a standard set of criteria when assessing participants scores on different features. This technique improves the reliability of responses across individuals but does not guarantee the validity of the responses in general.

A few studies compare the EDE interview with the corresponding self report version, the EDE-Q. The findings suggest that the interview and questionnaire correspond most closely for salient behavioral items (e.g., purging) and less so for more complex cognitive features (e.g., overconcern about shape and weight) (Black & Wilson, 1996; Fairburn & Belgin, 1994; Wilfley, Schwartz, Spurrell, & Fairburn, 1997).

THEORY AND RESEARCH ON RISK FACTORS AND VULNERABILITY

Models of the Etiology of Binge-Eating Disorder

When examining the literature on BED in adulthood, two models of etiology have received the most support: the dietary restraint model and the interpersonal vulnerability model (see Wilfley, Pike, & Striegel-Moore, 1997). Figure 18.1 outlines these models.

The Dietary Restraint Model

The dietary restraint model emphasizes the role of extreme dieting as an immediate precursor to the initiation of binge eating (Polivy & Herman,

RESTRAINT MODEL	INTERPERSONAL VULNERABILITY MODEL
EMPHASIS ON WEIGHT / SHAPE IN SOCIAL NETWORK	DISTURBANCE IN EARLY CHILD–CARETAKER RELATIONSHIP
↓	↓
INTERNALIZED SOCIAL EXPECTATIONS ABOUT THINNESS AND BEAUTY	INSECURE ATTACHMENT
↓	↓
BODY IMAGE CONCERNS	DISTURBANCE IN SELF (SOCIAL SELF DISTURBANCE) (LOW SELF-ESTEEM)
↓	↓
EXTREME DIETARY RESTRAINT	AFFECTIVE DYSREGULATION
↓	↓
BINGE EATING	BINGE EATING

FIGURE 18.1. Models of etiology of binge eating: Dietary restraint and interpersonal vulnerability. From Wilfley, Pike, and Striegel-Moore (1997). Copyright 1997 by Plenum Publishing Corp. Reprinted by permission.

1993). This model posits that individuals experience an emphasis on weight and shape in their social network, which they then internalize as priorities for themselves. These unrealistic pressures for thinness create body dissatisfaction, which individuals attempt to improve by overrestrictive dieting. Overrestrictive diets include behaviors such as skipping meals and completely avoiding certain foods and the belief that certain foods are "bad."

Diets that involve the complete avoidance of certain foods contribute to the likelihood of binge eating through the abstinence violation effect (Wilson, 1995a). The abstinence violation effect occurs when people decide to avoid a particular type of food (e.g., cake), and then find themselves in a situation in which eating that food feels unavoidable (e.g., a birthday party). After eating a normal portion of the food, they feel they have blown it and they may as well eat a lot of it. The binge eating behavior can be attributed to all-or-none thinking: "If I can't be perfect, I may as well not try to restrain at all." Another cognitive factor is the plan to resume the diet tomorrow; thus it makes sense to enjoy the forbidden foods today. After a binge eating event, the diet typically becomes even more rigid, which perpetuates the diet–binge cycle.

Wilfley, Pike, and Striegel-Moore (1997) present evidence in support of the dietary restraint model for each stage and explain that the primary strength of the model is that it describes a set of very specific risk variables. They add that the weakness of the model, however, is that each of the variables may be neither necessary nor sufficient to predict the development of an eating disorder. For example, many people diet yet only a minority develop eating disorders (see Wilson, 1995a). In addition, evidence presented later in this chapter demonstrates that among patients with BED, dieting does not always precede binge eating.

The Interpersonal Vulnerability Model

The interpersonal vulnerability model differs most clearly from the dietary restraint model in that dieting is not necessarily a precursor to binge eating. Rather, this model states that binge eating develops as a way of coping with affective distress. Wilfley, Pike, and Striegel-Moore (1997) present a detailed description of this model as well as the research findings that support it. To summarize, vulnerability begins in childhood with a disturbance in the individual's relationship with early caregivers. If caregivers are unable to meet the child's physical and emotional needs, the person develops an insecure attachment style. This leads to low self-esteem and social self-disturbance, which is defined as a heightened concern about how one is viewed by others, an excessive need for a positive self-presentation and social approval, and a feeling of inadequacy compared to others (Wilfley, Pike, & Striegel-Moore, 1997, p. 18). This impairment in social functioning then leads to affective dysregulation and depression, which the person tries to cope with by binge eating. The binge eating is presumed to help the person "numb out" these negative feelings and escape from self-awareness (Heatherton & Baumeister, 1991).

Historically, it is interesting to note that these models originated in the bulimia nervosa literature and emerged as a pair after the finding that bulimia nervosa patients responded equally well to interpersonal therapy and cognitive-behavioral therapy (Fairburn, Jones, Peveler, Hope, & O'Connor, 1993). These treatments were then adapted and tested with patients with BED and results suggest that both treatment approaches are effective in treating binge eating (Wilfley, 1999; Wilfley et al., 1993).

Treatments for Binge-Eating Disorder

The dietary restraint model and the interpersonal vulnerability model both provide a theoretical framework for two empirically validated treatments for binge eating: cognitive-behavioral therapy and interpersonal therapy. These two treatment approaches are summarized next (for detailed descriptions, see Wilfley, Grilo, & Rodin, 1997; Fairburn, Marcus, & Wilson, 1993). Each of these treatment protocols can be delivered in an individual or group format; however, the research on BED has primarily used group treatments (e.g., Wilfley, 1999).

Cognitive-Behavioral Therapy

Cognitive-behavioral therapy uses a short-term (typically 20 sessions) problem-directed approach focused on the present and future rather than the past. Clients are taught the cognitive-behavioral view of the etiology and maintenance of their eating disorder (i.e., the dietary restraint model). The goal of cognitive-behavioral therapy is to change the maladaptive behaviors and distorted cognitions that are associated with binge eating. Developmental and psychodynamic issues are not addressed, and interpersonal problems are addressed only to the extent that they are triggers for binge episodes.

The first stage of this treatment is the behavioral prescription to eat three meals a day plus one or two snacks. The purpose is to create a regular eating pattern and reduce the patterns of grazing all day or restricting all day and binge eating at night. Clients are taught about heart-healthy nutrition and are encouraged to make healthy food choices following the food guide pyramid. They learn how to self-monitor their food intake, where, when, and with whom they eat, and their speed of eating. This information is used to identify binge triggers, such as going too long without eating or eating late at night. The second stage of treatment is to identify the thoughts and feelings that lead up to a binge. The primary goal here is to challenge the belief that binge episodes occur randomly; instead, clients learn that they can predict when they are at risk for a binge by noticing the chain of events, thoughts, and feelings that occur first. As they identify those thoughts (e.g., all-or-nothing thinking and the abstinence violation effect), cognitive restructuring is used to challenge the dysfunctional beliefs. This strategy is also used to challenge dysfunctional cognitions regarding interpersonal events, which helps prevent interpersonal distress from becoming a binge trigger.

The final stage of cognitive-behavioral therapy focuses on relapse prevention. Clients learn how to maintain the changes they have made after treatment ends and to use problem-solving and coping skills when they encounter high-risk situations. One issue that is complicated for obese clients with BED is that they may have successfully been able to stop their binge eating but they are likely to still be significantly overweight. It is useful to help such clients set reasonable weight loss goals and to encourage them to continue to make healthy food choices and increase their exercise level.

Interpersonal Therapy

Interpersonal therapy was originally developed as a treatment for depression (Klerman, Weissman, Rounsaville, & Chevron, 1984) and has been adapted for eating disorders (see Wilfley, Grilo, & Rodin, 1997). It is designed as a short-term treatment that is problem focused and emphasizes the quality of current interpersonal relationships. The central premise is that binge eating is a maladaptive coping strategy used to manage negative affect linked to interpersonal distress, (i.e., the interpersonal vulnerability model). Past relationships are considered important information for the therapist to gather in the initial evaluation, but the treatment focuses on current relationships and changes that can be made in the here and now.

During the evaluation and first stage of treatment, each individual identifies his or her problem areas and how they are linked to binge eating. Klerman et al. (1984) outline four major interpersonal problem areas: (1) grief, (2) interpersonal disputes (e.g., with spouse, children), (3) role transitions (e.g., new job, relocation), and (4) interpersonal deficits (e.g., loneliness and social isolation). Among clients with BED, the most common problem areas are interpersonal deficits, followed by interpersonal disputes (Wilfley et al., 1993). In linking the problem area to eating, someone with *interpersonal deficits* may describe binge eating while feeling lonely and isolated on a weekend night. Someone with *interpersonal disputes* may describe binge eating at night while her husband is in the next room drinking alcohol and watching television (linking her binges to her anger with her husband about his drinking).

The second stage of treatment is to actively work to solve the problem that has been identified. For example, the first person's goal may be to reduce social isolation; thus the treatment would focus on strategies for forming new relationships. The second person's goal may be to open up communication with her husband about their relationship and see if resolution is possible; if not, she may need to move on to mourn the loss of the relationship.

The final stage of treatment addresses termination and preparation for the future. The end of the treatment is used as an opportunity to practice managing feelings of loss. Therapists emphasize the progress clients made during treatment and also anticipate future challenges and coping strategies. Clients are taught that they will probably always be vulnerable to eating problems when they are in distress. However, this can help them recognize when they are upset about something, so they can then use a more adaptive way of coping, such as turning to people for support rather than to food.

These brief outlines of cognitive-behavioral therapy and interpersonal therapy are presented to illustrate how the factors described in the two models of etiology (dietary restraint and interpersonal vulnerability) are translated into clinical practice. Because both these treatments have received significant empirical support as effective treatments for BED (Wilfley, 1999), we believe they address vulnerability factors (i.e., behavioral, cognitive, and interpersonal) that are central to the development of BED.

Biological Risk Factors

Within the framework of the dietary restraint and interpersonal vulnerability models, biological risk factors combine with environmental and psychological factors to make certain individuals more vulnerable to developing BED. Two such factors are childhood obesity and parental affective illness. Body weight is influenced by both genetics and the environment (Brownell & Wadden, 1992). Whereas having an obese parent places one at biological risk for obesity, the home environment may increase vulnerability to BED in a variety of ways (e.g., parents may model unhealthy eating habits and a sedentary lifestyle or children may observe overrestrictive dieting and learn about good vs. bad foods). Being overweight increases the likelihood of dieting and potentially getting caught in the diet–binge cycle.

Another biological risk factor is having a parent with an affective disorder, which increases one's own risk of developing an affective disorder through both genetic and environmental influences (Harrington, 1996; Marton & Maharaj, 1993; McGuffin & Katz, 1989). A child may be more vulnerable to BED if the parent's mental illness has an impact on the parent–child relationship. In the interpersonal vulnerability model, the first factor is a disturbance in the early child–caretaker relationship, which may be more likely if the parent is suffering from an affective disorder. In addition, if someone is suffering from an affective disorder, he or she may be more likely to use binge eating as a way to numb out negative feelings.

Childhood Obesity and Parental Affective Illness

Childhood obesity and parental affective illness are two of the specific vulnerability factors that emerged in Fairburn et al.'s (1998) study of risk factors for BED. This study used a case-control method to examine 52 female patients with BED and 104 healthy controls matched on sex, age, and socioeconomic status. The researchers also included comparisons with a slightly younger group of 102 patients with bulimia nervosa and 102 matched psychiatric controls. Data were collected through home interviews, and assessed exposure to risk factors for the period before onset of the disorder. This relevant period was defined as before the age at which the first significant behaviors began, such as sustained dieting, regular overeating episodes, self-induced vomiting, or laxative misuse. The control for each subject was interviewed for the same period in her life.

Risk factors were divided into categories: (1) personal vulnerability (i.e., childhood characteristics, premorbid psychiatric disorder, behavioral problems, and lifetime parental psychiatric disorder); (2) environmental factors (i.e., parental problems, disruptive events, parental psychiatric disorder, teasing and bullying, and sexual and physical abuse); (3) dieting vulnerability (i.e., dieting risk, obesity risk, and parental eating disorder); and (4) additional risk factors (i.e., age at menarche, pregnancy, parity, and abortion).

When compared to the normal control group, the participants with BED reported significantly higher levels of several personal vulnerability factors: (1) negative self-evaluation, (2) lifetime parental depression, (3) major depression, (4) marked conduct problems, and (5) deliberate self-harm. Of the environmental factors, participants with BED reported higher levels of (1) parental criticism, (2) high expectation, (3) minimal affection, (4) parental underinvolvement, (5) maternal low care, and (6) maternal high overprotection. The participants with BED were also more likely than controls to report sexual and repeated severe physical abuse and bullying.

There were fewer significant differences between participants with BED and the psychiatric control group. The participants with BED experienced (1) lower parental contact, (2) greater likelihood of childhood obesity, and (3) more critical comments by family about shape, weight, or eating. This is important as it begins to separate the general risk factors for psychiatric illness from the specific risk factors for BED.

This study suggests that childhood obesity and parental affective illness are two variables that place an individual at risk for the development of BED. Some of the environmental factors seem contradictory, however, such as parental high expectation and parental underinvolvement. One possibility is that the environmental and psychological mechanisms through which these biological risk factors lead to the development of BED may follow two paths: (1) childhood obesity leads to vulnerability as outlined by the dietary restraint model (which would include parental criticism and critical comments by family about shape, weight and eating) and (2) parental affective illness has an impact on vulnerability as outlined by the interpersonal vulnerability model (which would include lower parental contact, minimal affection, and major depression). Some of the factors that emerged in this study could fit into both models, such as negative self-evaluation and deliberate self-harm. This theory could by studied in the future by categorizing patients with BED by the two primary models of etiology and assessing their risk factors to see whether there are differences in the histories of the two groups, suggesting two risk profiles based on the two proposed models of etiology of BED.

Obesity and Psychological Distress

In addition to childhood obesity, current obesity may be a risk factor for an adult-onset eating disorder. Many studies have tested the hypothesis that individuals who are obese have greater levels of psychopathology than do individuals who are normal in weight. This hypothesis has received mixed support. Friedman and Brownell (1995) review this literature and present a model for research suggesting that obesity alone is not related to psychological distress; rather, additional variables combine to place specific individuals who are obese at higher risk of psychopathology. In this context, there is accumulating evidence that having BED is a mediating variable in the relationship between obesity and psychopathology.

Telch and Agras (1994) address this point in a study of 107 obese women with BED. They divided the sample into moderate or severe binge eaters and moderate or severe obesity. They then compared the groups on measures of depression, self-esteem, interpersonal problems, and general distress. They found that severity of binge eating, not level of obesity, accounted for the differences between groups on these psychological variables. This supports the view that binge eating is a mediator between obesity and psychopathology.

We do not yet understand, however, how binge eating mediates the link between obesity and psychological distress. One possibility is that the variables of weight, binge eating, and psychopathology form a destructive cycle. For example, some people are born with a genetic predisposition for becoming overweight. As they grow heavier, they attempt to diet, which leads to binge eating. As the binge eating worsens, their weight increases. At each step of this cycle, their cognitive style, personality, and psychological distress both contribute to and result from the fluctuation between the desire to diet and the desire to binge. The next section presents research on the role of dieting in the development of BED.

The Role of Dieting

Dieting and Binge Eating: Which Comes First?

Two studies have examined the sequence of dieting and binge eating in the history of patients with BED. This is an important question because according to the dietary restraint model, dietary restriction is a necessary precursor to binge eating, yet a significant number of patients with BED report that they began binge eating first. For example, Wilson, Nonas, and Rosenblum (1993) found that only 8.7% of 31 participants with BED reported having been on a strict diet when they began to binge eat.

Spurrell et al. (1997) interviewed 87 male and female patients with BED presenting for treatment at a university clinic. The average age at which participants were first overweight was 17 years old, and the age of their first diet was 17.6 years. Following that, the average age of their first binge was 18 years old. This suggests a general pattern of becoming overweight, dieting, and then binge eating within a 1-year span of time. When asked directly which came first, 55% reported binge eating first, while 45% reported dieting first. Binge-first individuals said they began this behavior on average at age 12.6, whereas the diet-first group said they began binge eating at age 24.9. These data suggest that dieting may be a greater risk factor for binge eating among adults, whereas, children and adolescents may binge eat in response to stressors apart from dietary restraint.

Spurrell et al. (1997) also looked at the age of onset of obesity as well as the individuals' perception of themselves as overweight as a child. There were no significant differences between the diet-first and binge-first groups in terms of age of onset of overweight (both groups reported becoming overweight in their mid to late teens), but binge-first participants were more likely to perceive themselves as overweight (even though they were not) between the ages of 6 and 12. Individuals in the binge-first group were also more likely to have a personality disorder and either a current or lifetime diagnosis of a substance use disorder. In addition, binge-first participants reported more sibling and family problems as well as more life events related to the onset of binge eating. These results suggest that adolescents who begin to binge eat before dieting may experience more environmental stress and are also more vulnerable to personality and substance use disorders than are adults who begin binge eating following a diet.

A second study, conducted by Abbott et al. (1998) had similar findings. They studied 92 overweight binge eaters seeking treatment and found that 39% binged first and 48% dieted first. The remainder (13%) said they began both behaviors at the same age, and were excluded from analyses. They also found that the binge-first group reported an average age of onset of binge eating in adolescence (age 11.8 years) as opposed to the diet-first group, which began binge eating as young adults (age 25.7 years). Consistent with the Spurrell et al. (1997) study, there was not a difference between the groups for age of onset of overweight, and there were trends in the expected direction of binge-first participants reporting higher levels of personality disorders, although the differences did not reach significance. In contrast to the Spurrell et al. (1997) study, however, the diet-first group reported higher rates of lifetime stimulant abuse than did the binge-first group.

The findings from these two studies suggest that there may be different vulnerability factors for the development of BED in childhood versus adulthood. There seem to be two sensitive times for the development of BED; the first is adolescence (which is clearly consistent with the other eating disorders), and the second is young adulthood (i.e., mid-20s). In the first case, it seems that dieting may not be a necessary precursor, whereas in the older group, dieting does seem to play a causal role in the development of BED.

Weight Cycling

Dieting appears to play in important role in the development of BED for some individuals but not others. In addition to looking at the first diet, research has also been done on the role of weight cycling (repeated weight losses followed by regain). One hypothesis is that the physiological and psychological effects of weight cycling increase vulnerability to an eating disorder (Brownell, 1995). To examine this question, a number of studies have measured the history of weight cycling in patients with BED and compared those histories to obese individuals without BED. Some have found that patients with BED have higher rates of weight cycling (e.g., de Zwann et al., 1994), whereas others have found that they do not differ significantly (e.g., Kuehnel & Wadden, 1994).

One issue in the weight cycling literature is the lack of consistency in how cycling is measured. Studies measure it as number of diets, number of pounds lost and regained, amount of weight regained after a specific weight loss attempt, or the belief or view of oneself as a weight cycler. There is evidence from a recent study that the measurement of the subjective experience of oneself as a weight cycler accounts for more variance in psychological variables (i.e., body satisfaction, life satisfaction, and self-esteem) than does the actual number of pounds lost and regained (Friedman, Schwartz, & Brownell, 1998). One hypothesis is that the role of weight cycling with eating disorders is cognitive; self-definition as a weight cycler may create a self-fulfilling prophecy of restriction, lapses, the abstinence violation effect, and binge eating.

CHARACTERISTICS OF INDIVIDUALS WITH BINGE-EATING DISORDER

One way to generate hypotheses about vulnerability processes is to ask what are the characteristics of people who develop BED? A growing number of studies have attempted to identify distinguishing characteristics of individuals who struggle with binge eating. Studies have looked at general cognitive styles and personality traits, as well as comorbid Axis I and Axis II diagnoses. The typical method is to assess women who present for weight loss treatment at a university clinic. These studies use correlation analyses to measure the relationships among variables and illustrate which characteristics seem to occur together. The limitation of this method is that they may be identifying risk factors rather than vulnerability processes (i.e., causal relationships between the feature and the development of BED). Another issue is that these variables may be both predisposing characteristics for binge eating as well as features that are secondary to the binge eating; in other words, they have a cyclical relationship with binge eating, both increasing the likelihood of and resulting from the problem behavior.

Personality and Cognitive Factors

In an early study of the relationship between personality and binge eating, Kolotkin, Revis, Kirkley, and Janik (1987) measured binge eating and personality (with the Minnesota Multiphasic Personality Inventory [MMPI]) in a sample of 207 obese women who presented for weight loss treatment at a university clinic. They found that psychological disturbance increased as binge severity increased. Specifically, the MMPI Psychasthenia scale (Pt) had the strongest relationship with binge eating, accounting for 23% of the variance. This scale measures self-derogation, obsessive-compulsive tendencies, anxiety, and perfectionism. In another study, de Zwaan et al. (1994) conducted interviews with 100 obese women presenting for weight loss treatment and divided the participants into four categories of binge eating severity: (1) full diagnostic criteria for BED ($n = 43$), (2) overeating plus loss of control ($n = 20$), (3) overeating without loss of control ($n = 15$), and (4) no overeating episodes ($n = 22$). They found that greater problems with binge eating were associated not only with dieting and weight variables but also with higher levels of ineffectiveness, perfectionism, and impulsivity. Binge eating was also associated with lower levels of self-esteem and interoceptive awareness.

Dysfunctional attitudes and automatic thoughts associated with binge eating have also been studied. Kuehnel and Wadden (1994) assessed 70 women who presented for weight loss at a university clinic. They compared patients with BED ($n = 11$) to those without BED ($n = 30$) and subclinical binge eaters ($n = 29$) and found that individuals with BED reported higher levels of depression and higher levels of depressotypic cognitions than did the other two groups. The participants with BED also had more dysfunctional attitudes (i.e., vulnerability, need for approval, need to please others, and imperatives) than did participants without BED. Kuehnel and Wallen

(1994) concluded that people with BED tend to "(1) lack confidence in their ability to deal effectively with a world they view as threatening and (2) use an external frame of reference in determining self-worth" (p. 326).

Taken together, these findings suggest that individuals with BED struggle with perfectionism and ineffectiveness. This is consistent with the cognitive style described in the dietary restraint model (i.e., I have to diet perfectly, but I can't diet perfectly, so I may as well binge). The tendency to see the world as a threatening place, low interoceptive awareness, and low self-esteem, seem like plausible precursors to turning to food as a means of coping. In addition, using an external frame of reference in determining self-worth may make some individuals more vulnerable to society's pressure for thinness as a sign of personal success, leading to distress about current weight and attempts at rigid, unhealthy eating behaviors.

Axis I and Axis II Disorders

Many studies that have found that binge eaters who are obese report significantly higher levels of psychopathology than do non-binge eaters. In a study using self-report measures, Marcus, Wing, and Hopkins (1988) studied obese women (35 binge eaters and 33 non-binge eaters) presenting for weight loss treatment and found that binge eaters reported higher levels of depression and global psychological distress than did non-binge eaters. Antony, Johnson, Carr-Nangle, and Abel (1994) did another assessment of depression, anxiety, and binge eating using self-report. Participants included 72 women who either presented for treatment for binge eating or responded to recruitment posters for a study on eating and emotions. They completed measures on binge eating, depression, and anxiety. Participants were divided into three groups: BED, subclinical binge eaters, and non-eating-disordered controls. They found that the group with BED reported significantly higher rates of depression, anxiety, and body dissatisfaction than did the normal controls; the subclinical binge eater scores fell in between.

In an interview study, Yanovski, Nelson, Dubbert, and Spitzer (1993) interviewed obese men (*n* = 39) and women (*n* = 89) recruited through either general advertisements for subjects or a weight loss program. They used an interview based on DSM-IV criteria to assess BED, the Structured Clinical Interview for DSM-III-R to assess Axis I diagnoses (SCID; Spitzer, Williams, Gibbon, & First, 1990a), and the Structured Clinical Interview for DSM-III-R Personality Disorders to assess Axis II diagnoses (SCID-II; Spitzer, Williams, Gibbon, & First, 1990b). They found that 34% of the participants met criteria for BED (43 women and 10 men) and the participants with BED had a greater prevalence of any lifetime Axis I or Axis II disorder. The specific disorders that were higher in the participants with BED were major depression, panic disorder, bulimia nervosa, borderline

personality disorder, and avoidant personality disorder. This study also found
that those with BED were more likely to have a family history of substance
abuse, but there were no differences for history of sexual abuse.

In a similar study, Specker, de Zwaan, Raymond, and Mitchell (1994)
assessed both Axis I and Axis II disorders among 100 obese women presenting for weight loss treatment and compared those who met full criteria for
BED (n = 43) with those who did not (n = 57). Participants with BED had
higher lifetime prevalence rates for any Axis I diagnosis, and specifically for
major depression and bulimia nervosa. Participants with BED also had higher
rates of Cluster B and Cluster C personality disorders. The three personality
disorders with the highest prevalence rates in the BED group were histrionic
personality disorder (47%), borderline personality disorder (30%), and
avoidant personality disorder (26%). These findings are consistent with those
of Yanovski et al. (1993), which found that patients with BED had significantly higher rates of borderline and avoidant personality disorder than did
obese individuals without BED.

Given the consistent finding that individuals with BED have higher
rates of depression than obese controls without BED, Mussell et al. (1995)
conducted a study to examine the temporal relationship of the ages of onset
of binge eating, dieting, obesity, BED, and affective disorders. They evaluated
30 female patients with BED participating in a treatment study. The majority of participants reported being normal weight as adolescents, and becoming overweight by age 20. Their obesity (body mass index [BMI] > 30) did
not occur until 10 years after the onset of BED. The mean age of onset for
binge eating in this sample was 18.0 (8.1) years, whereas the mean onset of
dieting was 22.0 (10.1). The pattern of age of onset for binge eating versus
dieting was similar to that described earlier in the Spurrell et al. (1997) and
Abbott et al. (1998) papers, with approximately half the participants reporting binge eating first and the remainder reporting dieting first or doing
both concurrently. This study did not compare the diet-first with the binge-
first subjects, as the focus was on the sequence of depression and BED. They
found that half of all their participants had a history of major depressive
disorder, and within this group, 60% reported developing BED before their
first major depressive episode. Taken together, these findings add to the
picture that there are subgroups of patients with BED who experience different sequences of events; some appear to binge first, others diet first, and
still others become depressed before the onset of eating symptoms. It is also
interesting to note that among some of these individuals, obesity appears to
be a consequence rather than a precursor to BED.

To summarize, individuals with BED have higher rates of affective disorders (primarily major depression) than do obese individuals without BED.
The rates of affective disorders ranges from 48 to 55% in the studies reviewed here; hence approximately half of obese patients with BED presenting for treatment suffer from an affective disorder as well as their eating
disorder. Whether the depression is a trigger for the binge eating, a conse-

quence of the binge eating, or both, these findings suggest the importance of addressing depression when treating patients with BED. In terms of etiology, the interpersonal vulnerability model posits that for some people, depression is a precursor to binge eating, and individuals use binge eating to numb out negative affect. This suggests that a history of depression may make one vulnerable to binge eating.

Second, individuals with BED are more likely than their obese counterparts without BED to have personality disorders. Specifically, they are more likely to have histrionic, borderline, or avoidant personality disorder. All three of these personality disorders have interpersonal features that link to the "disturbance of social self" described in the interpersonal vulnerability model. One of the features of borderline personality disorder is unstable and intense interpersonal relationships, a feature of histrionic personality disorder is that one considers relationships to be more intimate than they are, and a feature of avoidant personality disorder is an unwillingness to get involved with people due to a fear of rejection (American Psychiatric Association, 1994). The interpersonal vulnerability model posits that binge eating follows negative affect and low self-esteem due to interpersonal difficulty. This suggests that people with borderline, histrionic, or avoidant personality disorder may be vulnerable to the development of binge eating due to their experience of interpersonal distress.

One limitation of this research is that nearly all these studies used patients presenting for treatment. To address this issue, Telch and Stice (1998) examined obese participants with BED and without BED from a community sample of women. There were still some differences, primarily that participants with BED had a higher lifetime prevalence of major depression and of any Axis I disorder than did participants without BED. However, overall rates of comorbidity were lower than in studies using patient samples.

Mitchell and Mussell (1995) note the importance of understanding the sequence of events among patients with BED, as it may provide clues about to the causal relationship. Based on current findings, they suggest that there may be two types of patients with BED: (1) those who have early dietary chaos, suggesting the use of food to modulate affect, and (2) those who develop BED subsequent to restrictive eating. They pose the hypothesis that the first type may have higher levels of psychopathology. We agree that research on BED supports the view that there may be two distinct subgroups within this clinical population—those who binge first and those who diet first—and the degree of associated psychopathology appears to be higher in the first group.

Life Events That May Contribute to Vulnerability

It is our impression that a number of factors can contribute to weight gain in adulthood, which could then lead to dietary restraint and BED. In our clinical experience, we have observed events that precede weight gain and, subsequently, binge eating in some clients. These events are pregnancy, recovery from substance abuse, and beginning a neuroleptic medication.

Pregnancy

Pregnancy represents a time of significant physical and psychological changes. Salient features for many women are changes in eating, weight, and body shape. For some women, the postpartum period may be a vulnerable time for the development of an eating disorder.

The first aspect of pregnancy that may increase vulnerability is weight gain. It is now recommended that women gain between 15 and 40 pounds during their pregnancies, depending on their prepregnancy weight status (Moore & Greenwood, 1995). Although most women will slowly lose the majority of this excess weight during the postpartum year, the average woman will still weigh 3 pounds more than her prepregnancy weight at 1-year postpartum (Moore & Greenwood, 1995).

Many women experience a disturbance in body image during pregnancy. In a study of women's perceptions of their bodies 4 months into pregnancy, Slade (1977) found significantly overestimated body dimensions, particularly waist and stomach depth. Errors of the pregnant women were between those of anorexia nervosa patients and controls (i.e., nonpregnant and non-eating-disordered women) (Slade, 1977). Another method used to study women's feelings about their pregnant bodies involved having women describe their bodies and coding the types of words they use as positive or negative. Women tend to see themselves as less attractive the more pregnant they become (Fawcett, Bliss-Holtz, Haas, Leventhal, & Rubin, 1986; Moore, 1978). Another study had women rate how much they liked their bodies prepregnancy, during pregnancy, and 2 and 6 weeks postpartum and found that women liked their prepregnancy bodies the best, then postpartum, and pregnancy body least (Strang & Sullivan, 1985). These studies suggest that women misperceive themselves as being larger than they actually are during pregnancy and also dislike their bodies both during pregnancy and postpartum. One group at particular risk may be women with a history of dieting. Fairburn and Welch (1990) assessed the feelings of a sample of female dieters during pregnancy and found that they felt worse about their bodies during pregnancy than when they were not pregnant.

Several studies have examined how normal women experience changes in body image and eating changes during and following pregnancy. This research assesses dietary restriction, binge eating, and overconcern with eating, shape, and weight (Davies & Wardle, 1994; Fairburn, Stein, & Jones, 1992; Stein & Fairburn, 1996). Davies and Wardle (1994) compared pregnant to nonpregnant women on dieting, an eating disorder measure, and figure selections for ideal body and current body. Pregnant women were generally happier with their bodies and reported less body dissatisfaction than were the nonpregnant women, even though they showed a greater discrepancy between their "ideal" body size and current body size. This supports the idea that during pregnancy, some women feel more accepting of their larger bodies. Fairburn et al. (1992) assessed 100 pregnant women at 15 and 32 weeks of pregnancy and also administered an eating disorder interview the month before pregnancy. Women's scores of concern about eating, shape, and weight, as well as restraint, decreased from prepregnancy to 15 weeks but then went back up again by 32 weeks. This suggests that the early stages of pregnancy may provide an opportunity for dietary disinhibition and relaxed feelings about body shape and weight, but as the body becomes significantly different by the end of pregnancy, feelings of distress return.

Stein and Fairburn (1996) followed normal women's eating disorder symptoms at 3 months and 6 months postpartum using the EDE interview. There was an increase in dietary restraint and concerns about eating, shape, and weight at 3 months postpartum, but all but weight concern reached a plateau at 6 months. In the women for whom weight concern continued to rise, several cases turned into clinical eating disorders. Women who had retained the most weight were the ones experiencing the most eating disorder symptoms (Stein & Fairburn, 1996). This study provides the strongest evidence to date that the postpartum period is a vulnerable time for women, particularly those who have retained a significant portion of the weight they gained during pregnancy.

Substance Abuse

In our clinical practice, we have observed a number of patients who present for treatment of BED a year or two following recovery from substance abuse (primarily alcohol, cocaine and opiates). These patients describe a pattern of weight gain and binge eating following abstinence. This presents an interesting clinical picture, as complex biological, psychological, and environmental changes occur when someone recovers from alcohol and drugs. A combination of these factors may make some individuals vulnerable to the development of an eating disorder at that time.

The first relevant feature of recovering from drug and alcohol abuse is the likelihood of weight gain. There is evidence that individuals addicted to alcohol and drugs are lower weight than controls (e.g., Addolorato, Capristo, Greco, Stefanini, & Gasbarrini, 1998b) and are poorly nourished (Santolaria-Fernandez et al., 1995). As the person's body recovers from alcohol and drug use, there is evidence that metabolism improves and body weight increases (Addolorato et al., 1998a). Some individuals may react with distress at this weight gain and begin rigid dieting, which in turn may lead to binge eating.

A second pathway toward binge eating involves the use of food to manage negative affect. Initial stages of recovery may include major environmental shifts in one's social circle, employment, or residence. Some people may have used alcohol and drugs as a way to manage negative affect and interpersonal distress, and in their abstinence from alcohol and drugs, food may become an alternative way of coping. How often this phenomenon occurs is an interesting empirical question that warrants research; we know of no studies on the topic. It is interesting to note, however, that there is no evidence of this type of symptom substitution in the other direction: Individuals who have recovered from eating disorders do not show higher rates of turning to substance abuse (Wilson, 1995b).

Psychiatric Medications That Cause Weight Gain

We have also seen a number of patients with schizophrenia treated with neuroleptics who then reported significant weight gain while on these medications. They report that their distress over this weight gain has led to dietary restraint followed by binge eating. Weight gain is a well-known side effect of many neuroleptics (Casey, 1996; Umbricht & Kane, 1996). For example, in one study of 42 patients on clozapine, the average body mass index went from 23.2 to 29.1 in women and from 26.4 to 29.7 in men (Frankenburg, Zanarini, Kando, & Centorrino, 1998). In light of the World Health Organization guidelines that a body mass index of 25 suggests overweight and a BMI of 30 defines obesity, these patients are making a clinically significant shift toward obesity. In another study, Bustillo, Buchanan, Irish, and Breier (1996) found that 58% of patients on clozapine gained at least 10% of their body weight at 1-year follow-up. To address this problem, the literature on the adverse effects of medications such as olanzapine (Gupta, Droney, Al-Samarrai, Keller, & Frank, 1998), clozapine (Bustillo et al., 1996; Young, Bowers, & Mazure, 1998), and risperidone (Kelly, Conley, Love, Horn, & Ushachak, 1998) recommends dietary education and exercise as part of the drug treatment program.

In addition to neuroleptic medication, other psychotropic medications have been linked to weight gain. There is strong evidence that lithium can cause weight gain (Baptista et al., 1995). The evidence is less clear for antidepressant medications (i.e., tricyclics, selective serotonin reuptake inhibitors and monoamine oxidase inhibitors). Some studies have found associated weight gain, but this may be an effect of recovery from depression, not a pharmacological effect (see Benazzi, 1998).

We know of no study that has assessed the development of BED following the use of psychotropic medication. As hypothesized earlier with recovery from substance abuse, some individuals may develop binge eating because they gain weight, feel distress about this, engage in rigid dieting, and then as a result of this dietary restraint begin binge eating. Other individuals may turn to binge eating to manage negative feelings. Patients we have seen at our clinic are at a challenging crossroads in their treatment; the symptoms of their major mental illness may be controlled, but they face new challenges (e.g., trying to make friends, work at their jobs, or go to school). Both the new weight gain and the new interpersonal challenges may increase vulnerability to binge eating.

Individual Difference Variables as Risk Factors

A number of individual difference variables may be risk factors for eating disorders. Among those studied are gender, ethnicity, and sexual orientation.

Gender

Ninety percent of cases of anorexia nervosa and bulimia nervosa are female, making it a disorder clearly linked to gender. BED, in contrast, seems to affect more men than do the other eating disorders. Up to 40% of binge eaters may be male (Wilson et al., 1993), suggesting that it may not be linked to gender in the same ways as the other eating disorders.

Some preliminary work has compared men to women with BED, and it seems that there are both similarities and differences. Tanofsky, Wilfley, Spurrell, Welch, and Brownell (1997) compared 21 men with BED to 21 age-matched women with BED using interview measures of eating disorder psychopathology as well as Axis I and Axis II disorders. There were no significant differences in BMI, level of education, family income, or eating disorder features (dietary restraint, weight concern, shape concern, eating concern). Nor were there differences in self-esteem or number of interpersonal problems. One important difference between the sexes was that the men reported significantly more Axis I psychiatric disorders. When this was examined more closely, the difference emerged only for lifetime substance-related disorders, not mood or anxiety disorders. Fifteen men (12 lifetime, 3 current) were diagnosed with substance abuse compared to only 6 (5 lifetime, 1 current) women.

This study suggests that vulnerability factors for males may differ from that of females. It is possible that a history of substance abuse may be a particular vulnerability for binge eating for men. It is also possible that although fewer women with BED have a history of substance abuse, women recovering from abuse may be particularly vulnerable to binge eating. As discussed in the earlier section on substance abuse, we know of no research addressing this question; however, these findings suggest that sex would be an important variable to include in such a study.

Ethnicity

Eating disorders have historically been considered a problem that affects affluent, Caucasian women. With the emergence of BED as a diagnostic category, however, that stereotype is changing. In her review of the research on binge eating in ethnic minority groups, Smith (1995) notes accumulating evidence from both population-based studies and clinic-based studies that the prevalence of BED among African American and Hispanic women may be as high as it is among Caucasian women. In one recent study, Caldwell, Brownell, and Wilfley (1997) measured weight, body dissatisfaction, and self-esteem among African American and Caucasian women. All the women were either middle or high socioeconomic status and had a history of dieting. They found that the two racial groups were more similar than different on the variables measured. This was surprising given previous findings that African American women have lower levels of body concern than do Caucasian women. The authors suggest that previous findings may reflect class rather than race effects.

Sexual Orientation

One theory is that women develop eating disorders due to cultural pressures for thinness and the desire to attract men. A related theory is that gay men experience similar pressures to be physically attractive to men and therefore are also at risk for body dissatisfaction and eating disorders (Siever, 1994). There is some evidence to support this theory, as studies of males with eating disorders have found that a disproportionately high number of them are gay or struggling with their sexual orientation (e.g., Herzog, Norman, Gordon, & Pepose, 1984; Schneider & Agras, 1987). Asking the question another way, Siever (1994) found that gay men are at higher risk of eating disorders than are heterosexual men. He compared four groups of undergraduate students (i.e., lesbians, gay men, heterosexual women, and heterosexual men) on self-report measures of (1) the importance of physical attractiveness, (2) body satisfaction, and (3) eating disorders measures. Lesbian women were less concerned about physical attractiveness, were more satisfied with their bodies, and had lower eating disorder scores than did heterosexual women. Gay men were more concerned about physical attractiveness, were less satisfied with their bodies, and had higher eating disorder scores than did heterosexual men. He interpreted these findings as reflecting the degree to which people experience sexual objectification by their sexual partners, with heterosexual women and gay men experiencing this objectification more than lesbians and heterosexual men (Siever, 1994).

If being gay increases the risk of developing an eating disorder for a man, does it protect women? The studies examining this question have had conflicting findings. As stated previously, Siever (1994) found that lesbians had lower eating disorder scores than did heterosexual women. In contrast, Heffernan (1996) examined rates of bulimia nervosa and BED among lesbians and found that the rate of bulimia nervosa was the same as has been reported among heterosexual women, and the rate of BED was higher. Interestingly, among the lesbian group, eating as negative affect regulation predicted binge eating more strongly than did body dissatisfaction or dieting. In another study, Beren, Hayden, Wilfley, and Grilo (1996) compared four groups of people (gay and heterosexual men and women) and found that (1) gay men were more dissatisfied with their bodies than heterosexual men, but (2) lesbians and heterosexual women did not differ on the variables measured. To further understand these conflicting findings and the array of influences on lesbians' attitudes toward their bodies, Beren, Hayden, Wilfley, and Striegel-Moore (1997) conducted interviews with lesbian college students and found that many experienced a conflict between mainstream and lesbian values about the importance of weight and appearance. Their article illustrates the complexity of this question and suggests future directions for research. At this time, the findings from these studies suggest that gay men are at greater risk for eating disorders than heterosexual men, but lesbians are not protected from the effects of living in a society that idealizes thinness and are as likely to struggle with eating disorders as heterosexual women.

Bulimia Nervosa

Although this chapter has focused on the research on BED, two studies that include samples of patients with bulimia nervosa are relevant to this discussion of vulnerability during adulthood. The first study addresses characteristics of patients with late-onset bulimia; the second describes a sample of patients whose diagnoses changed from bulimia nervosa to BED.

Late-Onset Bulimia

One study has compared individuals with typical versus late onset of bulimia nervosa (Mitchell, Hatsukami, Pyle, Eckert, & Soll, 1987). The authors defined late onset as age 25 or older and typical onset as age 20 or earlier. The findings were that members of the late-onset group differed from those in the other group in several ways. First, they had higher rates of affective disorders (both current and lifetime) and were more likely to have received treatment for an affective disorder. Second, they were more likely to have made a suicide attempt. Third, they were more likely to report chemical dependency problems (both current and lifetime) and showed a trend toward higher rates of chemical dependency treatment. Taken together, these findings suggest that the late-onset group has higher rates of psychopathology than do typical onset bulimic patients. It is possible that their vulnerability to developing bulimia in adulthood is linked to their struggles with affective disorders and substance abuse.

As discussed earlier, affective disorders are common among individuals with eating disorders and many questions remain about the possible causal link between the two (e.g., Mitchell & Mussell, 1995). This study suggests that a current or past affective disorder may be a vulnerability factor for the development of bulimia nervosa in adulthood.

Substance abuse is also a common comorbid diagnosis for patients with bulimia nervosa, with patients with an eating disorder showing higher rates of past and present substance abuse than would be expected in the general population (see review by Wilson, 1995b). Although there is debate whether eating disorders can be considered an addictive disorder, this study does suggest that a history of substance abuse may increase vulnerability to the development of bulimia nervosa in adulthood.

Transition from Bulimia Nervosa to Binge-Eating Disorder

A subset of individuals with BED once had bulimia nervosa and have stopped purging. Thus, one vulnerability factor for developing BED as an adult may be a history of bulimia nervosa. A recent study of 63 individuals with BED divided participants into those having a history of purging (i.e., vomiting and laxative abuse) or no history of purging (Peterson et al., 1998). The groups were compared on measures of Axis I psychopathology, depression, body dissatisfaction, eating disorder symptoms, and self-esteem. Surprisingly, a history of purging was *not* related to any variable. The authors suggest that because they excluded people who had purged in the last 6 months, were currently in psychotherapy or on psychotropic medication, and experienced substance abuse or dependence within the last 6 months, they may have inadvertently excluded the people for whom a history of purging would be a meaningful subgroup classification and indicator of psychopathology. This study does not support the hypothesis that having a history of purging significantly distinguishes a subset of patients with BED.

A COMPREHENSIVE VIEW OF VULNERABILITY

This chapter reviews the literature on the characteristics of individuals with BED and the links among obesity, dieting, psychopathology, and binge eating. At this time, our understanding of causality among these factors is limited; rather, we know only that certain cognitive, personality, and psychopathological features tend to cluster in adults with eating disorders. To summarize, the cognitive and personality features of individuals with BED are perfectionism, low self-efficacy, an external frame of reference in determining self-worth, ineffectiveness, low self-esteem, high impulsivity, low interoceptive awareness, and excessive doubts, compulsions, obsessions, and unreasonable fears. The most common comorbid psychiatric problems of individuals with BED are affective disorders (primarily depression), anxiety disorders, and personality disorders (primarily histrionic, borderline, and avoidant). We have also hypothesized that certain life events may precede the onset of an eating disorder due to unexpected weight gain; these are pregnancy, recovery from substance abuse, and beginning a medication that is linked to weight gain.

The childhood environment of individuals with BED may contribute to their vulnerability. To summarize the findings of Fairburn et al. (1998) presented earlier, the parents of patients with BED were more likely than those of healthy controls to have been depressed and critical, and to have had high expectations. They were also underinvolved and less affectionate than the other parents. The patients with BED also reported higher rates of physical abuse, bullying, and sexual abuse. As these are the characteristics that distinguished the BED group from the healthy controls, these parental and environmental characteristics appear to place individuals at risk for developing some type of psychiatric illness, not necessarily an eating disorder. The interpersonal vulnerability model begins with a disturbance in the early child–caretaker relationship, and these parental characteristics (particularly parental depression) could impair the ability of the child to become securely attached to his or her caregiver. Insecure attachment may lead to a variety of types of psychopathology, including BED.

The specific factors that seem to distinguish the patients with BED from other psychiatric patients are childhood obesity, less parental contact, and more critical comments by family about shape, weight, or eating. This paints a much more detailed picture of vulnerability: an obese child with low overall parental contact who is criticized by his or her family about eating, body shape, and weight. These data suggest that when a child is obese and parental criticism is focused on eating, body shape, and weight, it may predispose the child to develop an eating disorder rather than another type of psychiatric problem.

Figure 18.2 summarizes all the variables reviewed in this chapter that may be vulnerability factors for the development of eating disorders in adulthood. To understand how these variables lead to an eating disorder, we have presented the two most widely used models of etiology of binge eating (dietary restraint and interpersonal vulnerability). We believe that each of these variables may make one more likely to experience the processes described in these models.

IMPLICATION FOR PREVENTION

The vulnerability processes reviewed in this chapter that have the strongest implications for prevention are the life events linked to weight gain. We

WEIGHT	ENVIRONMENTAL FACTORS	COGNITIVE STYLE AND PERSONALITY CHARACTERISTICS	LIFE EVENTS	PSYCHOLOGICAL FACTORS	BEHAVIOR
Childhood obesity	Family criticism for weight, shape, and eating	Perfectionism, external frame of reference in determining self-worth	Pregnancy	*Axis I* Depression Anxiety	Dieting
Recent weight gain	Low parental contact	Low self-efficacy, ineffectiveness, low self-esteem	Recovery from substance abuse	*Axis II* Histrionic Borderline Avoidant	
Current obesity		Impulsivity, low interoceptive awareness, doubts, compulsions, obsessions, unreasonable fears	Medication that causes weight gain	Interpersonal distress	

FIGURE 18.2. A comprehensive view of vulnerability.

named only three events (pregnancy, recovery from substance abuse, and beginning a neuroleptic medication) that we have observed clinically as precursors to binge eating; however, there are many events in adulthood that may lead to weight gain. We believe it is important for medical professionals to be aware of weight gain as a potential risk factor for the development of an eating disorder and to help patients anticipate their reactions to changes in body weight and potential changes in eating behavior.

First, health care professionals could regularly assess eating disorder symptoms (particularly over concern with shape and weight) in pregnant women to help predict those women who are more likely to have a difficult time with changes in body shape and weight. Once identified, these women could receive special attention to help them understand what to expect in terms of weight gain during pregnancy and how to set realistic goals for weight loss following delivery.

Second, substance abuse counselors can help individuals in the early stages of recovery to monitor their eating and exercise patterns in order to teach them to eat in a healthy manner and to provide early identification of binge eating episodes if they occur. If there has been weight loss associated with the use of the drug, the counselor can predict some weight gain as the person resumes normal eating patterns and is no longer under the influence of the drug.

Third, psychiatrists prescribing medications that are strongly associated with weight gain, such as neuroleptics, can provide guidance for the patient about healthy eating and exercise from the beginning of the medication trial. Just as certain medications require the avoidance of particular foods or alcohol, patients can be told that these medications require special attention to eating and exercise behaviors in order to avoid dangerous weight gain. Perhaps regular consultations with a nutritionist and exercise professional during the first few months of medication could help patients strive toward a healthy, realistic eating and exercise pattern.

Another finding with prevention implications is that patients with BED are more likely to have been obese as children and to have been criticized by family members about shape, weight, and eating (Fairburn et al., 1998). This suggests that efforts to prevent childhood obesity may subsequently prevent new cases of BED. There is a significant literature of behavioral programs that have been tested to treat childhood obesity (see reviews by Epstein, 1993; Epstein & Wing, 1987; Jelalian & Saelens, 1999), and the components of these programs can be used for prevention efforts. The most important elements appear to be parental involvement, increasing exercise (Epstein, 1993), and reducing time spent in sedentary activities (Epstein et al., 1995).

In addition to preventing childhood obesity, another important public health message is to prevent the criticism of overweight children by family members. Many parents may criticize their child out of worry or their own feelings of helplessness. While family-based treatments teach parents how to use positive reinforcement with their children, only a small percentage of parents with obese children in our country have the opportunity to participate in a treatment group. On a broader scale, public health education campaigns may be useful to help parents learn how to communicate with their children about eating, shape, and weight in a productive manner.

FUTURE DIRECTIONS FOR RESEARCH

One area for future research is to empirically test the suggestions described previously on implications for prevention. For example, multiple issues need to be covered with pregnant women, newly recovered substance abusers, and newly medicated psychotic patients, and addressing eating and weight issues may not be at the top of the priority list. Research testing the cost-effectiveness of providing an eating and weight intervention at these potentially vulnerable times would provide important information for practitioners and patients.

Second, although clinicians can teach parents one at a time how to help their overweight children, a public health campaign on how parents and teachers can facilitate weight loss, health, and self-esteem in children may be a more cost-effective approach. Developing and evaluating community-based interventions is an important area for further research.

A third area for future research is to further our understanding of the causal links among the variables that have been studied in the adult population with BED. One important individual factor to address is gender, as males have been excluded from much of the research on binge eaters. Other important variables are affective disorders and substance abuse (past and present), as these appear throughout the literature as frequent comorbid diagnoses with BED.

As illustrated in Figure 18.2, there are many different domains of functioning and experiences that are probably interrelated. It would be ideal to study individuals longitudinally to assess the sequence of development of cognitive, personality, eating, weight, and psychological variables. Another method would be to address these research questions through path analysis. By identifying the amount of variance accounted for in each variable by the others, we may be able to further our understanding of the strength and direction of the links between them. It would also be important to test the two distinct models of etiology, dietary restraint and interpersonal vulnerability to see whether the experience of individuals reliably reflects one of these pathways. With this knowledge, we can then develop interventions to break the cycle.

REFERENCES

Abbott, D. W., de Zwann, M., Mussell, M. P., Raymond, N. C., Seim, H. C., Crow, S. J., Crosby, R. D., & Mitchell, J. E. (1998). Onset of binge eating and dieting in overweight women: Implications for etiology, associated features and treatment. *Journal of Psychosomatic Research, 44*, 367–374.

Addolorato, G., Capristo, E., Greco, A. V., Caputo, F., Stefanini, G. F., & Gasbarrini, G. (1998a). Three months of abstinence from alcohol normalizes energy expenditure and substrate oxidation in alcoholics: A longitudinal study. *American College of Gastroenterology, 93*, 2476–2481.

Addolorato, G., Capristo, E., Greco, A. V., Stefanini, G. F., & Gasbarrini, G. (1998b). Influence of chronic alcohol abuse on body weight and energy metabolism: Is excess ethanol consumption a risk factor for obesity or malnutrition? *Journal of Internal Medicine, 244*, 387–395.

American Psychiatric Association. (1994). *Diagnostic and statistical manual of mental disorders* (4th ed.). Washington, DC: Author.

Antony, M. M., Johnson, W. G., Carr-Nangle, R. E., & Abel, J. L. (1994). Psychopathology correlates of binge eating and binge eating disorder. *Comprehensive Psychiatry, 35*, 386–392.

Baptista, T., Teneud, L., Contreras, Q., Alastre, T., Burguera, J. L., de Burguera, M., de Baptista, E., Weiss, S., & Hernandez, L. (1995). Lithium and body weight gain. *Pharmacophyschiatry, 28*, 35–44.

Belgin, S. J., & Fairburn, C. G. (1992). What is meant by the term "binge"? *American Journal of Psychiatry, 149*, 123–124.

Benazzi, F. (1998). Weight gain in depression remitted with antidepressants: Pharmacological or recovery effect? *Psychotherapy and Psychosomatics, 67*, 271–274.

Beren, S. E., Hayden, H. A., Wilfley, D. E., & Grilo, C. M. (1996). The influence of sexual orientation on body dissatisfaction in adult men and women. *International Journal of Eating Disorders, 20*, 135–141.

Beren, S. E., Hayden, H. A., Wilfley, D. E., & Striegel-Moore, R. H. (1997). Body dissatisfaction among lesbian college students: The conflict of straddling mainstream and lesbian cultures. *Psychology of Women Quarterly, 21*, 431–445.

Black, C. M., & Wilson, G. T. (1996). Assessment of eating disorders: Interview versus questionnaire. *International Journal of Eating Disorders, 20*, 43–50.

Brownell, K. D. (1995). Effects of weight cycling on metabolism, health, and psychological factors. In K. D. Brownell & C. G. Fairburn (Eds.), *Eating disorders and obesity: A comprehensive handbook* (pp. 56–60). New York: Guilford Press.

Brownell, K. D., & Wadden, T. A. (1992). Etiology and treatment of obesity: Understanding a serious, prevalent, and refractory disorder. *Journal of Consulting and Clinical Psychology, 60*, 505–517.

Bustillo, J. R., Buchanan, R. W., Irish, D., & Breier, A. (1996). Differential effect of clozapineon weight: A controlled study. *American Journal of Psychiatry, 153*, 817–819.

Caldwell, M. B., Brownell, K. D., & Wilfley, D. E. (1997). Relationship of weight, body dissatisfaction, and self-esteem in African American and White female dieters. *International Journal of Eating Disorders, 22*, 127–130.

Casey, D. E. (1996). Side effect profiles of new antipsychotic agents. *Journal of Clinical Psychiatry, 57,* 40–45.

Cooper, Z., & Fairburn, C. (1987). The Eating Disorder Examination: A semi-structured interview for the assessment of the specific psychopathology of eating disorders. *International Journal of Eating Disorders, 6,* 1–8.

Davies, K., & Wardle, J. (1994). Body image and dieting in pregnancy. *Journal of Psychosomatic Research, 38,* 787–799.

de Zwann, M., Mitchell, J. E., Seim, H. C., Specker, S. M., Pyle, R. L., Raymond, N. C., & Crosby, R. B. (1994). Eating related and general psychopathology in obese females with binge eating disorder. *International Journal of Eating Disorders, 15,* 43–52.

Epstein, L. H. (1993). Methodological issues and ten-year outcomes for obese children. *Annals of the New York Academy of Sciences, 699,* 237–249.

Epstein, L. H., Valoski, A. M., Vara, L. S., McCurley, J., Wisniewski, L., Kalarchian, M. A., Klein, K. R., & Shrager, L. R. (1995). Effects of decreasing sedentary behavior and increasing activity on weight change in children. *Health Psychology, 14,* 109–115.

Epstein, L. H., & Wing, R. R. (1987). Behavioral treatment of childhood obesity. *Psychological Bulletin, 101,* 331–342.

Fairburn, C. G., & Belgin, S. J. (1994). The assessment of eating disorders: Interview or self-report questionnaire? *International Journal of Eating Disorders, 16,* 363–370.

Fairburn, C. G., Doll, H., Welch, S., Hay, P. J., Davies, B. A., & O'Connor, M. E. (1998). Risk factors for binge eating disorder. *Archives of General Psychiatry, 55,* 425–432.

Fairburn, C. G., Jones, R., Peveler, R. C., Hope, R. A., & O'Connor, M. (1993). Psychotherapy and bulimia nervosa: The longer-term effects of interpersonal psychotherapy, behavior therapy and cognitive-behavior therapy. *Archives of General Psychiatry, 50,* 419–428.

Fairburn, C. G., Marcus, M. D., & Wilson, G. T. (1993). Cognitive-behavioral therapy for binge eating and bulimia nervosa: A comprehensive treatment manual. In C. G. Fairburn & G. T. Wilson (Eds.), *Binge eating: Nature, assessment, and treatment* (pp. 361–404). New York: Guilford Press.

Fairburn, C. G., Stein, A., & Jones, R. (1992). Eating habits and eating disorders during pregnancy. *Psychosomatic Medicine, 54,* 665–672.

Fairburn, C. G., & Welch, S. L. (1990). The impact of pregnancy on eating habits and attitudes to shape and weight. *International Journal of Eating Disorders, 9,* 153–160.

Fairburn, C. G., Welch, S. L., Doll, H. A., Davies, B. A., & O'Connor, M. E. (1997). Risk factors for bulimia nervosa: A community-based control study. *Archives of General Psychiatry, 54,* 509–517.

Fawcett, J., Bliss-Holtz, V. J., Haas, M. B., Leventhal, M., & Rubin, M. (1986). Spouses' body image changes during and after pregnancy: A replication and extension. *Nursing Research, 35,* 220–223.

Frankenburg, F. R., Zanarini, M. C., Kando, J., & Centorrino, F. (1998). Clozapine and body mass change. *Biological Psychiatry, 43,* 520–524.

Friedman, M. A., & Brownell, K. D. (1995). Psychological correlates of obesity: Moving to the next research generation. *Psychological Bulletin, 117,* 3–20.

Friedman, M. A., Schwartz, M. B., & Brownell, K. D. (1998). Psychological correlates of weight cycling. *Journal of Consulting and Clinical Psychology, 66,* 646–650.

Garner, D. M., Olmstead, M. P., & Polivy, J. (1983). Development and validation of a multidimensional Eating Disorder Inventory for anorexia nervosa and bulimia. *International Journal of Eating Disorders, 2,* 15–34.

Gormally, J., Black, S., Daston, S., & Rardin, D. (1982). The assessment of binge eating severity among obese persons. *Addictive Behaviors, 7,* 47–55.

Gupta, S., Droney, T., Al-Samarrai, S., Keller, P., & Frank, B. (1998). Olanzapine-induced weight gain. *Annals of Clinical Psychiatry, 10,* 39.

Harrington, R. (1996). Family-genetic findings in child and adolescent depressive disorders. *International Review of Psychiatry, 8,* 355–368.

Heatherton, T. F., & Baumeister, R. F. (1991). Binge eating as an escape from self-awareness. *Psychological Bulletin, 110,* 86–108.

Heffernan, K. (1996). Eating disorders and weight concern among lesbians. *International Journal of Eating Disorders, 19,* 127–138.

Herzog, D. B., Norman, D. K., Gordon, C., & Pepose, M. (1984). Sexual conflict and eating disorders in 27 males. *American Journal of Psychiatry, 141,* 989–990.

Jelalian, E., & Saelens, B. E. (1999). Empirically supported treatments in pediatric psychology: Pediatric obesity. *Journal of Pediatric Psychology, 24,* 223–248.

Kelly, D. L., Conley, R. R., Love, R. C., Horn, D. S., & Ushchak, C. M. (1998). Weight gain in adolescents treated with risperidone and conventional antipsychotics over six months. *Journal of Child and Adolescent Psychopharmacology, 8,* 151–159.

Klerman, G. L., Weissman, M. M., Rounsaville, B. J., & Chevron, E. S. (1984). *Interpersonal psychotherapy for depression.* New York: Basic Books.

Kolotkin, R. L., Revis, E. S., Kirkley, B. G., & Janik, L. (1987). Binge eating in obesity: Associated MMPI characteristics. *Journal of Consulting and Clinical Psychology, 55,* 872–876.

Kuehnel, R. H., & Wadden, T. A. (1994). Binge eating disorder, weight cycling, and psychopathology. *International Journal of Eating Disorders, 15,* 321–329.

Leon, G. R., Keel, P. K., & Fulkerson, J. A. (1997). The future of risk factor research in understanding the etiology of eating disorders. *Psychopharmacology Bulletin, 33,* 405–411.

Marcus, M. D., Wing, R. R., & Hopkins, J. (1998). Obese binge eaters: Affect, cognitions, and response to behavioral weight control. *Journal of Consulting and Clinical Psychology, 56,* 433–439.

Marton, P., & Maharaj, S. (1993). Family factors in adolescent unipolar depression. *Canadian Journal of Psychiatry, 38,* 373–382.

McGuffin, P., & Katz, R. (1989). The genetics of depression and manic–depressive disorder. *British Journal of Psychiatry, 155,* 294–304.

Mitchell, J. E., Hatsukami, D., Pyle, R. L, Eckert, E. D., & Soll, E. (1987). Late onset bulimia. *Comprehensive Psychiatry, 28,* 323-328.

Mitchell, J. E., & Mussell, M. P. (1995). Comorbidity and binge eating disorder. *Addictive Behaviors, 20,* 725–732.

Moore, B. J., & Greenwood, M. R. C. (1995). Pregnancy and weight gain. In K. D. Brownell & C. G. Fairburn (Eds.), *Eating disorders and obesity: A comprehensive handbook* (pp. 51–55). New York: Guilford Press.

Moore, D. S. (1978). The body image in pregnancy. *Journal of Nurse-Midwifery, 22,* 17–27.

Mussell, M. P., Mitchell, J. E., Weller, C. L., Raymond, N. C., Crow, S. J., & Crosby, R. D. (1995). Onset of binge eating, dieting, obesity, and mood disorders among subjects seeking treatment for binge eating disorder. *International Journal of Eating Disorders, 17,* 395–401.

Peterson, C. B., Mitchell, J. E., Engbloom, S., Nugent, S., Mussell, M. P., Crow, S. J., & Miller, J. P. (1998). Binge eating disorder with and without a history of purging symptoms. *International Journal of Eating Disorders, 24,* 251–256.

Pike, K. M., & Rodin, J. (1991). Mothers, daughters, and disordered eating. *Journal of Abnormal Psychology, 100,* 198–204.

Polivy, J., & Herman. C. P. (1993). Etiology of binge eating: Psychological mechanisms. In C. G. Fairburn & G. T. Wilson (Eds.), *Binge eating: Nature, assessment, and treatment* (pp. 173–205). New York: Guilford Press.

Robertson, D. N., & Palmer, R. L. (1997). The prevalence and correlated of binge eating in a British community sample of women with a history of obesity. *International Journal of Eating Disorders, 22,* 323–327.

Santolaria-Fernandez, F. J., Gomez-Sirvent, J. L., Gonzalez-Reimers, C. E., Batista-Lopez, J. N., Jorge-Hernandez, J. A., Rodriguez-Moreno, F., Martinez-Riera, A., & Hernandez-Garcia, M. T. (1995). Nutritional assessment of drug addicts. *Drug and Alcohol Dependence, 38,* 11–18.

Schneider, J. A., & Agras, W. S. (1987). Bulimia in males: A matched comparison with females. *International Journal of Eating Disorders, 6,* 235–242.

Schwartz, M. B., & Brownell, K. D. (1998, April). *How do clients match themselves to treatment?: A study of participants in Overeaters Anonymous and Jenny Craig.* Paper presented at the International Conference for Eating Disorders, New York.

Siever, M. D. (1994). Sexual orientation and gender as factors in socioculturally acquired vulnerability to body dissatisfaction and eating disorders. *Journal of Consulting Clinical Psychology, 62,* 252–260.

Slade, P. D. (1977). Awareness of body dimensions during pregnancy: An analogue study. *Psychological Medicine, 7,* 245–252.

Smith, D. E. (1995). Binge eating in ethnic minority groups. *Addictive Behaviors, 20,* 695–703.

Specker, S., de Zwaan, M., Raymond, N., & Mitchell, J. (1994). Psychopathology in subgroups of obese women with and without binge eating disorder. *Comprehensive Psychiatry, 35,* 185-190.

Spitzer, R. L., Devlin, M., Walsh, B. T., Hasin, D., Wing, R., Marcus, M., Stukard, A., Wadden, T., Yanovski, S., Agras, S., Mitchell, J., & Nonas, C. (1992). Binge eating disorder: A multisite field trial of the diagnostic criteria. *International Journal of Eating Disorders, 11,* 191–203.

Spitzer, R. L., Williams, J. B. W., Gibbon, M., & First, M. (1990a). *Structured Clinical Interview for DSM-IV-R* (SCID). Washington, DC: American Psychiatric Press.

Spitzer, R. L., Williams, J. B. W., Gibbon, M., & First, M. (1990b). *Structured Clinical Interview for DSM-IV-R Personality Disorders* (SCID-II). Washington, DC: American Psychiatric Press.

Spitzer, R. L., Yanovski, S., Wadden, T., Wing, R., Marcus, M., Stunkard, A., Devlin, M., Mitchell, J., Hasin, D., & Horne, R. L. (1993). Binge eating disorder: Its further validation in a multisite study. *International Journal of Eating Disorders, 13,* 137–153.

Spurrell, E. B., Wilfley, D. E., Tanofsky, M. C., & Brownell, K. D. (1997). Age of onset for binge eating: Are there different pathways to binge eating? *International Journal of Eating Disorders, 21*, 55–65.

Stein, A., & Fairburn, C. G. (1996). Eating habits and attitudes in the postpartum period. *Psychosomatic Medicine, 58*, 321–325.

Strang, V. R., & Sullivan, P. L. (1995). Body image attitudes during pregnancy and the postpartum period. *Journal of Obstetric, Gynecologic, and Neonatal Nursing, 14*, 332–336.

Striegel-Moore, R. H. (1993). Etiology of binge eating: A developmental perspective. In C. G. Fairburn & G. T. Wilson (Eds.), *Binge eating: Nature, assessment, and treatment* (pp. 144–172). New York: Guilford Press.

Striegel-Moore, R. H. (1995). A feminist perspective on the etiology of eating disorders. In K. D. Brownell & C. G. Fairburn (Eds.), *Eating disorders and obesity: A comprehensive handbook* (pp. 224–229). New York: Guilford Press.

Striegel-Moore, R. H., Silberstein, L., & Rodin, J. (1986). Toward an understanding of risk factors for bulimia. *American Psychologist, 41*, 246–263.

Stunkard, A. J. (1976). *The pain of obesity.* Palo Alto, CA: Bull.

Tanofsky, M. B., Wilfley, D. E., Spurell, E. B., Welch, R., & Brownell, K. (1997). Comparison of men and women with binge eating disorder. *International Journal of Eating Disorders, 21*, 49–54.

Telch, C. F., & Agras, W. S. (1994). Obesity, binge eating, and psychopathology: Are they related? *International Journal of Eating Disorders, 15*, 53–61.

Telch, C., & Stice, E. (1998). Psychiatric comorbidity in women with binge eating disorder: Prevalence rates from a non-treatment-seeking sample. *Journal of Consulting and Clinical Psychology, 66*, 768–776.

Umbricht, D., & Kane, J. M. (1996). Medical complications of new antipsychotic drugs. *Schizophrenia Bulletin, 22*, 475–483.

Wilfley, D. E. (1999, April). Treatment of BED: Research findings and clinical applications. In B. Timothy Walsh (Chair), *Integrating research and clinical practice.* Plenary session at the 4th annual International Conference for Eating Disorders, London.

Wilfley, D. E., Agras, W. S., Telch, C. F., Rossiter, E. M., Schneider, J. A., Cole, A. G., Sifford, L., & Raeburn, S. D. (1993). Group cognitive-behavioral therapy and group interpersonal psychotherapy for the nonpurging bulimic: A controlled comparison. *Journal of Consulting and Clinical Psychology, 61*, 296–305.

Wilfley, D. E., Grilo, C. M., & Rodin, J. (1997). Group psychotherapy for the treatment of bulimia nervosa and binge eating disorder: Research and clinical methods. In J. L. Spira (Ed.), *Group therapy for medically ill patients* (pp. 225–295). New York: Guilford Press.

Wilfley, D. E., Pike, K. M., & Striegel-Moore, R. H. (1997). Toward and integrated model of risk for binge eating disorder. *Journal of Gender, Culture, and Health, 2*, 1–32.

Wilfley, D. E., & Rodin, J. (1995). Cultural influences on eating disorders. In K. D. Brownell & C. G. Fairburn (Eds.), *Eating disorders and obesity: A comprehensive handbook* (pp. 78–82). New York: Guilford Press.

Wilfley, D. E., Schwartz, M. B., Spurrell, E. B., & Fairburn, C. G. (1997). Assessing the specific psychopathology of binge eating disorder: Interview or self-report? *Behaviour Research and Therapy, 35*, 1151–1159.

Wilson, G. T. (1993). Assessment of binge eating. In C. G. Fairburn & G. T. Wilson (Eds.), *Binge eating: Nature, assessment, and treatment* (pp. 227–249). New York: Guilford Press.

Wilson, G. T. (1995a). The controversy over dieting. In K. D. Brownell & C. G. Fairburn (Eds.), *Eating disorders and obesity: A comprehensive handbook* (pp. 87–92). New York: Guilford Press.

Wilson, G. T. (1995b). Eating disorders and addictive disorders. In K. D. Brownell & C. G. Fairburn (Eds.), *Eating disorders and obesity: A comprehensive handbook* (pp. 165–170). New York: Guilford Press.

Wilson, G. T., Nonas, C. A., & Rosenblum, G. D. (1993). Assessment of binge eating in obese patients. *International Journal of Eating Disorders, 13*, 25–33.

Yanovski, S. Z., Nelson, J. E., Dubbert, B. K., & Spitzer, R. L. (1993). Association of binge eating disorder and psychiatric comorbidity in obese subjects. *American Journal of Psychiatry, 150*, 1472–1479.

Young, C. R., Bowers, M. B., & Mazure, C. M. (1998). Management of the adverse effects of clozapine. *Schizophrenia Bulletin, 24*, 381.

19

Vulnerability to Eating Disorders across the Lifespan

PAMELA K. KEEL
MARLENE B. SCHWARTZ

This summary provides an integrated view of vulnerability factors for eating disorders across the lifespan. Review of Chapter 17 (Keel, Leon, & Fulkerson) and Chapter 18 (Schwartz & Brownell) reveals several commonalities and differences in understanding eating disorder vulnerability factors. First, we review apparent commonalities in risk factors for childhood/adolescence and adulthood. We follow this discussion with a review of differences in risk factors. Finally, we discuss how research endeavors can benefit from application of methods and perspectives employed within both domains.

Anorexia nervosa appears to be associated with the earliest age of onset with an initial peak age of 14 years, followed by a second peak at 18 years. Conversely, bulimia nervosa is associated with a peak age of onset around approximately 19 years of age and often develops in girls with a history of anorexia nervosa. Finally, binge-eating disorder (BED) appears to have a bimodal age of onset. One subgroup of individuals begins binge eating approximately at age 12 (before their first diet), and others begin at about age 25, (following the onset of dieting).

COMMON THEMES, ISSUES, AND VULNERABILITY FACTORS

Despite the apparent age-related differences in eating pathology, it is possible for a single individual to develop anorexia nervosa as she transitions from childhood to adolescence, to develop bulimia nervosa as she begins her transition from adolescence to adulthood, and finally to develop BED as she transitions fully to adulthood. Such a pattern suggests that certain vulnerability factors may form a common core from which disordered eating develops. For example, particular psychological features have been implicated as risk factors for eating disorders across the lifespan such as perfectionism, poor interoceptive awareness, low self-esteem, and negative affect. These core psychological features may then interact with life transitions that predispose individuals to present with somewhat distinct behavioral patterns. Research findings regarding these psychological factors are reviewed in detail within the preceding chapters. However, we discuss the potential roles of negative affect and low self-esteem as common vulnerability factors for eating disorders from childhood to adulthood.

Individuals who are vulnerable to developing eating disorders may have a temperamental style marked by negative affectivity—that is, the tendency to experience greater levels of dysphoria and anxiety and to find transitions particularly stressful. This temperamental style may contribute to or be exacerbated by disturbances in the individual's early relationships with caregivers. If caregivers are unable to meet their child's physical and emotional needs, the child is predisposed to experience greater levels of depression and low self-esteem due to both an insecure attachment style and her temperament. This pattern can contribute to a disturbance in the child's social self, characterized by a heightened concern for how she is perceived by others, an excessive need for social approval, and a feeling of inadequacy. This core can lead to disordered eating patterns such as severely restrictive dieting, purging, and binge eating. Binge eating may represent a means of coping with negative affect as suggested by the interpersonal vulnerability model. Alternatively, low self-esteem may increase an individual's likelihood of engaging in severely restrictive dieting in an attempt to gain social approval from others. Severely restrictive dieting could then produce anorexia nervosa or contribute to the onset of binge eating episodes according to the restraint hypothesis.

In Chapters 17 and 18, evidence supporting the relationship between strict dieting and disordered eating was presented, suggesting that strict dieting may represent a common vulnerability factor across the lifespan. In addition to contributing to the severe weight loss characterizing anorexia nervosa, strict dieting appears to increase the likelihood of developing binge eating episodes by contributing to an "all-or-nothing" cognitive style. Specifically, severely restrictive diets characterize foods as being either "good" or "bad" and often categorize important nutritional components (such as fat) as "unacceptable." If the rigid dietary rules are broken, the individual experiences the abstinence violation effect—a sense that she has failed completely. Moreover, 3 potato chips and a 12-ounce bag of potato chips represent the same level of failure; thus the person feels she might as well consume the entire bag of chips. This response is particularly likely if the individual anticipates returning to her severely restrictive diet the next day.

Across the lifespan, women are more likely to develop disordered eating than are men. The role of dietary restraint in the development of disordered eating may explain this overrepresentation of women. This difference is most salient in adolescence, where women make up 85 to 90% of individuals suffering with anorexia nervosa and bulimia nervosa. Among adults, women appear to be somewhat more likely than men to have BED potentially because they are more likely to report a loss of control over food. Because women are more likely than men to diet, it may not be surprising that they also are more likely to develop disordered eating.

Notably, across the lifespan, eating disorders are associated with increased comorbid depression, anxiety, and substance use problems. These patterns suggest that eating disorders share vulnerability factors with other disorders. Such factors appear to include a family history of affective disorders, poor family environment, and poor peer relationships. These factors are likely to be particularly influential in times of role transition, such as puberty, leaving the home environment, leaving a college environment, and pregnancy. With each transition, individuals face challenges requiring the ability to form new relationships. Where psychological (poor self-worth) and environmental (poor support in family relationships) factors impair interpersonal functioning, such transitions are likely to increase the potential for the development of psychopathology.

Biological factors, such as genetic predisposition for obesity, temperament, and neurotransmitter function, may represent stable factors that contribute to a vulnerability for disordered eating across the lifespan. Individuals with a high propensity to gain weight, high levels of negative emotionality, and poor impulse control may be more vulnerable to develop disordered eating as they encounter life transitions. Conversely, an individual with no tendency toward being overweight, low levels of negative emotionality, and good impulse control may find the transitions less stressful and may be able to cope adaptively with life changes.

DIFFERENCES IN VULNERABILITY FACTORS

Notable differences between childhood/adolescent eating pathology and adult eating pathology include the phenomenology and epidemiology of eating disorders. At younger ages, eating disorders could be characterized as dieting disorders, as key features of both anorexia nervosa and bulimia nervosa involve attempts to reduce or control weight through restrictive eating, purging, or excessive exercise. In addition, these disorders are far more common in females compared to males. Conversely, adults are more likely to have BED than anorexia nervosa or bulimia nervosa, and the role of dieting in the etiology and maintenance of BED is less clear. Although dieting may have preceded the onset of BED for a subset of individuals, there is also a group of individuals who began binge eating first. Unlike anorexia nervosa and bulimia nervosa, the use of strategies to control weight (i.e., dietary restraint or inappropriate compensatory behaviors) is not a diagnostic criterion for BED, nor is body image disturbance. Moreover, adults are less likely to use inappropriate compensatory behaviors following binge eating episodes. This may be due to decreased pressure to maintain an ultrathin physique in adulthood, as compared to adolescence. It also may be due to maturity and increased concern about the physical risks of self-induced vomiting or laxative abuse. Another difference between BED and the other eating disorders is that as many as 40% of individuals with BED appear to be male, representing a less extreme gender difference for this form of pathology in adults.

The decreased gender difference in the development of BED compared to anorexia nervosa and bulimia nervosa may be explained by the interpersonal vulnerability model. Men and women may share a similar liability to developing disordered eating under the interpersonal vulnerability model. This model could be applied to understanding the development of anorexia nervosa, bulimia nervosa, and BED as food intake may be used to cope with interpersonal difficulties in all three disorders. However, men may be less likely to starve themselves or compensate after binge eating episodes by purging, fasting, or excessive exercise because of the decreased societal pressure to maintain a thin physique. The apparent underrepresentation of boys in adolescent eating disordered samples may reflect a failure to study behaviors characteristic of BED rather than anorexia nervosa or bulimia nervosa in these studies. The accuracy of the interpersonal vulnerability model in explaining the decreased gender difference in the prevalence of BED could be explored through cross-cultural research. The presence of BED in societies that do not endorse a thin ideal may serve as an analogy to the presence of BED in men within our society. Such research might demonstrate that BED is represented cross-culturally. Moreover, seeking solace for emotional pain using food may represent a fairly universal coping mechanism given the association between food and nurturing.

The majority of eating disorders research has studied adolescent and young adult female populations to understand vulnerability factors. The focus on these populations grew from the understanding that anorexia nervosa and bulimia nervosa typically developed in these demographic groups. However, the recent delineation of BED has increased research focus on adult populations. As such, there is a lack of parity in study designs employed with populations of different ages. As noted by Schwartz and Brownell (Chapter 18), no longitudinal prospective studies have been conducted to detect risk factors for eating disorders in adult populations. Thus, many of the conclusions regarding risk factors that influence disordered eating among adults rest on correlational data. This approach seems somewhat short-sighted. Although anorexia nervosa and bulimia nervosa have been closely associated with adolescence, long-term follow-up studies suggest that these disorders can persist into middle age. Thus factors that contribute to the maintenance of disordered eating are not limited to adolescence. Furthermore, the disparity in research on eating disorders in females versus males is far greater than the actual disparity in the prevalence of eating disorders in females versus males. Unfortunately, a tendency to focus on female populations seems to have been adopted within studies of adult populations despite evidence that men represent a higher proportion of individuals with eating disorders in adulthood compared to childhood or adolescence. Given recent findings from both child/adolescent and adult literatures, there appears to be potential for cross-fertilization for the benefit of future research on eating disorders vulnerability factors.

FUTURE RESEARCH DIRECTIONS

Although longitudinal prospective designs are costly, the use of collaborative studies in which several forms of psychopathology are investigated seems to be a viable approach. For further efficiency in use of resources, community-based samples that were assessed during adolescence for the onset of anorexia nervosa and bulimia nervosa could be included in further follow-up to assess for the development of BED during adulthood. Such study samples offer careful assessment of numerous factors that may be important for understanding the development of disordered eating across the lifespan. For example, dieting history, weight, and problems in self-esteem and affect have been carefully documented in these samples, as they are relevant for onset of anorexia nervosa and bulimia nervosa. These variables appear to be important for understanding BED as well. Rather than relying on retrospective reports, which may suffer from a recall bias, future studies could assess adults who participated in assessments during pre- and early adolescence to determine how factors such as dieting and interpersonal difficulties are important in the development of all eating disorders. In this way, research on childhood/adolescent vulnerability factors may make significant contributions to understanding vulnerability factors associated with eating disorders in adulthood.

Conversely, research on childhood/adolescent vulnerability factors can benefit from perspectives taken within the adult literature. For example, more research on disordered eating in males seems justified considering that recurrent binge eating appears to be almost as common in males as in females and that these patterns may begin as early as 12 years of age. The adult literature has proposed the expansion of existing etiological models of eating disorders to account for the presence of BED in both men and women and Caucasians and minority groups. Although BED may simply differ from anorexia nervosa and bulimia nervosa on demographic variables, the diversity represented in clinical descriptions of BED highlights the need to revisit assumptions concerning who suffers from eating pathology throughout the lifespan.

In this summary, we sought to provide an integrated view of vulnerability factors for eating disorders across the lifespan. For a more in-depth treatment of the issues raised in this summary chapter and citations, readers are referred to Chapters 17 and 18. This summary chapter reveals a pattern of greater commonality rather than distinction in vulnerability factors for eating disorders across childhood/adolescence and adulthood. Recognition of common themes and issues will ideally contribute to ongoing research attempting to understand the etiology of eating pathology.

Part IV

SUMMARY AND FUTURE DIRECTIONS OF THE VULNERABILITY APPROACH

20

Future Directions in the Study of Vulnerability to Psychopathology

JOSEPH M. PRICE
RICK E. INGRAM

One of the primary objectives for this volume was to provide an overview of the research on vulnerability to several of the major forms of psychopathology as manifested in both childhood and adulthood and, in so doing, to shed some light on the status the field of vulnerability research. As is evident from the chapters in this volume, research on vulnerability to psychopathology is flourishing. In the three decades since Meehl (1962) first introduced the concept of vulnerability, a wide range of vulnerability processes has been identified and examined. Progress has been made in uncovering both genetic-based and environmentally based vulnerability processes. In addition, single-factor models of vulnerability to psychopathology have been replaced by diathesis–stress and developmental models of psychopathology. These more comprehensive and ecologically valid models view psychopathology as resulting from a complex and dynamic series of interactions between the characteristics of the individual, including his or her genotype, acquired cognitive, affective, and behavioral orientations, and the characteristics of the person's life experiences and stressors. Guided by these models, efforts have also been made to understand the interaction between vulnerability processes and environmental stressors and to determine the influence of this interaction on the emergence and maintenance of psychopathology. Yet in spite of these advances, unanswered questions and unresolved issues remain. In this final chapter, our goal is to propose several directions for future research on vulnerability to psychopathology, and to

455

do so by synthesizing the recommendations of the authors of chapters of this volume along with our own recommendations for the directions for future research.

UNDERSTANDING THE NATURE AND CHARACTERISTICS OF THE DISORDERS

Whereas for some disorders there appears to be at least some consensus as to the nature and defining characteristics of the disorder (e.g., depression), for other forms of psychopathology there appears to be less agreement as to the nature of the disorder, and whether the disorder is best conceptualized as a single unified condition or a heterogeneous disorder with various subgroups. Clearly, whether a given disorder is conceptualized as a single or a heterogeneous condition has important implications for research on the vulnerability processes associated with that particular disorder. In Chapter 15, Harvey argues that one of the impediments to the identification of causal processes in schizophrenia has been the tendency to view schizophrenia as a homogeneous rather than a heterogeneous disorder. Thus, Brennan and Harvey (Chapter 16) suggest that future efforts be made to define meaningful and etiologically distinct subgroups of individuals who have been diagnosed for schizophrenia. Similarly, Chassin, Collins, Ritter, and Shirley (Chapter 7) call for more research to explore the heterogeneity of substance abuse and dependence, especially among adolescent populations. The need for clearer and more precise conceptualizations of maladjustment and psychopathology is a theme that was repeatedly echoed by the authors in this volume.

In general, it appears that the nature and characteristics of disorders manifested during adulthood are better understood and more clearly defined than they are for disorders that appear in childhood and adolescence. For example, Malcarne and Handsdottir (Chapter 11) argue that the distinctions between anxiety disorders manifested during childhood are much less clear than when they are manifested during adulthood. Given the high degree of comorbidity among anxiety disorders during childhood, it is uncertain whether there are a shared set of core characteristics for all anxiety disorders and whether valid distinctions can be made between types of anxiety disorders. Similarly, in their chapter on vulnerability processes related to personality disorders, Geiger and Crick (Chapter 4) point out the ambiguity concerning the nature of personality disorders during childhood and adolescence.

Several possible explanations could be offered for this more limited understanding of the nature of childhood and adolescent disorders relative to adult disorders. First, in comparison to the research history of adult psychopathology, the history of research on child and adolescent psychopathology is shorter and less extensive. Second, dramatic developmental changes occur across all domains of functioning during childhood and adolescence, making it more difficult to determine commonality in a particular disorder across age groups. Third, development appears to proceed from undifferentiation among developmental processes toward differentiation and distinction between processes. Thus, during childhood one might expect less organization and cohesion in the symptoms of disorders than during adulthood. Future research directed toward delineating the nature and characteristics of childhood disorders should help to decrease the disparity between the child and adult literatures and also facilitate lifespan research on vulnerability processes.

One important avenue of research in this area will be determining the degree of commonality among the child, adolescent, and adult versions of particular disorders. In this volume, a number of possibilities were offered for the relation between childhood manifestations and adult manifestations of particular disorders. One proposed possibility is that there may be a high degree of similarity and commonality in a disorder across developmental periods, which McNally, Malcarne, and Hansdottir (Chapter 13) suggest is the case for certain phobias (e.g., blood or animal). Second, the childhood manifestation of a disorder might represent a developmental variant of an adult syndrome, as McNally, Malcarne, and Hansdottir contend is the connection between overanxious disorder in childhood and generalized disorder in adulthood. Third, for some disorders, while the underlying nature of the disorder may be the same across developmental periods, the behavioral manifestation may vary across developmental periods. Kagan (1971) suggests that although homotypical continuity, or the same behavioral manifestation of an underlying process at different points in development, can occur, it is likely to be rare. It is possible that heterotypical continuity, involving persistence in the underlying organization and meaning of behavior despite changing behavior manifestation, may more accurately represent the developmental nature of certain disorders. Finally, it is possible that the childhood manifestation of a particular disorder constitutes a different form of the disorder than does the adult version, as might be the case with schizophrenia.

Vulnerability research would likely benefit from taking a step back in the process of scientific inquiry and collecting additional descriptive and qualitative data on the nature and characteristics of various forms of psychopathology. This type of research would lead to the development of more accurate construct and operational definitions of disorders for use in future research. Vulnerability research would also likely gain from research directed toward better understanding the nature and characteristics of the vulnerability processes themselves. Such research on vulnerability processes is likely to play a pivotal role in helping us to understand the very nature of the disorders associated with these vulnerability processes.

CONTINUING THE SEARCH FOR VULNERABILITY FACTORS AND RELATIONS AMONG VULNERABILITY FACTORS

As is indicated in the chapters in this volume, over the past three decades an increasing number of biologically and environmentally based vulnerability processes have been identified. Recent advances in the biological and behavioral sciences are likely to help to continue this trend. Progress on the Human Genome project and advances in behavioral genetics promise to provide additional clues to potential sources of vulnerability processes that are rooted in hereditary processes. Advances in brain imaging techniques and neurophysiological assessments and the increased availability of such techniques will make it easier to assess neurological processes that may serve as vulnerability factors for certain disorders. In addition, recent research linking the characteristics of the prenatal environment with psychopathology (e.g., Brennan & Walker, Chapter 14) will broaden the definition and scope of environmentally based vulnerability factors. Finally, continued research on the impact of early social experiences on cognitive and affective processes related to psychopathology will increase our understanding of learning-based factors that may function as vulnerability processes.

Yet the identification of single vulnerability processes cannot be the end point of our efforts if we are to fully understand the role of vulnerability processes in the etiology and treatment of disorder. Many of the authors in this volume have called for the need to examine the role of combinations of vulnerability factors in the etiology of psychopathology. As noted by Rutter (1996), even in medicine, the search for multidimensional causality is the rule rather than the exception. As we move beyond models that assert that disorders arise from singular, endogenous pathogens, the need to investigate multiple determinants of psychopathology becomes more apparent. Furthermore, as is suggested by a developmental psychopathology perspective, the emergence of psychopathology is governed by the unique interaction of both vulnerability and protective factors. Therefore, an expanded form of this line of inquiry would be to examine how combinations of specific vulnerability and protective factors contribute to the onset, maintenance, and even remittance of specific forms of psychopathology. We now have at our disposal the statistical techniques and software programs that enable us to examine these various influences simultaneously.

In addition to expanding our knowledge base on the complexity of the nature of the etiological of psychopathology, another benefit of research on multiple vulnerability factors will be in making distinctions between true vulnerability factors, that is factors that play some sort of causal role in the development of the disorder, and factors that are merely markers of causal factors. Although correlational studies of the associations between vulnerability processes and psychopathology have been valuable in helping to identify potential vulnerability processes, such designs do not differentiate between true causal factors and factors that are associated with the disorder because of their relation to the vulnerability factor or some other correlated factor. Future efforts need to be directed toward identifying and understanding these important distinctions between true vulnerability processes and marker variables. An example of this kind of research is recent research that has identified deficiencies in smooth-pursuit eye movement as a maker of a genetic cause for schizophrenia (Brennan & Walker, Chapter 14; Harvey, Chapter 15).

Another important benefit of the inclusion of multiple vulnerability processes in future research will be helping to distinguish between factors that are involved in the onset of the disorder and factors that play an important role in the maintenance of the disorder. Not that a particular vulnerability process may not be simultaneously involved in both the onset and the maintenance of a disorder. As research on the cognitive vulnerabilities to depression suggests, it is certainly possible for a specific vulnerability process to contribute both to the emergence and clinical course of a disorder. Rather, for certain disorders, different vulnerability factors may serve different functions. Whereas one factor may play a crucial role in the emergence of the disorder, another may be more involved in the maintenance of the disorder. For example, hostile attributional biases appear to play a causal role in the development of certain forms of aggressive behavior in children, in particular reactive aggression (Dodge, Price, Bachorowski, & Newman, 1990). Thus, a hostile attributional bias could be conceptualized as an acquired vulnerability factor, perhaps as a result of physical abuse (Dodge, Bates, & Pettit, 1990). In contrast, peer rejection, which often results from displays of aggression toward peers, appears to play an important role in maintaining and perpetuating the aggressive child's antisocial tendencies (Price & Dodge, 1989).

Finally, multiple vulnerability and protective factors can be examined in relation to multiple forms of psychopathology to determine the degree to which a particular vulnerability factor or set of factors are *specific* to a particular disorder, as opposed to increasing the likelihood of disorder in general. Whereas some vulnerability factors may be specific to the development of a particular disorder, such as dopaminergic hyperactivity is to schizophrenia, other types of vulnerability factors may individually be related to a variety of disorders. For example, perceptions of lack of control appear to be associated with a variety of disorders, including anxiety, depression, and eating disorders. Likewise, an insecure attachment has been found to be linked to anxiety, depression, conduct disorder, and substance abuse. Thus, perceptions of lack of control and an insecure attachment may turn out to be vulnerability factors that are associated with psychopathology in general rather than any specific form of psychopathology. The challenge that remains is to determine the degree of specificity and globality of association of the various types of vulnerability factors identified in this volume with various forms of psychopathology (Ingram, 1990; Ingram & Malcarne, 1995). This can only be accomplished by examining multiple vulnerability processes in relation to multiple forms of psychopathology.

UNDERSTANDING CONTINUITY AND CHANGE IN VULNERABILITY PROCESSES ACROSS THE LIFESPAN

Another of our goals for this volume was to examine vulnerability processes associated with psychopathology across the lifespan. We chose to accomplish this goal by bringing together researchers from the fields of child and adult psychopathology, and by having them share their perspectives on their own and each other's fields of research. As we have seen in these chapters, there appears to be both continuity and discontinuity in the vulnerability processes across developmental periods, depending on the type and nature of the psychopathology being examined. Yet as beneficial as the discussion afforded by this volume is in shedding light on the continuity and change in vulnerability processes across the life cycle, there is a paucity of research that directly examines the continuity and discontinuity of vulnerability processes.

It is possible that certain disorders share vulnerability processes across both the child and adult manifestations of the disorder. For example, Keel and Schwartz (Chapter 19) hypothesize that a core set of vulnerability processes may underlie eating disorders that are manifested across developmental periods. They suggest that in the right cultural context, poor self-esteem and perfectionism may predispose an individual to anorexia in childhood and binge-eating disorders in adulthood. Thus, although the behavioral manifestation of the eating disorders may change across developmental periods, the underlying organization and influence of the vulnerability processes remains the same. In contrast, it might be the case that for some types of disorder, the earlier-onset version of the disorder is associated with different combinations of vulnerability processes than is the later-onset version. For example, antisocial behavior is more predictive of the onset of alcohol abuse during adolescence than it is for the onset of alcohol abuse in adulthood (Chassin, Collins, Ritter, & Shirley, Chapter 7).

Research on the continuity and discontinuity of vulnerability factors could also help to reveal distinctions between proximal and distal vulnerability factors. As defined by Ingram, Miranda, and Segal (1998), proximal factors are those that immediately precede the disorder and also occur temporally close to the disorder. As an example of a proximal vulnerability factor, these researchers note that dysfunctional cognitive interpretations of a recent event will result in depression. In contrast, distal vulnerability factors occur much earlier than the onset of the disorder. An example of a distal vulnerability factor might be the presence of a negative self-schema that has its origins in childhood. Thus, distal vulnerability factors might represent developmental antecedents for a particular disorder. Lifespan research on the continuity of vulnerability processes could help to identify important distinctions between proximal and distal causes of psychopathology.

In addition to these research directions, research on the continuity and change of vulnerability processes will naturally lead to the examination of the interaction between vulnerability factors and normal maturational processes (e.g., puberty). Research by Brennan and Walker (Chapter 14) suggests that early neurological deficits associated with schizophrenia may interact with hormonal changes in adolescence to contribute to the onset of the disorder in late adolescence and early adulthood. This research illustrates how endogenous vulnerability processes may interact with normal maturational processes to determine the conditions for the emergence of psychopathology.

Finally, research on the continuity and discontinuity in vulnerability processes across the lifespan can also provide insights into how vulnerability processes might interact with major life transitions to contribute to the development of disorder. For instance, with its associated stresses, the transition between adolescence and adulthood has been hypothesized to play a contributory role to the emergence to schizophrenia. It is possible that major life transitions such as the transition to elementary, middle, or high school; the transition to parenthood; or the transitions that result from disruptions in primary relationships may play a similar role in the onset of other forms of psychopathology.

Naturally, issues of the continuity and discontinuity of vulnerability processes implies the use of longitudinal or follow-up research designs. Specifically, these issues call for the use of longitudinal research across major periods of development. For example, research using longitudinal designs can help explain the linkage between early temperament (e.g., difficult temperament) and late adult personality (e.g., negative affectivity) and whether these personality constructs are related to a particular disorder in the same way across the lifespan. The specific developmental periods that should be included in such research depends on the type of disorder being examined. For some disorders, the most critical developmental periods might include the span of time between childhood and adolescence, whereas for other disorders the most informative developmental time span would range from childhood through adulthood.

As insightful as longitudinal research might be in addressing these issues, the drawbacks of longitudinal research are the time and expense involved in collecting the relevant data. As a way of facilitating the collection of longitudinal data, and of decreasing the time and costs involved, child and adult researchers might consider collaborating in studies that use follow-ups in adulthood on samples of children and/or adolescents for whom extensive data on vulnerability processes already exist. Keel and Schwartz (Chapter 19) suggest this strategy as a means of facilitating longitudinal research on eating disorders and bringing together researchers of child and adult eating disorders.

UNDERSTANDING THE INTERACTION BETWEEN VULNERABILITY PROCESSES AND THE ENVIRONMENTAL CONTEXT

Both diathesis–stress and developmental psychopathology perspectives emphasize the importance of the environmental context in the emergence of maladaptation and psychopathology. According to both perspectives, the characteristics of the individual, including endogenous vulnerability processes, interact with the specific characteristics of the individuals' environmental context to influence the trajectory either toward or away from maladjustment and psychopathology. Thus far, some of the environmental factors that have been identified include the quality of the person's interactions with significant relationship figures at a various developmental periods, socioeconomic conditions, cultural values and norms, and a wide range of stressors (e.g., violence, divorce, school, and work pressures). What has yet to be determined is which specific features of environmental contexts interact with which specific vulnerability processes to contribute to particular forms of psychopathology. Moreover, as Hammen and Garber (Chapter 10) suggest, the role of the transactional dynamics of the relation between the individual and his or her environment in the development of psychopathology has yet to be thoroughly examined.

Another direction for future research is to examine vulnerability to psychopathology across various environmental contexts. If, as is suggested by both diathesis–stress and developmental psychopathology models, vulnerability processes interact with environmental stressors and demands, then differences in environmental contexts may change the susceptibility to disorder and the defining features of the disorder. Unfortunately, there is a paucity of research on contextual differences in vulnerability to psychopathology, especially important social contexts such as culture. Not only will research on cultural differences in vulnerability to psychopathology help to extend the generalizability of current models of psychopathology to a wider range of cultural and ethnic groups, but it will also lead to interventions that are more sensitive to individual differences.

In addition to understanding the interaction between vulnerability processes and the environmental context, it is equally important to understand the changing influence of social contexts across the lifespan. Chassin et al. (Chapter 7) point out that with substance abuse disorders, the specific sources of influence may vary somewhat at different stages of development. During childhood, parents and family members may serve as models and socializers; during adolescence, peers are an increasingly important socialization context; and during adulthood, relationship partners become a more important influence. Similar developmental changes in social influences could be associated with other types of psychopathology as well.

UNDERSTANDING DEVELOPMENTAL PATHWAYS: THE IMPORTANCE OF INDIVIDUAL DIFFERENCES

Since the origins of risk research, the typical approach to examining vulnerability factors has been to use variable-oriented strategies that strive to identify the primary causal agents involved in the etiology of the psychopathology. These variable-oriented strategies are important because they reveal vulnerability and protective processes that contribute to psychopathology at the group level. This particular research approach also helps us to understand the average or most expected outcomes associated with particular vulnerability processes. In addition, the variable-oriented approach helps to establish relations between particular vulnerability and protective factors and particular forms of psychopathology within the general population. The limitation of this approach, however, is that it reveals little about individual patterns of psychopathology and the diversity of pathways that lead to psychopathology.

To gain a better understanding of the alternative pathways taken by individuals in route to psychopathology, Cicchetti and Rogosch (1996) advocate the use of a pathways, or person-oriented, approach. Such an approach to understanding psychopathology focuses on identifying the various routes or pathways taken by different individuals to particular maladaptive outcomes. For example, whereas for one individual the pathway to a borderline personality disorder might be rooted in an insecure attachment relationship during infancy, for someone else the same disordered personality structure might have its original trajectory determined by a chaotic home life during later childhood. A pathways approach also attends to common and uncommon outcomes associated with particular pathways. For instance, depending on the individual genotype and the availability of social support, the experience of early physical abuse might lead to depression in one person but to a conduct or antisocial personality disorder in another.

Sroufe (1997) has argued that if possible, developmental pathways should be traced from a point prior to the onset of disturbance. By tracing pathways from a point prior to the emergence of psychopathology it is possible to discover heterogeneity in disorder. Individuals who display similar "symptoms" may in fact be on different developmental pathways if examined longitudinally and may have predictably different outcomes.

Following the suggestion of Cicchetti and Rogosch (1996), one way to facilitate the transition between variable-oriented and person-oriented research in a particular area is to use homogeneous subgroups of the disorder to examine the diversity of vulnerability processes and psychopathology outcomes associated with the various subgroupings. Along these lines, Brennan and Harvey (Chapter 16) advocate identifying subgroups of schizophrenia based on common etiology. Chassin et al. (Chapter 7) also argue for the value of identifying subgroups of substance abuse among adolescents. However, as they point out, difficulties in subtyping may occur because some subcategories of a disorder may not develop until early adulthood. Thus, although it might be possible to identify subtypes of a particular disorder at one point in the lifespan (e.g., adulthood), the disorder might be manifest as a homogeneous and unified condition at another point (e.g., childhood).

Another avenue of research within a pathways perspective would be to examine the role of individual choices and actions in the development of psychopathology. With development, the individual plays an increasingly active role in adaptation, interpreting and creating experience as well as responding to a variety of internal and external changes. For example, the literature on depression suggests that by withdrawing from social interaction and failing to complete daily responsibilities, individuals who are depressed contribute to their own feelings of worthlessness, which, in turn, perpetuates their depressive state. However, to date, little research has been devoted to the examination of the role of individual choices and actions in the development of psychopathology, or to how the individual's choices and actions may interact with vulnerability processes and environmental stressors.

As the chapters in this volume reveal, for many forms of psychopathology a substantial empirical base has been acquired using variable-oriented strategies. Subgroup and pathways approaches can extend this knowledge base by examining the different types of pathways and vulnerability processes that could be associated with various forms of psychopathology. In turn, this information can be used to develop a wider range of intervention strategies that could be tailored to the specific needs of individuals.

UNDERSTANDING THE MALLEABILITY OF VULNERABILITY FACTORS AND PROCESSES

One of the core issues that remains to be adequately addressed in vulnerability research is the extent to which vulnerability processes are open to malleability and change (Ingram et al., 1998). It might be expected that biologically based vulnerability processes that are rooted in genotype or environmental trauma would be less open to change than vulnerability processes acquired through socialization and learning. However, the question of the extent to which both hereditary and learning-based vulnerability processes are malleable remains largely unanswered in the vulnerability literature. It may be possible that even hereditary-based biological vulnerabilities can be altered to some extent. Conversely, although learning-based vulnerabilities such as learned helplessness might be expected to be receptive to alteration, they may, nonetheless, be quite resistant to change. Many developmental theorists and researchers (e.g., Sroufe, 1997), contend that change in psychological processes may be constrained by prior adaptation. That is, the longer a maladaptive pathway has been followed, the less likely it is that the person will reclaim positive adaptation. Thus, even learning-based vulnerability processes (e.g., learned helplessness), if used consistently and over a long period, may be resistant to change.

A natural first step to addressing this issue would be to examine existing data from prevention and treatment intervention research literatures to determine the extent to which vulnerability processes have been able to be altered and whether the degree of change depends on developmental level. Data available from prevention projects could provide insights into the extent to which vulnerability processes can be altered prior to the onset of the disorder. Likewise, data available from treatment studies could be used to examine the degree to which vulnerability processes can be modified after the onset of disorder. The next step in the process of determining the extent to which vulnerability processes can be altered would be to design prevention and treatment studies with the explicate goal of targeting specific vulnerability processes for change.

SUMMARY

At the close of this volume, we stand in agreement with the other authors in calling for increased dialogue between child and adult researchers of vulnerability to psychopathology. As is evident from the summary chapters, such communication increases our overall understanding of the vulnerability processes that are associated with various forms of maladjustment and psychopathology as they occur across the lifespan. These discussions provide a rich context for the generation of new ideas and directions for future research. We also support the assertion made by many of the authors that a developmental perspective will greatly enhance our future research efforts in identifying and understanding vulnerability processes across the lifespan. Both general and specific developmental models of psychopathology exist to guide this line of research. In addition, sophisticated statistical procedures for analyzing longitudinal data with multiple variables (e.g., HLM and Liseral-based techniques) exist to facilitate more lifespan research. The current state of the field of vulnerability research provides a solid bedrock for launching a new and informative era for the study of vulnerability to psychopathology. Ideally, as investigators of childhood disorders and investigators of adult disorders increase their dialogue, the focus of this new era of research will be on vulnerability to psychopathology across the lifespan.

REFERENCES

Cicchetti, D., & Rogosch, F. A. (1996). Equifinality and multifinality in developmental psychopathology. *Development and Psychopathology, 8,* 597–600.

Dodge, K. A., Bates, J. E., & Pettit, G. S. (1990). Mechanisms in the cycle of violence. *Science, 250,* 1678–1683.

Dodge, K. A., Price, J. M., Bachorowski, J., & Newman, J. P. (1990). Hostile attributional biases in severely aggressive adolescents. *Journal of Abnormal Psychology, 99,* 385–392.

Ingram, R. E. (1990). Self-focused attention in clinical disorders: Review and a conceptual model. *Psychological Bulletin, 107,* 156–176.

Ingram, R. E., & Malcarne, V. L. (1995). Cognition in depression and anxiety: Same, different, or little of both? In K. D. Craig & K. S. Dobson (Eds.), *Anxiety and depression in adults and children* (pp. 37–56). Newbury Park, CA: Sage.

Ingram, R. E., Miranda, J., & Segal, Z. V. (1998). *Cognitive vulnerability to depression.* New York: Guilford Press.

Kagan, J. (1971). *Change and continuity in infancy.* New York: Wiley.

Meehl, P. E. (1962). Schizotaxia, schizotypy, and schizophrenia. *American Psychologist, 17,* 827–838.

Price, J. M., & Dodge, K. A. (1989). Peers' contributions to children's social maladjustment: Description and intervention. In T. J. Berndt & G. W. Ladd (Eds.), *Contributions of peer relationships to children's development* (pp. 341–370). New York: Wiley.

Rutter, M. (1996). Developmental psychopathology: Concepts and prospects. In M. Lenzenseger & J. Havguard (Eds.), *Frontiers of developmental psychopathology* (pp. 209–237). New York: Oxford University Press.

Sroufe, L. A. (1997). Psychopathology as an outcome of development. *Development and Psychopathology, 9,* 251–268.

Index

f indicates a figure; t indicates a table

Abuse; *see also* specific types
  personality disorders and, 84
Adolescence; *see also* Childhood/
    adolescence
  anxiety disorders in, 275
  behavior during, 57–58
Adulthood
  anxiety disorders in, 44–45,
      304–321; *see also* Anxiety
      disorders in adulthood
  definition of, 15–17
  depression in, 226–257; *see also*
      Depression, in adulthood
  disorders in, 40–46
    anxiety, 44–45
    eating-related, 41–42
    future research on, 51–52
    modification of, 48–49
    of mood/affect, 43
    rationale for studying, 46–51
    schizophrenia, 45–46
    substance-related, 40–41
    types of, 40–46
    unipolar, 43–44
    vulnerability to, 39–54, 46–49
  eating disorders in, 412–446; *see
      also* Eating disorders, in
      adulthood
  schizophrenia in, 355–381; *see also*
      Schizophrenia, in adulthood
  substance abuse disorders in, 135–
      164; *see also* Substance use
      disorders, in adulthood

Affect
  flat
    as precursor to personality
        disorders, 60t, 70–71
  negative, substance use disorders
      and, 116–119, 168–169
Aggression
  ADHD and, 73
  relational, 75–76
Agoraphobia
  in adult, 306–312
  anxiety sensitivity and, 306–309
  genetic factors in, 309–311
Alcohol, sensitivity to reinforcing
      effects of, substance use
      disorders and, 119–121
Alcohol disorders, genetic factors in,
      142–143
Alcohol intoxication, criteria for, 41
Alcohol use/abuse
  age at onset, 108
  brain-evoked potentials and, 143
  continuum of, 138–139
  demographic correlates of, 137–138
  enzyme activity and, 143–144
  models of, 139–141
Anhedonia, 177
Anorexia nervosa; *see also* Eating
      disorders
  binge eating/purging *versus*
      restricted, 42
  criteria for, 42
  in DSM-IV, 389

Antidepressants, 247–248
  for anxiety disorders, 293–294
  for depression, 263
Antisocial personality disorder, 72–73
Anxiety
  vulnerability factors in, 28*t*
  vulnerability studies and, 23–24
Anxiety disorders, 44–45
  across lifespan, 322–325
  in adulthood, 304–321
    obsessive–compulsive disorder,
      314–316
    panic disorder/agoraphobia, 306–
      312
    posttraumatic stress disorder,
      312–314
  in children/adolescents, 271–303
    biological processes in, 280–285
    cognitive processes in, 285–287
    comorbidity, 277–278
    developmental course/stability,
      273–277
    epidemiology of, 272–273
    future research directions, 294–
      295
    prevention and treatment, 291–
      294
    risk factors, 278–280
    social processes in, 287–291
    stability of, 275–277
  depression and, 178–179
  in DSM-IV, 271
Anxiety sensitivity, in panic disorder/
    agoraphobia, 306–309
Assessment tools, for pathological
    personality function, 63–65
Attachment relationships
  development of, 71
  insecure, 77
Attention, selective, schizophrenia and,
    369–370
Attention deficit
  in schizophrenia, 336–337
  schizophrenia and, 368–369
Attention-deficit/hyperactivity
    disorder
  criteria for, 72–73
  vulnerability factors in, 29*t*
Avoidant personality disorder, 79, 81

B

BED; *see* Binge-eating disorder
Behavioral factors, in schizophrenia,
    335–338, 370–371
Behavioral inhibition, characteristics
    of, 280–282
Behavioral inhibition system
  in anxiety disorders, 285–286
  temperamental differences and, 74
Behaviorally uninhibited,
    characteristics of, 281–282
Binge-eating disorder, 395–397; *see
    also* Eating disorders
  in adulthood
    characteristics associated with,
      425–435
    dieting and, 424–425
    history of approaches to, 414–416
    theory and research, 417–419,
      417*f*
    treatment of, 419–423
  definition of, 413
  DSM-IV criteria for, 413*t*
  models of
    dietary restraint, 417–418, 417*f*
    interpersonal vulnerability, 418–
      419
  prevalence of, 413–414
Biological factors
  in adult substance use, 141–144
  in anxiety disorders, 280–285
  in binge-eating disorder, 421–423
  in child/adolescent depression, 186–
    191
  in depression, 232–238
    brain changes, 236–237
    circadian rhythms, 237–238
    genetic, 233–234
    hormonal, 238
    neurotransmitters, 235–236
    psychoneuroendocrinological,
      234–235
  in substance abuse, 165–166
Bipolar disorder, 44
  modifying vulnerability to, 48
Borderline personality disorder, 63, 72
  emotion regulation and, 69
  personal relationships and, 75

Brain; *see also* Central nervous system
  abnormalities of
    in depression, 189–190
    in schizophrenia, 331–333
  changes in, in depression, 236–237
  in lifespan studies of depression, 261
Bulimia nervosa; *see also* Eating disorders
  binge-eating disorder and, 435–436
  criteria for, 42
  in DSM-IV, 389–390
  late-onset, 435–436
  subtypes of, 42
  transition to binge-eating disorder, 436

C

Cannabis intoxication, criteria for, 41
Car accidents, PTSD following, 314
Caregiver, characteristics of, 80
Causality
  defining, 3–4
  versus onset, 4
CBT intervention, for anxiety
    disorders, 292–293
Central nervous system; *see also* Brain
  in child/adolescent depression, 186
  emotional regulation by, 67–68
Child abuse, 81–82, 84
Childhood, definition of, 15–17
Childhood/adolescence
  anxiety disorders in, 271–303; *see
    also* Anxiety disorders, in
    children/adolescents
  depression in, 175–225; *see also*
    Depression, in children/
    adolescents
  eating disorders in, 389–411; *see
    also* Eating disorders, in
    children/adolescents
  psychopathology in
    comorbidity with, 22–23
    defining, 21–22
    defining vulnerability to, 25–26
    prevalence of, 22–23
    rationale for study of, 23–25
    research on vulnerability to, 26–34
  schizophrenia in, 329–354; *see also*
    Schizophrenia, in childhood/
    adolescence

substance use disorders in, 107–134;
    see also Substance use disorders,
    in children/adolescents
  vulnerability in, 20–38
Circadian rhythms, in depression, 237–
    238
Cognitive factors
  in anxiety disorders, 285–287
  in binge-eating disorder, 426–427
  in child/adolescent depression, 195–
    199
    cross-sectional studies of, 195–
      197
    offspring studies of, 198
    prevention studies of, 198–199
    prospective studies of, 197
  in depression, 238–241
  in lifespan studies of depression,
    261–263
  negative, in anxiety disorders, 286–
    287
  in schizophrenia, 368
  vulnerability studies and, 23–24
Cognitive therapy, for depression, 263
Cognitive-behavioral therapy, for
    binge-eating disorder, 419–
    420
Concentration problems, causes of,
    178
Conduct disorders
  alcohol use and, 147
  research on, 32
  vulnerability factors in, 28*t*, 29
Conduct problems, substance use
    disorders and, 112–116
Congenital factors, in schizophrenia,
    330–340
  physical/dermatoglyphic
    abnormalities, 333–335
  structural brain abnormalities, 331–
    333
Control, perceived, in anxiety
    disorders, 285–286
Cortisol, depression and, 187–188
Cultural factors; *see also* Ethnicity
  in eating disorders, 397–399
  substance abuse and, 166
Cultural influences, child–adult
    distinction and, 16

D

Delusions, 86–87
Dependence
  depression and, 245
  excessive, 75
  substance, 136
Dependent personality disorder, 81–82
Depression
  across lifespan, 258–270
    diagnostic and definitional issues,
      258–260
    intervention approaches, 263–264
    models of, 260–263
  in adulthood, 226–257
    biological vulnerability and, 232–
      238
    brain changes in, 236–237
    cognitive factors in, 238–241
    course of, 228–229
    definitions and characteristics,
      226–229
    epidemiology/demographics, 229
    future research directions, 248–249
    genetic vulnerability, 233–234
    historical approaches to, 229–230
    interpersonal approaches to, 244–
      247
    neurotransmitters and, 235–236
    personality and, 243
    prevention/treatment, 247–248
    psychoneuroendocrinology of,
      234–235
    stress sensitization and, 243–244
    stressful life events and, 241–242
    study methods, 230–231
    theory and research, 232–247
  with anxiety disorders, 277–278
  causality in, 4
  in children/adolescents, 175–225
    cognitive factors in, 195–199
    course and outcome, 179–181
    definitions and characteristics,
      175–182
    future research directions, 206–208
    gender factors and, 204–205
    genetic factors in, 183–186
    interpersonal perspectives on,
      199–204

  methods for studying, 182–183
  neurobiological factors in, 186–191
  phenomenology of, 175–179
  as predictor of adult depression,
    259–260
  prevalence of, 181–182
  and prior depressive symptoms,
    205–206
  stressful life events and, 191–195
  theory and research, 183–206
continuity of, 179
criteria for, 43–44
developmental differences in, 176–
  177
in DSM-IV, 175–176
effects on others, 244–245
epidemiological studies of, 181–182
maternal, 68
models of, 229–230
modifying vulnerability to, 48
symptoms of, 227
vulnerability factors in, 28*t*
vulnerability studies and, 23–24
vulnerability theory and, 51
Dermatoglyphic abnormalities, in
    schizophrenia, 333–335
Developmental pathways, vulnerability
    factors and, 463–464
Developmental stages,
    psychopathology and, 21–22
Deviance proneness, substance use
    disorders and, 112–116, 122–123
Dexamethasone suppression test, 187
*Diagnostic and Statistical Manual of
    Mental Disorders,* 4th ed.
  adult disorder in, 40
  anxiety disorders in, 271
  child *versus* adult distinction in, 15–16
  depression in, 175–176
  eating disorders in, 389, 412, 413*t*
  major depressive disorder in, 227
  personality disorders in, 58, 59, 60*t*–
    61*t*
  substance-related disorders in, 135–
    136
Diathesis–stress model, 33–34, 47
  of schizophrenia, 27, 329
Diathesis–stress relationship, 11–12,
    15*f*

Dieting
  binge-eating disorder and, 424–425
  chronic, 395–397
Dissociative identity disorder, 40
Distractibility, schizophrenia and, 369–370
Drinking restraint, substance abuse and, 149
Drug therapy
  for anxiety disorders, 293–294
  for depression, 247–248
Drugs, gateway, 107
Dysfunction
  concepts of, 5–6
  risk and, 13
Dyskinesia, schizophrenia and, 335–336

E

Eating disorders, 41–42
  across lifespan, 447–452
  in adulthood, 412–446; *see also* Binge-eating disorder
    future research directions, 440
    prevention of, 437, 439–440
  anorexia nervosa, 42
  binge; *see* Binge-eating disorder
  bulimia nervosa, 42
  in children/adolescents, 389–411
    biological factors in, 392–394
    biopsychosocial model of, 400–403
    developmental changes and, 399–400
    developmental course of, 391–392
    future research on, 403–404
    psychological factors in, 394–397
    risk factor research on, 390–391
    social factors in, 397–399
    treatment/prevention, 403
  definition of, 413
  in DSM-IV, 389, 412
Emotion
  CNS regulation of, 67–68
  inappropriate/intense, as precursor to personality disorders, 60t, 67–70
  negative, substance use disorders and, 116–119, 168–169

  poor skills for regulating, 69–70
  unresponsiveness in, 76–77
Environment, vulnerability factors and, 462–463
Environmental factors, 25–26
  in childhood vulnerability, 27
Epifinality, characteristics of, 30
Ethnicity; *see also* Cultural factors
  anxiety disorders and, 279–280
  binge-eating disorder and, 434
  substance use disorders and, 115
Eye movement, smooth-pursuit, abnormalities in schizophrenia, 337–338

F

Family, dysfunctional, personality disorders and, 69–70
Flat affect, as precursor to personality disorders, 60t, 70–71
Freud, S., vulnerability theory of, 49

G

Gender
  anxiety disorders and, 278–279
  binge-eating disorder and, 433, 439
  child/adolescent depression and, 204–205
  depression and, 204–205
  mental disorders and, 137
Generalized anxiety disorder, 271, 274–275
Genetic factors, 25–26
  in alcohol use, 142–143
  in anxiety disorders, 282–283
  in child/adolescent depression, 183–186
  in childhood vulnerability, 27
  in depression, 233–234
  in eating disorders, 392
  in lifespan studies of depression, 260–261
  in panic disorder/agoraphobia, 309–311
  in schizophrenia, 339–340, 360–362, 361t
  in substance abuse, 165–166
Growth hormone, depression and, 188

H

Hallucinations, 86
Hereditary factors; *see* Genetic factors
Histrionic personality disorder, 72
Hopelessness, 177–178
Hormones
  in depression, 238
  in schizophrenia, 342–344
Hostility, as precursor to personality
    disorders, 60*t,* 65–66
Hypersensitivity
  alcohol use and, 147
  as precursor to personality disorder,
    68–69
Hypothalamic–pituitary–adrenal axis
  abnormalities in, 187–188
  in anxiety disorders, 284

I

Impulsivity, as precursor to personality
    disorders, 60*t,* 71–73
Infants, anxiety disorders in, 273
Intelligence, social behavior and, 88
Interpersonal perspectives on
    depression, 199–204, 244–247
  cross-sectional studies of, 199–201
  offspring studies of, 202–203
  prevention studies of, 203–204
  prospective studies of, 201–202
Interpersonal therapy
  for binge-eating disorder, 420–421
  for depression, 264
Intervention programs, preventative,
    24–25
Intoxicated states, 40–41

K

Kindling, characteristics of, 48–49

L

Lifespan
  anxiety disorders across, 322–325
  continuity and change across, 460–
    462
  depression across, 258–270

eating disorders across, 447–452
  schizophrenia across, 382–388
  substance use disorders across, 165–
    174
Lithium carbonate, in control of
    vulnerability, 48

M

Major depressive disorder, 43–44; *see
    also* Depression
  in DSM-IV, 227
  rates of, 181
Maltreatment, child, 81–82, 84
Markers, of schizophrenia, 365–367
Medications, binge-eating disorder
    and, 432–433
Mood disorders, research on, 32
Mood/affective disorders, 43

N

Narcissistic personality disorder, 85
Neurobiology, of anxiety disorders,
    283–285
Neurochemical approaches, in lifespan
    studies of depression, 261
Neuromotor factors, in schizophrenia,
    335–336
Neuropsychology, of anxiety disorders,
    283–285
Neurotransmitters, depression and,
    188–189, 235–236
Not inhibited, characteristics of, 282

O

Obesity, binge-eating disorder and,
    427–429
  adult, 423
  in childhood, 422–423, 439–440
Obsessive–compulsive personality
    disorder, 74
  in adults, 314–316
Obstetric complications, in
    schizophrenia, 338–340
Onset, *versus* causality, 4
Overanxious disorder, 271, 274–275
  in adolescence, 275

P

Panic disorder
  in adult, 306–312
  anxiety sensitivity and, 306–309
  genetic factors in, 309–311
Paranoid world view, as precursor to
    personality disorders, 60*t*, 65–
    66
Parent–child relationships, in anxiety
    disorders, 287–290
Parenting
  anxiety disorders and, 291–292
  negative, 81–82, 89
    substance use disorders and, 113–
    114
Parents
  addicted, children of, 122
  affective illness of, binge-eating
    disorder and, 422–423
  depressed, children of, 183
Passivity, 77–78
Perfectionism, 74
Perinatal factors, in schizophrenia,
    338–340, 363–364
Personality
  binge-eating disorder and, 426–427
  schizophrenia and, 370–371
  substance abuse and, 144–149, 166
Personality disorders
  assessment and stability of, 62–65
  assessment tools for, 63–64
  childhood/adolescent precursors to,
    57–58, 65–89
    distant/avoidant relationships, 76–
    79
    emotional intensity, 66–70
    exaggerated sense of self, 85
    flat affect, 70–71
    future research directions, 91–93
    hostility/paranoia, 65–66
    impulsivity, 71–73
    indifferences to social norms/
    others' needs, 87–89
    individual differences in, 89–90
    intervention implications, 90–91
    lack of sense of self, 82–85
    negative sense of self, 79–82
    overly close relationships, 75–76

  peculiar thought processes/
    behaviors, 86–87
  rigidity, 73–75
  developmental approach to, 58–59,
    60*t*–61*t*, 62–63
  diagnosis of, 58–59, 60*t*–61*t*, 61
    inadequacies in, 58
  DSM-IV classification of, 58, 59,
    60*t*–61*t*
  vulnerability to, 57–102
Phobias
  in adults, 305
  in children/adolescents, 277
  specific, 272, 274
Posttraumatic stress disorder
  in adults, 305–306, 312–314
  vulnerability to, 47
Pregnancy, binge-eating disorder and,
    430–431
Prenatal factors, in schizophrenia,
    338–340, 362–363
Preschool children, anxiety disorders
    in, 273
Psychological factors
  in adult substance use, 144–149
  in eating disorders, 394–397
Psychoneuroendocrinology, 187–188
  of depression, 234–245
Psychopathology
  in children *versus* adults, 456–457
  definitions of, 5–7, 21
  development of, 3
  understanding characteristics of,
    456–457
  vulnerability to; *see* Vulnerability
Psychotherapy, interpersonal, for
    depression, 264
Psychotic thought processes, 86

R

Rape, PTSD following, 312–314
Rapid visual processing, in
    schizophrenia, 369
Reassurance seeking, depression and,
    245
Relationships
  distant/avoidant, 76–79
  dysfunctional, depression and, 245–246

Relationships(*continued*)
  enmeshed, 75–76
  overly close/distant, as precursor of
    personality disorders, 60*t*
Research
  on continuity and change across
    lifespan, 460–462
  on developmental pathways, 463–464
  diathesis–stress models of, 33–34;
    see also Diathesis–stress model
  future directions in, 455–466
  on interaction between vulnerability
    and environment, 462–463
  longitudinal, 32–33
  on malleability of vulnerability
    factors, 464–465
  on nature/characteristics of
    disorders, 456–457
  on personality disorders, 64–65, 91–
    93
  on relationships among vulnerability
    factors, 458–460
  risk, 33–34
  on vulnerability in children/
    adolescents, 23–25, 31–34
Resilience, *versus* vulnerability, 14
Rigidity, as precursor to personality
    disorders, 60*t*, 73–75
Risk
  research on, 33–34
  versus vulnerability, 12–14, 25

S

Schizoid personality disorders,
    precursors to, 70–71
Schizophrenia, 45–46
  across lifespan, 382–388
  in adulthood, 355–381
    general characteristics, 356–357
    markers of, 365–372
    prevention of, 372–373
    reconciling data on, 373–375
    vulnerability to, 357–365
  in children/adolescents, 329–354
    behavioral markers of, 335–338
    congenital vulnerability and, 330–
      340
    future research directions, 345–346

  hormonal factors in, 342–344
  interactional processes in
    development of, 340–344
  intervention, 344–345
  physical signs of, 331–335
  prenatal/perinatal factors in, 338–
    339
  diathesis–stress model of, 27, 329
  genetic factors in, 8
  heterogeneity of, 456
  neurodevelopmental perspective,
    329–330
  polythetic structure of, 355
  vulnerability factors in, 29*t*
  vulnerability theory and, 50–51
  vulnerability to, 23, 32–33
Schizotaxia, 50
  concept of, 8
Schizotypal personality disorder, 63,
    86–87
  precursors to, 70–71
Selective attention, schizophrenia and,
    369–370
Selective serotonin reuptake inhibitors,
    for depression, 263
Self, disturbed sense of, as precursor of
    personality disorders, 61*t*, 79–85
Self-restraint
  deficient, substance use disorders
    and, 113
  lack of, 72–73
Separation anxiety disorder, 271, 274
Serotonin, eating disorders and, 392–393
Serotonin reuptake inhibitors, for
    reducing depression, 189
Sexual orientation, binge-eating
    disorder and, 434–435
Sleep disturbances, depression and,
    190–191, 237–238
Smooth-pursuit eye movements,
    abnormalities in schizophrenia,
    337–338
Social factors
  in adult substance use, 149–152
  in anxiety disorders, 287–291
  in eating disorders, 397–399
  in lifespan studies of depression,
    261–263
  substance abuse and, 166

Social information, poor skills for processing, 66
Social norms, indifference to, as precursor of personality disorders, 61*t*
Socioeconomic factors, substance abuse and, 151–152
Socioeconomic status, anxiety disorders and, 280
Stability
    of personality disorders, 62–65
    of vulnerability, 7–9, 26
Stress
    definitions of, 11
    generation of, in depressed persons, 246
    hypersensitivity to, 24
    in schizophrenia, 340–341
    vulnerability and, 10–11
Stress sensitization, depression and, 243–244
Stress–diathesis relationship, 11–12, 15*f*
Stressful life events
    in anxiety disorders, 290–291
    binge-eating disorder and, 429–433
    in child/adolescent depression, 191–195
    in depression, 262
    depression and, 191–195, 241–243
        cross-sectional studies of, 191–192
        offspring studies of, 193–194
        prevention studies of, 194–195
        prospective studies of, 192–193
    substance abuse and, 148
Stressors, highly traumatic, 312–313
Substance abuse
    binge-eating disorder and, 431–432, 439
    defined, 135
Substance use disorders, 40–41
    across lifespan, 165–174
        future research on, 169–170
    in adulthood, 135–164
        approaches to, 138–139
        biological vulnerability and, 141–144
        classification/assessment, 139–141
        definitions and prevalence, 135–138

future research, 154–156
        prevention and treatment, 152–154
        psychological vulnerability and, 144–149
        social aspects of, 149–152
    in children/adolescents, 107–134
        future research on, 123–125
        identifying pathways to, 111–112
        prevention of, 123
        research and methodology, 109–111
        research on, prevention and, 121–123
        through deviance proneness and conduct problems, 112–116
        through negative affect, 116–119
        through sensitivity to reinforcing effects, 119–121
    at different developmental periods, 167–169
    and heterogeneity of abusers, 168
    models of, 139–141
    vulnerability to, in childhood and adolescence, 107–134
Suicide, depressive disorders and, 43–44
Suicide risk, psychoneuroendocrinological assessment of, 187

T

Temperament
    anxiety disorders and, 280–282
    behavioral inhibition system and, 74
    eating disorders and, 393–394
    styles of, 68–69
    substance use disorders and, 112–113, 166
Theoretical models, of vulnerability in childhood/adolescence, 26–31, 28*t*, –29*t*
Thought processes, peculiar, as precursor of personality disorders, 61*t*
Trauma, PTSD following, 312; *see also* Posttraumatic stress disorder
Treatment, vulnerability processes and, 3–4

Tricyclic antidepressants, 247–248
  for anxiety disorders, 293–294
  for depression, 263

U

Unipolar disorder, major depressive
  episode, 43–44

V

Visual processing, rapid, in
  schizophrenia, 369
Vulnerability
  adult, 39–54, 46–49
    disorders involving, 40–46
    future research on, 51–52
    rationale for studying, 46–51
  affective, 28t–29t, 29–30
  biological, 28t–29t, 29–30
  changes in, 9
  child–adult classification and, 15–17
  in children/adolescents, 20–38
    theoretical models of, 26–31, 28t–
      29t
  cognitive, 28t–29t, 29–30
  core features of, 7–12
  definitions of, 7
  developmental pathways and, 463–464

endogenous nature of, 10
environmental context and, 462–463
future research directions, 455–466
hereditary *versus* environmental
  factors in, 25–26, 27
intensification of, 48–49
latency of, 10
lifespan perspective on, 52
malleability of factors in, 464–465
multiple manifestations of, 34–35
reducing, 49
relationships among factors in, 458–
  460
versus resilience, 14
versus risk, 12–14, 25
role of, 3–19
social/behavioral, 28t–29t, 29–30
as stable trait, 7–9, 26
stress and, 10–11
treatment and, 3–4

W

Weight cycling, binge-eating disorder
  and, 425
Withdrawal, types of, 77–78
World view, hostile, paranoid, as
  precursor to personality
  disorders, 65–66